Infant & Toddler Health Sourcebook

Infectious Diseases Sourcebook

Injury & Trauma Sourcebook

Learning Disabilities Sourcebook,
2nd Edition

Leukemia Sourcebook

Liver Disorders Sourcebook

Lung Disorders Sourcebook

Medical Tests Sourcebook, 2nd Edition

Men's Health Concerns Sourcebook,
2nd Edition

Mental Health Disorders Sourcebook,
3rd Edition

Mental Retardation Sourcebook

Movement Disorders Sourcebook

Muscular Dystrophy Sourcebook

Obesity Sourcebook

Osteoporosis Sourcebook

Pain Sourcebook, 2nd Edition

Pediatric Cancer Sourcebook

Physical & Mental Issues in Aging
Sourcebook

Podiatry Sourcebook, 2nd Edition

Pregnancy & Birth Sourcebook,
2nd Edition

Prostate Cancer Sourcebook

Prostate & Urological Disorders
Sourcebook

Public Health Sourcebook

Reconstructive & Cosmetic Surgery
Sourcebook

Rehabilitation Sourcebook

Respiratory Diseases & Disorders
Sourcebook

Sexually Transmitted Diseases
Sourcebook, 3rd Edition

Sleep Disorders Sourcebook,
2nd Edition

Smoking Concerns Sourcebook

Sports Injuries Sourcebook, 2nd Edition

Stress-Related Disorders Sourcebook

Stroke Sourcebook

Substance Abuse Sourcebook

Surgery Sourcebook

Thyroid Disorders Sourcebook

Transplantation Sourcebook

Traveler's Health Sourcebook

Urinary Tract & Kidney Diseases &
Disorders Sourcebook, 2nd Edition

Vegetarian Sourcebook

Women's Health Concerns Sourcebook,
2nd Edition

Workplace Health & Safety Sourcebook

Worldwide Health Sourcebook

Teen Health Series

Alcohol Information for Teens

Allergy Information for Teens

Asthma Information for Teens

Cancer Information for Teens

Complementary & Alternative
Medicine Information for
Teens

Diabetes Information for Teens

Diet Information for Teens,
2nd Edition

Drug Information for Teens,
2nd Edition

Eating Disorders Information
for Teens

Fitness Information for Teens

Learning Disabilities Information
for Teens

Mental Health Information for
Teens, 2nd Edition

Sexual Health Information for
Teens

Skin Health Information for
Teens

Sports Injuries Information
for Teens

Suicide Information for Teens

Tobacco Information for Teens

Cancer
SOURCEBOOK
Fifth Edition

Health Reference Series

Fifth Edition

Cancer
SOURCEBOOK

*Basic Consumer Health Information about Major Forms
and Stages of Cancer, Featuring Facts about Head and
Neck Cancers, Lung Cancers, Gastrointestinal Cancers,
Genitourinary Cancers, Lymphomas, Blood Cell
Cancers, Endocrine Cancers, Skin Cancers, Bone
Cancers, Metastatic Cancers, and More*

*Along with Facts about Cancer Treatments, Cancer Risks
and Prevention, a Glossary of Related Terms, Statistical
Data, and a Directory of Resources for Additional
Information*

Edited by
Karen Bellenir

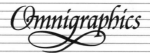

Omnigraphics

615 Griswold Street • Detroit, MI 48226

Bibliographic Note

Because this page cannot legibly accommodate all the copyright notices, the Bibliographic Note portion of the Preface constitutes an extension of the copyright notice.

Edited by Karen Bellenir

Health Reference Series

Karen Bellenir, *Managing Editor*
David A. Cooke, M.D., *Medical Consultant*
Elizabeth Collins, *Research and Permissions Coordinator*
Cherry Stockdale, *Permissions Assistant*
EdIndex, Services for Publishers, *Indexers*

* * *

Omnigraphics, Inc.

Matthew P. Barbour, *Senior Vice President*
Kay Gill, *Vice President—Directories*
Kevin Hayes, *Operations Manager*
David P. Bianco, *Marketing Director*

* * *

Peter E. Ruffner, *Publisher*

Frederick G. Ruffner, Jr., *Chairman*

Copyright © 2007 Omnigraphics, Inc.

ISBN 978-0-7808-0947-5

Library of Congress Cataloging-in-Publication Data

Cancer sourcebook : basic consumer health information about major forms and stages of cancer, featuring facts about head and neck cancers, lung cancers, gastrointestinal cancers, genitourinary cancers, lymphomas, blood cell cancers, endocrine cancers, skin cancers, bone cancers, metastatic cancers, and more; along with facts about cancer treatments, cancer risks and prevention, a glossary of related terms, statistical data, and a directory of resources for additional information / edited by Karen Bellenir. -- 5th ed.
    p. cm. -- (Health reference series)
   Summary: "Provides basic consumer health information about risks, prevention, and treatment of major forms of cancer. Includes index, glossary of related terms, and other resources"--Provided by publisher.
   Includes bibliographical references and index.
   ISBN 978-0-7808-0947-5 (hardcover : alk. paper) 1. Cancer--Popular works. 2. Cancer--Handbooks, manuals, etc. I. Bellenir, Karen.
   RC263.C294 2007
   616.99'4--dc22
                                                                                    2007003054

This book is printed on acid-free paper meeting the ANSI Z39.48 Standard. The infinity symbol that appears above indicates that the paper in this book meets that standard.

Printed in the United States

Table of Contents

Visit www.healthreferenceseries.com to view *A Contents Guide to the Health Reference Series*, a listing of more than 13,000 topics and the volumes in which they are covered.

Part II: Types of Cancer

Part III: Understanding Cancer Treatments

Preface

About This Book

In recent years, major advances have been made in the early detection, diagnosis, and treatment of cancer. The result has been declining death rates for the four most common cancers, as well as for all cancers combined. In fact, between the years 1993 and 2002, cancer death rates dropped 1.1 percent per year. In addition, the numbers of new cancer cases have been relatively stable since the 1990s.

In announcing the *Annual Report to the Nation on the Status of Cancer, 1975–2002*, which was published in the fall of 2005, Julie Gerberding, M.D., Director of the Centers for Disease Control and Prevention claimed, "Day by day we are winning the war against cancer as more people than ever before are being screened and are receiving treatments necessary for them to lead healthy and productive lives."

While cancer research has yielded significant progress, much work remains to be done. Cancer is still the second leading cause of death among Americans, surpassed only by heart disease. Incidence rates for some types of cancer—including breast cancer and lung cancer in women, cancers of the prostate and testes in men, leukemia, non-Hodgkin lymphoma, myeloma, melanoma, and cancers of the thyroid, kidney, and esophagus—are rising. Costs associated with cancer treatment continue to escalate, and racial and socioeconomic disparities in cancer rates and deaths remain unexplained.

Cancer Sourcebook, Fifth Edition provides updated information to help readers understand cancer risk factors, cancer prevention efforts, and the ongoing effort to develop better treatments. It offers descriptions of the major forms and stages of cancers affecting specific organs and the respiratory, nervous, lymphatic, circulatory, skeletal, gastrointestinal, and reproductive systems. It also describes special concerns related to metastatic, recurrent, and advanced cancers. A glossary of cancer terms and directories of organizations able to provide additional information are also included.

Readers seeking information about concerns encountered throughout the entire continuum of cancer care, including tips for maintaining wellness during and after cancer treatment, may wish to consult *Cancer Survivorship Sourcebook*, a separate volume within the *Health Reference Series*. In addition, some specific forms of cancer are discussed in a more in-depth manner in other *Health Reference Series* books:

- Breast cancer: *Breast Cancer Sourcebook, Second Edition*
- Childhood cancers: *Pediatric Cancer Sourcebook*
- Gynecological cancers: *Cancer Sourcebook for Women, Third Edition*
- Leukemia: *Leukemia Sourcebook*
- Prostate cancer: *Prostate Cancer Sourcebook* and *Prostate and Urological Disorders Sourcebook*
- Thyroid cancer: *Thyroid Disorders Sourcebook*

How to Use This Book

This book is divided into parts and chapters. Parts focus on broad areas of interest. Chapters are devoted to single topics within a part.

Part I: Cancer Risk Factors and Cancer Prevention describes how cancers get started and how they grow. It discusses factors known—or suspected—to increase a person's risk for cancer, including lifestyle choices and environmental exposures, and it outlines steps that can be taken to reduce cancer risks.

Part II: Types of Cancer begins with an overview of statistical information about cancers of all types. It continues with a detailed description of the symptoms, diagnosis, and treatment options for a wide variety of the most common cancers. These include head, neck, and eye cancers, brain and nerve cell cancers, lung cancers, gastrointestinal cancers, urinary tract cancers, reproductive and gender-linked cancers, blood cell and immune system cancers, endocrine cancers, skin cancers, sarcomas, and metastatic cancers.

Part III: Understanding Cancer Treatments explains the most commonly used standard cancer treatments, including chemotherapy, radiation therapy, and bone marrow transplantation. It also explains the use of cryosurgery and laser therapy, and it explains newer and experimental treatments such as biological therapy, photodynamic therapy, targeted therapies, and proton therapy. The part concludes with a chapter that discusses the uses of complementary and alternative medicine in cancer care.

Part IV: Special Concerns Related to Recurrent or Advanced Cancer discusses the unique cares, worries, and problems people face if they learn that cancer has come back after a time of remission. It also addresses patients who have been told that their cancer is not responding to treatment and that long-term remission is no longer likely. In addition, it provides facts for caregivers and offers patients suggestions for remaining in control of treatment choices and medical actions during end-of-life care.

Part V: Additional Help and Information includes a glossary of terms related to cancer and directories for more information about cancer. It also offers facts about obtaining cancer-related information in Spanish.

Bibliographic Note

This volume contains documents and excerpts from publications issued by the following U.S. government agencies: Center for Food Safety and Applied Nutrition; Centers for Disease Control and Prevention (CDC); National Cancer Institute; National Center for Chronic Disease Prevention and Health Promotion; Office of the Surgeon General; Surveillance Epidemiology and End Results (SEER); U.S. Department of Health and Human Services; and the U.S. Food and Drug Administration (FDA).

In addition, this volume contains copyrighted documents from the following organizations and individuals: A.D.A.M. Inc.; Alabama Cooperative Extension System (Alabama A&M and Auburn Universities); American Association of Neurological Surgeons; American Cancer Society; American Lung Association; American Thyroid Association, Inc.; Bascom Palmer Eye Institute; CancerHelp UK; Cincinnati Children's Hospital Medical Center; Gynecologic Cancer Foundation; Hirshberg Foundation for Pancreatic Cancer Research; Hormone Foundation; Leukemia and Lymphoma Society; Lymphoma Research Foundation; Multiple Myeloma Research Foundation; Timothy G. Murray. M.D.; National

Academy of Sciences; National Association for Proton Therapy; National Marrow Donor Program; Nature Publishing Group; Nemours Foundation; New York State Department of Health; New Zealand Dermatological Society; Novartis Pharmaceuticals Corporation; Orthopedic Oncology, New York University Medical Center Hospital for Joint Diseases; Oxford University Press, Inc.; Skin Cancer Foundation; Thyroid Foundation of America; University of Iowa Cancer Information Service; University of Texas, M.D. Anderson Cancer Center; and Wellsource, Inc.

Full citation information is provided on the first page of each chapter or section. Every effort has been made to secure all necessary rights to reprint the copyrighted material. If any omissions have been made, please contact Omnigraphics to make corrections for future editions.

Acknowledgements

In addition to the organizations, agencies, and individuals who have contributed to this *Sourcebook*, special thanks go to editorial assistants Nicole Salerno and Elizabeth Bellenir, research and permissions coordinator Liz Collins, and permissions assistant Cherry Stockdale.

About the Health Reference Series

The *Health Reference Series* is designed to provide basic medical information for patients, families, caregivers, and the general public. Each volume takes a particular topic and provides comprehensive coverage. This is especially important for people who may be dealing with a newly diagnosed disease or a chronic disorder in themselves or in a family member. People looking for preventive guidance, information about disease warning signs, medical statistics, and risk factors for health problems will also find answers to their questions in the *Health Reference Series*. The *Series*, however, is not intended to serve as a tool for diagnosing illness, in prescribing treatments, or as a substitute for the physician/patient relationship. All people concerned about medical symptoms or the possibility of disease are encouraged to seek professional care from an appropriate health care provider.

A Note about Spelling and Style

Health Reference Series editors use *Stedman's Medical Dictionary* as an authority for questions related to the spelling of medical terms and the *Chicago Manual of Style* for questions related to grammatical structures, punctuation, and other editorial concerns. Consistent adherence is not always possible, however, because the individual volumes within the *Series* include many documents from a wide variety of different producers and copyright holders, and the editor's primary goal is to present material from each source as accurately as is possible following the terms specified by each document's producer. This sometimes means that information in different chapters or sections may follow other guidelines and alternate spelling authorities. For example, occasionally a copyright holder may require that eponymous terms be shown in possessive forms (Crohn's disease *vs.* Crohn disease) or that British spelling norms be retained (leukaemia *vs.* leukemia).

Locating Information within the Health Reference Series

The *Health Reference Series* contains a wealth of information about a wide variety of medical topics. Ensuring easy access to all the fact sheets, research reports, in-depth discussions, and other material contained within the individual books of the *Series* remains one of our highest priorities. As the *Series* continues to grow in size and scope, however, locating the precise information needed by a reader may become more challenging.

A Contents Guide to the Health Reference Series was developed to direct readers to the specific volumes that address their concerns. It presents an extensive list of diseases, treatments, and other topics of general interest compiled from the Tables of Contents and major index headings. To access *A Contents Guide to the Health Reference Series*, visit www.healthreferenceseries.com.

Medical Consultant

Medical consultation services are provided to the *Health Reference Series* editors by David A. Cooke, M.D. Dr. Cooke is a graduate of Brandeis University, and he received his M.D. degree from the University of Michigan. He completed residency training at the University of Wisconsin Hospital and Clinics. He is board-certified in Internal Medicine. Dr. Cooke currently works as part of the University of Michigan Health System and practices in Brighton, MI. In his free time, he enjoys writing, science fiction, and spending time with his family.

Our Advisory Board

We would like to thank the following board members for providing guidance to the development of this *Series*:

- Dr. Lynda Baker, Associate Professor of Library and Information Science, Wayne State University, Detroit, MI
- Nancy Bulgarelli, William Beaumont Hospital Library, Royal Oak, MI
- Karen Imarisio, Bloomfield Township Public Library, Bloomfield Township, MI
- Karen Morgan, Mardigian Library, University of Michigan-Dearborn, Dearborn, MI
- Rosemary Orlando, St. Clair Shores Public Library, St. Clair Shores, MI

Health Reference Series *Update Policy*

The inaugural book in the *Health Reference Series* was the first edition of *Cancer Sourcebook* published in 1989. Since then, the *Series* has been enthusiastically received by librarians and in the medical community. In order to maintain the standard of providing high-quality health information for the layperson the editorial staff at Omnigraphics felt it was necessary to implement a policy of updating volumes when warranted.

Medical researchers have been making tremendous strides, and it is the purpose of the *Health Reference Series* to stay current with the most recent advances. Each decision to update a volume is made on an individual basis. Some of the considerations include how much new information is available and the feedback we receive from people who use the books. If there is a topic you would like to see added to the update list, or an area of medical concern you feel has not been adequately addressed, please write to:

Editor
Health Reference Series
Omnigraphics, Inc.
615 Griswold Street
Detroit, MI 48226
E-mail: editorial@omnigraphics.com

Part One

Cancer Risk Factors and Cancer Prevention

Chapter 1

Cancer: An Overview

Cancer begins in cells, the building blocks that form tissues. Tissues make up the organs of the body.

Normally, cells grow and divide to form new cells as the body needs them. When cells grow old, they die, and new cells take their place.

Sometimes, this orderly process goes wrong. New cells form when the body does not need them, and old cells do not die when they should. These extra cells can form a mass of tissue called a growth or tumor.

Tumors can be benign or malignant:

- Benign tumors are not cancer:

    - Benign tumors are rarely life-threatening.

    - Generally, benign tumors can be removed, and they usually do not grow back.

    - Cells from benign tumors do not invade the tissues around them.

    - Cells from benign tumors do not spread to other parts of the body.

- Malignant tumors are cancer:

From "What You Need to Know About™ Cancer—An Overview," National Cancer Institute, June 2005. The complete text of this document, including links to additional resources, is available online at http://www.cancer.gov/cancertopics/wyntk/overview.

- Malignant tumors are generally more serious than benign tumors. They may be life-threatening.

- Malignant tumors often can be removed, but sometimes they grow back.

- Cells from malignant tumors can invade and damage nearby tissues and organs.

- Cells from malignant tumors can spread (metastasize) to other parts of the body. Cancer cells spread by breaking away from the original (primary) tumor and entering the bloodstream or lymphatic system. The cells can invade other organs, forming new tumors that damage these organs. The spread of cancer is called metastasis.

Most cancers are named for where they start. For example, lung cancer starts in the lung, and breast cancer starts in the breast. Lymphoma is cancer that starts in the lymphatic system. And leukemia is cancer that starts in white blood cells (leukocytes).

When cancer spreads and forms a new tumor in another part of the body, the new tumor has the same kind of abnormal cells and the same name as the primary tumor. For example, if prostate cancer spreads to the bones, the cancer cells in the bones are actually prostate cancer cells. The disease is metastatic prostate cancer, not bone cancer. For that reason, it is treated as prostate cancer, not bone cancer. Doctors sometimes call the new tumor "distant" or metastatic disease.

Risk Factors

Doctors often cannot explain why one person develops cancer and another does not. But research shows that certain risk factors increase the chance that a person will develop cancer. These are the most common risk factors for cancer:

- **Growing older:** The most important risk factor for cancer is growing older. Most cancers occur in people over the age of 65. But people of all ages, including children, can get cancer, too.

- **Tobacco:** Tobacco use is the most preventable cause of death. Each year, more than 180,000 Americans die from cancer that is related to tobacco use. Using tobacco products or regularly being around tobacco smoke (environmental or secondhand smoke) increases the risk of cancer. Smokers are more likely than nonsmokers to develop cancer of the lung, larynx (voice box), mouth, esophagus, bladder, kidney, throat, stomach, pancreas, or cervix. They also are more likely to develop acute myeloid leukemia (cancer that starts in blood cells). People who use smokeless tobacco (snuff or chewing tobacco) are at increased risk of cancer of the mouth.

- **Sunlight:** Ultraviolet (UV) radiation comes from the sun, sunlamps, and tanning booths. It causes early aging of the skin and skin damage that can lead to skin cancer.

- **Ionizing radiation:** Ionizing radiation can cause cell damage that leads to cancer. This kind of radiation comes from rays that enter the Earth's atmosphere from outer space, radioactive fallout, radon gas, x-rays, and other sources. Medical procedures are a common source of radiation.

- **Certain chemicals and other substances:** People who have certain jobs (such as painters, construction workers, and those in the chemical industry) have an increased risk of cancer. Many studies have shown that exposure to asbestos, benzene, benzidine, cadmium, nickel, or vinyl chloride in the workplace can cause cancer.

- **Some viruses and bacteria:** Being infected with certain viruses or bacteria may increase the risk of developing cancer:

  - **Human papillomaviruses (HPVs):** HPV infection is the main cause of cervical cancer. It also may be a risk factor for other types of cancer.

  - **Hepatitis B and hepatitis C viruses:** Liver cancer can develop after many years of infection with hepatitis B or hepatitis C.

  - **Human T-cell leukemia/lymphoma virus (HTLV-1):** Infection with HTLV-1 increases a person's risk of lymphoma and leukemia.

  - **Human immunodeficiency virus (HIV):** HIV is the virus that causes AIDS. People who have HIV infection are at greater risk of cancer, such as lymphoma and a rare cancer called Kaposi sarcoma.

  - **Epstein-Barr virus (EBV):** Infection with EBV has been linked to an increased risk of lymphoma.

- **Human herpesvirus 8 (HHV8):** This virus is a risk factor for Kaposi sarcoma.

- *Helicobacter pylori:* This bacterium can cause stomach ulcers. It also can cause stomach cancer and lymphoma in the stomach lining.

Many of these risk factors can be avoided. Others, such as family history, cannot be avoided. People can help protect themselves by staying away from known risk factors whenever possible.

Screening

Some types of cancer can be found before they cause symptoms. Checking for cancer (or for conditions that may lead to cancer) in people who have no symptoms is called screening.

Screening can help doctors find and treat some types of cancer early. Generally, cancer treatment is more effective when the disease is found early.

Screening tests are used widely to check for cancers of the breast, cervix, colon, and rectum:

- **Breast:** A mammogram is the best tool doctors have to find breast cancer early. A mammogram is a picture of the breast made with x-rays. The NCI recommends that women in their forties and older have mammograms every one to two years. Women who are at higher-than-average risk of breast cancer should talk with their health care provider about whether to have mammograms before age 40 and how often to have them.

- **Cervix:** The Pap test (sometimes called Pap smear) is used to check cells from the cervix. The doctor scrapes a sample of cells from the cervix. A lab checks the cells for cancer or changes that may lead to cancer (including changes caused by human papillomavirus, the most important risk factor for cancer of the cervix). Women should begin having Pap tests three years after they begin having sexual intercourse, or when they reach age 21 (whichever comes first). Most women should have a Pap test at least once every three years.

- **Colon and rectum:** A number of screening tests are used to detect polyps (growths), cancer, or other problems in the colon and rectum. People aged 50 and older should be screened.

People who have a higher-than-average risk of cancer of the colon or rectum should talk with their doctor about whether to have screening tests before age 50 and how often to have them.

- **Fecal occult blood test:** Sometimes cancer or polyps bleed. This test can detect tiny amounts of blood in the stool.

- **Sigmoidoscopy:** The doctor checks inside the rectum and lower part of the colon with a lighted tube called a sigmoidoscope. The doctor can usually remove polyps through the tube.

- **Colonoscopy:** The doctor examines inside the rectum and entire colon using a long, lighted tube called a colonoscope. The doctor can usually remove polyps through the tube.

- **Double-contrast barium enema:** This procedure involves several x-rays of the colon and rectum. The patient is given an enema with a barium solution, and air is pumped into the rectum. The barium and air improve the x-ray images of the colon and rectum.

- **Digital rectal exam:** A rectal exam is often part of a routine physical exam. The health care provider inserts a lubricated, gloved finger into the rectum to feel for abnormal areas. A digital rectal exam allows for examination of only the lowest part of the rectum.

You may have heard about other tests to check for cancer in other parts of the body. At this time, we do not know whether routine screening with these other tests saves lives. The NCI is supporting research to learn more about screening for cancers of the breast, cervix, colon, lung, ovary, prostate, and skin.

Doctors consider many factors before they suggest a screening test. They weigh factors related to the test and to the cancer that the test can detect. They also pay special attention to a person's risk for developing certain types of cancer. For example, doctors think about the person's age, medical history, general health, family history, and lifestyle. They consider how accurate the test is. In addition, doctors keep in mind the possible harms of the screening test itself. They also look at the risk of follow-up tests or surgery that the person might need to see if an abnormal test result means cancer. Doctors also think about the risks and benefits of treatment if testing finds cancer. They consider how well the treatment works and what side effects it causes.

You may want to talk with your doctor about the possible benefits and harms of being checked for cancer. The decision to be screened, like many other medical decisions, is a personal one. Each person should decide after learning about the pros and cons of screening.

You may want to ask the doctor the following questions about screening:

- Which tests do you recommend for me? Why?
- How much do the tests cost? Will my health insurance help pay for screening tests?
- Do the tests hurt? Are there any risks?
- How soon after the tests will I learn the results?
- If the results show a problem, how will you learn if I have cancer?

Symptoms

Cancer can cause many different symptoms. These are some of them:

- A thickening or lump in the breast or any other part of the body
- A new mole or a change in an existing mole
- A sore that does not heal
- Hoarseness or a cough that does not go away
- Changes in bowel or bladder habits
- Discomfort after eating
- A hard time swallowing
- Weight gain or loss with no known reason
- Unusual bleeding or discharge
- Feeling weak or very tired

Most often, these symptoms are not due to cancer. They may also be caused by benign tumors or other problems. Only a doctor can tell for sure. Anyone with these symptoms or other changes in health should see a doctor to diagnose and treat problems as early as possible.

Usually, early cancer does not cause pain. If you have symptoms, do not wait to feel pain before seeing a doctor.

Diagnosis

If you have a symptom or your screening test result suggests cancer, the doctor must find out whether it is due to cancer or to some other cause. The doctor may ask about your personal and family medical history and do a physical exam. The doctor also may order lab tests, x-rays, or other tests or procedures.

Lab Tests

Tests of the blood, urine, or other fluids can help doctors make a diagnosis. These tests can show how well an organ (such as the kidney) is doing its job. Also, high amounts of some substances may be a sign of cancer. These substances are often called tumor markers. However, abnormal lab results are not a sure sign of cancer. Doctors cannot rely on lab tests alone to diagnose cancer.

Imaging Procedures

Imaging procedures create pictures of areas inside your body that help the doctor see whether a tumor is present. These pictures can be made in several ways:

- **X-rays:** X-rays are the most common way to view organs and bones inside the body.

- **CT scan (computed tomography scan):** An x-ray machine linked to a computer takes a series of detailed pictures of your organs. You may receive a contrast material (such as dye) to make these pictures easier to read.

- **Radionuclide scan:** You receive an injection of a small amount of radioactive material. It flows through your bloodstream and collects in certain bones or organs. A machine called a scanner detects and measures the radioactivity. The scanner creates pictures of bones or organs on a computer screen or on film. Your body gets rid of the radioactive substance quickly.

- **Ultrasound:** An ultrasound device sends out sound waves that people cannot hear. The waves bounce off tissues inside your body like an echo. A computer uses these echoes to create a picture called a sonogram.

- **MRI (magnetic resonance imaging):** A strong magnet linked to a computer is used to make detailed pictures of areas in your

9

body. Your doctor can view these pictures on a monitor and can print them on film.

- **PET scan (positron emission tomography scan):** You receive an injection of a small amount of radioactive material. A machine makes pictures that show chemical activities in the body. Cancer cells sometimes show up as areas of high activity.

Biopsy

In most cases, doctors need to do a biopsy to make a diagnosis of cancer. For a biopsy, the doctor removes a sample of tissue and sends it to a lab. A pathologist looks at the tissue under a microscope. The sample may be removed in several ways:

- **With a needle:** The doctor uses a needle to withdraw tissue or fluid.

- **With an endoscope:** The doctor uses a thin, lighted tube (an endoscope) to look at areas inside the body. The doctor can remove tissue or cells through the tube.

- **With surgery:** Surgery may be excisional or incisional.

  - In an *excisional biopsy*, the surgeon removes the entire tumor. Often some of the normal tissue around the tumor also is removed.

  - In an *incisional biopsy*, the surgeon removes just part of the tumor.

You may want to ask the doctor these questions before having a biopsy:

- Where will I go for the biopsy?

- How long will it take? Will I be awake? Will it hurt?

- Are there any risks? What are the chances of infection or bleeding after the procedure?

- How soon will I know the results?

- If I do have cancer, who will talk to me about the next steps? When?

Staging

To plan the best treatment for cancer, the doctor needs to know the extent (stage) of your disease. For most cancers (such as breast, lung, prostate, or colon cancer), the stage is based on the size of the tumor and whether the cancer has spread to lymph nodes or other parts of the body. The doctor may order x-rays, lab tests, and other tests or procedures to learn the extent of the disease.

Treatment

Many people with cancer want to take an active part in making decisions about their medical care. It is natural to want to learn all you can about your disease and treatment choices. However, shock and stress after the diagnosis can make it hard to think of everything you want to ask the doctor. It often helps to make a list of questions before an appointment.

To help remember what the doctor says, you may take notes or ask whether you may use a tape recorder. Some people also want to have a family member or friend with them when they talk to the doctor— to take part in the discussion, to take notes, or just to listen.

You do not need to ask all your questions at once. You will have other chances to ask the doctor or nurse to explain things that are not clear and to ask for more information.

Your doctor may refer you to a specialist, or you may ask for a referral. Specialists who treat cancer include surgeons, medical oncologists, hematologists, and radiation oncologists.

Getting a Second Opinion

Before starting treatment, you may want a second opinion about your diagnosis and treatment plan. Many insurance companies will cover a second opinion if your doctor requests it. It may take some time and effort to gather medical records and arrange to see another doctor. Usually it is not a problem to take several weeks to get a second opinion. In most cases, the delay in starting treatment will not make treatment less effective. But some people with cancer need treatment right away. To make sure, you should discuss this delay with your doctor.

There are a number of ways to find a doctor for a second opinion:

• Your doctor may refer you to one or more specialists. At cancer centers, several specialists often work together as a team.

- NCI's Cancer Information Service, at 800-4-CANCER, can tell you about nearby treatment centers. Information Specialists also can provide online assistance through LiveHelp at http://www.cancer.gov.

- A local or state medical society, a nearby hospital, or a medical school can usually provide the names of specialists.

- The American Board of Medical Specialties (ABMS) has a list of doctors who have had training and passed exams in their specialty. You can find this list in the Official ABMS Directory of Board Certified Medical Specialists. This directory is in most public libraries. Also, ABMS offers this information at http://www.abms.org. (Click on "Who's Certified.")

- The NCI provides a fact sheet called "How to Find a Doctor or Treatment Facility If You Have Cancer."

- Nonprofit organizations with an interest in cancer may be of help. See the NCI fact sheet "National Organizations That Offer Services to People with Cancer and Their Families."

Treatment Methods

The treatment plan depends mainly on the type of cancer and the stage of the disease. Doctors also consider the patient's age and general health. Often, the goal of treatment is to cure the cancer. In other cases, the goal is to control the disease or to reduce symptoms for as long as possible. The treatment plan may change over time.

Most treatment plans include surgery, radiation therapy, or chemotherapy. Some involve hormone therapy or biological therapy. In addition, stem cell transplantation may be used so that a patient can receive very high doses of chemotherapy or radiation therapy.

Some cancers respond best to a single type of treatment. Others may respond best to a combination of treatments.

Treatments may work in a specific area (local therapy) or throughout the body (systemic therapy):

- Local therapy removes or destroys cancer in just one part of the body. Surgery to remove a tumor is local therapy. Radiation to shrink or destroy a tumor also is usually local therapy.

- Systemic therapy sends drugs or substances through the bloodstream to destroy cancer cells all over the body. It kills or slows the growth of cancer cells that may have spread beyond the original tumor. Chemotherapy, hormone therapy, and biological therapy are usually systemic therapy.

Your doctor can describe your treatment choices and the expected results. You and your doctor can work together to decide on a treatment plan that is best for you.

Because cancer treatments often damage healthy cells and tissues, side effects are common. Side effects depend mainly on the type and extent of the treatment. Side effects may not be the same for each person, and they may change from one treatment session to the next.

Before treatment starts, the health care team will explain possible side effects and suggest ways to help you manage them. This team may include nurses, a dietitian, a physical therapist, and others.

At any stage of cancer, supportive care is available to relieve the side effects of therapy, to control pain and other symptoms, and to ease emotional and practical problems. Information about supportive care is available on NCI's Web site at http://www.cancer.gov/cancertopics/coping and from Information Specialists at 800-4-CANCER.

You may want to ask the doctor these questions before treatment begins:

- What is my diagnosis?

- Has the cancer spread? If so, where? What is the stage of the disease?

- What is the goal of treatment? What are my treatment choices? Which do you recommend for me? Why?

- What are the expected benefits of each kind of treatment?

- What are the risks and possible side effects of each treatment? How can side effects be managed?

- Will infertility be a side effect of my treatment? Can anything be done about that? Should I consider storing sperm or eggs?

- What can I do to prepare for treatment?

- How often will I have treatments? How long will my treatment last?

- Will I have to change my normal activities? If so, for how long?

- What is the treatment likely to cost? Will my insurance cover the costs?

- What new treatments are under study? Would a clinical trial be appropriate for me?

Surgery

In most cases, the surgeon removes the tumor and some tissue around it. Removing nearby tissue may help prevent the tumor from growing back. The surgeon may also remove some nearby lymph nodes.

The side effects of surgery depend mainly on the size and location of the tumor, and the type of operation. It takes time to heal after surgery. The time needed to recover is different for each type of surgery. It is also different for each person. It is common to feel tired or weak for a while.

Most people are uncomfortable for the first few days after surgery. However, medicine can help control the pain. Before surgery, you should discuss the plan for pain relief with the doctor or nurse. The doctor can adjust the plan if you need more pain relief.

Some people worry that having surgery (or even a biopsy) for cancer will spread the disease. This seldom happens. Surgeons use special methods and take many steps to prevent cancer cells from spreading. For example, if they must remove tissue from more than one area, they use different tools for each one. This approach helps reduce the chance that cancer cells will spread to healthy tissue.

Similarly, some people worry that exposing cancer to air during surgery will cause the disease to spread. This is not true. Air does not make cancer spread.

Radiation Therapy

Radiation therapy (also called radiotherapy) uses high-energy rays to kill cancer cells. Doctors use several types of radiation therapy. Some people receive a combination of treatments:

- **External radiation:** The radiation comes from a large machine outside the body. Most people go to a hospital or clinic for treatment five days a week for several weeks.

- **Internal radiation (implant radiation or brachytherapy):** The radiation comes from radioactive material placed in seeds, needles, or thin plastic tubes that are put in or near the tissue. The patient usually stays in the hospital. The implants generally remain in place for several days.

- **Systemic radiation:** The radiation comes from liquid or capsules containing radioactive material that travels throughout the body. The patient swallows the liquid or capsules or receives an injection. This type of radiation therapy can be used to treat cancer or control pain.

The side effects of radiation therapy depend mainly on the dose and type of radiation you receive and the part of your body that is treated. For example, radiation to your abdomen can cause nausea, vomiting, and diarrhea. Your skin in the treated area may become red, dry, and tender. You also may lose your hair in the treated area.

You may become very tired during radiation therapy, especially in the later weeks of treatment. Resting is important, but doctors usually advise patients to try to stay as active as they can.

Fortunately, most side effects go away in time. In the meantime, there are ways to reduce discomfort. If you have a side effect that is especially severe, the doctor may suggest a break in your treatment.

Chemotherapy

Chemotherapy is the use of drugs that kill cancer cells. Most patients receive chemotherapy by mouth or through a vein. Either way, the drugs enter the bloodstream and can affect cancer cells all over the body.

Chemotherapy is usually given in cycles. People receive treatment for one or more days. Then they have a recovery period of several days or weeks before the next treatment session.

Most people have their treatment in an outpatient part of the hospital, at the doctor's office, or at home. Some may need to stay in the hospital during chemotherapy.

Side effects depend mainly on the specific drugs and the dose. The drugs affect cancer cells and other cells that divide rapidly:

- **Blood cells:** When drugs damage healthy blood cells, you are more likely to get infections, to bruise or bleed easily, and to feel very weak and tired.

- **Cells in hair roots:** Chemotherapy can cause hair loss. Your hair will grow back, but it may be somewhat different in color and texture.

- **Cells that line the digestive tract:** Chemotherapy can cause poor appetite, nausea and vomiting, diarrhea, or mouth and lip sores.

15

Some drugs can affect fertility. Women may be unable to become pregnant, and men may not be able to father a child.

Although the side effects of chemotherapy can be distressing, most of them are temporary. Your doctor can usually treat or control them.

Hormone Therapy

Some cancers need hormones to grow. Hormone therapy keeps cancer cells from getting or using the hormones they need. It is systemic therapy. Hormone therapy uses drugs or surgery:

- **Drugs:** The doctor gives medicine that stops the production of certain hormones or prevents the hormones from working.

- **Surgery:** The surgeon removes organs (such as the ovaries or testicles) that make hormones.

The side effects of hormone therapy depend on the type of therapy. They include weight gain, hot flashes, nausea, and changes in fertility. In women, hormone therapy may make menstrual periods stop or become irregular and may cause vaginal dryness. In men, hormone therapy may cause impotence, loss of sexual desire, and breast growth or tenderness.

Biological Therapy

Biological therapy is another type of systemic therapy. It helps the immune system (the body's natural defense system) fight cancer. For example, certain patients with bladder cancer receive bacille Calmette-Guérin (BCG) solution after surgery. The doctor uses a catheter to put the solution in the bladder. The solution contains live, weakened bacteria that stimulate the immune system to kill cancer cells. BCG can cause side effects. It can irritate the bladder. Some people may have nausea, a low-grade fever, or chills.

Most other types of biological therapy are given through a vein. The biological therapy travels through the bloodstream. Some people get a rash where the therapy is injected. Some have flu-like symptoms such as fever, chills, headache, muscle aches, fatigue, weakness, and nausea. Biological therapy also can cause more serious side effects, such as changes in blood pressure and breathing problems. Biological therapy is usually given at the doctor's office, clinic, or hospital.

Stem Cell Transplantation

Transplantation of blood-forming stem cells enables patients to receive high doses of chemotherapy, radiation, or both. The high doses destroy both cancer cells and normal blood cells in the bone marrow. After the treatment, the patient receives healthy, blood-forming stem cells through a flexible tube placed in a large vein. New blood cells develop from the transplanted stem cells. Stem cells may be taken from the patient before the high-dose treatment, or they may come from another person. Patients stay in the hospital for this treatment.

The side effects of high-dose therapy and stem cell transplantation include infection and bleeding. In addition, graft-versus-host disease (GVHD) may occur in people who receive stem cells from a donor. In GVHD, the donated stem cells attack the patient's tissues. Most often, GVHD affects the liver, skin, or digestive tract. GVHD can be severe or even fatal. It can occur any time after the transplant, even years later. Drugs may help prevent, treat, or control GVHD.

Complementary and Alternative Medicine

Some people with cancer use complementary and alternative medicine (CAM). An approach is generally called complementary medicine when it is used along with standard treatment. An approach is called alternative medicine when it is used instead of standard treatment.

Acupuncture, massage therapy, herbal products, vitamins or special diets, visualization, meditation, and spiritual healing are types of CAM.

Many people say that CAM helps them feel better. However, some types of CAM may change the way standard treatment works. These changes could be harmful. Other types of CAM could be harmful even if used alone.

Some types of CAM are expensive. Health insurance may not cover the cost.

Follow-up Care

Advances in early detection and treatment mean that many people with cancer are cured. But doctors can never be certain that the cancer will not come back. Undetected cancer cells can remain in the body after treatment. Although the cancer seems to be completely removed or destroyed, it can return. Doctors call this a recurrence.

To find out whether the cancer has returned, your doctor may do a physical exam and order lab tests, x-rays, and other tests. If you have a recurrence, you and your doctor will decide on new treatment goals and a new treatment plan.

During follow-up exams, the doctor also checks for other problems, such as side effects from cancer therapy that can arise long after treatment. Checkups help ensure that changes in health are noted and treated if needed. Between scheduled visits, you should contact the doctor if any health problems occur.

Chapter 2

Cancer Screening and Symptoms Suspicious of Cancer

How Cancers Start

Cancer does not develop all at once in a cell. Several changes must occur in the genetic information (DNA) carried in a single cell before it can become a cancer cell and multiply into a tumor. Cells change their abnormal growth properties one step at a time; each genetic change pushes the cell further along the spectrum of abnormal growth. Not all cells acquire the same genetic changes nor can anyone predict when the changes will occur. That explains to some extent why some cancers develop and grow rapidly and cause death in months; other cancers may grow so slowly that the person eventually dies from a cause other than cancer.

Stages of Cancer

- In stage I, cancer cells can be distinguished from normal cells. The cancer cells are still localized (usually referred to as cancer in situ) and surgical removal of the tumor usually results in a cure.

This chapter includes "How Cancers Start," "Detecting Cancer," and "Cancer-Focused Exams," from the *Understanding Cancer* series produced by Novartis Oncology. © 2006 Novartis Pharmaceuticals Corporation. All rights reserved. Reprinted with permission. For additional information visit http://www.us.novartisoncology.com.

- In stage II, tumor size is increased. The cancer cells may or may not have spread to the lymph nodes, and begun encroaching on nearby tissue.

- By stage III, the cancer cells have continued to grow and extend into the area around the tumor.

- In stage IV, tumors have spread to other parts of the body.

Symptoms Suspicious of Cancer

In its early stages, cancer typically does not have any symptoms. However, here are some important body signals that might indicate the presence of cancer and should be brought to the attention of your doctor:

- **Any changes in bowel habits:** If you've always had normal bowel movements but suddenly develop constipation that continues for two weeks or more, especially if it's accompanied by intermittent attacks of diarrhea, let your doctor know. Cancer of the bowel often presents itself in this way. Blood in the stool, even if you would like to attribute it to your hemorrhoids, should also be checked out because hemorrhoids can coexist with more serious colon problems. Finally, if your normally bulky stool has become thin and ribbon-like, the reduced caliber may be due to a growth that's narrowing a portion of the colon.

- **An open sore or a persistent rash** that does not clear up may reflect skin cancer.

- **Blood or discharge** from any body orifice—vomited, coughed up, in the urine, from the vagina, or in the stool—must be explained.

- **Show your doctor any persistent bump or lump** anywhere you find it—in the breast, on the skin, in the testicle, under your arms, in your neck, your groin, or in your abdomen.

- **Pain in your stomach**, either when you're hungry or after you eat, indigestion, or difficulty swallowing, may all be important danger signals.

- **A chronic, nagging cough**, with or without sputum and especially (but not necessarily) accompanied by any amount of blood, however small, is an ominous sign—especially in smokers. So is persistent hoarseness.

- **A low-grade fever** without an obvious cause (doctors called it FUO—fever of unknown origin) that continues for longer than a week or two warrants a visit to your doctor. It may be due to something as innocuous as an infection behind a tooth or an allergic response to some medication you're taking, but it may also reflect a serious process such as a diseased heart valve, an abscess somewhere in the body—or a hidden malignancy.

- **If you're losing weight** for no apparent reason, you should have a thorough checkup. The problem may be some medication you're taking (a notorious culprit is digitalis, widely used for treating various heart conditions), an overactive thyroid, an undiagnosed infection, or a hidden cancer.

Although these signs may be symptoms of other conditions, you should not ignore any of these signs simply because they are not causing you any pain—at the moment. Cancers often don't hurt in the early stages.

Detecting Cancer

A checkup is a fishing expedition for the earliest evidence of any silent disease or disorder, including cancer. The focus of the routine physical depends on your age, vulnerability, and sex. If you have specific symptoms, fears, or susceptibility, your doctor will perform a targeted exam. But don't wait until you're sick. Get your physical while you're still healthy.

During a general checkup, your doctor should obtain a detailed medical history so that he or she can pay special attention to areas of potential disease. Most doctors spend less time with their presumably healthy patients, that instead of asking you these questions face to face, they give you a printed form to answer. Don't gloss over it. Think carefully about each question; it may remind you of something you've forgotten to tell the doctor or didn't think was important. And be sure to discuss any query to which you answered yes.

A careful, total body physical exam is extremely important. Beware of any doctor who examines you while you're partially dressed; you should be wearing nothing so that every part of your body is visible. No exam is complete without an examination of all your lymph glands—in the neck, the armpit, and the groin—as well as a digital evaluation of the rectum and, in women, a pelvic exam too.

After the physical, you should have your urine checked for evidence of infection, blood, and abnormal proteins; your stool should be analyzed for the presence of blood (it's not always visible to the naked eye); and your blood should be drawn for a spectrum of tests. Government legislation prohibits Medicare from reimbursing you for screening blood tests if you have no specific complaints. However, it is important to be tested because early diagnosis and treatment cost much less than waiting for trouble to appear. Over the years, many have been diagnosed from a host of unexpected abnormalities: cancer (from the chemical detection of blood in the stool); thyroid underfunction (from a routine blood test in patients who believed they were simply 'tired'); diabetes (from urine or blood of patients who never suspected that their sugar was elevated); kidney trouble; liver disease; abnormal cholesterol and other blood-fat levels; tumors of the parathyroid gland (when the only abnormality was a high calcium level in the blood); and hepatitis C. If you're in the Medicare age group, or if you're younger and your insurance carrier or managed-care company won't pay for routine blood tests, then talk with your doctor and have them arranged anyway.

In order to detect early cancer, certain tests should routinely be done at varying intervals depending on your age, sex, and the type of cancer (or other disease) to which you are especially susceptible. This might mean more frequently then just annually.

Although x-rays of the upper gastrointestinal tract and barium enemas are still widely used, newer techniques are often preferred when there is a suspicious finding. For example, the CT scan is a special procedure in which a computer is hooked up to an x-ray machine and a series of detailed pictures is taken at different levels or 'cuts' of the tissue being examined. This provides an in-depth analysis of a particular region of the body, such as the chest or the abdomen. Endoscopy allows the doctor to view the interior of the body through a thin tube with a light and a little snare at its end. (Such an exam is named for the organ being studied: a colonoscopy looks inside the colon; gastroscopy views the stomach; and bronchoscopy visualizes the respiratory system.) Looking directly at these tissues makes it possible to remove a polyp or to snip a piece off any suspicious tissue that is present and send it to the lab for analysis. The pathologist stains the cells, looks at them under the microscope, and can tell whether they're cancerous, and, if so, whether they are likely to grow slowly or quickly.

Radionuclear scanning is a noninvasive procedure in which you are given a mildly radioactive substance orally or by injection. A scanner measures the radioactivity level of the area or organ being evaluated and prints a picture of it on paper or film. The radioactive uptake pattern reveals the presence of growths and other abnormalities in the target tissue.

Ultrasound is a useful diagnostic procedure that is usually done to clarify a suspicious finding in the physical exam. High-frequency sound waves that cannot be heard by humans are directed toward the organ in question. Their 'echo' bounces back to produce a picture called a sonogram, which appears on a monitor, and is then printed on paper for a permanent record. Sonograms are especially valuable in the diagnosis of heart disease. However, they also reveal cancers in the abdomen that the doctor cannot feel, for example, in the pancreas, gallbladder, or liver.

Magnetic resonance imaging (MRI) involves the use of a powerful magnet linked to a computer that gives detailed pictures of various areas of the body. There is no radiation involved; the derived information is viewed on a monitor, and then printed out. With the exception of endoscopy, the MRI probably yields more information about cancer than any of the other diagnostic procedures described above.

Cancer-Focused Exams

On what aspects of the checkup should the doctor concentrate when looking for cancer? Listed below are some of the cancer-focused exams that you should have on a regular basis in order to detect the disease at an early stage.

Breast cancer: Women over the age of sixty-five who are at greatest risk for breast cancer should take the following three steps to ensure its early detection:

1. A mammogram: Properly done and carefully interpreted, this x-ray procedure identifies a breast tumor as early as two years before it can be felt.

2. Self-examination of your own breasts every month: Learn the right way to do it either from your doctor or by phoning the National Cancer Institute at 800-422-6237 (800-4-CANCER).

3. A breast exam by your doctor during your regular checkup or at least every year.

Uterine and cervical cancer: As a woman grows older, her risk of cancer of the uterus and cervix increases. Some women stop seeing their gynecologist after menopause because they think that since their periods have ended, there are no more potential "female" problems. This is not true. A gynecologist or your family doctor should do a pelvic exam and Pap test once a year regardless of how old you are. Although some doctors believe that if you have had a normal Pap test for three consecutive years after menopause, you may skip it, annually is still recommend.

Cancer of the colon and rectum are also more common in older persons. Three tests can detect this malignancy:

1. The guaiac stool test (also called the fecal, or stool, occult test, or hemoccult test) reveals the presence of traces of blood in the stool not visible to the naked eye. You can do this one yourself with a kit available at all pharmacies. It comes with explicit instructions. A chemical is added to the specimen, and a change in color indicates the presence of blood.

2. An annual rectal exam, in which the doctor feels for any bumps or irregular areas of the rectum.

3. Colonoscopy every three to five years beginning at age fifty. A long thin tube is inserted into the rectum and threaded the entire length of the colon. (Sigmoidoscopy is a similar procedure, but the instrument doesn't reach nearly as far.) This allows the doctor to inspect the lining of the bowel and detect any polyps or growths.

Prostate cancer is the most common malignancy among American men, 80 percent of whom are sixty-five and older.

Skin cancer: Your doctor should inspect your skin carefully in the course of every routine physical exam. Some "blemishes" can be tricky and your doctor might refer you a dermatologist once a year to have your entire body surface checked for malignant or premalignant lesions. You can improve the chances of finding one early in the game by inspecting your skin yourself. Look for and report anything that's suspicious to you, especially if it's changed in size, texture, color, its borders have become irregular, or is a sore that doesn't heal.

Look specifically for moles or pigmented spots on the skin. (Doctors call them nevi.) They first appear as small, flat, tan or brown spots that slowly become raised. In time, they can flatten again, become flesh-colored, and disappear. Nevi are specific cells in the skin (melanocytes) that have heaped up in a cluster instead of spreading out evenly. (Melanocytes give the skin its natural color. When you sit in the sun, your melanocytes produce more pigment, darkening and tanning the skin.) Most people normally have anywhere from ten to forty nevi, and develop new ones from time to time until approximately age forty. At least one of every ten of them is dysplastic, an unusual-looking or atypical mole different from the rest. Dysplastic nevi are more likely than the others to develop into a melanoma. (However, most don't.) Any skin lesion that's the least bit suspicious looking should be biopsied. That's the only way to be sure it isn't malignant.

You should check your mouth at regular intervals, and so should your doctor and dentist. Look for changes in the color of your lips and tongue. Then inspect the inner cheeks; search everywhere for scabs, cracks, sores, white patches, swelling, or bleeding. Report what you find to your doctor.

Skin cancer is the most common tumor in this country, in both men and women. Fortunately, most skin cancers, such as the basal or squamous cell types, are localized, easily removable, and rarely life-threaten. However, a malignant melanoma is potentially fatal and must be removed early—before it spreads through the body. This cancer is caused by exposure to ultraviolet radiation from the sun, sunlamps, and tanning booths. People at greatest risk for melanomas are those who have already had melanomas, who have close relatives with it, who were badly sunburned as children or teenagers, or whose skin is fair and burns or freckles easily. The incidence of malignant melanoma rose almost 80 percent between 1973 and 1988, and it continues to do so—more than any other cancer.

Chapter 3

What Causes Cancer?

Cancer has many causes. There are about 200 different types of cancer affecting all the different body tissues. What affects one body tissue may not affect another. For example, tobacco smoke that you breathe in may help to cause lung cancer. Over exposing your skin to the sun could give you a melanoma on your leg. But the sun won't give you lung cancer and smoking won't give you melanoma.

Apart from infectious diseases, most illnesses are multifactorial. Cancer is no exception. Multifactorial means that there are many factors involved. In other words, there is no single cause for any one type of cancer.

Carcinogens: A carcinogen is something that can help to cause cancer. Tobacco smoke is a powerful carcinogen. But not everyone who smokes gets lung cancer. So there must be other factors at work.

Age: Most types of cancer become more common as we get older. This is because the changes that cause a cell to become cancerous in the first place take a long time to develop. There have to be a number of changes to the genes within a cell before it turns into a cancer cell. The changes can happen by accident when the cell is dividing.

This chapter begins with "What Causes Cancer?" and also includes "Why Don't We All Get Cancer?" and "How Cancer Starts" from the "About Cancer" section of the CancerHelp UK website. Reprinted with permission of CancerHelp UK, the patient information website of Cancer Research UK (www.cancerhelp .org.uk). © 2006 Cancer Research UK.

Or they can happen because the cell has been damaged by carcinogens and the damage is then passed on to future "daughter" cells when that cell divides. The longer we live, the more time there is for us to accumulate these genetic mistakes in our cells.

Genetic make up: There have to be a number of genetic mutations within a cell before it becomes cancerous. Sometimes we are born with one of these mutations already. This does not mean we will get cancer. But with one mutation from the outset, it makes it more likely statistically that we will. Doctors call this genetic predisposition.

The BRCA1 and BRCA2 breast cancer genes are examples of genetic predisposition. Women who carry one of these faulty genes have a higher chance of developing breast cancer than women who do not.

The BRCA genes are good examples for another reason. Most women with breast cancer do not have a mutated BRCA1 or BRCA 2 gene. Less than 5% of all breast cancer is due to these genes. So although women with one of these genes are individually more likely to get breast cancer, most breast cancer is not caused by a high risk inherited gene fault.

This is true of other common cancers where some people have a genetic predisposition, for example colon (large bowel) cancer.

Researchers are looking at the genes of people with cancer in a study called SEARCH. They also hope to find out more about how other factors might interact with genes to increase the risk of cancer. Information about this study can be found on the CancerHelp website at www.cancerhelp.org.

Immune system: People who have problems with their immune systems are more likely to get some forms of cancer. This group includes the following groups of people:

- People who have had organ transplants and take drugs to suppress their immune systems to stop organ rejection
- People who have AIDS
- People who are born with rare medical syndromes which affect their immunity

The kinds of extra cancers that affect these groups of people fall into two, overlapping groups:

- Cancers that are caused by viruses, such as cervical cancer
- Lymphomas

Chronic infections or transplanted organs can continually stimulate cells to divide. This continual cell division means that immune cells are more likely to acquire mutations and develop into lymphomas.

Diet: Cancer experts estimate that changes to our diet could prevent about one in three cancer deaths. In the western world, many people eat too many animal fats and not enough fresh fruit and vegetables. This type of diet is known to increase your risk of cancer. But how exactly we should alter our diets is not clear.

Sometimes foods or food additives are blamed for directly causing cancer and described as carcinogenic. This is often a distortion of the truth. Sometimes a food is found to contain a substance that can cause cancer but in such small amounts that we could never eat enough of it to do any harm. And some additives may actually protect us.

Day-to-day environment: There are several things around you each day that may help to cause cancer. This could include the following:

- Tobacco smoke
- The sun
- Natural and man made radiation
- Work place hazards
- Asbestos

Some of these are avoidable and some aren't. Most are only contributing factors to causing cancers—part of the jigsaw puzzle that scientists are still trying to put together.

Viruses: Viruses can help to cause some cancers. But this does not mean that these cancers can be caught like an infection. What happens is that the virus can cause genetic changes in cells that make them more likely to become cancerous.

These cancers and viruses are linked:

- Cervical cancer and the genital wart virus, HPV
- Primary liver cancer and the hepatitis B virus
- T cell leukemia in adults and the human T cell leukemia virus

There will be people with primary liver cancer and with T cell leukemia who haven't had the related virus. But infection may increase their risk of getting that particular cancer. With cervical cancer, scientists now believe that everyone with an invasive cervical cancer will have had an HPV infection beforehand.

Many people can be infected with a cancer-causing virus, and never get cancer. The virus only causes cancer in certain situations. Many women get a high risk HPV infection but never develop cervical cancer. Another example is Epstein-Barr virus (EBV). These are some facts about this common virus:

- Most people are infected with EBV.

- People who catch it late get glandular fever but this does not cause cancer.

- In sub-Saharan Africa, EBV infection and repeated attacks of malaria together cause a cancer called Burkitt lymphoma that affects children.

- In China, EBV infection (together with other unknown factors) causes naso-pharyngeal cancer.

- In AIDS patients and transplant patients EBV can cause lymphoma.

- In the UK, about 4 out of 10 cases of Hodgkin disease seem to be related to EBV infection.

Why Don't We All Get Cancer?

This section tells you about why some people get cancer and some don't, even though they may live very similar lives. If you have read through "What causes cancer?" you may be forgiven for thinking that with that number of potential causes, everyone will get cancer. But not everyone does. So why do some people get it and others don't?

The clues are all there in "What causes cancer?" As ever, there are a number of different factors working together.

"Risky" behavior: This just means indulging in something that increases your risk. It may be smoking or drinking too much or eating a very unhealthy diet. Some of us look after ourselves better than others. And this can have a real effect on our health. But some people look after themselves really well and still get cancer. While others don't seem to look after themselves at all and never do.

30

Genetic predisposition: You may hear doctors or scientists talk about genetic predisposition to cancer. This means your genetic make up makes it more likely that you will develop cancer.

It is not common, but there are such things as cancer families. These families have a much higher incidence of cancer than one would normally expect. This may be particular types of cancer. But some families have all sorts of different cancers turning up in their family tree. They probably have a mutation in a gene that is crucial in the development of many different cancers. Researchers often ask such families to help them in their research. Their genetic make up provides clues that help show which genes are the most important in causing cancer.

For most people who may have a general susceptibility to getting cancer, then it is not that obvious. Many of us probably have particular genes that are not that important in cancer development, but may increase our risk a little. For example, the cells of the respiratory system may be more likely to be damaged by cigarette smoke for person "A" compared to person "B." It is more likely that person "A" will develop a cancer than person "B" who does not have that affected gene, even if they both smoke.

Cancer specialists believe that the younger someone is when they develop an "adult" cancer, the more likely it is that there are genetic factors at work.

Chance: Many changes in genes are accidental. Cells divide, and each time they do they have to copy their genetic code completely. Sometimes mistakes happen. Many of these would be fatal and cause the daughter cell to die. Sometimes the damage is repaired. Some changes wouldn't make that much difference to how the cell worked. But they may take that cell one step further along the road to becoming cancerous.

Many people with cancer, and their families, find this aspect of their disease very difficult to come to terms with. It somehow makes cancer easier to deal with if you understand why you have it.

Your immune system: The balance between the immune system and cancer is complicated. There is more about this in the section on the immune system in "What Causes Cancer?"

Age: Some doctors say that if all men lived long enough they would get prostate cancer. It is true that the longer we live, the more likely we are to gather enough genetic damage to start a cancer off. Most of us just die of something else before we get to that point.

How Cancer Starts

Doctors and scientists now know that each cancer starts with one cell. Usually many years before you can feel a lump, or a doctor can see it on a scan, that cell has started to reproduce itself uncontrollably.

You can see from the differences between normal cells and cancer cells that the cancer cell seems to have lost a number of vital control systems. What has happened is that some of the genes in the cell have been damaged or lost. Scientists call this mutation.

Genes and Mutation

Genes are coded messages inside a cell that tell it how to behave. The genes are codes that tell the cell how to make many different proteins. One gene codes for one protein.

Proteins are the building blocks that make up a cell. Some proteins act as "on/off" switches that help to control how a cell behaves. For example, a hormone signal acts on a protein in or on the cell. The protein then sends a signal down a chain of switches. The final signal tells the cell to reproduce by dividing into two.

Mutation means a gene has been damaged or lost. A mutation may mean that too much protein is made. Or that a protein is not made at all. For example, a signaling protein may be permanently switched on. Other proteins, whose job is to control and limit cell division, may be permanently switched off.

Something that damages a cell and makes it more likely to be cancerous is called a carcinogen. There are carcinogens in cigarette smoke for example.

Identifying Abnormal Genes

There are three different types of genes that are important in making a cell cancerous:

- Genes that encourage the cell to multiply
- Genes that stop the cell multiplying
- Genes that repair the other damaged genes

Oncogenes: Some genes encourage cells to multiply or "double." Normally, in adults, this would not happen very often. Cells would only multiply to repair damage (for example, after a wound or operation). But if these genes become abnormal, they tell the cell to multiply all the time. Scientists call these genes oncogenes. This really means "cancer genes."

Tumour suppressor genes: Some genes are in the cell specifically to stop the cell multiplying or doubling. They act as the brake to the oncogene's accelerator. If one of these "tumour suppressor genes" becomes damaged and stops working, then the cell may carry on and on multiplying. In other words it becomes immortal, which is one of the properties of a cancer cell. The best known tumour suppressor gene is called p53. This gene normally stops cells with other damaged genes from reproducing and encourages them to commit suicide (apoptosis). p53 is damaged or missing in most human cancers.

Genes that repair other damaged genes: These genes normally repair any damage to the DNA that the cell's genes are made of. If these genes are damaged, then other mutations are not repaired and the cell can reproduce the mutations in its daughter cells. These genes have been found to be damaged in some human cancers, including bowel cancer.

How Mutations Happen

Mutations can happen by chance when a cell is reproducing. It is not easy for a normal cell to turn into a cancer cell. There have to be about half a dozen different mutations before this happens. Cells often self destruct if they carry a mutation. Or they might be recognized by the immune system as abnormal and killed. This means most precancerous cells die before they can cause disease. Only a few turn into a cancer.

It can take a long time before enough mutations happen for a cell to become cancerous. This is why many cancers are more common in older people. There has been more time to be exposed to carcinogens and more time for accidents when cells reproduce.

Some people are said to have a genetic predisposition to a type of cancer. This means they are more likely to develop that type of cancer than most people because they have been born with one of the mutations that makes a cell cancerous. They do not actually have the cancer because more than one mutation is necessary. But they are naturally further along the road towards getting cancer than people without that mutation.

Chapter 4

Cancer Clusters

Defining Disease Clusters

A disease cluster is the occurrence of a greater than expected number of cases of a particular disease within a group of people, a geographic area, or a period of time. Clusters of various diseases have concerned scientists for centuries. Some recent disease clusters include the initial cases of a rare type of pneumonia among homosexual men in the early 1980s that led to the identification of the human immunodeficiency virus (HIV) and acquired immunodeficiency syndrome (AIDS); the outbreak in 2003 of a respiratory illness, later identified as severe acute respiratory syndrome (SARS), caused by a previously unrecognized virus; and periodic outbreaks of food poisoning caused by eating food contaminated with bacteria.

Cancer clusters may be suspected when people report that several family members, friends, neighbors, or coworkers have been diagnosed with the same or related cancer(s). In the 1960s, one of the best known cancer clusters emerged, involving many cases of mesothelioma (a rare cancer of the lining of the chest and abdomen). Researchers traced the development of mesothelioma to exposure to asbestos, a fibrous mineral that was used heavily in shipbuilding during World War II and has also been used in manufacturing industrial and consumer products. Working with asbestos is the major risk factor for mesothelioma.

From "Cancer Clusters," National Cancer Institute, February 2004. The complete text of this document, including links to additional resources, is available online at http://www.cancer.gov/cancertopics/factsheet/Risk/clusters.

Facts about Cancer Clusters

Reported disease clusters of any kind, including suspected cancer clusters, are investigated by epidemiologists (scientists who study the frequency, distribution, causes, and control of diseases in populations). Epidemiologists use their knowledge of diseases, environmental science, lifestyle factors, and biostatistics to try to determine whether a suspected cluster represents a true excess of cancer cases.

Epidemiologists have identified certain circumstances that may lead them to suspect a potential common source or cause of cancer among people thought to be part of a cancer cluster. A suspected cancer cluster is more likely to be a true cluster, rather than a coincidence, if it involves:

- a large number of cases of a specific type of cancer, rather than several different types;

- a rare type of cancer, rather than common types; or

- an increased number of cases of a certain type of cancer in an age group that is not usually affected by that type of cancer.

Before epidemiologists can accurately assess a suspected cancer cluster, they must determine whether the type of cancer involved is a primary (original) cancer or a cancer that has spread from another organ (metastasis). This is important to know because scientists consider only the primary cancer when they investigate a possible cancer cluster. Epidemiologists also try to establish whether the suspected exposure has the potential to cause the reported cancer, based on what is known about that cancer's likely causes and what is known about the cancer-causing potential of the exposure.

In addition, epidemiologists must show that the number of cancer cases which have occurred is significantly greater than the expected number of cases, given the age, gender, and racial distribution of the group of people at risk of developing the disease. They must also determine if the cancer cases could have occurred by chance. Epidemiologists often test for "statistical significance," which is a measure of the likelihood that the observed association could simply have been due to chance. In common practice, a statistically significant finding means that there is a five percent or less chance that the observed number of cases could have happened by chance. For instance, if one examines the number of cancer cases in 100 neighborhoods, and cancer cases are occurring randomly, one should expect to find about five neighborhoods with statistically significant elevations. In other words, some amount of clustering within the same family or neighborhood may occur simply by chance.

Another difficulty epidemiologists face when investigating a possible cancer cluster is accurately defining the group of people who should be considered "at risk." One of the greatest pitfalls of defining clusters is the tendency to extend the geographic borders of the cluster to include additional cases of the suspected disease as they are discovered. The tendency to define the borders of a cluster on the basis of where known cases are located, rather than to first define the population and then determine if the number of cancers is excessive, creates many "clusters" that are not genuine.

Epidemiologists must also consider that a confirmed cancer cluster may not be the result of any single, external cause or hazard. A cancer cluster could be the result of chance, miscalculation of the expected number of cancer cases, or differences in the case definition (the criteria that determine whether or not the cases being investigated are related to the cluster) between observed cases and expected cases. Moreover, because people change residence from time to time, it can be difficult for epidemiologists to identify previous exposures and find the records that are needed to determine the kind of cancer a person had—or if it was cancer at all.

Because a variety of factors often work together to create the appearance of a cluster where nothing abnormal is occurring, most reports of suspected cancer clusters are not shown to be true clusters. Many reported clusters do not include enough cases for epidemiologists to arrive at any conclusions. Sometimes, even when a suspected cluster has enough cases for study, a greater than expected number of cases (a true statistical excess) cannot be demonstrated. Other times, epidemiologists find a true excess of cases, but they cannot find an explanation for it. For example, a suspected carcinogen may cause cancer only under certain circumstances, making its impact difficult to detect.

Genetics and Environment

Because most cancers are likely to be caused by a combination of factors related to genetics and environment (including behavior and lifestyle), studies of suspected cancer clusters usually focus on these two issues. However, establishing significant and valid evidence that a specific genetic factor leads to an increased chance that a specific environmental exposure will result in cancer (called a gene-environment interaction) requires studies of large populations over long periods of time. Researchers are just beginning to learn about the roles heredity and environmental exposures play in carcinogenesis. Some of their discoveries are outlined in the following text.

Genetics

- All cancers develop because of genetic alterations of one kind or another. An alteration is a change or mutation in the physical structure of a gene that interferes with the gene's normal functions.

- Some alterations that increase the risk of cancer are present at birth in the genes of all cells in the body, including reproductive cells. These alterations, which are called germline alterations, can be passed from parent to child. This type of alteration is known as an inherited susceptibility and is uncommon as a cause of cancer.

- Most cancers are not due to an inherited susceptibility but result from genetic changes that occur during one's lifetime within the cells of a particular organ. These genetic changes are called somatic alterations.

- Familial cancer clusters (multiple cases among relatives) have been reported for many types of cancer. Because cancer is a common disease, it is not unusual for several cases to occur within a family.

- Familial cancer clusters are sometimes linked to inherited susceptibility, but environmental factors and chance may also be involved.

- Having an inherited susceptibility for a type of cancer does not guarantee that the cancer will occur; it means there is an increased chance of developing cancer if other factors that promote the development of cancer are present or later develop.

Environment

- The term environment includes not only air, water, and soil, but also substances and conditions in the home and workplace. It also includes diet; the use of tobacco, alcohol, or drugs; exposure to chemicals; and exposure to sunlight and other forms of radiation.

- People are exposed to a variety of environmental factors for varying lengths of time, and these factors interact in ways that are still not fully understood. Further, individuals have varying levels of susceptibility to these factors.

- Because some workers may have greater and more prolonged exposures to hazardous chemicals that are found widely at lower levels in the general environment, positive findings from studies in the workplace provide important leads regarding causes of cancer in other settings. In fact, occupational studies have identified many specific chemical carcinogens and have provided direction for prevention activities to reduce or eliminate cancer-causing exposures in the workplace and elsewhere.

Reporting Suspected Cancer Clusters

Concerned individuals may report a suspected cancer cluster to their state or local health department. State and local health departments use established criteria to investigate reports of cancer clusters. When a suspected cancer cluster is first reported, the health department gathers information about the suspected cluster and gives the inquirer general information about cancer clusters. Although health departments may use different processes, most follow a basic procedure in which increasingly specific information is obtained and analyzed in stages. Health departments are likely to request the following:

- Information about the potential cluster: type(s) of cancer, number of cases, suspected exposure(s), and suspected geographic area/time period.

- Information about each person with cancer in the potential cluster: name, address, telephone number, gender, race, age, occupation(s), and area(s) lived in/length of time.

- Information about each case of cancer: type of cancer, date of diagnosis, age at diagnosis, possible causes, metastatic sites, and physician contact.

Between 75 and 80 percent of reports of suspected cancer clusters are resolved at this initial contact because concerned individuals realize that what seemed like a cancer cluster is not a true cluster. If further evaluation is needed, the health department will take the following steps to investigate a possible cancer cluster:

- Attempt to verify the reported diagnoses by contacting patients and relatives, and obtaining medical records.

- Compare the number of cases in the suspected cancer cluster with information in census data and cancer registries.

- Review the scientific literature to establish whether the reported cancer(s) has been linked to the suspected exposure.

- Work with federal agencies, if necessary, to gather additional information to help decide whether to conduct a comprehensive epidemiological study.

Most state health departments report that fewer than five percent of cancer cluster investigations are determined to require a comprehensive study.

Chapter 5

Tobacco and Cancer Risk

Chapter Contents

Section 5.1

Cigarette Smoking and Cancer

Excerpted from "Cigarette Smoking and Cancer: Questions and Answers," National Cancer Institute, November 2004. The complete text of this document, including references, can be found online at http://www.cancer.gov.

Tobacco use, particularly cigarette smoking, is the single most preventable cause of death in the United States. Cigarette smoking alone is directly responsible for approximately 30 percent of all cancer deaths annually in the United States. Cigarette smoking also causes chronic lung disease (emphysema and chronic bronchitis), cardiovascular disease, stroke, and cataracts. Smoking during pregnancy can cause stillbirth, low birthweight, sudden infant death syndrome (SIDS), and other serious pregnancy complications. Quitting smoking greatly reduces a person's risk of developing the diseases mentioned, and can limit adverse health effects on the developing child.

What are the effects of cigarette smoking on cancer rates?

Cigarette smoking causes 87 percent of lung cancer deaths. Lung cancer is the leading cause of cancer death in both men and women. Smoking is also responsible for most cancers of the larynx, oral cavity and pharynx, esophagus, and bladder. In addition, it is a cause of kidney, pancreatic, cervical, and stomach cancers, as well as acute myeloid leukemia.

What harmful chemicals are found in cigarette smoke?

Cigarette smoke contains about 4,000 chemical agents, including over 60 carcinogens. In addition, many of these substances, such as carbon monoxide, tar, arsenic, and lead, are poisonous and toxic to the human body. Nicotine is a drug that is naturally present in the tobacco plant and is primarily responsible for a person's addiction to tobacco products, including cigarettes. During smoking, nicotine is absorbed quickly into the bloodstream and travels to the brain in a matter of seconds. Nicotine causes addiction to cigarettes and other tobacco products that is similar to the addiction produced by using heroin and cocaine.

How does exposure to tobacco smoke affect the cigarette smoker?

Smoking harms nearly every major organ of the body. The risk of developing smoking-related diseases, such as lung and other cancers, heart disease, stroke, and respiratory illnesses, increases with total lifetime exposure to cigarette smoke. This includes the number of cigarettes a person smokes each day, the intensity of smoking (for example, the size and frequency of puffs), the age at which smoking began, the number of years a person has smoked, and a smoker's secondhand smoke exposure.

How would quitting smoking affect the risk of developing cancer and other diseases?

Smoking cessation has major and immediate health benefits for men and women of all ages. Quitting smoking decreases the risk of lung and other cancers, heart attack, stroke, and chronic lung disease. The earlier a person quits, the greater the health benefit. For example, research has shown that people who quit before age 50 reduce their risk of dying in the next 15 years by half compared with those who continue to smoke. Smoking low-yield cigarettes, as compared to cigarettes with higher tar and nicotine, provides no clear benefit to health.

Section 5.2

The Truth about "Light" Cigarettes

"The Truth about 'Light' Cigarettes: Questions and Answers," produced by a joint effort of the Office on Smoking and Health at the Centers for Disease Control and Prevention and the National Cancer Institute, August 2004.

Many smokers choose "low-tar," "mild," "light, " or "ultra-light" cigarettes because they think that these cigarettes may be less harmful to their health than "regular" or "full-flavor" cigarettes. Although smoke from light cigarettes may feel smoother and lighter on the throat and chest, light cigarettes are not healthier than regular cigarettes. The truth is that light cigarettes do not reduce the health risks of smoking. The only way to reduce a smoker's risk, and the risk to others, is to stop smoking completely.

What about the lower tar and nicotine numbers on light and ultra-light cigarette packs and in ads for these products?

- These numbers come from smoking machines, which "smoke" every brand of cigarettes exactly the same way.

- These numbers do not really tell how much tar and nicotine a particular smoker may get because people do not smoke cigarettes the same way the machines do. And no two people smoke the same way.

How do light cigarettes trick the smoking machines?

- Tobacco companies designed light cigarettes with tiny pinholes on the filters. These "filter vents" dilute cigarette smoke with air when light cigarettes are "puffed" on by smoking machines, causing the machines to measure artificially low tar and nicotine levels.

- Many smokers do not know that their cigarette filters have vent holes. The filter vents are uncovered when cigarettes are smoked on smoking machines. However, filter vents are placed just millimeters from where smokers put their lips or fingers when smoking. As a result, many smokers block the vents—which actually turns the light cigarette into a regular cigarette.

- Some cigarette makers increased the length of the paper wrap covering the outside of the cigarette filter, which decreases the number of puffs that occur during the machine test. Although tobacco under the wrap is still available to the smoker, this tobacco is not burned during the machine test. The result is that the machine measures less tar and nicotine levels than is available to the smoker.

- Because smokers, unlike machines, crave nicotine, they may inhale more deeply; take larger, more rapid, or more frequent puffs; or smoke a few extra cigarettes each day to get enough nicotine to satisfy their craving. This is called "compensating," and it means that smokers end up inhaling more tar, nicotine, and other harmful chemicals than the machine-based numbers suggest.

What is the scientific evidence about the health effects of light cigarettes?

- The federal government's National Cancer Institute (NCI) has concluded that light cigarettes provide no benefit to smokers' health.

- According to the NCI monograph *Risks Associated with Smoking Cigarettes with Low Machine-Measured Yields of Tar and Nicotine*, people who switch to light cigarettes from regular cigarettes are likely to inhale the same amount of hazardous chemicals, and they remain at high risk for developing smoking-related cancers and other diseases.

- Researchers also found that the strategies used by the tobacco industry to advertise and promote light cigarettes are intended to reassure smokers, to discourage them from quitting, and to lead consumers to perceive filtered and light cigarettes as safer alternatives to regular cigarettes.

- There is also no evidence that switching to light or ultra-light cigarettes actually helps smokers quit.

Have the tobacco companies conducted research on the amount of tar and nicotine people actually inhale while smoking light cigarettes?

- The tobacco industry's own documents show that companies are aware that smokers of light cigarettes compensate by taking bigger puffs.

- Industry documents also show that the companies are aware of the difference between machine-measured yields of tar and nicotine and what the smoker actually inhales.

What is the bottom line for smokers who want to protect their health?

- There is no such thing as a safe cigarette. The only proven way to reduce the risk of smoking-related disease is to quit smoking completely.

- Smokers who quit live longer than those who continue to smoke. In addition, the earlier smokers quit, the greater the health benefit. Research has shown that people who quit before age 30 eliminate almost all of their risk of developing a tobacco-related disease. Even smokers who quit at age 50 reduce their risk of dying from a tobacco-related disease.

- Quitting also decreases the risk of lung cancer, heart attacks, stroke, and chronic lung disease.

Section 5.3

Cigar Smoking and Cancer

"Questions and Answers about Cigar Smoking and Cancer,"
National Cancer Institute, March 2000.

What are the health risks associated with cigar smoking?

Scientific evidence has shown that cancers of the oral cavity (lip, tongue, mouth, and throat), larynx, lung, and esophagus are associated with cigar smoking. Furthermore, evidence strongly suggests a link between cigar smoking and cancer of the pancreas. In addition, daily cigar smokers, particularly those who inhale, are at increased risk for developing heart and lung disease.

Like cigarette smoking, the risks from cigar smoking increase with increased exposure. For example, compared with someone who has never smoked, smoking only one to two cigars per day doubles the risk for oral and esophageal cancers. Smoking three to four cigars daily can increase the risk of oral cancers to more than eight times the risk for a nonsmoker, while the chance of esophageal cancer is increased to four times the risk for someone who has never smoked. Both cigar and cigarette smokers have similar levels of risk for oral, throat, and esophageal cancers.

The health risks associated with occasional cigar smoking (less than daily) are not known. About three-quarters of cigar smokers are occasional smokers.

What is the effect of inhalation on disease risk?

One of the major differences between cigar and cigarette smoking is the degree of inhalation. Almost all cigarette smokers report inhaling while the majority of cigar smokers do not because cigar smoke is generally more irritating. However, cigar smokers who have a history of cigarette smoking are more likely to inhale cigar smoke. Cigar smokers experience higher rates of lung cancer, coronary heart disease, and chronic obstructive lung disease than nonsmokers, but not as high as the rates for cigarette smokers. These lower rates for cigar smokers are probably related to reduced inhalation.

47

How are cigars and cigarettes different?

Cigars and cigarettes differ in both size and the type of tobacco used. Cigarettes are generally more uniform in size and contain less than 1 gram of tobacco each. Cigars, on the other hand, can vary in size and shape, and can measure more than 7 inches in length. Large cigars typically contain between 5 and 17 grams of tobacco. It is not unusual for some premium cigars to contain the tobacco equivalent of an entire pack of cigarettes. U.S. cigarettes are made from different blends of tobaccos, whereas most cigars are composed primarily of a single type of tobacco (air-cured or dried burley tobacco). Large cigars can take between one and two hours to smoke, whereas most cigarettes on the U.S. market take less than ten minutes to smoke.

How are the health risks associated with cigar smoking different from those associated with smoking cigarettes?

Health risks associated with both cigars and cigarettes are strongly linked to the degree of smoke exposure. Since smoke from cigars and cigarettes are composed of many of the same toxic and carcinogenic (cancer causing) compounds, the differences in health risks appear to be related to differences in daily use and level of inhalation.

Most cigarette smokers smoke every day and inhale. In contrast, as many as three-quarters of cigar smokers smoke only occasionally, and the majority do not inhale.

All cigar and cigarette smokers, whether or not they inhale, directly expose the lips, mouth, tongue, throat, and larynx to smoke and its carcinogens. Holding an unlit cigar between the lips also exposes these areas to carcinogens. In addition, when saliva containing smoke constituents is swallowed, the esophagus is exposed to carcinogens. These exposures probably account for the fact that oral and esophageal cancer risks are similar among cigar smokers and cigarette smokers.

Cancer of the larynx occurs at lower rates among cigar smokers who do not inhale than among cigarette smokers. Lung cancer risk among daily cigar smokers who do not inhale is double that of nonsmokers, but significantly less than the risk for cigarette smokers. However, the lung cancer risk from moderately inhaling smoke from five cigars a day is comparable to the risk from smoking up to one pack of cigarettes a day.

What are the hazards for nonsmokers exposed to cigar smoke?

Environmental tobacco smoke (ETS), also known as secondhand or passive smoke, is the smoke released from a lit cigar or cigarette.

The ETS from cigars and cigarettes contains many of the same toxins and irritants (such as carbon monoxide, nicotine, hydrogen cyanide, and ammonia), as well as a number of known carcinogens (such as benzene, nitrosamines, vinyl chloride, arsenic, and hydrocarbons). Because cigars contain greater amounts of tobacco than cigarettes, they produce greater amounts of ETS.

There are, however, some differences between cigar and cigarette smoke due to the different ways cigars and cigarettes are made. Cigars go through a long aging and fermentation process. During the fermentation process, high concentrations of carcinogenic compounds are produced. These compounds are released when a cigar is smoked. Also, cigar wrappers are less porous than cigarette wrappers. The nonporous cigar wrapper makes the burning of cigar tobacco less complete than cigarette tobacco. As a result, compared with cigarette smoke, the concentrations of toxins and irritants are higher in cigar smoke. In addition, the larger size of most cigars (more tobacco) and longer smoking time produces higher exposures to nonsmokers of many toxic compounds (including carbon monoxide, hydrocarbons, ammonia, cadmium, and other substances) than a cigarette. For example, measurements of the carbon monoxide (CO) concentration at a cigar party and a cigar banquet in a restaurant showed indoor CO levels comparable to those measured on a crowded California freeway. Such exposures could place nonsmoking workers attending such events at significantly increased risk for cancer as well as heart and lung diseases.

What are the benefits of quitting?

There are many health benefits to quitting cigar smoking. The likelihood of developing cancer decreases. Also, when someone quits, an improvement in health is seen almost immediately. For example, blood pressure, pulse rate, and breathing patterns start returning to normal soon after quitting. People who quit will also see an improvement in their overall quality of life. People who decide to quit have many options available to them. Some people choose to quit all at once. Other options gaining popularity in this country are nicotine replacement products, such as patches, gum, and nasal sprays. If considering quitting, ask your doctor to recommend a plan that could best suit you and your lifestyle.

Section 5.4

Smokeless Tobacco and Cancer

"Smokeless Tobacco and Cancer: Questions and Answers,"
National Cancer Institute, May 2003.

What is smokeless tobacco?

There are two types of smokeless tobacco—snuff and chewing tobacco. Snuff, a finely ground or shredded tobacco, is packaged as dry,
moist, or in sachets (tea bag-like pouches). Typically, the user places
a pinch or dip between the cheek and gum. Chewing tobacco is available in loose leaf, plug (plug-firm and plug-moist), or twist forms, with
the user putting a wad of tobacco inside the cheek. Smokeless tobacco
is sometimes called "spit" or "spitting" tobacco because people spit out
the tobacco juices and saliva that build up in the mouth.

What harmful chemicals are found in smokeless tobacco?

- Chewing tobacco and snuff contain 28 carcinogens. The most
  harmful carcinogens in smokeless tobacco are the tobacco-specific
  nitrosamines (TSNAs). They are formed during the growing, cur-
  ing, fermenting, and aging of tobacco. TSNAs have been detected
  in some smokeless tobacco products at levels many times higher
  than levels of other types of nitrosamines that are allowed in
  foods, such as bacon and beer.

- Other cancer-causing substances in smokeless tobacco include
  N-nitrosamino acids, volatile N-nitrosamines, benzo(a)pyrene,
  volatile aldehydes, formaldehyde, acetaldehyde, crotonaldehyde,
  hydrazine, arsenic, nickel, cadmium, benzopyrene, and polonium-
  210.

- All tobacco, including smokeless tobacco, contains nicotine,
  which is addictive. The amount of nicotine absorbed from smokeless tobacco is 3 to 4 times the amount delivered by a cigarette.
  Nicotine is absorbed more slowly from smokeless tobacco than
  from cigarettes, but more nicotine per dose is absorbed from

smokeless tobacco than from cigarettes. Also, the nicotine stays in the bloodstream for a longer time.

What cancers are caused by or associated with smokeless tobacco use?

- Smokeless tobacco users increase their risk for cancer of the oral cavity. Oral cancer can include cancer of the lip, tongue, cheeks, gums, and the floor and roof of the mouth.

- People who use oral snuff for a long time have a much greater risk for cancer of the cheek and gum than people who do not use smokeless tobacco.

- The possible increased risk for other types of cancer from smokeless tobacco is being studied.

What are some of the other ways smokeless tobacco can harm users' health?

Some of the other effects of smokeless tobacco use include addiction to nicotine, oral leukoplakia (white mouth lesions that can become cancerous), gum disease, and gum recession (when the gum pulls away from the teeth). Possible increased risks for heart disease, diabetes, and reproductive problems are being studied.

Is smokeless tobacco a good substitute for cigarettes?

In 1986, the Surgeon General concluded that the use of smokeless tobacco "is not a safe substitute for smoking cigarettes. It can cause cancer and a number of non-cancerous conditions and can lead to nicotine addiction and dependence." Since 1991, NCI has officially recommended that the public avoid and discontinue the use of all tobacco products, including smokeless tobacco. NCI also recognizes that nitrosamines, found in tobacco products, are not safe at any level. The accumulated scientific evidence does not support changing this position.

What about using smokeless tobacco to quit cigarettes?

Because all tobacco use causes disease and addiction, NCI recommends that tobacco use be avoided and discontinued. Several non-tobacco methods have been shown to be effective for quitting cigarettes. These methods include pharmacotherapies such as nicotine replacement therapy and bupropion SR, individual and group counseling, and telephone quitlines.

Section 5.5

Secondhand Smoke and Cancer

Excerpted from "Secondhand Smoke: Questions and Answers," National Cancer Institute, February 2005. The complete text of this document, including references, can be found online at http://www.cancer.gov.

What is secondhand smoke?

Secondhand smoke, also called environmental tobacco smoke (ETS), is the combination of two forms of smoke from burning tobacco products: sidestream smoke and mainstream smoke. Sidestream smoke, which makes up about half of all secondhand smoke, comes from the burning end of a cigarette, cigar, or pipe. Mainstream smoke is exhaled by the smoker. Exposure to secondhand smoke is also called involuntary smoking or passive smoking.

What chemicals are present in secondhand smoke?

Many factors affect what chemicals are present in secondhand smoke. These factors include the type of tobacco, the chemicals added to the tobacco, how the product is smoked, and the paper in which the tobacco is wrapped. More than 4,000 chemicals have been identified in mainstream tobacco smoke; however, the actual number may be more than 100,000. Of the chemicals identified in secondhand smoke, at least 60 are carcinogens, such as formaldehyde. Six others are substances that interfere with normal cell development, such as nicotine and carbon monoxide.

Some of the compounds present in secondhand smoke become carcinogenic only after they are activated by specific enzymes (proteins that control chemical reactions) in the body. After these compounds are activated, they can then become part of a cell's DNA and may interfere with the normal growth of cells. In 1993, the U.S. Environmental Protection Agency (EPA) determined that there is sufficient evidence that secondhand smoke causes cancer in humans and classified it as a Group A carcinogen. In 2000, the U.S. Department of Health and Human Services (DHHS) formally listed secondhand smoke as a known human carcinogen in The U.S. National Toxicology Program's *10th Report on Carcinogens*.

Scientists do not know what amount of exposure to secondhand smoke, if any, is safe. Because it is a complex mixture of chemicals, measuring secondhand smoke exposure is difficult and is usually determined by testing blood, saliva, or urine for the presence of nicotine, particles inhaled from indoor air, or cotinine (the primary product resulting from the breakdown of nicotine in the body). Nicotine, carbon monoxide, and other evidence of secondhand smoke exposure have been found in the body fluids of nonsmokers exposed to secondhand smoke. Nonsmokers who live with smokers in homes where smoking is allowed are at the greatest risk for suffering the negative health effects of secondhand smoke exposure.

What cancer risks are associated with exposure to secondhand smoke?

Secondhand smoke exposure is a known risk factor for lung cancer. Approximately 3,000 lung cancer deaths occur each year among adult nonsmokers in the United States as a result of exposure to secondhand smoke. Secondhand smoke is also linked to nasal sinus cancer. Some research suggests an association between secondhand smoke and cancers of the cervix, breast, and bladder. However, more research is needed in order to confirm a link to these cancers.

Section 5.6

There Is No Risk-Free Level of Exposure to Secondhand Smoke

From "The Health Consequences of Involuntary Exposure to Tobacco Smoke: A Report of the Surgeon General," U.S. Department of Health and Human Services, June 2006. For more information, visit www.cdc.gov/tobacco.

The U.S. Surgeon General has concluded that breathing even a little secondhand smoke poses a risk to your health. Scientific evidence indicates that there is no risk-free level of exposure to secondhand smoke.

Secondhand smoke causes lung cancer.

- Secondhand smoke is a known human carcinogen and contains more than 50 chemicals that can cause cancer.

- Concentrations of many cancer-causing and toxic chemicals are potentially higher in secondhand smoke than in the smoke inhaled by smokers.

Secondhand smoke causes heart disease.

- Breathing secondhand smoke for even a short time can have immediate adverse effects on the cardiovascular system, interfering with the normal functioning of the heart, blood, and vascular systems in ways that increase the risk of heart attack.

- Even a short time in a smoky room can cause your blood platelets to become stickier, damage the lining of blood vessels, decrease coronary flow velocity reserves, and reduce heart rate variability.

- Persons who already have heart disease are at especially high risk of suffering adverse affects from breathing secondhand smoke, and should take special precautions to avoid even brief exposure.

Secondhand smoke causes acute respiratory effects.

- Secondhand smoke contains many chemicals that can quickly irritate and damage the lining of the airways.

- Even brief exposure can trigger respiratory symptoms, including cough, phlegm, wheezing, and breathlessness.

- Brief exposure to secondhand smoke can trigger an asthma attack in children with asthma.

- Persons who already have asthma or other respiratory conditions are at especially high risk for being affected by secondhand smoke, and should take special precautions to avoid secondhand smoke exposure.

Secondhand smoke can cause sudden infant death syndrome and other health consequences in infants and children.

- Smoking by women during pregnancy has been known for some time to cause SIDS.

- Infants who are exposed to secondhand smoke after birth are also at greater risk of SIDS.

- Children exposed to secondhand smoke are also at an increased risk for acute respiratory infections, ear problems, and more severe asthma. Smoking by parents causes respiratory symptoms and slows lung growth in their children.

Separating smokers from nonsmokers, cleaning the air, and ventilating buildings cannot eliminate secondhand smoke exposure.

- The American Society of Heating, Refrigerating and Air-Conditioning Engineers (ASHRAE), the preeminent U.S. standard-setting body on ventilation issues, has concluded that ventilation technology cannot be relied on to completely control health risks from secondhand smoke exposure.

- Conventional air cleaning systems can remove large particles, but not the smaller particles or the gases found in secondhand smoke.

- Operation of a heating, ventilating, and air conditioning system can distribute secondhand smoke throughout a building.

Chapter 6

Questions and Answers about Obesity and Cancer Risk

What is obesity?

People who are obese have an abnormally high and unhealthy proportion of body fat. To measure obesity, researchers commonly use a formula based on weight and height known as the body mass index (BMI). BMI is the ratio of weight (in kilograms) to height (in meters) squared. BMI provides a more accurate measure of obesity or being overweight than does weight alone.

Guidelines established by the National Institutes of Health (NIH) place adults age 20 and older into one of four categories based on their BMI:

- Less than 18.5: underweight
- 18.5 to 24.9: healthy
- 25.0 to 29.9: overweight
- Greater than 30.0: obese

Figure 6.1 can be used to determine BMI category. (Find the height, and move across the chart to the appropriate weight.)

Excerpted from "Obesity and Cancer: Questions and Answers," National Cancer Institute, reviewed March 16, 2004. The complete text of this document, including references, is available online at http://www.cancer.gov/cancertopics/fact sheet/Risk/obesity.

BMI	19	20	21	22	23	24	25	26	27	28	29	30	31	32	33	34	35

Height   Body Weight (pounds)
(inches)

Height	19	20	21	22	23	24	25	26	27	28	29	30	31	32	33	34	35
58	91	96	100	105	110	115	119	124	129	134	138	143	148	153	158	162	167
59	94	99	104	109	114	119	124	128	133	138	143	148	153	158	163	168	173
60	97	102	107	112	118	123	128	133	138	143	148	153	158	163	168	174	179
61	100	106	111	116	122	127	132	137	143	148	153	158	164	169	174	180	185
62	104	109	115	120	126	131	136	142	147	153	158	164	169	175	180	186	191
63	107	113	118	124	130	135	141	146	152	158	163	169	175	180	186	191	197
64	110	116	122	128	134	140	145	151	157	163	169	174	180	186	192	197	204
65	114	120	126	132	138	144	150	156	162	168	174	180	186	192	198	204	210
66	118	124	130	136	142	148	155	161	167	173	179	186	192	198	204	210	216
67	121	127	134	140	146	153	159	166	172	178	185	191	198	204	211	217	223
68	125	131	138	144	151	158	164	171	177	184	190	197	203	210	216	223	230
69	128	135	142	149	155	162	169	176	182	189	196	203	209	216	223	230	236
70	132	139	146	153	160	167	174	181	188	195	202	209	216	222	229	236	243
71	136	143	150	157	165	172	179	186	193	200	208	215	222	229	236	243	250
72	140	147	154	162	169	177	184	191	199	206	213	221	228	235	242	250	258
73	144	151	159	166	174	182	189	197	204	212	219	227	235	242	250	257	265
74	148	155	163	171	179	186	194	202	210	218	225	233	241	249	256	264	272
75	152	160	168	176	184	192	200	208	216	224	232	240	248	256	264	272	279
76	156	164	172	180	189	197	205	213	221	230	238	246	254	263	271	279	287

BMI	36	37	38	39	40	41	42	43	44	45	46	47	48	49	50	51	52	53	54
58	172	177	181	186	191	196	201	205	210	215	220	224	229	234	239	244	248	253	258
59	178	183	188	193	198	203	208	212	217	222	227	232	237	242	247	252	257	262	267
60	184	189	194	199	204	209	215	220	225	230	235	240	245	250	255	261	266	271	276
61	190	195	201	206	211	217	222	227	232	238	243	248	254	259	264	269	275	280	285
62	196	202	207	213	218	224	229	235	240	246	251	256	262	267	273	278	284	289	295
63	203	208	214	220	225	231	237	242	248	254	259	265	270	278	282	287	293	299	304
64	209	215	221	227	232	238	244	250	256	262	267	273	279	285	291	296	302	308	314
65	216	222	228	234	240	246	252	258	264	270	276	282	288	294	300	306	312	318	324
66	223	229	235	241	247	253	260	266	272	278	284	291	297	303	309	315	322	328	334
67	230	236	242	249	255	261	268	274	280	287	293	299	306	312	319	325	331	338	344
68	236	243	249	256	262	269	276	282	289	295	302	308	315	322	328	335	341	348	354
69	243	250	257	263	270	277	284	291	297	304	311	318	324	331	338	345	351	358	365
70	250	257	264	271	278	285	292	299	306	313	320	327	334	341	348	355	362	369	376
71	257	265	272	279	286	293	301	308	315	322	329	338	343	351	358	365	372	379	386
72	265	272	279	287	294	302	309	316	324	331	338	346	353	361	368	375	383	390	397
73	272	280	288	295	302	310	318	325	333	340	348	355	363	371	378	386	393	401	408
74	280	287	295	303	311	319	326	334	342	350	358	365	373	381	389	396	404	412	420
75	287	295	303	311	319	327	335	343	351	359	367	375	383	391	399	407	415	423	431
76	295	304	312	320	328	336	344	353	361	369	377	385	394	402	410	418	426	435	443

Table 6.1. *Body Mass Index Table (Source: Excerpted from "The Practical Guide: Identification, Evaluation, and Treatment of Overweight and Obesity in Adults," National Heart, Lung, and Blood Institute (NHLBI), NIH Publication Number 00-4084, October 2000.)*

How many people get cancer by being overweight or obese? How many die?

In 2002, about 41,000 new cases of cancer in the United States were estimated to be due to obesity. This means that about 3.2 percent of all new cancers are linked to obesity. In 2003, a report estimated that, in the United States, 14 percent of deaths from cancer in men and 20 percent of deaths in women were due to overweight and obesity.

Does obesity increase the risk of breast cancer?

The effect of obesity on breast cancer risk depends on a woman's menopausal status. Before menopause, obese women have a lower risk of developing breast cancer than do women of a healthy weight. However, after menopause, obese women have 1.5 times the risk of women of a healthy weight.

Obese women are also at increased risk of dying from breast cancer after menopause compared with lean women. Scientists estimate that about 11,000 to 18,000 deaths per year from breast cancer in U.S. women over age 50 might be avoided if women could maintain a BMI under 25 throughout their adult lives.

Obesity seems to increase the risk of breast cancer only among postmenopausal women who do not use menopausal hormones. Among women who use menopausal hormones, there is no significant difference in breast cancer risk between obese women and women of a healthy weight.

Both the increased risk of developing breast cancer and dying from it after menopause are believed to be due to increased levels of estrogen in obese women. Before menopause, the ovaries are the primary source of estrogen. However, estrogen is also produced in fat tissue and, after menopause, when the ovaries stop producing hormones, fat tissue becomes the most important estrogen source. Estrogen levels in postmenopausal women are 50 to 100 percent higher among heavy versus lean women. Estrogen-sensitive tissues are therefore exposed to more estrogen stimulation in heavy women, leading to a more rapid growth of estrogen-responsive breast tumors.

Another factor related to the higher breast cancer death rates in obese women is that breast cancer is more likely to be detected at a later stage in obese women than in lean women. This is because the detection of a breast tumor is more difficult in obese versus lean women.

Studies of obesity and breast cancer in minority women in the United States have been limited. There is some evidence that, among

59

African American women, the risk associated with obesity may be absent or less than that of other populations. However, in 2002 a report showed that African American women who have a high BMI are more likely to have an advanced stage of breast cancer at diagnosis. Another report showed that obese Hispanic white women were twice as likely to develop breast cancer as non-obese Hispanics, but the researchers did not detect a difference in risk for obese Hispanic women before and after menopause.

Weight gain during adulthood has been found to be the most consistent and strongest predictor of breast cancer risk in studies in which it has been examined. The distribution of body fat may also affect breast cancer risk. Women with a large amount of abdominal fat have a greater breast cancer risk than those whose fat is distributed over the hips, buttocks, and lower extremities. Results from studies on the effect of abdominal fat are much less consistent than studies on weight gain or BMI.

Does obesity increase the risk of cancer of the uterus?

Obesity has been consistently associated with uterine (endometrial) cancer. Obese women have two to four times greater risk of developing the disease than do women of a healthy weight, regardless of menopausal status. Increased risk has also been demonstrated among overweight women. Obesity has been estimated to account for about 40 percent of endometrial cancer cases in affluent societies.

It is unclear why obesity is a risk factor for endometrial cancer; however, it has been suggested that lifetime exposure to hormones and high levels of estrogen and insulin in obese women may be contributing factors.

Does obesity increase the risk of colon cancer?

Colon cancer occurs more frequently in people who are obese than in those of a healthy weight. An increased risk of colon cancer has been consistently reported for men with high BMIs. The relationship between BMI and risk in women, however, has been found to be weaker or absent.

Unlike for breast and endometrial cancer, estrogen appears to be protective for colon cancer for women overall. However, obesity and estrogen status also interact in influencing colon cancer risk. Women with a high BMI who are either premenopausal or postmenopausal and taking estrogens have an increased risk of colon cancer similar to that found for men with a high BMI. In contrast, women with a high BMI who are postmenopausal and not taking estrogens do not have an increased risk of colon cancer.

There is some evidence that abdominal obesity may be more important in colon cancer risk. In men, a high BMI tends to be associated with abdominal fat. In women, fat is more likely to be distributed in the hips, thighs, and buttocks. Thus, two measures of abdominal fat, waist-to-hip ratio or waist circumference, may be better predictors of colon cancer risk. Few studies have yet compared waist-to-hip ratios to colon cancer risk in women. One study that did find an increased risk of colon cancer among women with high waist-to-hip ratios found that the association was present only among inactive women, suggesting that high levels of physical activity may counteract the effects of increased abdominal fat.

A number of mechanisms have been proposed for the adverse effect of obesity on colon cancer risk. One of the major hypotheses is that high levels of insulin or insulin-related growth factors in obese people may promote tumor development.

Does obesity increase the risk of kidney cancer?

Studies have consistently found a link between a type of kidney cancer (renal cell carcinoma) and obesity in women, with some studies finding risk among obese women to be two to four times the risk of women of a healthy weight.

Results of studies including men have been more variable, ranging from an association similar to that seen in women, to a weak association, to no association at all. A meta-analysis (where several studies are combined into a single report), which found an equal association of risk among men and women, estimated the kidney cancer risk to be 36 percent higher for an overweight person and 84 percent higher for an obese person compared to those with a healthy weight.

The mechanisms by which obesity may increase renal cell cancer risk are not well understood. An increased exposure to sex steroids, estrogen and androgen, is one possible mechanism.

Does obesity increase the risk of cancer of the esophagus or stomach?

Overweight and obese individuals are two times more likely than healthy weight people to develop a type of esophageal cancer called esophageal adenocarcinoma. A smaller increase in risk has been found for gastric cardia cancer, a type of stomach cancer that begins in the area of the stomach next to the esophagus. Most studies have not observed increases in risk with obesity in another type of esophageal cancer, squamous cell cancer. An increased risk of esophageal adenocarcinoma has also been associated with weight gain, smoking, and being younger than age 59.

The mechanisms by which obesity increases risk of adenocarcinoma of the esophagus and gastric cardia are not well understood. One of the leading mechanisms proposed has been that increases in gastric reflux due to obesity may increase risk. However, in the few studies that have examined this issue, risk associated with BMI was similar for those with and without gastric reflux.

Does obesity increase the risk of prostate cancer?

Of the more than 35 studies on prostate cancer risk, most conclude that there is no association with obesity. Some report that obese men are at higher risk than men of healthy weight, particularly for more aggressive tumors. One study found an increased risk among men with high waist-to-hip ratios, suggesting that abdominal fat may be a more appropriate measure of body size in relation to prostate cancer.

Despite the lack of association between obesity and prostate cancer incidence, a number of studies have examined potential biological factors that are related to obesity, such as insulin-related growth factors, leptin, and other hormones. Results of these studies are inconsistent, but generally, risk has been linked to men with higher levels of leptin, insulin, and IGF–1 (insulin-like growth factor-1).

Is there any evidence that obesity is linked to cancer of the gallbladder, ovaries, or pancreas?

An increased risk of gallbladder cancer has been found to be associated with obesity, particularly among women. This may be due to the higher frequency of gallstones in obese individuals, as gallstones are considered a strong risk factor for gallbladder cancer. However, there is not enough evidence to draw firm conclusions.

It is unclear whether obesity affects ovarian cancer risk. Some studies report an increased risk among obese women, whereas others have found no association. In 2003, a report found an increased risk in women who were overweight or obese in adolescence or young adulthood; no increased risk was found in older obese women.

Studies evaluating the relationship between obesity and pancreatic cancer have been inconsistent. One study conducted in 2001, found that obesity increases the risk of pancreatic cancer only among those who are not physically active. A recent meta-analysis reported that obese people may have a 19 percent higher risk of pancreatic cancer than those with a healthy BMI. The results, however, were not conclusive.

Does avoiding weight gain decrease the risk of cancer?

The most conclusive way to test if avoiding weight gain will decrease the risk of cancer is through a controlled clinical trial. There have been no controlled clinical trials on the effect on cancer related to avoiding weight gain. However, many observational studies have shown that avoiding weight gain lowers the risk of cancers of the colon, breast (postmenopausal), endometrium, kidney, and esophagus. There is limited evidence for thyroid cancers, and no substantial evidence for all other cancers.

Does losing weight lower the risk of cancer?

There is insufficient evidence that intentional weight loss will affect cancer risk for any cancer. A very limited number of observational studies have examined the effect of weight loss, and a few found some decreased risk for breast cancer among women who have lost weight. However, most of these studies have not been able to evaluate whether the weight loss was intentional or related to other health problems.

In 2003, one study examined the effect of intentional weight loss and found that women who experienced intentional weight loss of 20 or more pounds and were not currently overweight had cancer rates at the level of healthy women who never lost weight. However, unintentional weight loss episodes were not associated with decreased cancer risk.

Does regular physical activity lower the risk of cancer?

There have been no controlled clinical trials on the effect of regular physical activity on the risk of developing cancer. However, observational studies have examined the possible association between physical activity and a lower risk of developing colon or breast cancer:

- **Colon cancer:** In 2002, a major review of observational trials found that physical activity reduced colon cancer risk by 50 percent. This risk reduction occurred even with moderate levels of physical activity. For example, one study showed that even moderate exercise, such as brisk walking for 3 to 4 hours per week, can lower colon cancer risk. A limited number of studies have examined the effect of physical activity on colon cancer risk for both lean and obese people. Most of these studies have found a protective effect of physical activity across all levels of BMI.

- **Breast cancer:** The pattern of the association between physical activity and breast cancer risk is somewhat different. Most studies on breast cancer have focused on postmenopausal women. A recent study from the Women's Health Initiative found that physical activity among postmenopausal women at a level of walking about 30 minutes per day was associated with a 20 percent reduction in breast cancer risk. However, this reduction in risk was greatest among women who were of normal weight. For these women, physical activity was associated with a 37 percent decrease in risk. The protective effect of physical activity was not found among overweight or obese women.

What biological mechanisms are thought to be involved in explaining the link between obesity and cancer?

The biological mechanism that explains how obesity increases cancer risk may be different for different cancers. The exact mechanisms are not known for any of the cancers. However, possible mechanisms include alterations in sex hormones (for example, estrogen, progesterone, and androgens), and insulin and IGF–1 in obese people that may account for their increased risk for cancers of the breast, endometrium, and colon. Sex-hormone binding globulin, the major carrier protein for certain sex hormones in the plasma, may also be involved in the altered risk for these cancers in obese people.

Chapter 7

Physical Activity May Help Prevent Cancer

What is physical activity?

Physical activity is any bodily movement produced by skeletal muscles; such movement results in an expenditure of energy. Physical activity is a critical component of energy balance, a term used to describe how weight, diet, and physical activity influence health, including cancer risk.

How is physical activity related to health?

Researchers have established that regular physical activity can improve health in the following ways:

- Helping to control weight

- Maintaining healthy bones, muscles and joints

- Reducing the risk of developing high blood pressure and diabetes

- Promoting psychological well-being

- Reducing the risk of death from heart disease

- Reducing the risk of premature death

Excerpted from "Physical Activity and Cancer: Fact Sheet," National Cancer Institute, March 29, 2004. The complete text of this document, including references, can be found online at http://www.cancer.gov.

In addition to these health benefits, researchers are learning that physical activity can also affect the risk of cancer. There is convincing evidence that physical activity is associated with a reduced risk of cancers of the colon and breast. Several studies also have reported links between physical activity and a reduced risk of cancers of the prostate, lung and lining of the uterus (endometrial cancer). Despite these health benefits, recent studies have shown that more than 60 percent of Americans do not engage in enough regular physical activity.

How much physical activity do adults need?

The Centers for Disease Control and Prevention (CDC) recommend that adults: "engage in moderate-intensity physical activity for at least 30 minutes on five or more days of the week," or "engage in vigorous-intensity physical activity for at least 20 minutes on three or more days of the week."

What is the relationship between physical activity and colon cancer risk?

Individuals who are physically active can reduce their risk of developing colon cancer by 40 to 50 percent, with the greatest reduction in risk among those who are most active. A decreased risk of colon cancer has been consistently reported for physically active men. Many studies have reported a reduction in colon cancer risk for physically active women. The relationship between physical activity and risk in women, however, has been less consistent. Physical activity most likely influences the development of colon cancer through multiple, perhaps overlapping, biological pathways. Many researchers believe physical activity aids in regular bowel movements, which may decrease the time the colon is exposed to potential carcinogens. Increased physical activity also causes changes in insulin resistance, metabolism, and hormone levels, which may help prevent tumor development. Physical activity has also been found to alter a number of inflammatory and immune factors, some of which may influence colon cancer risk.

How can physical activity reduce breast cancer risk?

Physically active women have up to a 40 percent reduced risk of developing breast cancer. Most evidence suggests that physical activity reduces breast cancer risk in both premenopausal and postmenopausal women. Although a lifetime of regular, vigorous activity is thought to be of greatest benefit, women who occasionally engage in physical activity also experience a reduced risk compared to inactive women. A number of studies also suggest that the effect of physical activity may be different across levels of BMI (body mass index), with the greatest benefit seen in women in the normal weight range (generally a BMI under 25 kg/m^2). For example, a major report from the Women's Health Initiative found that among postmenopausal women, walking 30 minutes per day was associated with a 20 percent reduction in breast cancer risk. The health benefits of physical activity were greatest among women who were of normal weight; they experienced a 37 percent decrease in risk. The protective effect of physical activity was not found among overweight or obese women. Researchers have proposed several biological mechanisms that may explain the relationship between physical activity and breast cancer development. Physical activity causes changes in hormone metabolism, body mass, and immune function, which may prevent tumor development.

How might physical activity reduce prostate cancer risk?

Physical activity probably reduces men's risk for prostate cancer by 10 to 30 percent. The likely association between physical activity and prostate cancer is based on a small number of studies that evaluated the role of physical activity in men who developed prostate cancer. Most of these studies indicate that inactive men have higher rates of prostate cancer compared to men who are very physically active. While it is probable that men who are physically active experience a reduction in risk for prostate cancer, the potential biological mechanisms that may explain this association are unknown.

How might physical activity reduce endometrial cancer risk?

Studies also suggest that women who are physically active have a 30 to 40 percent reduced risk of endometrial cancer, with the greatest reduction in risk among those who are most active. The possible association between physical activity and endometrial cancer is based on a limited number of studies, some of which indicate that inactive women have higher rates of endometrial cancer compared to physically active women. Changes in body mass and alterations in level and metabolism of sex hormones, such as estrogen, are the major biological mechanisms thought to explain the association between physical activity and endometrial cancer. A few studies have examined whether the effect of physical activity varies according to the weight of the woman, but the results have been inconsistent.

How might physical activity reduce lung cancer risk?

It is possible that individuals who are physically active have a 30 to 40 percent reduced risk of developing lung cancer. The possible link between physical activity and lung cancer is based on a limited number of studies that have found higher rates of lung cancer among those who are physically inactive compared to those who are active, after accounting for smoking status. The relationship between physical activity and lung cancer risk is less clear for women than it is for men.

However, the results of many of these studies are difficult to interpret because smokers who are able to engage in physical activity may have much better lung function. Investigators hypothesize that improvements in pulmonary function and ventilation in active, compared to inactive individuals, may explain the possible association between lung cancer and reduced physical activity.

Is the National Cancer Institute exploring the role of physical activity in the quality of life and prognosis of cancer patients?

National Cancer Institute (NCI)-funded studies are exploring the ways in which physical activity may improve the quality of life of cancer patients and survivors. One study is examining the feasibility and benefits of a home-based moderate exercise program among breast cancer survivors. Another is testing the effectiveness of a nurse-directed walking exercise program to mitigate fatigue and maintain physical functioning during treatment for prostate, breast, or colorectal cancer.

What are some examples of NCI studies investigating the role of physical activity in cancer risk?

A number of NCI-funded studies are answering questions about the relationship between physical activity and the risk of developing cancer. For example, one study is investigating whether women who engage in moderate and strenuous physical activity have a reduced risk of endometrial and ovarian cancer, and if strenuous physical activity reduces this risk more than moderate physical activity. Another is examining the effect of one year of moderate aerobic and strength training exercise among patients with colorectal polyps.

Do any of these studies focus on special populations who are at increased risk of cancer?

NCI funds a number of research projects and interventions aimed at helping vulnerable populations reduce their risk for cancer by becoming more active, changing their nutritional behavior, and/or maintaining an optimal weight. Populations included in these projects include multiethnic working poor populations, African American women, African American church communities, rural church communities, overweight women, overweight men, and adolescents. For example, one study involving rural churches is exploring methods of helping participants to change their nutrition, activity, and exercise patterns to meet cancer risk reduction guidelines.

NCI is supporting national and regional surveys to gain more accurate information on physical activity across all age groups and diverse populations as defined by race, ethnicity, income, and other factors known to influence levels of physical activity. This information will help identify groups who may benefit from programs to increase physical activity.

Chapter 8

Dietary Choices and Cancer Risk

Chapter Contents

Section 8.1

Alcohol and Cancer

"Alcohol and Cancer," reprinted with permission from the University of Iowa Cancer Information Service. Copyright © 2006 The University of Iowa.

Over the past few years, scientists have studied alcohol intake and its relationship to developing cancer. Drinking alcohol increases the risk of the following cancers in men and women:

- mouth and throat
- voice box or larynx
- esophagus (food tube)
- liver
- breast cancer in women

Scientists know that alcohol damages cells. It is this cell damage that causes cancer. Alcohol also depletes vitamin A and selenium, nutrients that may have a protective effect against cancer. Alcohol decreases the body's ability to fight off cancer by compromising the immune system. It also irritates the lining of internal organs.

In general the cancer risk increases after two drinks a day for males and one drink per day for women. One drink equals the following:

- 12 ounces of beer
- 5 ounces of wine
- 1.5 ounces (1 shot) of 80 proof liquor

For women, two drinks daily increases the risk of getting breast cancer by about 25%.

The chances of getting liver cancer increase markedly with five or more drinks per day. Heavy alcohol use may also increase the risk of colorectal cancer and leads to greater increases in risk for most of the alcohol-related cancers. The earlier that long-term, heavy alcohol use begins, the greater the cancer risk. Also, using alcohol with tobacco is riskier than using either alone, because it further increases the chances of getting cancers of the mouth, throat, and esophagus.

Section 8.2

Heterocyclic Amines in Cooked Meats May Increase Cancer Risk

From "Heterocyclic Amines in Cooked Meats," National Cancer Institute, reviewed September 15, 2004. The complete text of this document, including references, can be found online at http://www.cancer.gov.

Research has shown that cooking certain meats at high temperatures creates chemicals that are not present in uncooked meats. A few of these chemicals may increase cancer risk. For example, heterocyclic amines (HCAs) are the carcinogenic chemicals formed from the cooking of muscle meats such as beef, pork, fowl, and fish. HCAs form when amino acids (the building blocks of proteins) and creatine (a chemical found in muscles) react at high cooking temperatures. Researchers have identified 17 different HCAs resulting from the cooking of muscle meats that may pose human cancer risk.

Research conducted by the National Cancer Institute (NCI) as well as by Japanese and European scientists indicates that heterocyclic amines are created within muscle meats during most types of high temperature cooking.

Recent studies have further evaluated the relationship associated with methods of cooking meat and the development of specific types of cancer. One study conducted by researchers from NCI's Division of Cancer Epidemiology and Genetics found a link between individuals with stomach cancer and the consumption of cooked meats. The researchers assessed the diets and cooking habits of 176 people diagnosed with stomach cancer and 503 people without cancer. The researchers found that those who ate their beef medium-well or well-done had more than three times the risk of stomach cancer than those who ate their beef rare or medium-rare. They also found that people who ate beef four or more times a week had more than twice the risk of stomach cancer than those consuming beef less frequently. Additional studies have shown that an increased risk of developing colorectal, pancreatic, and breast cancer is associated with high intakes of well-done, fried, or barbecued meats.

Four factors influence HCA formation: type of food, cooking method, temperature, and time. HCAs are found in cooked muscle meats. Other sources of protein (milk, eggs, tofu, and organ meats such as liver) have very little or no HCA content naturally or when cooked. Temperature is the most important factor in the formation of HCAs. Frying, broiling, and barbecuing produce the largest amounts of HCAs because the meats are cooked at very high temperatures. One study conducted by researchers showed a threefold increase in the content of HCAs when the cooking temperature was increased from 200° to 250° C (392° to 482° F). Oven roasting and baking are done at lower temperatures, so lower levels of HCAs are likely to form, however, gravy made from meat drippings does contain substantial amounts of HCAs. Stewing, boiling, or poaching are done at or below 100° C (212° F); cooking at this low temperature creates negligible amounts of the chemicals. Foods cooked a long time ("well-done" instead of "medium") by other methods will also form slightly more of the chemicals.

Meats that are partially cooked in the microwave oven before cooking by other methods also have lower levels of HCAs. Studies have shown that microwaving meat prior to cooking helps to decrease mutagens by removing the precursors. Meats that were microwaved for 2 minutes prior to cooking had a 90-percent decrease in HCA content. In addition, if the liquid that forms during microwaving is poured off before further cooking, the final quantity of HCAs is reduced.

One study has evaluated the content of HCAs in fast food restaurants. After evaluating five kinds of meat products from various fast food restaurant chains, the study concluded that there were low levels of HCAs found in fast food meat products due to factors such as cooking temperature and time. The study suggested that greater exposure to HCAs stems from home cooking and cooking in non-fast-food restaurants where food may be cooked to order and where a larger amount of meat is consumed.

Studies are being conducted to assess the amount of HCAs in the average American diet, but at present the maximum daily intake of HCAs in food has not been established. At the moment, no federal agency monitors the HCA content of cooked meats (how much a person could be eating), there is no good measure of how much HCAs would have to be eaten to increase cancer risk, and there are no guidelines concerning consumption of foods with HCAs. Further research is needed before such recommendations can be made.

However, concerned individuals can reduce their exposure to HCAs by varying methods of cooking meats; microwaving meats more often, especially before frying, broiling, or barbecuing; and refraining from making gravy from meat drippings.

Section 8.3

Does Acrylamide in Food Increase Cancer Risk?

Excerpted from "Acrylamide in Foods: Fact Sheet," National Cancer Institute, November 22, 2002. The complete text of this document can be found online at http://www.cancer.gov.

What is acrylamide?

Acrylamide is a chemical compound that occurs as a solid crystal or in liquid solution. Its primary use is to make polyacrylamide and acrylamide copolymers. Trace amounts of the original (unreacted) acrylamide generally remain in these products. Polyacrylamide and acrylamide copolymers are used in many industrial processes, including production of paper, dyes, and plastics, and the treatment of drinking water, sewage, and waste. They are also present in consumer products such as caulking, food packaging, and some adhesives.

Does acrylamide increase the risk of cancer?

Acrylamide has not been shown to cause cancer in humans. However, the relationship between acrylamide and cancer has not been studied extensively in humans. Because it has been shown to cause cancer in laboratory rats when given in the animals' drinking water, both the Environmental Protection Agency (EPA) and the International Agency for Research on Cancer (IARC) in Lyon, France, consider acrylamide to be a probable human carcinogen. The National Toxicology Program's

Ninth Report on Carcinogens states that acrylamide can be "reasonably anticipated to be a human carcinogen."

Is there acrylamide in food?

Recent studies by research groups in Sweden, Switzerland, Norway, Britain, and the United States have found acrylamide in certain foods. It has been determined that heating some foods to a temperature of 120° C (248° F) can produce acrylamide. Potato chips and french fries have been found to contain relatively high levels of acrylamide compared to other foods with lower levels also present in bread and cereals. A joint World Health Organization and Food and Agriculture Organization (WHO/FAO) consultation in June 2002 concluded that the levels of acrylamide in foods pose a major concern and called for more research to determine what the risk is and what should be done.

How does cooking produce acrylamide?

In September 2002, researchers discovered that the amino acid asparagine, which is present in many vegetables, with higher amounts in some varieties of potatoes, can form acrylamide when heated to high temperatures in the presence of certain sugars. High-heat cooking methods, such as frying, baking, or broiling, are most likely to result in acrylamide formation. Boiling and microwaving appear less likely to form acrylamide. Longer cooking times increase the amount of acrylamide produced when the temperature is high enough.

Should I change my diet?

The best advice at this early stage in our understanding of this complex issue is to follow established dietary guidelines and eat a healthy, balanced diet that is low in fat and rich in high-fiber grains, fruits, and vegetables.

What research is needed?

The WHO/FAO consultation concluded that further research is necessary to determine how acrylamide is formed during the cooking process and whether acrylamide is present in foods other than those already tested. They also recommended population-based studies of those cancers that could potentially develop due to exposure to acrylamide.

Section 8.4

Is There a Link between Artificial Sweeteners and Cancer Risk?

Excerpted from "Artificial Sweeteners and Cancer: Questions and Answers," National Cancer Institute (NCI), reviewed February 17, 2006. Additional information about aspartame and the NIH-AARP Diet and Health Study is excerpted from "Aspartame and Cancer: Questions and Answers," NCI, September 12, 2006. For more information, visit http://www.cancer.gov.

What are artificial sweeteners and how are they regulated in the United States?

Artificial sweeteners, also called sugar substitutes, are substances that are used instead of sucrose (table sugar) to sweeten foods and beverages. Because artificial sweeteners are many times sweeter than table sugar, smaller amounts are needed to create the same level of sweetness. Artificial sweeteners are regulated by the U.S. Food and Drug Administration (FDA). The FDA, like the National Cancer Institute (NCI), is an agency of the Department of Health and Human Services. The FDA regulates food, drugs, medical devices, cosmetics, biologics, and radiation-emitting products. The Food Additives Amendment to the Food, Drug, and Cosmetic Act, which was passed by Congress in 1958, requires the FDA to approve food additives, including artificial sweeteners, before they can be made available for sale in the United States. However, this legislation does not apply to products that are "generally recognized as safe." Such products do not require FDA approval before being marketed.

Is there an association between artificial sweeteners and cancer?

Questions about artificial sweeteners and cancer arose when early studies showed that cyclamate in combination with saccharin caused bladder cancer in laboratory animals. However, results from subsequent carcinogenicity studies (studies that examine whether a substance can

77

cause cancer) on these sweeteners and other approved sweeteners have not provided clear evidence of an association between artificial sweeteners and cancer in people.

What have studies shown about a possible association between specific artificial sweeteners and cancer?

Saccharin: Studies in laboratory rats during the early 1970s linked saccharin with the development of bladder cancer. For this reason, Congress mandated that further studies of saccharin be performed and required that all food containing saccharin bear the following warning label: "Use of this product may be hazardous to your health. This product contains saccharin, which has been determined to cause cancer in laboratory animals." Subsequent studies in rats showed an increased incidence of urinary bladder cancer at high doses of saccharin consumption, especially in male rats. However, mechanistic studies (studies that examine how a substance works in the body) have shown that these results apply only to rats. Human epidemiology studies (studies of patterns, causes, and control of diseases in groups of people) have shown no consistent evidence that saccharin is associated with bladder cancer incidence.

Because the bladder tumors seen in rats are due to a mechanism not relevant to humans, and because there is no clear evidence that saccharin causes cancer in humans, saccharin was delisted in 2000 from the U.S. National Toxicology Program's *Report on Carcinogens*, where it had been listed since 1981 as a substance reasonably anticipated to be a human carcinogen (a substance known to cause cancer). More information about the delisting of saccharin is available at http://ntp .niehs.nih.gov/ntp/roc/eleventh/append/appb.pdf. The delisting led to legislation, which was signed into law on December 21, 2000, repealing the warning label requirement for products containing saccharin.

Aspartame: Aspartame, distributed under several trade names (for example, NutraSweet® and Equal®), was approved in 1981 by the FDA after numerous tests showed that it did not cause cancer or other adverse effects in laboratory animals. Questions regarding the safety of aspartame were renewed by a 1996 report suggesting that an increase in the number of people with brain tumors between 1975 and 1992 might be associated with the introduction and use of this sweetener in the United States. However, an analysis of then-current NCI statistics showed that the overall incidence of brain and central nervous system cancers began to rise in 1973, eight years prior to the approval of aspartame, and continued to rise until 1985. Moreover, increases in overall brain cancer incidence occurred primarily in people age 70 and older, a group that was not exposed to the highest doses of aspartame since its introduction. These data do not establish a clear link between the consumption of aspartame and the development of brain tumors. More information about aspartame can be found in the *FDA Statement on Aspartame*, which is available at http://www.cfsan.fda.gov/~lrd/tpaspart.html.

A study of about half a million people, published in 2006, compared people who drank aspartame-containing beverages with those who did not. National Cancer Institute researchers examined data from the NIH-AARP Diet and Health Study to investigate questions about aspartame and risk for lymphoma, leukemia, and brain cancers. The NIH-AARP Diet and Health Study is an observational study where people provide information on a questionnaire about their recent intake of various foods and then are followed up for subsequent development of cancer. Specifically, about half a million AARP members (285,079 men and 199,905 women) who were 50 to 71 years old and living in eight study areas across the U.S. were given a questionnaire in 1995 and 1996. The participants were followed until the end of 2000 by linkage of their records with cancer registries that track the occurrence of new cancers.

The questionnaire inquired about consumption frequency and diet drink-type preference for three potentially aspartame-containing beverages (soda, fruit drinks, and iced tea), as well as aspartame added to coffee and hot tea. The researchers then computed daily consumption of aspartame, taking into account aspartame content, portion size, and consumption frequency of each beverage. The estimated aspartame intake was next compared with the occurrence of 1,888 lymphomas or leukemias and 315 malignant brain cancers to see if there was any correlation between intake and cancer. Results of the study showed that increasing levels of consumption were not associated with any risk of lymphomas, leukemias, or brain cancers in men or women.

Acesulfame potassium, sucralose, and neotame: In addition to saccharin and aspartame, there are three other artificial sweeteners currently permitted for use in food in the United States. Acesulfame potassium (also known as ACK, Sweet One®, and Sunett®) was approved by the FDA in 1988 for use in specific food and beverage categories, and was later approved as a general purpose sweetener (except in meat and poultry) in 2002. Sucralose (also known as Splenda®) was approved by the FDA as a tabletop sweetener in 1998, followed by approval as a general purpose sweetener in 1999. Neotame, which is similar to aspartame, was approved by the FDA as a general purpose sweetener (except in meat and poultry) in 2002. Before approving these sweeteners, the FDA reviewed more than 100 safety studies that were conducted on each sweetener, including studies to assess cancer risk. The results of these studies showed no evidence that these sweeteners cause cancer or pose any other threat to human health.

Cyclamate: Because the findings in rats suggested that cyclamate might increase the risk of bladder cancer in humans, the FDA banned the use of cyclamate in 1969. Upon the reexamination of cyclamate carcinogenicity and the evaluation of additional data, scientists concluded that cyclamate was not a carcinogen or a co-carcinogen (a substance that enhances the effect of a cancer-causing substance). A food additive petition is currently filed with FDA for the reapproval of cyclamate. The FDA's concerns about cyclamate are not cancer related.

Section 8.5

Can Fluoridated Water Cause Cancer?

Excerpted from "Fluoridated Water: Questions and Answers," National Cancer Institute, reviewed June 29, 2005. The complete text of this document can be found online at http://cancer.gov.

What is fluoride?

Fluoride is the name given to a group of compounds that are composed of the naturally occurring element fluorine and one or more other elements. Fluorides are present naturally in water and soil.

What is fluoridated water?

Virtually all water contains some amount of fluoride. Water fluoridation is the process of adding fluoride to the water supply so that the level reaches approximately 1 part fluoride per million parts water (ppm) or 1 milligram fluoride per liter of water (mg/L); this is the optimal level for preventing tooth decay.

Why fluoridate water?

In the early 1940s, scientists discovered that people who lived where drinking water supplies had naturally occurring fluoride levels of approximately 1.0 ppm had fewer dental caries (cavities). Many more recent studies have supported this finding.

Fluoride can prevent and even reverse tooth decay by enhancing remineralization, the process by which fluoride "rebuilds" tooth enamel that is beginning to decay.

Can fluoridated water cause cancer?

The possible relationship between fluoridated water and cancer has been debated at length. The debate resurfaced in 1990 when a study by the National Toxicology Program, part of the National Institute of Environmental Health Sciences, showed an increased number of osteosarcomas (bone tumors) in male rats given water high in fluoride for two years. However, other studies in humans and in animals have not shown an association between fluoridated water and cancer.

In a February 1991 Public Health Service (PHS) report, the agency said it found no evidence of an association between fluoride and cancer in humans. The report, based on a review of more than 50 human epidemiological (population) studies produced over the past 40 years, concluded that optimal fluoridation of drinking water "does not pose a detectable cancer risk to humans" as evidenced by extensive human epidemiological data reported to date.

In one of the studies reviewed for the PHS report, scientists at the National Cancer Institute evaluated the relationship between the fluoridation of drinking water and the number of deaths due to cancer in the United States during a 36-year period, and the relationship between water fluoridation and number of new cases of cancer during a 15-year period. After examining more than 2.2 million cancer death records and 125,000 cancer case records in counties using fluoridated water, the researchers found no indication of increased cancer risk associated with fluoridated drinking water.

In 1993, the Subcommittee on Health Effects of Ingested Fluoride of the National Research Council, part of the National Academy of Sciences, conducted an extensive literature review concerning the association between fluoridated drinking water and increased cancer risk. The review included data from more than 50 human epidemiological studies and six animal studies. The Subcommittee concluded that none of the data demonstrated an association between fluoridated drinking water and cancer. A 1999 report by the CDC supported these findings. The report concluded that studies to date have produced "no credible evidence" of an association between fluoridated drinking water and an increased risk for cancer.

Section 8.6

No Link between Microwave Cooking and Cancer

An Alabama Cooperative Extension food scientist has this advice for people disturbed by a widely forwarded e-mail claiming that microwave cooking of food in plastic wrap causes cancer: Relax.

In fact, if you're really intent on reducing potentially harmful trace amounts of carcinogens in your food during cooking, she advises giving your frying pan a rest instead.

The e-mail, which has since proven to be largely a hoax, claims a seventh-grade Arkansas student discovered that two supposedly cancer-causing substances, DEHA and dioxin, leach into food from plastic wrap during microwave cooking.

Part of this is true. A seventh-grade Arkansas student named Claire Nelson was, in fact, curious to learn whether potentially harmful chemicals released from heated plastic during microwave cooking ended up in food.

It's also true that Nelson, working with the FDA-affiliated Center for Toxicological Research in Jonesboro, Arkansas, tested the effects on olive oil enclosed in plastic wrap during microwave cooking. Her testing revealed that one of the substances, known by its initials DEHA, turned up in trace amounts in the oil after cooking and migrated into the oil at between 200 parts and 500 parts per million. The current FDA standard for DEHA is 0.05 parts per billion.

DEHA is a phthalate, one of many types of plasticizers commonly added to plastics to enhance their flexibility.

Likewise, xenoestrogens, believed to reduce sperm-count levels in men and cause breast cancer in women, also were found in oil. However, it was difficult for Nelson to determine how much was too much, since there currently are no FDA guidelines establishing tolerance levels for xenoestrogens in foods. This much is true.

What is not true is that DEHA is a known cancer-causing agent or that dioxin was one of the substances uncovered during testing, says Dr. Jean Weese, an Alabama Cooperative Extension System food scientist.

"While some forms of phthalates have been shown to cause health effects, including cancer, in laboratory mice and rats, DEHA isn't one of them," Weese says.

"In fact, the most recent studies involving DEHA and some other phthalates have shown no link with cancer," she adds, stressing that the EPA and the European Union agencies currently do not recognize DEHA as a known carcinogen.

Equally untrue is the claim that dioxin is produced from plastic wraps during microwave cooking. While dioxin is a serious health risk, causing a variety of health problems, including cancer, Nelson's studies turned up no evidence that dioxin was released into food during microwave cooking.

"It is true that dioxins are produced by the burning of plastics, especially polyvinyl chloride, but to my knowledge, no scientific study has ever shown that dioxins are formed in plastics heated by microwaves," Weese says.

Indeed, frying is the only form of cooking that has ever been associated with the production of trace amounts of dioxins in food. The problem stems from the fact that oils and fats typically used in frying contain triglycerides.

"Once these substances reach high temperatures from frying, the fats attached to this glycerol backbone begin breaking down into peroxide and other substances, including, in some cases, dioxins and PCBs, another known carcinogen," Weese says.

Under the circumstances, she says, consumers would be better off putting away the frying pan and broiling your food instead.

She also offers this advice to consumers who still harbor any lingering concerns about using plastics in the microwave:

- First, use only cookware that is labeled for use in the microwave oven.

- Second, avoid using plastic storage containers such as margarine tubs, takeout containers, and other one-time use containers, all of which can melt or warp when heated.

- Third, never use thin plastic storage bags, brown paper, plastic grocery bags, newspaper, or aluminum foil in the microwave oven.

On the other hand, microwave plastic wraps, wax paper, cooking bags, parchment paper, and white microwave-safe paper towels are safe to use.

Chapter 9

Dietary Choices and Cancer Prevention

Chapter Contents

Section 9.1

Does Garlic Prevent Cancer?

"Garlic and Cancer Prevention: Fact Sheet,"
National Cancer Institute, November 27, 2002.

Garlic is the edible bulb from a plant in the lily family. Garlic, onions, leeks, scallions, shallots, and chives are classified as members of the Allium genus. Thus, they are commonly described as Allium vegetables.

Does garlic prevent cancer?

A host of studies provide compelling evidence that garlic and its organic allyl sulfur components are effective inhibitors of the cancer process. These studies reveal that the benefits of garlic are not limited to a specific species, to a particular tissue, or to a specific carcinogen. Of 37 observational studies in humans using garlic and related allyl sulfur components, 28 studies showed some cancer preventive effect. The evidence is particularly strong for a link between garlic and prevention of prostate and stomach cancers. However, all of the available information comes from observational studies comparing cancer incidence in populations who consume or do not consume garlic (epidemiologic studies), animal models, or observations with cells in culture. These findings have not yet been verified by clinical trials in humans.

Although health benefits of garlic are frequently reported, excessive intake can have harmful effects. Studies have reported symptoms including garlic odor on breath and skin, occasional allergic reactions, stomach disorders and diarrhea, decrease in serum protein and calcium levels, association with bronchial asthma, and contact dermatitis, and possible associations with production of sperm in males. Garlic preparations vary in concentration and in the number of active compounds they contain. Thus, quality control is an important consideration when foods such as garlic are considered for use as a cancer-fighting agent.

How might garlic prevent cancer?

Several compounds are involved in garlic's possible anticancer effects. Garlic contains allyl sulfur and other compounds that slow or prevent the growth of tumor cells. Allyl sulfur compounds, which occur naturally in garlic and onions, make cells vulnerable to the stress created by products of cell division. Because cancer cells divide very quickly, they generate more stressors than most normal cells. Thus, cancer cells are damaged by the presence of allyl sulfur compounds to a much greater extent than normal cells.

The chemistry of garlic is complicated. As a result, the quality of garlic products depends on the manufacturing process. Peeling garlic and processing garlic into oil or powder can increase the number and variety of active compounds. Peeling garlic releases an enzyme called allinase and starts a series of chemical reactions that produce diallyl disulfide (DADS). DADS is also formed when raw garlic is cut or crushed. However, if garlic is cooked immediately after peeling, the allinase is inactivated and the cancer-fighting benefit of DADS is lost. Scientists recommend waiting 15 minutes between peeling and cooking garlic to allow the allinase reaction to occur.

Processing garlic into powder or garlic oil releases other cancer-fighting agents. The inconsistent results of garlic research may be due, at least in part, to problems standardizing all of the active compounds within garlic preparations. Some of the garlic compounds currently under investigation are: allin (responsible for the typical garlic odor), alline (odorless compound), ajoene (naturally occurring disulfide), diallyl sulfide (DAS), diallyl disulfide (DADS), diallyl trisulfide (DAT), S-allylcysteine (SAC), organosulfur compounds, and allyl sulfur compounds.

Section 9.2

Does Red Wine Inhibit Cancer Development?

"Red Wine and Cancer Prevention: Fact Sheet,"
National Cancer Institute, November 27, 2002.

Red wine is a rich source of biologically active phytochemicals, chemicals found in plants. Particular compounds called polyphenols found in red wine—such as catechins and resveratrol—are thought to have antioxidant or anticancer properties.

What are polyphenols and how do they prevent cancer?

Polyphenols are antioxidant compounds found in the skin and seeds of grapes. When wine is made from these grapes, the alcohol produced by the fermentation process dissolves the polyphenols contained in the skin and seeds. Red wine contains more polyphenols than white wine because the making of white wine requires the removal of the skins after the grapes are crushed. The phenols in red wine include catechin, gallic acid, and epicatechin.

Polyphenols have been found to have antioxidant properties. Antioxidants are substances that protect cells from oxidative damage caused by molecules called free radicals. These chemicals can damage important parts of cells, including proteins, membranes, and DNA. Cellular damage caused by free radicals has been implicated in the development of cancer. Research on the antioxidants found in red wine has shown that they may help inhibit the development of certain cancers.

What is resveratrol and how does it prevent cancer?

Resveratrol is a type of polyphenol called a phytoalexin, a class of compounds produced as part of a plant's defense system against disease. It is produced in the plant in response to an invading fungus, stress, injury, infection, or ultraviolet irradiation. Red wine contains high levels of resveratrol, as do grapes, raspberries, peanuts, and other plants.

Resveratrol has been shown to reduce tumor incidence in animals by affecting one or more stages of cancer development. It has been shown to inhibit growth of many types of cancer cells in culture. Evidence also exists that it can reduce inflammation. It also reduces activation of NF kappa B, a protein produced by the body's immune system when it is under attack. This protein affects cancer cell growth and metastasis. Resveratrol is also an antioxidant.

What have red wine studies found?

The cell and animal studies of red wine have examined effects in several cancers including leukemia, skin, breast, and prostate cancers. Scientists are studying resveratrol to learn more about its cancer preventive activities. Recent evidence from animal studies suggests this anti-inflammatory compound may be an effective chemopreventive agent in three stages of the cancer process: initiation, promotion, and progression.

Research studies published in the *International Journal of Cancer* show that drinking a glass of red wine a day may cut a man's risk of prostate cancer in half and that the protective effect appears to be strongest against the most aggressive forms of the disease. It was also seen that men who consumed four or more 4-ounce glasses of red wine per week have a 60 percent lower incidence of the more aggressive types of prostate cancer.

However, studies of the association between red wine consumption and cancer in humans are in their initial stages. Although consumption of large amounts of alcoholic beverages may increase the risk of some cancers, there is growing evidence that the health benefits of red wine are related to its nonalcoholic components.

Section 9.3

Vitamin D and Cancer Risk

This text is by Larry Axmaker, EdD, PhD.
© 2006 Wellsource, Inc. Reprinted with permission.

Researchers from the Moores Cancer Center at the University of California San Diego Medical Center are recommending that everyone get 1000 International Units (IU) (25 micrograms) of vitamin D on a daily basis. Their study—a systematic review of 63 prior studies involving vitamin D—indicates that sufficient amounts of vitamin D can reduce the risk of colon, breast, and ovarian cancer up to 50 percent.

Vitamin D Deficiency

Vitamin D deficiency is common, especially in areas with less sunshine (such as in the northeastern U.S.) and in individuals with more skin pigment. Those with low levels of vitamin D are at risk for broken bones, osteoporosis, muscle pains, and some cancers. Vitamin D deficiency has been estimated to affect between 21 percent and 58 percent of Americans. Rates will vary depending on age, gender, racial background, and geographical location.

Previous Recommendations

The Institute of Medicine (IOM) has recommended that: people from birth to 50 years old receive 200 IUs per day; adults ages 51 to 70 receive 400 IUs per day; and adults 71 and over should receive 600 IUs per day. Some experts, including the researchers at the San Diego Medical Center, cite evidence that the amount should be even higher, especially for older people. 1000 IU a day has been determined to be a safe dosage by the National Academy of Sciences.

Spending 15 to 20 minutes a day in the sunshine is a good source of vitamin D for most people, but may not meet total vitamin D needs. Sunshine also has some risks, however, such as skin damage through sunburn. Sunscreen, while protecting skin, prevents absorption of UV rays that help produce vitamin D. In some climates there is very little sunshine during winter months.

A multiple vitamin usually includes 400 IU of vitamin D. A glass of milk contains 100 IU. Other good sources of vitamin D are cod liver oil, orange juice, yogurt, cheese, salmon, cod, and shrimp.

Bottom Line

Based on their review of vitamin D studies, the authors recommend that everyone eat vitamin D-rich foods and take a vitamin supplement containing vitamin D to help insure they get enough to help maintain bone strength, muscle health, and be preventive of some cancers and other diseases.

Section 9.4

Omega-3 Fatty Acids Unlikely to Prevent Cancer

National Cancer Institute (NCI), reprinted
from *NCI Cancer Bulletin*, vol. 3/no. 5, Jan. 31, 2006.

An analysis of numerous, large population cohort studies did not detect evidence of a significant link between dietary intake of omega-3 fatty acids (found in fish) and the incidence of several major cancer types, according to a review study published in the January 25, 2006, issue of the *Journal of the American Medical Association*.

The reviewers analyzed 38 articles covering 20 population cohorts that included more than 700,000 individuals. The participants were studied for the effects of consuming omega-3—either in fish, dietary supplements, or both—on the incidence of 11 different types of cancer, although more than half of the reports were for either breast, colorectal, or prostate cancers.

The combined studies provided 65 estimates of associations between omega-3 and cancer incidence, but "only ten were statistically significant," reported the researchers led by Dr. Catherine H. MacLean with RAND Health. Significant associations between omega-3 fatty acid consumption and cancer risk were reported for breast, colorectal, lung, prostate, and skin cancers. "However, for breast, lung, and prostate cancer, there were significant associations for both increased risk and decreased risk and far more estimates that did not demonstrate any association," the researchers noted.

Across the cohorts, no trend was found linking omega-3 fatty acids with a reduced overall cancer risk. "Likewise, there is little to suggest that omega-3 fatty acids reduce the risk of any single type of cancer," the authors wrote.

Chapter 10

Sunshine, Tanning, and Cancer Risk

Chapter Contents

Section 10.1

Questions and Answers about Sunshine and Cancer

"Questions and Answers," Cancer Prevention and Control, National Center for Chronic Disease Prevention and Health Promotion, Centers for Disease Control and Prevention, February 2006.

When do I need to protect myself from sun exposure?

Protection from sun exposure is important all year round, not just during the summer or at the beach. Any time the sun's ultraviolet (UV) rays are able to reach the earth, you need to protect yourself from excessive sun exposure. UV rays can cause skin damage during any season or temperature.

Relatively speaking, the hours between 10 AM and 4 PM during daylight savings time (9 AM–3 PM during standard time) are the most hazardous for UV exposure in the continental United States. UV radiation is the greatest during the late spring and early summer in North America.

Remember: UV rays reach you on cloudy and hazy days, as well as on bright and sunny days. UV rays will also reflect off any surface like water, cement, sand, and snow.

What exactly are "ultraviolet rays"?

Ultraviolet (UV) rays are a part of sunlight that is an invisible form of radiation. UV rays can penetrate and change the structure of skin cells.

There are three types of UV rays: ultraviolet A (UVA), ultraviolet B (UVB), and ultraviolet C (UVC). UVA is the most abundant source of solar radiation at the earth's surface and penetrates beyond the top layer of human skin. Scientists believe that UVA radiation can cause damage to connective tissue and increase a person's risk for developing skin cancer.

UVB rays are less abundant at the earth's surface than UVA because a significant portion of UVB rays is absorbed by the ozone layer.

UVB rays penetrate less deeply into the skin than do UVA rays, but also can be damaging.

UVC radiation is extremely hazardous to skin, but it is completely absorbed by the stratospheric ozone layer and does not reach the surface of the earth.

How can I protect myself from the sun's UV rays?

When possible, avoid outdoor activities during midday, when the sun's rays are strongest. This usually means the hours between 10 AM and 4 PM. You can also wear protective clothing, such as a wide-brimmed hat, long-sleeved shirt, and long pants.

For eye protection, wear wrap-around sunglasses that provide 100 percent UV ray protection. And always wear a broad-spectrum (protection against both UVA and UVB rays) sunscreen and lipscreen with a sun protection factor (SPF) of at least 15. Remember to reapply as indicated by the manufacturer's directions.

Also, check the sunscreen's expiration date. Sunscreen without an expiration date has a shelf life of no more than three years. Exposure to extreme temperatures can shorten the expiration date or shelf life of sunscreen.

What can excessive exposure to UV rays do to my health?

UV exposure appears to be the most important environmental factor in the development of skin cancer and a primary factor in the development of lip cancer.

Although getting some sun exposure can yield a few positive benefits, excessive and unprotected exposure to the sun can result in premature aging and undesirable changes in skin texture. Such exposure has been associated with various types of skin cancer, including melanoma, one of the most serious and deadly forms. UV rays also have been found to be associated with various eye conditions, such as cataracts.

What is the UV Index?

The UV Index was developed by the National Weather Service and the Environmental Protection Agency (EPA). It provides a forecast of the expected risk of overexposure to UV rays and indicates the degree of caution you should take when working, playing, or exercising outdoors.

The UV Index predicts exposure levels on a 0–10+ scale, where 0 indicates a low risk of overexposure and 10+ means a very high risk of overexposure. Calculated on a next-day basis for dozens of cities across the U.S., the UV Index takes into account clouds and other local conditions that affect the amount of UV radiation reaching the ground.

The level of danger calculated for the basic categories of the index are for a person with Type II skin. For a person with type II skin, for example, an Index value of 5 or 6 represents a moderate possibility of UV overexposure.

More information about the UV Index is available at the EPA website: http://www.epa.gov/sunwise/uvindex.html. You can also call the Environmental Protection Agency (EPA) hotline at 800-296-1996 for more information on the UV Index.

What does a suntan indicate? Why does the skin tan when exposed to the sun?

The penetration of UV rays to the skin's inner layer results in the production of more melanin. That melanin eventually moves toward the outer layers of the skin and becomes visible as a tan.

A suntan is not an indicator of good health. Some physicians consider the skin's tanning a response to injury because it appears after the sun's UV rays have killed some cells and damaged others.

Not everyone burns or tans in the same manner. Are there ways to classify different skin types?

Whether individuals burn or tan depends on a number of factors, including their skin type, the time of year, and the amount of sun exposure they have received recently. The skin's susceptibility to burning can be classified on a five-point scale as outlined in Table 10.1.

Though everyone is at risk for damage as a result of excessive sun exposure, people with skin types I and II are at the highest risk.

Does it matter what kind of sunscreen I use?

Sunscreens come in a variety of forms such as lotions, gels, and sprays, so there are plenty of different options. There are also sunscreens made for specific purposes, such as the scalp, sensitive skin, and for use on babies. Regardless of the type of sunscreen you choose, be sure that you use one that blocks both UVA and UVB rays and that it offers at least SPF 15.

What does a sunscreen's SPF rating mean?

Sunscreens are assigned a sun protection factor (SPF) number according to their effectiveness in offering protection from UV rays. Higher numbers indicate more protection. As a rule of thumb, you should always use a sunscreen with at least SPF 15.

Do sunscreens need to be reapplied during the course of a day?

You should follow the manufacturer's directions regarding reapplication or you risk not getting the protection that you might think you are getting. Though recently developed sunscreens are more resistant to loss through sweating and getting wet than previous sunscreens were, you should still reapply frequently, especially during peak sun hours or after swimming or sweating.

Table 10.1. Skin Type and Burning Susceptibility

Skin Type	Tanning and Sunburning History
I	Always burns, never tans, sensitive to sun exposure
II	Burns easily, tans minimally
III	Burns moderately, tans gradually to light brown
IV	Burns minimally, always tans well to moderately brown
V	Rarely burns, tans profusely to dark
VI	Never burns, deeply pigmented, least sensitive

How do sunscreens work?

Most sun protection products work by absorbing, reflecting, or scattering the sun's rays. Such products contain chemicals that interact with the skin to protect it from UV rays. Sunscreens help prevent problems related to sun exposure, such as aging skin and precancerous growths.

Keep in mind that sunscreen is not meant to allow you to spend more time in the sun than you would otherwise. That's why it is important to complement sunscreen use with other sun protection options: cover up, wear a hat and sunglasses, and seek shade.

Some cosmetic products claim to protect you from UV rays. Can they?

There are cosmetics and lip protectors that contain some of the same protective chemicals used by sunscreens on the market. However, not all of these products meet the standard of having at least SPF 15, and therefore do not offer sufficient protection by themselves.

What kinds of clothing best protect my skin from UV rays?

Clothing that covers your skin protects against the sun's UV rays. Loose-fitting long-sleeved shirts and long pants made from tightly woven fabric offer the best protection. A wet T-shirt offers you much less UV protection than does a dry one.

If wearing this type of clothing isn't practical, at least try to wear a T-shirt or a beach cover-up. Keep in mind, however, that a typical T-shirt actually has an SPF rating substantially lower than the recommended SPF 15, so double-up on protection by using sunscreen with at least SPF 15 (and UVA and UVB protection) and staying in the shade when you can.

Does protective clothing have to be a certain color?

Wearing clothing made of tightly-woven fabric is best for protecting your skin, regardless of the color. Darker colors, though, may offer more protection than lighter colors.

It gets so hot here in the summer, there's no way I could be comfortable in long pants and a long-sleeved shirt. So, what else can I do to protect my skin?

Protecting yourself from the sun's UV rays doesn't have to be a major chore; it's just a matter of knowing your options and using them. Wearing a dry T-shirt is a good start, but it is not enough if you are going to be outside for more than a few minutes.

If you can't wear long pants and a long-sleeved shirt, you can boost your protection by seeking shade whenever possible and by always wearing sunscreen with at least SPF 15.

Will a hat help protect my skin? Are there recommended styles for the best protection?

Hats can help shield your skin from the sun's UV rays. Choose a hat that provides shade for all of your head and neck. For the most protection, wear a hat with a brim all the way around that shades your face, ears, and the back of your neck.

If you choose to wear a baseball cap, you should also protect your ears and the back of your neck by wearing clothing that covers those areas, using sunscreen with at least SPF 15, or by staying in the shade.

For the best protection, what material should I look for in a hat?

A tightly woven fabric, such as canvas, works best to protect your skin from UV rays. When possible, avoid straw hats with holes that let sunlight through.

Does the color of my hat matter?

The amount of shade offered by a particular hat appears to be its most important prevention characteristic. If a darker hat is an option, though, it may offer even more UV protection.

Are sunglasses an important part of my sun protection plan?

Yes. Sunglasses protect your eyes from UV rays and reduce the risk of cataracts. They also protect the tender skin around your eyes from sun exposure.

What type of sunglasses best protects my eyes from UV rays?

Sunglasses that block both UVA and UVB rays offer the best protection. The majority of sunglasses sold in the United States, regardless of cost, meet this standard. Wrap-around sunglasses work best because they block UV rays from sneaking in from the side.

Is there any particular time I should try to stay in the shade?

The sun's UV rays are strongest and do the most damage during midday, so it's best to avoid direct exposure between 10:00 AM and 4:00 PM. You can reduce your risk of skin damage and skin cancer by seeking shade under an umbrella, tree, or other shelter before you need relief from the sun.

I work outdoors all summer and can't stay in the shade. What can I do to protect my skin?

If you can't avoid the sun, you can protect your skin by wearing a wide-brimmed hat, wraparound sunglasses that block both UVA and UVB rays, long-sleeved shirt, and long pants. You can also wear a sunscreen and lipscreen with at least SPF 15 and UVA and UVB protection and reapply according to the manufacturer's directions. When you can, take your breaks and your lunch in the shade.

If I stay in the shade, should I still use sunscreen and wear a hat?

UV rays can reflect off virtually any surface (including sand, snow and concrete) and can reach you in the shade. Your best option to protect your skin and lips is to use sunscreen or wear protective clothing when you're outside—even when you're in the shade.

Section 10.2

Sunscreens and Tanning Products

Excerpted from "Sunscreens, Tanning Products, and Sun Safety," U. S. Food and Drug Administration, Center for Food Safety and Applied Nutrition, Office of Cosmetics and Colors Fact Sheet, June 27, 2000; revised April 30, 2003.

The following information on sunscreens and tanning products is intended to help consumers make informed decisions about sun protection and tanning.

Sunscreens

Sunscreens play an important role as one part of a total program to reduce the harmful effects of the sun, which first includes limiting sun exposure and wearing protective clothing. FDA regulates sunscreens as over-the-counter (OTC) drugs. Cosmetic products that are marketed with sun-protection claims are regulated as both drugs and cosmetics.

To help consumers select products that best suit their needs, sunscreens are labeled with SPF numbers. SPF stands for "Sun Protection Factor." The higher the SPF number, the more sunburn protection the product provides. Experts recommend using sunscreens with an SPF number of 15 or higher that also provide protection from UVA rays. Remember, sunscreen use alone will not prevent all of the possible harmful effects of the sun.

The effectiveness of a sunscreen is reduced if it is not applied in adequate amounts or it is washed off, rubbed off, sweated off, or otherwise removed. For maximum effectiveness, apply a sunscreen liberally before going outside and reapply it frequently on all sun-exposed skin. Unless otherwise stated on the label, 30 minutes before going outside and at least every two hours thereafter is a general rule of thumb. About one ounce of sunscreen should be used per application on the average adult.

Label Warning Requirement for Suntanning Products without Sunscreen

FDA is concerned about the health hazards associated with suntanning products that do not contain sunscreen ingredients. Such suntanning products must bear the following warning statement:

"Warning—This product does not contain a sunscreen and does not protect against sunburn. Repeated exposure of unprotected skin while tanning may increase the risk of skin aging, skin cancer, and other harmful effects to the skin even if you do not burn." (Title 21 of the Code of Federal Regulations, Section 740.19)

Tanning Accelerators

Lotions and pills marketed as "tanning accelerators" often contain tyrosine (an amino acid), often in combination with other substances. Tanning accelerators may be marketed with the claim that they enhance tanning by stimulating and increasing melanin formation. FDA has concluded that these "tanning accelerators" are actually unapproved drugs, and the agency has issued warning letters to several manufacturers of these products. There is a lack of scientific data showing that they work; in fact, at least one study has found them ineffective.

Tanning Pills

Pills that contain large doses of canthaxanthin are sometimes marketed as "tanning pills." Although FDA has approved canthaxanthin for use as a color additive in foods, where it is used in small amounts, its use as a tanning agent is not approved. Imported tanning pills containing canthaxanthin are subject to import detention as products containing non-permitted color additives.

When a person ingests canthaxanthin in large quantities, the substance is deposited in various parts of the body, including the skin, where it imparts a color ranging from orange to brownish. Tanning pills have been associated with side effects, particularly a condition called "canthaxanthin retinopathy," the formation of yellow deposits in the retina of the eye.

Sunless Tanners and Bronzers

Sunless tanners, sometimes referred to as self-tanners or tanning extenders, are promoted as a way to get tan without the sun. They produce a tanned appearance by interacting with amino acids on the skin's surface. The only color additive currently approved by FDA for this purpose is dihydroxyacetone (DHA). These products can be difficult to apply and the chemicals may react differently on various areas of your body, resulting in uneven coloring.

The term "bronzer" refers to a variety of products used to achieve a temporary tanned appearance. Some are applied topically to stain the skin temporarily. Usually, soap and water will remove them. They may streak after application and, when wet, some may stain clothing.

Among other products marketed as bronzers are tinted moisturizers and brush-on powders. These also produce a temporary effect, similar to other types of makeup. Still others are combination products that also contain DHA.

Sunless tanners and bronzers may or may not contain sunscreen ingredients or be labeled with SPF numbers. Consumers are advised to read the labeling carefully to determine whether or not these products provide protection from the sun.

Section 10.3

Artificial Tanning Booths and Cancer

From "NCI Health Information Tip Sheet for Writers: Artificial Tanning Booths and Cancer," National Cancer Institute, August 2004.

What is the problem?

Long-term exposure to artificial sources of ultraviolet rays like tanning beds (or to the sun's natural rays) increases both men and women's risk of developing skin cancer. In addition, exposure to tanning salon rays increases damage caused by sunlight because ultraviolet light actually thins the skin, making it less able to heal. Women who use tanning beds more than once a month are 55 percent more likely to develop malignant melanoma, the most deadly form of skin cancer.

According to the National Cancer Institute, more than one million people are diagnosed with non-melanoma skin cancer in the United States every year. In fact, non-melanoma skin cancer is the most common type of cancer in the country. 40 to 50 percent of Americans who live to age 65 will have this form of skin cancer at least once. These are startling statistics for a cancer that can, for the most part, be prevented.

Who is at risk?

Almost everyone who frequently uses a tanning salon or exposes themselves to the sun is putting themselves at risk for skin cancer. The risk is greatest for people with fair skin; blonde, red, or light hair; and blue, green, or gray eyes. Artificial tanning can also be more dangerous for those who burn easily, have already been treated for skin cancer, or have a family member who has had skin cancer. In addition, women have a higher risk of contracting skin cancer on their legs, and men have a higher risk of getting it on their backs.

Can it be prevented?

There are various things than one can do to prevent their exposure to artificial sources of ultraviolet rays:

- Avoid tanning beds and booths.

- Instead of going to a tanning salon, try tanning sprays. In fact, some salons now provide only tanning spray services.

- Regardless of your exposure to natural or artificial UV rays, conduct a monthly skin self-exam looking for any abnormalities (like bumps or sores that don't heal) or moles that have changed size, color or shape. Be sure to check all areas. Have a friend or family member check your back.

- Visit your physician or a dermatologist to get annual exams. If caught early skin cancer is now almost 100 percent curable.

What's the bottom line?

Long-term exposure to artificial (or natural) sources of ultraviolet rays increases one's risk of developing skin cancer. However there are alternatives one can take to minimize the risk associated with artificial rays such as using sunless tanning lotions or sprays in concert with regular skin checks by your physician or dermatologist.

Chapter 11

Questions and Answers about Radon and Cancer Risk

What is radon?

Radon is a radioactive gas released from the normal decay of uranium in rocks and soil. It is an invisible, odorless, tasteless gas that seeps up through the ground and diffuses into the air. In a few areas, depending on local geology, radon dissolves into ground water and can be released into the air when the water is used. Radon gas usually exists at very low levels outdoors. However, in areas without adequate ventilation, such as underground mines, radon can accumulate to levels that substantially increase the risk of lung cancer.

How is the general population exposed to radon?

Radon is present in nearly all air. Everyone breathes radon in every day, usually at very low levels. However, people who inhale high levels of radon are at an increased risk for developing lung cancer.

Radon can enter homes through cracks in floors, walls, or foundations, and collect indoors. It can also be released from building materials, or from water obtained from wells that contain radon. Radon levels can be higher in homes that are well insulated, tightly sealed, or built on uranium-rich soil. Because of their closeness to the ground, basement and first floors typically have the highest radon levels.

"Radon and Cancer: Questions and Answers," National Cancer Institute, July 2004.

How does radon cause cancer?

Radon decays quickly, giving off tiny radioactive particles. When inhaled, these radioactive particles can damage the cells that line the lung. Long-term exposure to radon can lead to lung cancer, the only cancer proven to be associated with inhaling radon.

How many people develop lung cancer because of exposure to radon?

Cigarette smoking is the most common cause of lung cancer. Radon represents a far smaller risk for this disease, but it is the second leading cause of lung cancer in the United States. Scientists estimate that approximately 15,000 to 22,000 lung cancer deaths per year are related to radon.

Although the association between radon exposure and smoking is not well understood, exposure to the combination of radon gas and cigarette smoke creates a greater risk for lung cancer than either factor alone. The majority of radon-related cancer deaths occur among smokers.

How did scientists discover that radon plays a role in the development of lung cancer?

Radon was identified as a health problem when scientists noted that underground uranium miners who were exposed to it died of lung cancer at high rates. Results of miner studies have been confirmed by experimental animal studies, which show higher rates of lung tumors among rodents exposed to high radon levels.

What have scientists learned about the relationship between radon and lung cancer?

Scientists agree that radon causes lung cancer in humans. Recent research has focused on specifying the effect of residential radon on lung cancer risk. In these studies, scientists measure radon levels in the homes of people who have lung cancer and compare them to the levels of radon in the homes of people who have not developed lung cancer.

One of these studies, funded by the National Institute of Environmental Health Sciences, examined residential radon exposure in Iowa among females who had lived in their current home for at least 20 years. This study included 413 females with lung cancer and 614 females without lung cancer. During the study, radon levels were tested in homes, lung cancer tissues were examined, and the scientists collected information about home characteristics and other topics. Results from this study suggested a link between exposure to radon and lung cancer.

Scientists have conducted more studies like this in other regions of the United States and around the world. Many of these studies have demonstrated an association between residential exposure to radon and lung cancer, but this finding has not been observed in all studies. The inconsistencies between studies are due in part to the small size of some studies, the varying levels of radon in many homes, and the difficulty of measuring a person's exposure to radon over time.

Researchers have combined and analyzed data from all radon studies conducted in Canada and the United States. By combining the data from these studies, scientists were able to analyze data from thousands of people. The results of this analysis demonstrated a slightly increased risk of lung cancer associated with exposure to household radon. This increased risk was consistent with the level of risk estimated based on studies of underground miners.

Researchers are also investigating more precise ways to measure a person's exposure to radon over time. In a study published in 2002, scientists examined radon exposure among people in Sweden who had not smoked daily for more than a year. This study included 110 people with lung cancer and 231 people without lung cancer. As with previous studies, the scientists measured radon levels of indoor air. The researchers also used a new technique of analyzing glass to estimate radon exposure over time. Using this technique, the scientists took measurements from glass in an object (e.g., a mirror or picture frame) that was at least 15 years old and had been in the person's home throughout that time, even if the person had moved from one home to another. In this study, both of the techniques for measuring radon demonstrated a relationship between long-term exposure to radon and lung cancer, and supported the results of previous studies.

How can people know if they have an elevated level of radon in their homes?

Testing is the only way to know if a person's home has elevated radon levels. Indoor radon levels are affected by the soil composition under and around the house, and the ease with which radon enters the house. Homes that are next door to each other can have different indoor radon levels, making a neighbor's test result a poor predictor of radon risk. In addition, precipitation, barometric pressure, and other influences can cause radon levels to vary from month to month or day to day, which is why both short-term and long-term tests are available.

Short-term detectors measure radon levels for 2 days to 90 days, depending on the device. Long-term tests determine the average concentration for more than 90 days. Because radon levels can vary from day to day and month to month, a long-term test is a better indicator of average radon level. Both tests are relatively easy to use and inexpensive. A state or local radon official can explain the differences between testing devices and recommend the most appropriate test for a person's needs and conditions.

The U.S. Environmental Protection Agency (EPA) recommends taking action to reduce radon in homes that have a radon level at or above 4 picocuries per liter (pCi/L). About 1 in 15 U.S. homes is estimated to have radon levels at or above this EPA action level. Scientists estimate that lung cancer deaths could be reduced by two to four percent, or about 5,000 deaths, by lowering radon levels in homes exceeding the EPA's action level.

The cost of a radon reduction depends on the size and design of a home and the radon reduction methods that are needed. These costs typically range from $800 to $2,500, with an average cost of $1,200.

Where can people find more information about radon?

The following organizations can provide additional resources that readers may find helpful:

- The EPA website contains news, information, and publications on radon. It is located at http://www.epa.gov/iaq/radon on the internet.

- The National Safety Council (NSC), in partnership with the EPA, operates a Radon Hotline.

  - To reach an automated system for ordering materials and listen to informational recordings, call 800-SOS-RADON (800-767-7236).

  - To contact an information specialist, dial 800-55-RADON (800-557-2366) or send an e-mail to airqual@nsc.org.

  - More information about radon and its testing can be found on the NSC's website at http://www.nsc.org/ehc/radon.htm on the internet.

- The Indoor Air Quality Information Clearinghouse (IAQ INFO) is operated by the EPA. To order publications or contact an information specialist, call 800-438-4318. Alternatively, IAQ INFO can be reached by e-mail at iaqinfo@aol.com, by fax at 703-356-5386, or by mail at Post Office Box 37133, Washington, DC 20013-7133.

- The National Hispanic Indoor Air Quality Helpline is a service of the National Alliance for Hispanic Health, in partnership with the EPA. The Helpline provides bilingual (Spanish/English) information about indoor air pollutants. To speak with an information specialist, call 800-SALUD-12 (800-725-8312).

Selected References

1. Darby S, Hill D, Doll R. Radon: A likely carcinogen at all exposures. *Annals of Oncology* 2001; 12(10):1341–1351.

2. Field RW. A review of residential radon case-control epidemiologic studies performed in the United States. *Reviews on Environmental Health* 2001; 16(3):151–167.

3. Field RW, Steck DJ, Smith BJ, et al. Residential radon gas exposure and lung cancer: The Iowa Radon Lung Cancer Study. *American Journal of Epidemiology* 2000; 151(11):1091–1102.

4. Frumkin H, Samet JM. Radon. CA: *A Cancer Journal for Clinicians* 2001; 51(6):337–344.

5. Lagarde F, Falk R, Almren K, et al. Glass-based radon-exposure assessment and lung cancer risk. *Journal of Exposure Analysis and Environmental Epidemiology* 2002; 12(5):344–354.

6. National Research Council. Committee on Health Risks of Exposure to Radon: BEIR VI. *Health Effects of Exposure to Radon.* Washington, DC: National Academy Press, 1999.

7. U.S. Environmental Protection Agency (May 2002). A Citizen's Guide to Radon: The Guide to Protecting Yourself and Your Family From Radon (4th ed.). Retrieved July 13, 2004, from: http://www.epa.gov/iaq/radon/pubs/citguide.html.

Chapter 12

Radiation and Cancer Risk

Chapter Contents

Section 12.1

Radiation and Health

Radiation and radioactive materials are part of our environment. The radiation in the environment comes from both cosmic radiation that originates in outer space and from radioactive materials that occur naturally in the earth and in our own bodies. Together, these are known as background radiation. Everyone is exposed to background radiation daily. In addition, radiation and radioactive materials are produced by many human activities. Radiation is produced by x-ray equipment and by particle accelerators used in research and medicine. Radioactive materials are also produced in nuclear reactors.

Today, radiation is a common and valuable tool in medicine, research, and industry. It is used in medicine to diagnose illnesses, and in high doses, to treat diseases such as cancer. Also, high doses of radiation are used to kill harmful bacteria in food and to extend the shelf life of fresh produce. Radiation produces heat that is used to generate electricity in nuclear power reactors. Radioactive materials are used in a number of consumer products, such as smoke detectors and exit signs, and many other research and industrial purposes.

What is radiation?

Radiation is energy that moves through space or matter at a very high speed. This energy can be in the form of particles, such as alpha or beta particles, which are emitted from radioactive materials, or waves such as light, heat, radiowaves, microwaves, x-rays, and gamma rays. Radioactive materials, also known as radionuclides or radioisotopes, are atoms that are unstable. In nature, there is a tendency for unstable atoms to change into a stable form. As they change form, they release radiation.

Radiation that can produce ions when it interacts with matter is called ionizing radiation. Ions are the charged particles that are produced when electrons are removed from their positions in the atoms.

Alpha particles, beta particles, x-rays, and gamma rays are forms of ionizing radiation. On the other hand, radiation that is not capable of producing ions in matter is known as nonionizing radiation. Radiowaves, microwaves, heat waves, visible light, and ultraviolet radiation are forms of non-ionizing radiation. This chapter focuses on the health effects of ionizing radiation.

How does ionizing radiation affect health?

Ionizing radiation affects health when it causes changes in the cells of the human body. It does this by breaking the chemical bonds that hold together groups of atoms called molecules. For example, DNA molecules, which contain a person's genetic information, control the chemical and physical functions of human cells. If damaged, the DNA molecules are able to repair the damage in most cases; but in some instances, damage to DNA molecules will affect the ability of the cells to do their work and to pass information to new cells.

How is the radiation dose measured?

As radiation moves through matter, some of its energy is absorbed into the material. The amount of radiation energy deposited per unit of mass of matter is known as the absorbed dose. The unit of measurement for an absorbed dose of radiation is the rad. When radiation is absorbed by living tissue, the type of radiation, in addition to the absorbed dose, is important in determining the degree of damage that may occur. Alpha radiation, which is heavier and carries more electric charge, causes more damage than beta or gamma radiation. To account for this difference and to give the dose from all types of radiation a common measure, a quantity known as dose equivalent is used. The dose equivalent is found by multiplying the absorbed dose (in rads) by a "quality factor" for the specific type of radiation. The unit for this measurement is called the rem. In many cases, the amount of radiation dose equivalent is much less than one rem. So, a smaller unit, the millirem, is used (1 rem = 1,000 millirem).

What is the dose equivalent in the U.S. from all radiation sources?

In the United States, the annual absorbed dose includes exposure to background radiation, indoor radon, and different radiation sources (for example, industrial and medical). The annual dose to individuals varies by where they live and whether they had medical x-ray or nuclear medicine procedures in the past year. On the average, the dose equivalent in the United States from all sources is about 360 millirem per year.

People are exposed to various levels of radon gas which occurs naturally in the air that we breathe. Radon in indoor air results in a dose equivalent of about 200 millirem annually, on the average, but can be much higher or lower depending on the radon level in a person's home. Besides radon, the average dose equivalent from background radiation to residents of the United States is about 100 millirem per year. About 40 percent of this dose comes from radioactive materials that occur naturally in our bodies. The rest comes from outer space, cosmic radiation, or from radioactive materials in the ground.

Another common source of radiation dose is medical x-rays. The dose equivalent from this source varies with the type of examination one receives. For example, a chest x-ray results in a dose equivalent of about 10 millirem; a mammogram about 200-300 millirem; an abdominal examination about 400 millirem); and a CT examination (computed tomography, also called "CAT scan"), between 2,000 and 10,000 millirem. When radiation therapy is used to treat cancer, a very large dose of radiation, about 5,000,000 millirem (or 5,000 rem) is delivered to the tumor site.

Fallout from nuclear weapons tests is another source of radiation exposure. The exposure from this source has decreased with time since atmospheric testing was stopped in the United States in 1962. Now it contributes less than 1 millirem per year.

What health effects can be caused by radiation?

A great deal is known about health effects caused by large doses of radiation received in a short period of time. At high radiation doses, a human cell can be damaged so severely that it will die. At lower doses, the cell can repair the damage and survive. If the repair is faulty, however, the cell could give incorrect information to the new cells it produces.

Exposure to radiation may lead to different health effects. The type and probability of the effects produced generally depend on the radiation dose received. This could result in health problems for the exposed individuals or in genetic defects that may show up in their descendants.

Background radiation is an example of a low dose of radiation and of a low dose rate. A low dose rate occurs when exposure to radiation is spread over a long period of time. Exposure to radiation delivered at low dose rates is generally less dangerous than when the same dose is given all at once because the cell has more time to repair damage to the DNA molecule.

Generally speaking, there are two types of health effects from radiation—threshold and non-threshold effects.

Threshold effects: High doses of radiation received in a short period of time result in effects that are noticeable soon after exposure. These are known as threshold effects. A certain dose range must be exceeded before they can occur. These effects include radiation sickness and death, cataracts, sterility, loss of hair, reduced thyroid function, and skin radiation burns. The severity of these effects increases with the size of the dose.

- **Radiation Sickness:** At doses of about 60 rem, 5% of exposed individuals may vomit. This increases to about 50% at 200 rem. At doses between 300 and 400 rem and without medical treatment, there is a 50% chance that a person will die within 60 days. With proper medical care, however, some people exposed to 1,000 rem could survive.

- **Cataracts:** A single exposure between 200 and 500 rem could cause cataracts (clouding of the lens of the eye). If an exposure took place over a period of months, however, it would take about a total of 1,000 rem to produce a cataract.

- **Sterility:** In men, a single dose of 15 rem can cause temporary sterility, and a single dose between 400 and 500 rem can cause permanent sterility. In women, a total dose of 400 rem received over two or three exposures has been known to cause permanent sterility.

- **Fetal effects:** A number of threshold effects can result from high doses, depending on the stage of development of the fetus. Fetal death is most likely in the first two weeks after conception. During this period, a dose of 10 rem may increase the risk of a fetal death by about 0.1 to 1 percent. Cataracts, malformations, and mental and growth retardation can occur as a result of high radiation doses received three to seven weeks after conception. These effects were not observed at doses of 10 rem or less. Exposures eight to 15 weeks after conception may lead to mental retardation if the total dose is more than 20 rem. Also, a study of atomic bomb survivors in Japan showed that exposure between

115

eight and 15 weeks after conception resulted in lower IQ scores in the exposed children. It is estimated that an absorbed dose of 100 rads lowers the IQ score by about 30 points.

Non-threshold effects: There are other health effects of radiation that generally do not appear until years after an exposure. It is assumed that there are no threshold doses for these effects and that any radiation exposure can increase a person's chances of having these effects. These are called non-threshold effects. While the chances of these delayed effects occurring increase with the size of the dose, the severity does not. They can occur in the person who receives the radiation dose or in that person's offspring. In the latter case, they are known as genetic effects.

- **Genetic effects:** No increase of genetic effects from radiation exposure have been found in humans. However, there have been a number of animal studies that have shown that exposure to fairly high doses of radiation increases the chances of genetic effects in the offspring of the exposed animals. They also indicate that radiation does not cause any unique effects. Rather, it increases the number of genetic effects that are normally seen in unexposed animals. Even though genetic effects have not been found to increase in exposed human populations, it is safer to assume that there is an increased chance of these effects, even at low radiation doses.

- **Fetal effects:** The embryo/fetus is particularly sensitive to radiation. Some studies have shown increases in the rates of childhood cancer in children exposed to radiation before birth.

- **Cancer:** Cancer is the most common non-threshold effect of high radiation doses in humans. The cancers caused by radiation are no different from cancers due to other causes.

What is the source of information on radiation-induced cancer?

Estimates of cancer risk for specific doses of radiation are based on many studies of groups of people who were exposed to high doses of radiation. These include the survivors of the atomic bombings in Japan, people who were exposed to radiation for medical reasons, and workers who were exposed to high doses of radiation on the job.

The survivors of the World War II atomic bomb explosions in Hiroshima and Nagasaki were exposed to an average radiation dose equivalent of 24 rem, and their health has been carefully studied since 1950. This study is the most important source of information on the risk of cancer from radiation exposure because it involves a large number of individuals who received whole body radiation exposure. It provides information on the risk of increased cancer to all organs and on the variation of risk with age at the time of exposure.

Are all tissues and organs equally sensitive to radiation?

Radiation has been found to induce cancer in most body tissues and organs. Different tissues and organs, however, show varying degrees of sensitivity. The tissues and organs showing high sensitivity include bone marrow (leukemia), breasts, thyroid glands and lungs. In contrast, there is no clear evidence that radiation causes cancer of the cervix or prostate. The following list ranks human tissues and organs by their sensitivity to radiation induced cancer:

- **High:** bone marrow, breast (premenopausal), thyroid (child), lung
- **Moderate:** stomach, ovary, colon, bladder, skin
- **Low:** brain, bone, uterus, kidney, esophagus, liver

Are all people at equal risk?

Some people are more sensitive to harmful effects of radiation than others. There are a number of factors that influence an individual's sensitivity to radiation. These factors include age, gender, other exposures, and genetic factors.

Age: In general, exposed children are more at risk than adults. Breast cancer risk among women exposed to radiation is greatest among women who were exposed before age 20, and least when exposure occurred after menopause. Also, exposed children are at greater risk of radiation-induced thyroid cancer than adults.

Gender: In women, the risk of breast and ovarian cancers from radiation is high, but there is no clear evidence that radiation causes breast or prostate cancers in men. Females are also seen to have more radiation induced thyroid cancer than males.

Other exposures: Underground miners exposed to high levels of radon have increased risk of lung cancer, and those who smoke have an even greater risk. Exposure to ultraviolet radiation from the sun following the use of x-rays to treat scalp ringworm conditions increases the risk of developing skin cancer in the area of the skin exposed to both types of radiation.

Genetic factors: Individuals with certain pre-existing genetic diseases have increased sensitivity to radiation, especially if they receive radiation therapy. For example, children genetically predisposed to cancer of the retina (retinoblastoma) and who are treated with radiation are at increased risk of developing bone cancer following treatment. Patients with ataxia telangiectasia (AT), a rare genetic disorder, are unusually sensitive to tissue damage from radiation therapy, but there is no clear evidence that they are at increased risk of radiation induced cancer.

What is the risk of death from cancers caused by radiation exposure?

In the 1990 report *Health Effects of Exposures to Low Levels of Ionizing Radiation - BEIR V*, The National Research Council estimated that the excess lifetime risk of fatal cancer following a single exposure to 10 rem would be 0.8 percent. This means that if 1,000 people were exposed to 10 rem each, 8 would be expected to die of cancer induced by the radiation. These deaths are in addition to about 220 cancer deaths that result from other causes. If the 10 rem were received over a period of weeks or months, the extra lifetime risk could be reduced to 0.5 percent. These risk factors are average values for a population similar to that of the United States.

These percentages are not precise predictions of risk, especially at low radiation doses and dose rates. At doses comparable to natural background radiation (0.1 rem per year), the risk could be higher than these estimates, but it could also be lower or even non-existent.

Is there a cancer risk from any radiation exposure?

The risk of increased cancer incidence is well established for doses above 10 rem. For low doses, it has not been possible to scientifically determine if an increased risk exists, but many scientists believe that small doses of radiation do lead to increased cancer risk and that the degree of risk is directly proportional to the size of the dose. Risk estimates from low doses are obtained by extrapolation from high dose observations.

How is the public protected from radiation risks?

Because of the potential for harm from exposure to radiation, radiation protection programs are designed to protect both workers and the general public, their descendants, and the environment, while still allowing society to benefit from the many valuable uses of radiation. Current radiation protection systems are based on the following principles:

• The benefit must outweigh the risk. Radiation exposure must produce a net positive benefit.

• The amount of exposure must be limited. Radiation doses to individuals cannot exceed limits set by state and federal agencies.

• All radiation exposures and releases to the environment must be kept as low as reasonably achievable, below regulatory limits.

What can an individual do to reduce radiation exposure?

Exposure to indoor radon contributes a large portion of the total average dose. Exposure can be reduced by testing the home for radon and implementing measures to reduce radon levels, if necessary.

Also, a person should receive only x-ray examinations that his or her health care provider thinks are truly necessary for an accurate diagnosis. Alternative, non-x-ray tests should be used instead, if available. However, one should not refuse an x-ray examination that a doctor feels is necessary.

Are there new areas of research that will add to our knowledge of radiation risks?

Recent advances in molecular genetics and microbiology have increased our understanding of cancer development. It is hoped that further research will provide additional information on the risk of radiation-induced cancer and genetic effects, especially at low doses.

Section 12.2

Low Levels of Ionizing Radiation May Cause Harm

From "Low Levels of Ionizing Radiation May Cause Harm," June 25, 2005. © 2005 National Academy of Sciences. Reprinted with permission.

A preponderance of scientific evidence shows that even low doses of ionizing radiation, such as gamma rays and x-rays, are likely to pose some risk of adverse health effects, says a new report from the National Academies' National Research Council.

The report's focus is low-dose, low-LET (linear energy transfer) ionizing radiation that is energetic enough to break biomolecular bonds. In living organisms, such radiation can cause DNA damage that eventually leads to cancers. However, more research is needed to determine whether low doses of radiation may also cause other health problems, such as heart disease and stroke, which are now seen with high doses of low-LET radiation.

The study committee defined low doses as those ranging from nearly zero to about 100 millisievert (mSv)—units that measure radiation energy deposited in living tissue. The radiation dose from a chest x-ray is about 0.1 mSv. In the United States, people are exposed on average to about 3 mSv of natural "background" radiation annually.

The committee's report develops the most up-to-date and comprehensive risk estimates for cancer and other health effects from exposure to low-level ionizing radiation. In general, the report supports previously reported risk estimates for solid cancer and leukemia, but the availability of new and more extensive data have strengthened confidence in these estimates.

Specifically, the committee's thorough review of available biological and biophysical data supports a "linear, no-threshold" (LNT) risk model, which says that the smallest dose of low-level ionizing radiation has the potential to cause an increase in health risks to humans. In the past, some researchers have argued that the LNT model exaggerates adverse health effects, while others have said that it underestimates the harm.

The preponderance of evidence supports the LNT model, this new report says.

"The scientific research base shows that there is no threshold of exposure below which low levels of ionizing radiation can be demonstrated to be harmless or beneficial," said committee chair Richard R. Monson, associate dean for professional education and professor of epidemiology, Harvard School of Public Health, Boston. "The health risks—particularly the development of solid cancers in organs—rise proportionally with exposure. At low doses of radiation, the risk of inducing solid cancers is very small. As the overall lifetime exposure increases, so does the risk." The report is the seventh in a series on the biological effects of ionizing radiation.

Assessing Health Risks

The committee's risk models for exposure to low-level ionizing radiation were based on a sex and age distribution similar to that of the entire U.S. population, and refer to the risk that an individual would face over his or her life span. These models predict that about one out of 100 people would likely develop solid cancer or leukemia from an exposure of 0.1 sievert (Sv; 100 mSv). About 42 additional people in the same group would be expected to develop solid cancer or leukemia from other causes. Roughly half of these cancers would result in death. These particular estimates are uncertain, however, because of limitations in the data used to develop risk models.

Survivors of atomic bombings in Hiroshima and Nagasaki, Japan, were the primary sources of data for estimating risks of most solid cancers and leukemia from exposure to ionizing radiation. The committee's review included an examination of updated cancer-incidence data from tumor registries of the survivors, and of research data on solid cancer deaths—which is now more abundant because the number of deaths available for analysis has nearly doubled since the Research Council published its previous report on this topic in 1990. The committee combined this information with data on people who had been medically exposed to radiation to estimate risks of breast cancer in women and thyroid cancer. Data from additional medical studies and from studies of people exposed to radiation through their occupations also were evaluated and found to be compatible with the committee's statistical models. Follow-up studies should continue for the indefinite future, the report says.

Adverse hereditary health effects that could be attributed to radiation have not been found in studies of children whose parents were exposed to radiation from the atomic bombs. However, studies of mice and other organisms have produced extensive data showing that radiation-induced cell mutations in sperm and eggs can be passed on to offspring, the report says. There is no reason to believe that such mutations could not also be passed on to human offspring. The failure to observe such effects in Hiroshima and Nagasaki probably reflects an insufficiently large survivor population.

Follow-up studies of people who receive computed tomography (CT) scans, especially children, should be conducted, the report adds. Also needed are studies of infants who are exposed to diagnostic radiation because catheters have been placed in their hearts, as well as infants who receive multiple x-rays to monitor pulmonary development. CT scans, often referred to as whole body scans, result in higher doses of radiation than typically experienced with conventional x-rays.

Sources of Ionizing Radiation

People are exposed to natural background ionizing radiation from the universe, the ground, and basic activities such as eating, drinking, and breathing. These sources account for about 82 percent of human exposure.

Nationwide, man-made radiation comprises 18 percent of human exposure. In this overall category, medical x-rays and nuclear medicine account for about 79 percent, the report says. Elements in consumer products—such as tobacco, tap water, and building materials—account for another 16 percent. Occupational exposure, fallout, and the use of nuclear fuel constitute roughly 5 percent of the man-made component nationwide.

Factors that could increase exposure include greater use of radiation for medical purposes, working around radioactive materials, and smoking tobacco. Living at low altitudes, where there is less cosmic radiation, and living and working on the upper floors of buildings, where there is less radon gas—a primary source of natural ionizing radiation—are factors that could decrease exposure.

The report was sponsored by the U.S. departments of Defense, Energy, and Homeland Security, the U.S. Nuclear Regulatory Commission, and the U.S. Environmental Protection Agency. The National Research Council is the principal operating arm of the National Academy of Sciences and the National Academy of Engineering. It is a private, nonprofit institution that provides science and technology advice under a congressional charter.

Copies of *Health Risks from Exposure to Low Levels of Ionizing Radiation (BEIR VII - Phase 2)* are available from the National Academies Press (202-334-3313 or 800-624-6242) or on the internet at http://www.nap.edu.

Section 12.3

X-Rays and Cancer Risk

"Cancer Radiation Risk Estimated," by Helen R. Pilcher, published online January 30, 2004. Reprinted with permission from News@Nature.com. © 2004 Nature Publishing Group. All rights reserved.

A British study has quantified the cancer risk from diagnostic x-rays. Radiation from medical and dental scans is thought to cause about 700 cases of cancer per year in Britain and more than 5,600 cases in the United States.[1]

The benefits of using x-rays still far outweigh the potential increase in cancer risk, says Amy Berrington de González from Oxford University, UK, who coordinated the study. But it's important to know what that risk is, she says, so doctors can weigh up the pros and cons of using the technique.

X-rays and their computerized cousin, CT scans, are routinely used to diagnose cancer and examine bone breaks. But the radiation can penetrate through cells and damage DNA. In some people, this can trigger cancer.

To minimize the risks, doctors use low doses. A chest x-ray, for example, delivers just three days' worth of low, background radiation. But x-rays are commonplace in hospitals and huge numbers of people receive them—there are 500 x-rays for every 1,000 people every year in Britain.

Attempts to quantify the risk of x-rays have been made before. The most recent previous estimate, made in 1981, found that x-rays probably accounted for 0.5% of cancer cases in the United States.

The new study, using more data from 15 different countries, is a much-needed update on those risk estimates, says Berrington de González, particularly because many more x-rays are done today than

20 years ago. The study estimates that diagnostic x-rays account for 0.9% of cancer cases in the United States, although the authors caution that their methodology is very different from that used previously, making it hard to compare the results.

Working Backwards

To make their calculations, Berrington de González and colleague Sarah Darby assessed the relationship between high levels of radiation exposure and cancer. This included information on survivors of the Hiroshima bomb, who were exposed to radiation levels far greater than the normal x-ray exposure. The duo then worked backwards to work out the risks from lower doses.

Scaling down from large exposures to small ones is a difficult and controversial calculation, however. So the pair also used a complex computer model to try and weed out the effects of lower doses of radiation.

They found that about 0.6% of cancer cases in Britain are currently caused by x-rays. Poland, Sweden, Kuwait, and the Netherlands have similar rates. The highest rate—3%—was found in Japan, where x-ray use is more common.

X-rays are not the only diagnostic tool available to doctors, says Paul Dubbins, dean of the UK-based Royal College of Radiologists. Ultrasound can be used to image a baby in the womb, for example. But ultrasound doesn't travel well through air, so is rarely used for lung examinations. Magnetic resonance imaging (MRI) can be used to study brain activity, but is not very good at imaging bones. "We don't use x-rays unless they're absolutely necessary," says Dubbins.

It's not possible to predict who will develop cancer as a result of x-ray exposure, or what type of cancer they will get, says Berrington de González. Radiation can trigger many different types of the disease. On the other hand, not all cancers are caused by radiation—diet and genetics, for example, also play a role.

Reference

1.   Berrington de González, A. and Darby, S. Risk of cancer from diagnostic X-rays: estimates for the UK and 14 other countries. *The Lancet*, 363, 345–351 (2003).

Section 12.4

Pediatric Computed Tomography: Special Concerns about Cancer-Related Risks

From "Radiation Risks and Pediatric Computed Tomography (CT): A Guide for Health Care Providers," National Cancer Institute (NCI), August 20, 2002. The complete text of this document, including references, is available online through the NCI website at http://www.cancer.gov.

The use of pediatric computed tomography (CT), a valuable imaging tool, has been increasing rapidly. Because of the growing use of CT and the potential for increased radiation exposure to children undergoing these scans, pediatric CT has become a public health concern. This section discusses the value of CT and the importance of minimizing the radiation dose, especially in children.

CT as a Diagnostic Tool

CT is an extremely valuable tool for diagnosing illness and injury in children. For an individual child, the risks of CT are small and the individual risk-benefit balance almost always favors the benefit. Approximately 2–3 million CT examinations are performed annually on children in the U.S. The use of CT in adults and children has increased about 7-fold in the past 10 years. Much of this increase is due to increased availability, technical improvements, and utility for common diseases. The newest technology, multidetector (or multislice) CT, provides even greater imaging opportunities in both adults and children. Despite the many benefits of CT, a disadvantage is the inevitable radiation exposure. Although CT scans comprise about 10% of diagnostic radiological procedures in large U.S. hospitals, it is estimated that CT scans contribute approximately 65% of the effective radiation dose from all medical x-ray examinations to the population.

Unique Considerations for Radiation Exposure in Children

Radiation exposure is a concern in both adults and children. However, there are two unique considerations in children:

- Children are considerably more sensitive to radiation than adults, as demonstrated in epidemiologic studies of exposed populations.

- Children also have a longer life expectancy, resulting in a larger window of opportunity for expressing radiation damage.

As an example, compared with a 40-year old, the same radiation dose given to a neonate is several times more likely to produce a cancer over the child's lifetime.

Moreover, the same exposure parameters used for a child and an adult will result in larger doses to the child. There is no need for these larger doses to children, and CT settings can be reduced significantly while maintaining diagnostic image quality. Therefore, children should not be scanned using adult CT exposure parameters. Currently, adjustments are not frequently made in the exposure parameters that determine the amount of radiation children receive from CT, resulting in a greater radiation dose than necessary.

Radiation Risks from CT in Children: A Public Health Issue

Major national and international organizations responsible for evaluating radiation risks agree there probably is no low-dose radiation "threshold" for inducing cancers (that is, no amount of radiation should be considered absolutely safe). Recent data from the atomic bomb survivors and medically irradiated populations demonstrate small, but significant, increases in cancer risk even at the low levels of radiation that are relevant to pediatric CT scans. Doses from a single pediatric CT scan can range from about 5 mSv to 60 mSv. Among children who have undergone CT scans, approximately one-third have had at least three scans. Multiple scans present a particular concern. For example, three scans would be expected to triple the cancer risk of a single scan.

Although the benefits of properly performed CT examinations almost always outweigh the risks for an individual child, unnecessary exposure is associated with unnecessary risk. Minimizing radiation exposure from pediatric CT, whenever possible, will reduce the projected number of CT-related cancer deaths.

Immediate Measures to Minimize CT Radiation Exposure in Children

Physicians, other pediatric health care providers, CT technologists, CT manufacturers, and various medical and governmental organizations share the responsibility to minimize CT radiation doses to children. Several immediate steps can be taken to reduce the amount of radiation that children receive from CT examinations:

- Perform only necessary CT examinations. Communication between pediatric health care providers and radiologists can determine the need for CT and the technique to be used. Although there are standard indications for CT in children, radiologists should review reasons prior to every pediatric scan and be available for consultation when indications are uncertain. Consider other modalities such as ultrasound or magnetic resonance imaging, which do not use ionizing radiation.

- Adjust exposure parameters for pediatric CT based on child size, region scanned, organ systems scanned, and scan resolution.

- Minimize the CT examinations that use multiple scans obtained during different phases of contrast enhancement (multiphase examinations). These multiphase examinations are rarely necessary, especially in body (chest and abdomen) imaging, and result in a considerable increase in dose.

Issues to discuss with parents:

- Is CT the best examination to diagnose conditions in the child?

- Will the CT examination be adjusted based on the size of the child?

- Will a radiologist be responsible for performing and interpreting the child's CT exam?

Conclusion

While CT remains a crucial tool for pediatric diagnosis, it is important for the health care community to work together to minimize the radiation dose to children. Radiologists must continually think about reducing exposure as low as reasonably achievable (ALARA), by using exposure settings customized for children. All physicians who prescribe pediatric CT should continually assess its use on a case-by-case basis. Used prudently and optimally, CT is one of our most valuable imaging modalities for both children and adults.

Section 12.5

Radioactive Iodine-131 from Nuclear Fallout

From "Get the Facts about Exposure to I-131 Radiation,"
National Cancer Institute, September 2002.

During the Cold War in the 1950s and early 1960s, the U.S. government conducted about one hundred nuclear weapons (atomic bomb) tests in the atmosphere at a test site in Nevada. The radioactive substances released by these tests are known as "fallout." They were carried thousands of miles away from the test site by winds. As a result, people living in the United States at the time of the testing were exposed to varying levels of radiation.

Among the numerous radioactive substances released in fallout, there has been a great deal of concern about and study of one radioactive form of iodine—called iodine-131, or I-131. I-131 collects in the thyroid gland. People exposed to I-131, especially during childhood, may have an increased risk of thyroid disease, including thyroid cancer. Thyroid cancer is uncommon and is usually curable. Typically, it is a slow-growing cancer that is highly treatable. About 95 out of 100 people who are diagnosed with thyroid cancer survive the disease for at least five years after diagnosis.

The thyroid controls many body processes, including heart rate, blood pressure, and body temperature, as well as childhood growth and development. It is located in the front of the neck, just above the top of the breastbone and overlying the windpipe.

Although the potential of developing thyroid cancer from exposure to I-131 is small, it is important for Americans who grew up during the atomic bomb testing between 1951 and 1963 to be aware of risks.

How Americans Were Exposed to I-131

During the Cold War, the United States developed and tested nuclear weapons in an effort to deter and to be fully prepared for nuclear attacks from other nations. Most of the aboveground U.S. nuclear tests were conducted in Nevada from 1951 to 1963. As a result of these tests, potentially health-harming radioactive materials were released into the atmosphere and produced fallout.

I-131 was among the radioactive materials released by the atomic bomb tests. It was carried thousands of miles away from the test areas on the winds. Because of wind and rainfall patterns, the distribution of fallout varied widely after each test. Therefore, although all areas of the U.S. received fallout from at least one nuclear weapons test, certain areas of North America received more fallout than others.

Scientists estimate that the larger amounts of I-131 fell over some parts of Utah, Colorado, Idaho, Nevada, and Montana. But I-131 traveled to all states, particularly those in the Midwestern, Eastern, and Northeastern United States. Some of the I-131 collected on pastures and on grasses, where it was consumed by cows and goats. When consumed by cows or goats, I-131 collects in the animals' milk. Eating beef from cows exposed to I-131 carried little risk. Much of the health risk associated with I-131 occurred among milk-drinkers—usually children. From what is known about thyroid cancer and radiation, scientists think that people who were children during the period of atomic bomb testing are at higher risk for developing thyroid cancer.

In addition to nuclear testing in Nevada, Americans were exposed to I-131 through:

- Nuclear testing elsewhere in the world (mainly in the 1950s and 1960s)

- Nuclear power plant accidents (such as the Chernobyl accident in 1986)

- Releases from atomic weapons production plants (such as the Hanford facility in Washington state from 1944 to 1957)

Scientists are working to find out more about ways to measure and address potential I-131 exposure from other sources. Scientists are also working to find out more about other radioactive substances released by fallout and about their possible effects on human health.

The Search for Answers

Congress directed government health agencies to investigate the I-131 problem many years ago, and to make recommendations to Americans who might have related health risks. Gathering information turned out to be very complicated. Record-keeping was incomplete at the time of the bomb testing. Much of the information needed to calculate an individual's dose of I-131 and associated risk is either unreliable or unavailable.

Despite such challenges, government agencies organized expert scientific teams that have devoted many years to learning more about I-131. Reports were published in 1997 and 1999.

I-131's Rapid Breakdown

Like all radioactive substances, I-131 releases radiation as it breaks down. It is this radiation that can injure human tissues. But I-131's steady breakdown means that the amount of I-131 present in the environment after a bomb test steadily decreased. Therefore, farm animals that grazed in fields within a few days after a test would have consumed higher levels of I-131 than animals grazing later.

The Milk Connection

People younger than 15 at the time of aboveground testing (between 1951 and 1963) who drank milk, and who lived in the Mountain West, Midwestern, Eastern, and Northeastern United States, probably have a higher thyroid cancer risk from exposure to I-131 in fallout than other people. Their thyroid glands were still developing during the testing period. And they were more likely to have consumed milk contaminated with I-131. The amount of I-131 people absorbed depends on the following:

- Their age during the testing period (between 1951 and 1963)
- The amount and source of milk they drank in those years
- Where they lived during the testing period

Age and residence during the Cold War years are usually known. But few people can recall the exact amounts or sources of the milk they drank as children. While the amount of milk consumed is important in determining exposure to I-131, it is also important to know the source of the milk. Fresh milk from backyard or farm cows and goats usually contained more I-131 than store-bought milk. This is because processing and shipping milk allowed more time for the I-131 to break down.

About Thyroid Disease

There are two main types of thyroid diseases: noncancerous thyroid disease and thyroid cancer.

Noncancerous thyroid disease: Some thyroid diseases are caused by changes in the amount of thyroid hormones that enter the body from the thyroid gland. Doctors can screen for these with a simple blood test. Noncancerous thyroid disease also includes lumps, or nodules, in the thyroid gland that are benign and not cancerous.

Thyroid cancer: Thyroid cancer occurs when a lump, or nodule, in the thyroid gland is cancerous.

Thyroid and I-131

Exposure to I-131 may increase a person's risk of developing thyroid cancer. It is thought that risk is higher for people who have had multiple exposures and for people exposed at a younger age. Thyroid cancer accounts for less than 2 percent of all cancers diagnosed in the United States. Typically, it is a slow-growing cancer that is highly treatable and usually curable. About 95 out of 100 people who are diagnosed with thyroid cancer survive the disease for at least five years, and about 92 out of 100 people survive the disease for at least 20 years after diagnosis.

The cause of most cases of thyroid cancer is not known. Exposure to I-131 can increase the risk of thyroid cancer. But even among people who have documented exposures to I-131, few develop this cancer. It is known that children have a higher-than-average risk of developing thyroid cancer many years later if they were exposed to radiation. This knowledge comes from studies of people exposed to x-ray treatments for childhood cancer or noncancerous head and neck conditions, or as a result of direct radiation from the atomic bombings of Hiroshima and Nagasaki.

The thyroid gland in adults, however, appears to be more resistant to the effects of radiation. There appears to be little risk of developing thyroid cancer from exposure to I-131 or other radiation sources as an adult.

There is no single or specific symptom of thyroid cancer. Doctors screen for thyroid cancer by feeling the gland, to check for a lump or nodule. If a doctor feels a nodule, it does not mean cancer is present. Most thyroid nodules found during a medical exam are not cancer.

If thyroid cancer is found, it is treated by removing the thyroid gland. People who undergo surgery will need to take thyroid hormone replacement pills for the rest of their lives. Although this is inconvenient and expensive, cancer survival rates are excellent. In fact, the cause of death among people who once had thyroid cancer is rarely the result of the return or spread of the same cancer.

Living with a serious disease like thyroid cancer isn't easy. A cancer diagnosis can be devastating. Some people find they need help coping with the emotional and practical aspects of their disease. Doctors and other health professionals can help with concerns about treatment and managing side effects. Support groups can help also. The National Cancer Institute's Cancer Information Service can help put you in touch with support groups in your community. Call 800-4-CANCER for more information.

Chapter 13

Electromagnetic Energy: Questions about Possible Cancer Risks

Magnetic Field Exposure and Cancer: Questions and Answers

What are electric and magnetic fields?

Electricity is the movement of electrons, or current, through a wire. The type of electricity that runs through power lines and in houses is alternating current (AC). AC power produces two types of fields (areas of energy)—an electric field and a magnetic field. An electric field is produced by voltage, which is the pressure used to push the electrons through the wire, much like water being pushed through a pipe. As the voltage increases, the electric field increases in strength. A magnetic field results from the flow of current through wires or electrical devices and increases in strength as the current increases. These two fields together are referred to as electric and magnetic fields, or EMFs.

Both electric and magnetic fields are present around appliances and power lines. However, electric fields are easily shielded or weakened by walls and other objects, whereas magnetic fields can pass through buildings, humans, and most other materials. Since magnetic fields are most likely to penetrate the body, they are the component of EMFs that are usually studied in relation to cancer.

This chapter includes text from "Magnetic Field Exposure and Cancer: Questions and Answers," April 2005, and "Cellular Telephone Use and Cancer: Questions and Answers," September 2005. Both documents are publications of the National Cancer Institute.

Examples of devices that emit these fields includes power lines and electrical appliances, such as electric shavers, hair dryers, computers, televisions, electric blankets, and heated waterbeds. Most electrical appliances have to be turned on to produce a magnetic field. The strength of a magnetic field decreases rapidly with increased distance from the source.

Is there a link between magnetic field exposure at home and cancer in children?

Numerous epidemiological (population) studies and comprehensive reviews have evaluated magnetic field exposure and risk of cancer in children.[1, 2] Since the two most common cancers in children are leukemia and brain tumors, most of the research has focused on these two types. A study in 1979 pointed to a possible association between living near electric power lines and childhood leukemia.[3] Among more recent studies, findings have been mixed. Some have found an association; others have not. These studies are discussed in the following paragraphs. In 2002, researchers concluded that there is limited evidence that magnetic fields from power lines cause childhood leukemia, and that there is inadequate evidence that these magnetic fields cause other cancers in children.[2] Researchers have not found a consistent relationship between magnetic fields from power lines or appliances and childhood brain tumors.

In one large study by the National Cancer Institute (NCI) and the Children's Oncology Group, researchers measured magnetic fields directly in homes.[4] This study found that children living in homes with high magnetic field levels did not have an increased risk of childhood acute lymphoblastic leukemia. The one exception may have been children living in homes that had fields greater than 0.4 microtesla (µT), a very high level that occurs in few residences. Another study conducted by NCI researchers reported that children living close to overhead power lines based on distance measurements were not at greater risk of leukemia.[5]

To estimate more accurately the risks of leukemia in children from magnetic fields resulting from power lines, researchers pooled (combined) data from many studies. In one pooled study that combined nine well-conducted studies from several countries, including a study from the NCI, a twofold excess risk of childhood leukemia was associated with exposure to magnetic fields above 0.4 µT.[6] In another pooled study that combined 15 studies, a similar increased risk was seen above 0.3 µT.[7] It is difficult to determine if this level of risk represents a real increase or if it results from study bias. Such study bias can be related to the selection of study subjects or possibly to other factors that relate to levels of magnetic field exposure. If magnetic fields caused childhood leukemia, certain patterns would have been found such as increasing risk with increasing levels of magnetic field exposure.

Another way that people can be exposed to magnetic fields is from household electrical appliances. Several studies have investigated this relationship.[2] Although magnetic fields near many electrical appliances are higher than near power lines, appliances contribute less to a person's total exposure to magnetic fields. This is because most appliances are used only for short periods of time, and most are not used close to the body, whereas power lines are always emitting magnetic fields.

In a detailed evaluation, investigators from NCI and the Children's Oncology Group examined whether the use of household electrical appliances by the mother while pregnant and later by the child increased the risk of childhood leukemia. Although some appliances were associated with childhood leukemia, researchers did not find any consistent pattern of increasing risk with increasing years of use or how often the appliance was used.[8] A few other studies have reported mostly inconsistencies or no relation between appliances and risk of childhood cancer.

Occupational exposure of mothers to high levels of magnetic fields during pregnancy has been associated with childhood leukemia in a Canadian study.[9] Similar studies need to be done in other populations to see if this is indeed the case.

Is there a link between magnetic field exposure in the home and cancer in adults?

Although several studies have looked into the relationship of leukemia, brain tumors, and breast cancer in adults exposed to magnetic fields in the home, there are only a few large studies with long-term, magnetic field measurements. No consistent association between magnetic fields and leukemia or brain tumors has been established.

The majority of epidemiological studies have shown no relationship between breast cancer in women and magnetic fields from electrical appliances. Recent studies of breast cancer and magnetic fields in the home have included direct and indirect magnetic field measurements. These studies mostly found no association between breast cancer in females and magnetic fields from power lines or electric blankets.[10, 11, 12, 13] A Norwegian study found a risk for exposure to magnetic fields in the home,[14] and a study in African American women found that use of electric bedding devices may increase breast cancer risk.[15]

Is there a link between magnetic field exposure at work and cancer in adults?

Several studies conducted in the 1980s and early 1990s reported that people who worked in some electrical occupations (such as power station operators and phone line workers) had higher than expected rates of some types of cancer, particularly leukemia, brain tumors, and male breast cancer.[2] Some occupational studies showed very small increases in risk for leukemia and brain cancer, but these results were based on job titles and not actual measurements. More recently conducted studies that have included both job titles and individual exposure measurements have no consistent finding of an increasing risk of leukemia, brain tumors, or female breast cancer with increasing exposure to magnetic fields at work.[14, 16, 17, 18]

What have scientists learned from animal experiments about the relationship between magnetic field exposure and cancer?

Animal studies have not found that magnetic field exposure is associated with increased risk of cancer.[2] The absence of animal data supporting carcinogenicity makes it biologically less likely that magnetic field exposures in humans, at home or at work, are linked to increased cancer risk.

Where can people find additional information on EMFs?

The National Institute of Environmental Health Sciences (NIEHS) website has information about EMFs and cancer, as well as information and publications related to the EMF Research and Public Information Dissemination (RAPID) Program. NIEHS can be contacted at:

National Institute of Environmental Health Sciences
Post Office Box 12233
Research Triangle Park, NC 27709
Phone: 919-541-3345
TTY: 919-541-0731
E-mail: webcenter@niehs.nih.gov
Website: http://www.niehs.nih.gov

Selected References

1. Ahlbom A, Cardis E, Green A, Linet M, Savitz D, Swerdlow A. Review of the epidemiologic literature on EMF and health. *Environmental Health Perspectives* 2001; 109(6): 911–933.

2. World Health Organization, International Agency for Research on Cancer. Volume 80: *Non-ionizing radiation, Part 1, Static and extremely low-frequency (ELF) electric and magnetic fields*. IARC Working Group on the Evaluation of Carcinogenic Risks to Humans. 2002: Lyon, France.

3. Wertheimer N, Leeper E. Electrical wiring configurations and childhood cancer. *American Journal of Epidemiology* 1979; 109(3): 273–284.

4. Linet MS, Hatch EE, Kleinerman RA, et al. Residential exposure to magnetic fields and acute lymphoblastic leukemia in children. *The New England Journal of Medicine* 1997; 337(1): 1–7.

5. Kleinerman RA, Kaune WT, Hatch EE, et al. Are children living near high voltage power lines at increased risk of acute lymphocytic leukemia? *American Journal of Epidemiology* 2000; 15: 512–515.

6. Ahlbom A, Day N, Feychting M, et al. A pooled analysis of magnetic fields and childhood leukaemia. *British Journal of Cancer* 2000; 83(5): 692–698.

7. Greenland S, Sheppard AR, Kaune WT, Poole C, Kelsh MA. A pooled analysis of magnetic fields, wire codes, and childhood leukemia. Childhood Leukemia-EMF Study Group. *Epidemiology* 2000; 11(6): 624–634.

8. Hatch EE, Linet MS, Kleinerman RA, et al. Association between childhood acute lymphoblastic leukemia and use of electrical appliances during pregnancy and childhood. *Epidemiology* 1998; 9(3): 234–245.

9. Infante-Rivard C, Deadman JE. Maternal occupational exposure to extremely low frequency magnetic fields during pregnancy and childhood leukemia. *Epidemiology* 2003; 14: 437–441.

10. Schoenfeld ER, O'Leary ES, Henderson K, et al. Electromagnetic fields and breast cancer on Long Island: A case-control study. *American Journal of Epidemiology* 2003; 158: 47–58.

11. London SJ, Pagoda JM, Hwang KL et al. Residential magnetic field exposure and breast cancer risk: A nested case-control study from a multi-ethnic cohort in Los Angeles, California. *American Journal of Epidemiology* 2003; 158: 969–980.

12. Davis S, Mirick DK, Stevens RG. Residential magnetic fields and the risk of breast cancer. *American Journal of Epidemiology* 2002; 155: 446–454.

13. Kabat GC, O'Leary ES, Schoenfeld ER, et al. Electric blanket use and breast cancer on Long Island. *Epidemiology* 2003; 14(5): 514–520.

14. Kliukiene J, Tynes T, Andersen A. Residential and occupational exposures to 50-Hz magnetic fields and breast cancer in women: A population-based study. *American Journal of Epidemiology* 2004; 159(9): 852–861.

15. Zhu K, Hunter S, Payne-Wilks K, et al. Use of electric bedding devices and risk of breast cancer in African American women. *American Journal of Epidemiology* 2003; 158: 798–806.

16. Tynes T, Haldorsen T. Residential and occupational exposure to 50 Hz magnetic fields and hematological cancers in Norway. *Cancer Causes & Control* 2003; 14: 715–720.

17. Labreche F, Goldberg MS, Valois M-F, et al. Occupational exposures to extremely low frequency magnetic fields and post-menopausal breast cancer. *American Journal of Industrial Medicine* 2003; 44: 643–652.

18. Willett E, McKinney PA, Fear NT, et al. Occupational exposure to electromagnetic fields and acute leukaemia: Analysis of a case-control study. *Occupational and Environmental Medicine* 2003; 60: 577–583.

Cellular Telephone Use and Cancer: Questions and Answers

Why is there concern that cellular telephones may cause cancer?

There are three main reasons why people are concerned that cellular telephones (also known as "wireless" or "mobile" telephones) may cause certain types of cancer.

- Cellular telephones emit radiofrequency (RF) energy, a form of radiation, which is under investigation for its effects on the human body.[1]

- Cellular telephone technology is relatively new and is still changing, so there are no long-term studies of the effects of RF energy from cellular telephones on the human body.[1]

- The number of cellular telephone users is increasing rapidly. According to the Cellular Telecommunications and Internet Association (CTIA), there are now more than 180 million subscribers to cellular telephone service in the United States. Experts estimate that by 2010, there will be 2.2 billion subscribers worldwide.

For these reasons, it is important to learn whether RF energy affects human health, and to provide reassurance if it does not.

What is RF energy and how can it affect the body?

RF energy, also called radio waves, is a form of electromagnetic radiation. Electromagnetic radiation can be ionizing (high-frequency) or non-ionizing (low-frequency).[2] RF energy belongs to the non-ionizing type of electromagnetic radiation. It is known that ionizing radiation, such as that produced by x-ray machines, can present a health risk at high levels of exposure. However, it is not yet known whether non-ionizing radiation poses a cancer risk.[2]

The most important use of RF energy is for telecommunications.[2] In the United States, cellular telephones operate in a frequency ranging from about 1,800 to 2,200 megahertz (MHz).[1] In that range, the radiation produced is in the form of non-ionizing RF energy. AM/FM radios, VHF/UHF televisions, and cordless telephones (telephones that have a base unit connected to the telephone wiring in a house) operate at somewhat lower radio frequencies than cellular telephones; microwave ovens, radar, and satellite stations operate at somewhat higher radio frequencies.[2]

RF energy produces heat, which can increase body temperature and damage those parts exposed to it.[1,2] It is generally agreed that the amount of RF energy encountered by the general public is too low to produce significant tissue heating or an increase in body temperature. However, it is also agreed that further research is needed to determine what effects, if any, low-level non-ionizing RF energy has on the body and whether it is dangerous to people.[2]

139

How much RF energy are cellular telephone users exposed to?

A cellular telephone user's level of exposure to RF energy depends on several factors. These include the number and duration of calls, the amount of cellular telephone traffic at a given time, the distance from the nearest cellular base station (a low-powered radio transmitter that communicates with a user's cellular telephone), the quality of the transmission, how far the antenna is extended, and the size of the handset.

A cellular telephone's main source of RF energy is its antenna. The antenna of hand-held cellular telephones is in the handset, which is typically held against the side of the head while the telephone is in use. The closer the antenna is to the head, the greater a person's expected exposure to RF energy. The amount of RF energy absorbed decreases rapidly with increasing distance between the antenna and the user.

Hands-free kits are a relatively recent feature that can be used with cellular telephones for convenience and comfort. These systems reduce the amount of RF energy exposure to the head because the phone, which is the source of RF energy, is not placed against the head.[2] However, most studies conducted on cellular telephone use and cancer risk have focused on hand-held models not equipped with hands-free systems, since they deliver the most RF energy to the user.

The intensity of RF energy emitted by cellular telephones depends on the level of the signal sent to or from the nearest base station.[1] A geographic area serviced by a base unit is often referred to as a "cell," which is why these devices are called "cellular" telephones.

When a call is placed from a cellular telephone, a signal is sent from the antenna of the phone to the nearest base station antenna. The base station routes the call through a switching center, where the call can be transferred to another cellular telephone, another base station, or to the local land-line telephone system. The farther a cellular telephone is from the base station antenna, the higher the power level needed to maintain the connection. This distance, in part, determines the amount of RF energy exposure to the user.

What parts of the body may be affected during cellular telephone use?

Because hand-held cellular telephones are used close to the head, there is concern that the RF energy produced by these devices may affect the brain and nervous system tissue in the head. Researchers have focused on whether RF energy can cause malignant (cancerous) brain tumors such as gliomas (cancers of the brain that begin in the glial cells, which are cells that surround and support nerve cells), as well as benign (non-cancerous) tumors, such as acoustic neuromas (tumors that arise in the cells of the nerve that supplies the ear) and meningiomas (tumors that occur in the meninges, which are the membranes that cover and protect the brain and spinal cord).[1]

What studies have been done? What do they show?

Many studies have already been done, and research is ongoing. A study funded by Wireless Technology Research LLC and the National Cancer Institute (NCI) was conducted in five academic medical centers in the United States. The study analyzed the possible link between brain cancer and cellular telephone use between 1994 and 1998. The study compared a group of 469 men and women with brain cancer to a group of 422 men and women who did not have brain cancer. Results of the study, published in 2000, found that the use of hand-held cellular telephones was unrelated to the risk of brain cancer, but additional studies covering longer periods of cellular telephone use were recommended.[3]

The results of another large NCI-funded study of cellular telephones and brain tumors were published in 2001. It focused on 782 patients with one of three types of brain tumors (glioma, meningioma, or acoustic neuroma) at three medical centers between 1994 and 1998. The control group consisted of 799 patients at the same hospitals who did not have brain tumors. The researchers did not find an increased risk of brain cancer among cellular telephone users. The results showed no evidence of increasing risk with increasing years of use, or average minutes of use per day. The study also found that brain tumors did not occur more often than expected on the side of the head on which participants reported using their phone.[4]

In 2005, a series of multinational case-control studies (studies that compare two groups of people: those with the disease or condition under study [cases], and a very similar group of people who do not have the disease or condition [controls]), collectively called INTERPHONE, have been developed and are being coordinated by the International Agency for Research on Cancer (IARC). The primary objective of these studies is to assess whether RF energy exposure from cellular telephones is associated with an increased risk of cancer. The participating scientists are also exploring other possible causes of brain tumors besides RF energy, including external (environmental) and internal (endogenous) risk factors. Genetic (inherited) factors will be studied in collaboration with the NCI consortium of brain cancer studies. Participating

141

countries include Australia, Canada, Denmark, Finland, France, Germany, Israel, Italy, Japan, New Zealand, Norway, Sweden, and the United Kingdom.[5]

The first two articles of the INTERPHONE study, both published in November 2004, examine the use of cellular telephones and the risk of the benign tumor acoustic neuroma. A Danish study compared 106 individuals having acoustic neuroma with a control group of 212 people without this condition. The study showed no increased risk of acoustic neuroma in long-term (10 years or more) cellular telephone users when compared to short-term users. Additionally, there was no increase in the incidence of tumors on the side of the head where the phone was usually held.[6] A Swedish study, however, compared 148 individuals with acoustic neuroma to 604 healthy individuals. This study suggests there is an increased risk of acoustic neuroma in long-term cellular telephone users, but not in short-term users.[7]

Other studies from INTERPHONE investigated whether there is a relationship between cellular telephone use and the risk of the brain tumors meningioma and glioma. A Danish study, published in 2005, compared 175 people with meningioma and 252 people with glioma to a control group of 822 disease-free individuals. This study demonstrated no link between meningioma or glioma and cellular telephone use.[8] A Swedish study, published in 2005, compared 273 individuals with meningioma and 371 people with gliomas to 674 people who did not have these conditions. This study also showed that people who use cellular telephones are not at an increased risk of meningioma or glioma.[9]

Overall, research has not consistently demonstrated a link between cellular telephone use and cancer or any other adverse health effect.

Why aren't the results of the studies consistent?

Scientists have had to assess how much RF energy people have been exposed to by interviewing individuals involved in a particular study about their cellular telephone habits (including frequency of use and duration of calls). Because of this, the accuracy of the data collected is subject to the memory of the people interviewed. Recently, however, RF-energy-measurement meters have been developed that will accurately measure RF energy exposure.[1]

Additionally, cellular telephones have only been widely available for a relatively short period of time (since the 1990s), and cellular technology continues to change.[1] For example, older studies evaluated RF exposure from analog telephones; today, most cellular telephones use digital technology. (Analog and digital telephones operate at different frequencies and power levels.) Another new technology is Bluetooth, a wireless technology that allows devices, such as cellular telephones and headsets, to communicate with each other using short-range radio frequency.

Furthermore, brain tumors develop over many years. Scientists have been unable to follow cellular telephone users consistently for the amount of time it might take for a brain tumor to develop.[1]

Although research has not consistently demonstrated a link between cellular telephone use and cancer, scientists still caution that more research needs to be done before conclusions can be drawn about the risk of cancer from cellular telephones.[1]

Do children have a higher risk of developing cancer due to cellular telephone use than adults?

There is no evidence that cellular telephone use poses more of a threat to children than to adults.[2] However, no study populations to date have included children, who are increasingly heavy users of cellular telephones and are likely to accumulate many years of exposure during their lives.[1]

In addition, children are at greatest risk from agents known to cause brain and nervous system cancers because their nervous systems are still developing. If RF energy from cellular telephones is proven to cause cancer, researchers would expect children to be more susceptible than adults. Again, however, there is no evidence of this to date.[1]

What can cellular telephone users do to reduce their exposure to RF?

The U.S. Food and Drug Administration (FDA) has suggested some steps that cellular telephone users can take if they are concerned about potential health risks from cellular telephones:

- Reserve the use of cellular telephones for shorter conversations, or for when a conventional phone is not available.

- Switch to a type of cellular telephone with a hands-free device that will place more distance between the antenna and the phone user.

Additionally, the Federal Communications Commission (FCC), which regulates interstate and international communications by radio, television, wire, satellite, and cable, provides consumers with information on human exposure to RF energy from cellular telephones and other devices at http://www.fcc.gov/oet/rfsafety on the internet. This webpage allows consumers to find information about the specific absorption rate (SAR) of cellular telephones produced and marketed within the last one to two years. The SAR corresponds to the relative amount of RF energy absorbed into the head of a cellular telephone user. Consumers can access this information using the phone's FCC ID number, which is usually located on the case of the phone.

Selected References

1. Ahlbom A, Green A, Kheifets L, et al. Epidemiology of health effects on radiofrequency exposure. *Environmental Health Perspectives* 2004; 112(14):1741–1754.

2. Food and Drug Administration (2003). *Cell Phone Facts: Consumer Information on Wireless Phones.* Retrieved May 10, 2005, from http://www.fda.gov/cellphones/qa.html.

3. Muscat JE, Malkin MG, Thompson S, et al. Handheld cellular telephone use and risk of brain cancer. *Journal of the American Medical Association* 2000; 284(23):3001–3007.

4. Inskip PD, Tarone RE, Hatch EE, et al. Cellular-telephone use and brain tumors. *New England Journal of Medicine* 2001; 344(2):79–86.

5. International Agency for Research on Cancer (2004). *The INTERPHONE Study.* Lyon, France: International Agency for Research on Cancer. Retrieved May 10, 2005, from http://www.iarc.fr/ENG/Units/RCAd.html.

6. Christensen HC, Schuz J, Kosteljanetz M, et al. Cellular telephone use and risk of acoustic neuroma. *American Journal of Epidemiology* 2004; 159(3):277–283.

7. Lonn S, Ahlbom A, Hall P, Feychting M. Mobile phone use and the risk of acoustic neuroma. *Epidemiology* 2004; 15(6):653–659.

8. Christensen HC, Schuz J, Kosteljanetz M, et al. Cellular telephones and risk for brain tumors: A population-based, incident case-control study. *Neurology* 2005; 64(7): 1189–1195.

9. Lonn S, Ahlbom A, Hall P, et al. Long-term mobile phone use and brain tumor risk. *American Journal of Epidemiology* 2005; 161(6):526–535.

Chapter 14

Cancer Risks Associated with Pregnancy Issues and Sexual Health

Chapter Contents

145

Section 14.1

Pregnancy and Breast Cancer Risk

Excerpted from "Pregnancy and Breast Cancer Risk,"
a National Cancer Institute fact sheet, reviewed December 30, 2003.

Pregnancy-Related Factors that Protect against Breast Cancer

Some factors associated with pregnancy are known to reduce a woman's chance of developing breast cancer later in life:

- The younger a woman has her first child, the lower her risk of developing breast cancer during her lifetime.

- A woman who has her first child after the age of 35 has approximately twice the risk of developing breast cancer as a woman who has a child before age 20.

- A woman who has her first child around age 30 has approximately the same lifetime risk of developing breast cancer as a woman who has never given birth.

- Having more than one child decreases a woman's chances of developing breast cancer. In particular, having more than one child at a younger age decreases a woman's chances of developing breast cancer during her lifetime.

- Although not fully understood, research suggests that pre-eclampsia, a pathologic condition that sometimes develops during pregnancy, is associated with a decrease in breast cancer risk in the offspring, and there is some evidence of a protective effect for the mother.

- After pregnancy, breastfeeding for a long period of time (for example, a year or longer) further reduces breast cancer risk by a small amount.

Pregnancy-Related Factors that Increase Breast Cancer Risk

Some factors associated with pregnancy are known to increase a woman's chances of developing breast cancer:

- After a woman gives birth, her risk of breast cancer is temporarily increased. This temporary increase lasts only for a few years.

- A woman who during pregnancy took DES (diethylstilbestrol), a synthetic form of estrogen that was used between the early 1940s and 1971, has a slightly higher risk of developing breast cancer. (So far, research does not show an increased breast cancer risk for their female offspring who were exposed to DES before birth. Those women are sometimes referred to as "DES daughters.")

Misunderstandings about Breast Cancer Risk Factors

There are a number of misconceptions about what can cause breast cancer. These include, but are not limited to, using deodorants or antiperspirants, wearing an under-wire bra, having a miscarriage or induced abortion, or bumping or bruising breast tissue. Even though doctors can seldom explain why one person gets cancer and another does not, it is clear that none of these factors increase a woman's risk of breast cancer. In addition, cancer is not contagious; no one can "catch" cancer from another person.

Preventing Breast Cancer

There are some things women can do to reduce their breast cancer risk.

Because some studies suggest that the more alcoholic beverages a woman drinks the greater her risk of breast cancer, it is important to limit alcohol intake. Maintaining a healthy body weight is important because being overweight increases risk of postmenopausal breast cancer. New evidence suggests that being physically active may also reduce risk. Physical activity that is sustained throughout lifetime or, at a minimum, performed after menopause, may be particularly beneficial in reducing breast cancer risk. Eating a diet high in fruits and vegetables, and energy and fat intake balanced to energy expended in exercise are useful approaches to avoiding weight gain in adult life.

147

Detecting Breast Cancer

A woman can be an active participant in improving her chances for early detection of breast cancer. NCI recommends that, beginning in their 40s, women have a mammogram every year or two. Women who have a higher than average risk of breast cancer (for example, women with a family history of breast cancer) should seek expert medical advice about whether they should be screened before age 40, and how frequently they should be screened.

Section 14.2

Abortion, Miscarriage, and Breast Cancer Risk

Excerpted from a National Cancer Institute Fact Sheet, updated May 30, 2003. The complete text of this document and links to related materials are available online at http://www.cancer.gov.

The relationship between induced and spontaneous abortion and breast cancer risk has been the subject of extensive research beginning in the late 1950s. Until the mid-1990s, the evidence was inconsistent. Findings from some studies suggested there was no increase in risk of breast cancer among women who had had an abortion, while findings from other studies suggested there was an increased risk. Most of these studies, however, were flawed in a number of ways that can lead to unreliable results. Only a small number of women were included in many of these studies, and for most, the data were collected only after breast cancer had been diagnosed, and women's histories of miscarriage and abortion were based on their "self-report" rather than on their medical records. Since then, better-designed studies have been conducted. These newer studies examined large numbers of women, collected data before breast cancer was found, and gathered medical history information from medical records rather than simply from self-reports, thereby generating more reliable findings. The newer studies consistently showed no association between induced and spontaneous abortions and breast cancer risk.

In February 2003, the National Cancer Institute (NCI) convened a workshop of over 100 of the world's leading experts who study pregnancy and breast cancer risk. Workshop participants reviewed existing population-based, clinical, and animal studies on the relationship between pregnancy and breast cancer risk, including studies of induced and spontaneous abortions. They concluded that having an abortion or miscarriage does not increase a woman's subsequent risk of developing breast cancer.

Section 14.3

Diethylstilbestrol (DES): Questions and Answers about Cancer Risk

Excerpted from "DES: Questions and Answers," National Cancer Institute, April 15, 2003. The complete text of this document, including references, is available online at http://www.cancer.gov.

What is DES?

DES (diethylstilbestrol) is a synthetic form of estrogen, a female hormone. It was prescribed between 1940 and 1971 to help women with certain complications of pregnancy. Use of DES declined in the 1960s after studies showed that it is not effective in preventing pregnancy complications. When given during the first five months of a pregnancy, DES can interfere with the development of the reproductive system in a fetus. For this reason, although DES and other estrogens may be prescribed for some medical problems, they are no longer used during pregnancy.

What health problems might DES-exposed daughters have?

In 1971, DES was linked to an uncommon cancer (called clear cell adenocarcinoma) in a small number of daughters of women who had used DES during pregnancy. This cancer of the vagina or cervix usually occurs after age 14, with most cases found at age 19 or 20 in DES-exposed daughters. Some cases have been reported in women in their

149

thirties and forties. The risk to women older than age 40 is still unknown, because the women first exposed to DES *in utero* are just reaching their fifties, and information about their risk has not been gathered. The overall risk of an exposed daughter to develop this type of cancer is estimated to be approximately 1/1000 (0.1 percent). Although clear cell adenocarcinoma is extremely rare, it is important that DES-exposed daughters be aware of the risk and continue to have regular physical examinations.

Scientists found a link between DES exposure before birth and an increased risk of developing abnormal cells in the tissue of the cervix and vagina. Physicians use a number of terms to describe these abnormal cells, including dysplasia, cervical intraepithelial neoplasia (CIN), and squamous intraepithelial lesions (SIL). These abnormal cells resemble cancer cells in appearance; however, they do not invade nearby healthy tissue as cancer cells do. These abnormal cellular changes usually occur between the ages of 25 and 35, but may appear in exposed women of other ages as well. Although this condition is not cancer, it may develop into cancer if left untreated. DES-exposed daughters should have a yearly Pap test and pelvic exam to check for abnormal cells. DES-exposed daughters also may have structural changes in the vagina, uterus, or cervix. They also may have irregular menstruation and an increased risk of miscarriage, tubal (ectopic) pregnancy, infertility, and premature births.

What health problems might DES-exposed sons have?

There is some evidence that DES-exposed sons may have testicular abnormalities, such as undescended testicles or abnormally small testicles. The risk for testicular or prostate cancer is unclear; studies of the association between DES exposure *in utero* and testicular cancer have produced mixed results. In addition, investigations of abnormalities of the urogenital system among DES-exposed sons have not produced clear answers.

What health problems might DES-exposed mothers have?

Women who used DES may have a slightly increased risk of breast cancer. Current research indicates that the risk of breast cancer in DES-exposed mothers is approximately 30 percent higher than the risk for women who have not been exposed to this drug. This risk has been stable over time, and does not seem to increase as the mothers become older. Additional research is needed to clarify this issue and whether DES-exposed mothers are at higher risk for any other types of cancer.

How can people find out if they took DES during pregnancy or were exposed to DES in utero?

It has been estimated that 5 to 10 million people were exposed to DES during pregnancy. Many of these people are not aware that they were exposed. A woman who was pregnant between 1940 and 1971 and had problems or a history of problems during pregnancy may have been given DES or a similar drug. Women who think they used a hormone such as DES during pregnancy, or people who think that their mother used DES during pregnancy, can contact the attending physician or the hospital where the delivery took place to request a review of the medical records. If any pills were taken during pregnancy, obstetrical records should be checked to determine the name of the drug. Mothers and children have a right to this information.

However, finding medical records after a long period of time can be difficult. If the doctor has retired or died, another doctor may have taken over the practice as well as the records. The county medical society or health department may know where the records have been stored. Some pharmacies keep records for a long time and can be contacted regarding prescription dispensing information. Military medical records are kept for 25 years. In many cases, however, it may be impossible to determine whether DES was used.

What should DES-exposed daughters do?

It is important for women who believe they may have been exposed to DES before birth to be aware of the possible health effects of DES and inform their doctor of their exposure. It is important that the physician be familiar with possible problems associated with DES exposure, because some problems, such as clear cell adenocarcinoma, are likely to be found only when the doctor is looking for them. A thorough examination may include the following:

- **Pelvic examination:** A physical examination of the reproductive organs. An examination of the rectum also should be done.

- **Palpation:** As part of a pelvic examination, the doctor feels the vagina, uterus, cervix, and ovaries for any lumps. Often palpation provides the only evidence that an abnormal growth is present.

- **Pap test:** A routine cervical Pap test is not adequate for DES-exposed daughters. The cervical Pap test must be supplemented with a special Pap test of the vagina called a "four-quadrant" Pap test, in which cell samples are taken from all sides of the upper vagina.

- **Iodine staining of the cervix and vagina:** An iodine solution is used to temporarily stain the linings of the cervix and vagina to detect adenosis (a non-cancerous but abnormal growth of glandular tissue) or other abnormal tissue.

- **Colposcopy:** In colposcopy, a magnifying instrument is used to view the vagina and cervix. Some doctors do not perform colposcopy routinely. However, if the Pap test result is not normal, it is very important to check for abnormal tissue.

- **Biopsy:** Small samples of any tissue that appears abnormal on colposcopy are removed and examined under a microscope to see whether cancer cells are present.

- **Breast examinations:** Researchers are studying whether DES-exposed daughters have a higher risk of breast cancer than unexposed daughters; therefore, DES-exposed daughters should continue to follow the routine breast cancer screening recommendations for their age group.

What should DES-exposed mothers do?

A woman who took DES while pregnant (or suspects she may have taken it) should inform her doctor. She should try to learn the dosage, when the medication was started, and how it was used. She also should inform her children who were exposed before birth so that this information can be included in their medical records. DES-exposed mothers should have regular breast cancer screening and yearly medical checkups that include a pelvic examination and a Pap test.

What should DES-exposed sons do?

DES-exposed sons should inform their physician of their exposure and be examined periodically. While the level of risk of developing testicular cancer is unclear among DES-exposed sons, males with undescended testicles or unusually small testicles have an increased risk of developing testicular cancer, whether or not they were exposed to DES.

Is it safe for DES-exposed daughters to use oral contraceptives or hormone replacement therapy?

Each woman should discuss this important question with her doctor. Although studies have not shown that the use of birth control pills or hormone replacement therapy are unsafe for DES-exposed daughters, some doctors believe these women should avoid these medications because they contain estrogen. Structural changes in the vagina or cervix should cause no problems with the use of other forms of contraception, such as diaphragms or spermicides.

Section 14.4

Menopausal Hormone Use and Cancer

Excerpted from "Menopausal Hormone Use and Cancer: Questions and Answers," National Cancer Institute, reviewed July 18, 2005. The complete text of this document, including references, is available online at http://www.cancer.gov.

What is menopause?

Menopause is the time in a woman's life when menstruation ends. It is part of a biological process that begins, for most women, in their mid-thirties. During this time, the ovaries gradually produce lower levels of natural sex hormones—estrogen and progesterone. Estrogen promotes the normal development of a woman's breasts and uterus, controls the cycle of ovulation (when an ovary releases an egg into a fallopian tube), and affects many aspects of a woman's physical and emotional health. Progesterone controls menstruation (having a period) and prepares the lining of the uterus to receive the fertilized egg.

"Natural menopause" occurs when a woman has her last menstrual period, or stops menstruating, and is considered complete when menstruation has stopped for one year. This usually occurs between ages 45 and 55, with variations in timing from woman to woman. Women who undergo surgery to remove both ovaries (an operation called bilateral oophorectomy) experience "surgical menopause"—an immediate end to menstruation caused by lack of hormones produced by the ovaries.

By the time a woman has reached natural menopause, estrogen output has decreased significantly. Even though low levels of this hormone are produced by other organs after menopause, they are only about one-tenth of the level found in premenopausal women. Progesterone is nearly absent in menopausal women.

What are menopausal hormones and why are they used?

Doctors may recommend menopausal hormones to counter some of the problems often associated with the onset of menopause (hot flashes, night sweats, sleeplessness, and vaginal dryness) or to prevent some long-term conditions that are more common in postmenopausal women, such as osteoporosis. Menopausal hormone use (sometimes referred to as hormone replacement therapy or postmenopausal hormone use) usually involves treatment with either estrogen alone or estrogen in combination with progesterone or progestin, a synthetic hormone with effects similar to those of progesterone. Among women who are prescribed menopausal hormones, women who have undergone hysterectomy (surgery to remove the uterus) are generally given estrogen alone. Women who have not undergone this surgery are given estrogen plus progestin, which is known to have a lower risk of causing endometrial cancer (cancer of the lining of the uterus).

What has medical research found out about the risks and benefits of hormone use after menopause?

The most comprehensive evidence about the risks and benefits of taking menopausal hormones to prevent disease after menopause comes from the Women's Health Initiative (WHI) Hormone Program, which was sponsored by the National Heart, Lung, and Blood Institute (NHLBI) and the National Cancer Institute (NCI), parts of the National Institutes of Health (NIH). This research program examined the effects of menopausal hormones on women's health. The WHI Hormone Program involved two studies—the use of estrogen plus progestin for women with a uterus (the Estrogen-plus-Progestin study), and the use of estrogen alone for women without a uterus (the Estrogen Alone study). In both hormone therapy studies, women were randomly assigned to receive either the hormone medication being studied or the placebo.

The WHI Estrogen-plus-Progestin study was stopped in July 2002, when investigators reported that the overall risks of estrogen plus progestin, specifically Prempro™, outweighed the benefits. The researchers found that use of this estrogen plus progestin pill increased the risk of heart disease, stroke, and blood clots, as well as breast cancer. The findings also showed fewer cases of colorectal cancer among women using estrogen plus progestin than in those taking the placebo.

The WHI Estrogen-Alone study, which involved Premarin™, was stopped in February 2004 when the researchers concluded that estrogen alone increased the risk of stroke and blood clots. In contrast with the WHI Estrogen-plus-Progestin study, the use of estrogen alone had no significant effect on the risk of breast or colorectal cancer.

How does menopausal hormone use affect breast cancer risk and survival?

The WHI Estrogen-plus-Progestin study concluded that combination therapy increases the risk of invasive breast cancer. After five years of follow-up, women taking these hormones had a 26 percent increase in breast cancer risk compared with women taking the placebo. The increase amounted to an additional eight cases of breast cancer for every 10,000 women taking estrogen plus progestin for one year compared with 10,000 nonusers.

A more detailed analysis showed that, among women taking estrogen plus progestin, the breast cancers were slightly larger and diagnosed at more advanced stages compared with breast cancers in women taking the placebo. Among women taking these hormones, 25.4 percent of the cancers had spread outside the breast to nearby organs or lymph nodes compared with 16.0 percent among nonusers. Breast cancer that has spread to other parts of the body (metastatic breast cancer) is more difficult to treat. Earlier studies had suggested that, although estrogen plus progestin increased risk, the breast cancers that were diagnosed in women taking the combination had features associated with good prognoses (likelihood of recovery). The WHI Estrogen-plus-Progestin study showed that not to be the case.

The WHI Estrogen-Alone study did not find a significant increase in the risk of breast cancer during the seven years the study was conducted. Although fewer cases of breast cancer were reported in study participants using estrogen alone, than in those taking the placebo, the findings were not significant enough for researchers to make definite conclusions.

The WHI supported the conclusion from observational data that hormone use is associated with an increased risk of breast cancer, with the greatest risk among women using estrogen plus progestin. In the Million Women Study, which was published in 2003, British researchers found that current use of estrogen, estrogen plus progestin, or other hormone preparations significantly increased the risk of breast cancer in women ages 50 to 64. Women using estrogen plus progestin were at greater risk than those using other hormone preparations. Current hormone users were also more likely to die from breast cancer than women who did not use them. Within about five years of stopping use, increased risk largely disappeared for women who took estrogen alone.

What are the effects of hormone use on the risk of endometrial cancer?

Studies have shown that long-term exposure of the uterus to estrogen alone increases a woman's risk of endometrial cancer. The risk associated with estrogen plus progestin appears to be much less, but some data suggest that the risk is still increased compared with non-users. The long-term effects of estrogen plus progestin on endometrial cancer risk remain uncertain.

The WHI Hormone Program showed that endometrial cancer rates for women taking estrogen plus progestin daily were the same as or possibly less than those for women taking the placebo pill. Uterine bleeding, however, was a common side effect, leading to more frequent biopsies and ultrasounds for women taking combined hormones compared with those taking a placebo.

The Million Women Study confirmed a lower risk of endometrial cancer in women taking combined hormones compared with those taking estrogen only or tibolone, a synthetic steroid that is not available in the United States. More studies are needed to assess the effects of estrogen plus progestin on endometrial cancer.

How does menopausal hormone use affect the risk of ovarian cancer?

Several observational studies have found that the use of estrogen alone is associated with a slightly increased risk of ovarian cancer for women who used this hormone for 10 or more years. One observational study that followed 44,241 menopausal women for approximately 20 years concluded that women who used estrogen alone for ten or more years were twice as likely to develop ovarian cancer compared with women who did not use menopausal hormones. Another large observational study also found an association between estrogen use and death due to ovarian cancer. In this study, the increased risk appeared to be limited to women who used estrogen for ten or more years.

Data from the WHI Estrogen-plus-Progestin study indicate that there may be an increased risk of ovarian cancer with combined hormone use. After 5.6 years of follow-up, a 58 percent increased risk of ovarian cancer was reported in women using estrogen plus progestin compared with nonusers, but the increased risk was not statistically significant. One observational study suggested that combined estrogen-progestin regimens do not increase the risk of ovarian cancer if progestin is used for more than 15 days per month, but this study was too small to draw firm conclusions. More research is needed to clarify the relationship between menopausal hormone use, particularly for combined therapy, and the risk of ovarian cancer.

How does menopausal hormone use affect the risk of colorectal cancer?

After five years of follow-up of women taking estrogen plus progestin, the WHI Estrogen-plus-Progestin study reported a 37 percent reduction in colorectal cancer cases compared with women taking the placebo. On average, the researchers found that if a group of 10,000 women takes estrogen plus progestin for a year, six fewer cases of colon cancer will occur than in nonusers. The WHI Estrogen-Alone study concluded that estrogen alone had no significant effect on colorectal cancer risk. However, this data is not consistent with those from observational studies. More research is needed.

What are the risks of menopausal hormones for women who have a history of cancer?

One of the roles of naturally occurring estrogen is to promote the normal growth of cells in the breast and uterus. For this reason, there is concern that menopausal estrogen use by women who have had cancer may promote further tumor growth. The U.S. Food and Drug Administration (FDA) advises women with a history of cancer not to take menopausal hormones containing estrogen and progestin. The effect of menopausal estrogen use after endometrial and breast cancer remains uncertain. Little research has been done on the risks associated with menopausal hormone use by women who have had endometrial cancer. A few small studies have found no evidence that hormone use has a negative effect on survival or recurrence of the disease in these women. However, no large, long-term studies have compared the potential benefits, such as protection against osteoporosis, with the potential cancer risks.

One observational study of breast cancer patients, most of whom were using estrogen alone, reported no increase in recurrence or mortality among women who continued hormone use after their diagnosis. Another study of breast cancer patients showed that users of estrogen had lower mortality rates from breast cancer than patients who did not use estrogen. Most of these patients stopped using estrogen at the time of diagnosis. However, the benefit of prior estrogen use diminished with time.

What should women do if they are concerned about taking menopausal hormones?

Although menopausal hormones have short-term benefits such as relief from hot flashes and vaginal dryness, several health concerns are associated with their use. Women should discuss with their health care provider whether to take menopausal hormones and what alternatives may be appropriate for them. The FDA currently advises women to use menopausal hormones for the shortest time and at the lowest dose possible to control symptoms.

Section 14. 5

Vasectomy and Cancer Risk

From a National Cancer Institute Fact Sheet, reviewed June 24, 2003. The complete text of this document, including references, can be found online at http://www.cancer.gov.

Some studies have raised questions about a possible relationship between vasectomy (an operation to cut or tie off the two tubes that carry sperm out of the testicles) and the risk of developing cancer, particularly prostate and testicular cancer. Such a relationship, if proven, would be of importance because about one in six men over age 35 in the United States has had a vasectomy.

Prostate Cancer

Prostate cancer is the most common cancer in American men and the second leading cause of cancer death in American men, after lung cancer. In March 1993, the National Institute of Child Health and Human Development (NICHD) convened a conference, cosponsored by the National Cancer Institute (NCI) and the National Institute of Diabetes and Digestive and Kidney Diseases, to clarify the available evidence on the relationship between vasectomy and prostate cancer. Scientists reviewed and carefully weighed all of the data available at that time, including results from published and unpublished studies.

They determined that the results of research on the association between vasectomy and prostate cancer were not consistent. In addition, the scientists could not find any convincing biological explanation for a link between vasectomy and an increased risk of prostate cancer. Based on these findings, the expert panel concluded that even if having a vasectomy can increase a man's risk of developing prostate cancer, the increase in risk is relatively small.

In 1997, the NCI convened the prostate cancer Progress Review Group (PRG), a committee that included members from the scientific, medical, industrial, and advocacy communities. This group was charged with developing a national plan to outline scientific efforts involving prostate cancer research. The PRG's final report, published

159

in August 1998, concluded that the evidence supporting a role for vasectomy in the development of prostate cancer is weak.

Researchers continue to investigate the possible relationship between vasectomy and prostate cancer. The majority of studies conducted thus far have upheld the conclusions made at the 1993 NICHD conference. Although a few studies have reported a link between vasectomy and prostate cancer, it is possible that other factors, including chance, may be responsible for the association suggested in these studies.

Testicular Cancer

Testicular cancer is much less common than prostate cancer, accounting for approximately one percent of all cancers in American men. This type of cancer is most often found in men ages 15 to 35. A few studies have suggested a link between vasectomy and an increased risk of testicular cancer, but the evidence is inconsistent and the association in some studies may be due to factors other than vasectomy. It is also possible that the vasectomy procedure increases the rate at which an existing, but undetected, testicular cancer will progress. At this time, it is believed that there is either no association or a weak association between vasectomy and testicular cancer; although more research is needed before definitive conclusions can be reached.

Men concerned about prostate cancer or testicular cancer should talk to their doctor about the symptoms to watch for and an appropriate schedule for checkups.

Section 14.6

Human Papillomaviruses and Cancer

Excerpted from "Human Papillomaviruses and Cancer: Questions and Answers," National Cancer Institute, updated May 17, 2005. The complete text of this document, including references, is available online at http://www.cancer.gov.

What are human papillomaviruses, and how are they transmitted?

Human papillomaviruses (HPVs) are a group of more than 100 types of viruses. They are called papillomaviruses because certain types may cause warts, or papillomas, which are benign (non-cancerous) tumors. The HPVs that cause the common warts which grow on hands and feet are different from those that cause growths in the throat or genital area. Some types of HPVs are associated with certain types of cancer.

Of the more than 100 types of HPVs, over 30 types can be passed from one person to another through sexual contact. Although HPVs are usually transmitted sexually, doctors cannot say for certain when infection occurred. Most HPV infections come and go over the course of a few years. However, sometimes HPV infection persists for many years, with or without causing cell abnormalities.

What are genital warts?

Some types of HPVs may cause warts to appear on or around the genitals or anus. Genital warts (technically known as condylomata acuminatum) are most commonly associated with two HPV types, HPV-6 and HPV-11. Warts may appear within several weeks after sexual contact with a person who is infected with HPV, or they may take months or years to appear, or they may never appear. HPVs may also cause flat, abnormal growths in the genital area and on the cervix (the lower part of the uterus that extends into the vagina). However, HPV infections usually do not cause any symptoms.

What is the association between HPV infection and cancer?

HPVs are now recognized as the major cause of cervical cancer. Studies also suggest that HPVs may play a role in cancers of the anus, vulva, vagina, and some cancers of the oropharynx (the middle part of the throat that includes the soft palate, the base of the tongue, and the tonsils). Data from several studies also suggest that infection with HPV is a risk factor for penile cancer (cancer of the penis).

Are there specific types of HPVs that are associated with cancer?

Some types of HPVs are referred to as "low-risk" viruses because they rarely develop into cancer. HPVs that are more likely to lead to the development of cancer are referred to as "high-risk." Both high-risk and low-risk types of HPVs can cause the growth of abnormal cells, but generally only the high-risk types of HPVs may lead to cancer. Sexually transmitted, high-risk HPVs include types 16, 18, 31, 33, 35, 39, 45, 51, 52, 56, 58, 59, 68, 69, and possibly a few others. These high-risk types of HPVs cause growths that are usually flat and nearly invisible, as compared with the warts caused by types HPV-6 and HPV-11. It is important to note, however, that the majority of high-risk HPV infections go away on their own and do not cause cancer.

What are the risk factors for HPV infection and cervical cancer?

Having many sexual partners is a risk factor for HPV infection. Although most HPV infections go away on their own without causing any type of abnormality, infection with high-risk HPV types increases the chance that mild abnormalities will progress to more severe abnormalities or cervical cancer. Still, of the women who do develop abnormal cell changes with high-risk types of HPVs, only a small percentage would develop cervical cancer if the abnormal cells were not removed. Studies suggest that whether a woman develops cervical cancer depends on a variety of factors acting together with high-risk HPVs. The factors that may increase the risk of cervical cancer in women with HPV infection include smoking and having many children.

How are HPV infections detected?

Testing samples of cervical cells is an effective way to identify high-risk types of HPVs that may be present. The U.S. Food and Drug

Administration (FDA) has approved an HPV test that can identify 13 of the high-risk types of HPVs associated with the development of cervical cancer. This test, which looks for viral DNA, is performed by collecting cells from the cervix and then sending them to a laboratory for analysis. The test can detect high-risk types of HPVs even before there are any conclusive visible changes to the cervical cells.

How are cervical cell abnormalities classified?

A Pap test is used to detect abnormal cells in the cervix. It involves the collection of cells from the cervix for examination under the microscope. Various terms have been used to describe the abnormal cells that may be seen in Pap tests.

The major system used to report the results of Pap tests in the United States is the Bethesda System. In this system, samples with cell abnormalities are divided into the following categories:

- **ASC (atypical squamous cells):** Squamous cells are the thin, flat cells that form the surface of the cervix. The Bethesda System divides this category into two groups:

  1. *ASC-US (atypical squamous cells of undetermined significance):* The squamous cells do not appear completely normal, but doctors are uncertain what the cell changes mean. Sometimes the changes are related to HPV infection. An HPV test may be done to clarify the findings.

  2. *ASC-H (atypical squamous cells cannot exclude a high-grade squamous intraepithelial abnormality):* Intraepithelial refers to the layer of cells that forms the surface of the cervix. The cells do not appear normal, but doctors are uncertain what the cell changes mean. ASC-H may be at higher risk of being precancerous compared with ASC-US.

- **AGC (atypical glandular cells):** Glandular cells are mucus-producing cells found in the endocervical canal (opening in the center of the cervix) or in the lining of the uterus. The glandular cells do not appear normal, but doctors are uncertain what the cell changes mean.

- **AIS (endocervical adenocarcinoma in situ):** Precancerous cells are found in the glandular tissue.

- **LSIL (low-grade squamous intraepithelial lesion):** Low-grade means there are early changes in the size and shape of the cells. The word "lesion" refers to an area of abnormal tissue. LSILs are considered mild abnormalities caused by HPV infection and are a common condition, especially among young women. The majority of LSILs return to normal over months to a few years.

- **HSIL (high-grade squamous intraepithelial lesion):** High-grade means that the cells look very different in size and shape from normal cells. HSILs are more severe abnormalities and may eventually lead to cancer if left untreated.

Pap test results may also be described using an older set of categories called the "dysplasia scale." Dysplasia is a term used to describe abnormal cells. Although dysplasia is not cancer, it may develop into very early cancer of the cervix. The cells look abnormal under the microscope, but they do not invade nearby healthy tissue.

There are four degrees of dysplasia: mild, moderate, severe, and carcinoma in situ. Carcinoma in situ is a precancerous condition that involves only the layer of cells on the surface of the cervix, and has not spread to nearby tissues. In the Bethesda System, mild dysplasia is classified as LSIL; moderate or severe dysplasia and carcinoma in situ are combined into HSIL.

Cervical intraepithelial neoplasia (CIN) is another term that is sometimes used to describe abnormal tissue findings. Neoplasia means an abnormal growth of cells. The term CIN along with a number (1, 2, or 3) describes how much of the thickness of the lining of the cervix contains abnormal cells. CIN-3 is considered to be a precancerous condition that includes carcinoma in situ.

What tests are used to screen for and diagnose precancerous cervical conditions?

A Pap test is the standard way to check for any cervical cell changes. A Pap test is usually done as part of a gynecologic exam. The U.S. Preventive Services Task Force guidelines recommend that women have a Pap test at least once every three years, beginning about three years after they begin to have sexual intercourse, but no later than age 21.

Because the HPV test can detect high-risk types of HPVs in cervical cells, the FDA approved this test as a useful addition to the Pap test to help health care providers decide which women with ASC-US need further testing, such as colposcopy and biopsy of any abnormal areas. (Colposcopy is a procedure in which a lighted magnifying instrument called a colposcope is used to examine the vagina and cervix.

Biopsy is the removal of a small piece of tissue for diagnosis.) In addition, the HPV test may be a helpful addition to the Pap test for general screening of women age 30 and over.

What are the treatment options for HPV infection?

Although there is currently no medical cure for papillomavirus infection, the lesions and warts these viruses cause can be treated. Methods commonly used to treat lesions include cryosurgery (freezing that destroys tissue), LEEP (loop electrosurgical excision procedure, the removal of tissue using a hot wire loop), and conventional surgery. Similar treatments may be used for external genital warts. In addition, some drugs may be used to treat external genital warts.

What research is being done on HPV-related cancers?

Researchers at the National Cancer Institute (NCI) and elsewhere are studying how HPVs cause precancerous changes in normal cells and how these changes can be prevented. They are using HPVs grown in the laboratory to find ways to prevent the infection and its associated disease and to create vaccines against the viruses. Vaccines for certain papillomaviruses are being studied in clinical trials for the prevention of cervical cancer. One promising vaccine targets HPV types 16 and 18, which account for approximately 70 percent of cervical cancer cases worldwide. Early findings have shown that this vaccine protects against persistent infection over a two to four year period. Large-scale phase III trials are under way to confirm these early findings and to determine the efficacy of the vaccine in protecting against CIN. Results are expected within the next two to three years. Information about clinical trials is available from the NCI's Cancer Information Service (CIS) (see below) or on the clinical trials page of the NCI's website at http://www.cancer.gov/clinicaltrials/ on the internet.

Laboratory research has indicated that HPVs produce proteins known as E5, E6, and E7. These proteins interfere with the cell functions that normally prevent excessive growth. For example, HPV E6 interferes with the human protein p53. This protein is present in all people and acts to keep tumors from growing. This research is being used to develop ways to interrupt the process by which HPV infection can lead to the growth of abnormal cells.

Chapter 15

Asbestos Exposure and Cancer Risk

What is asbestos?

"Asbestos" is the name given to a group of minerals that occur naturally as bundles of fibers which can be separated into thin threads. These fibers are not affected by heat or chemicals and do not conduct electricity. For these reasons, asbestos has been widely used in many industries. Four types of asbestos have been used commercially:

- Chrysotile, or white asbestos
- Crocidolite, or blue asbestos
- Amosite, which usually has brown fibers
- Anthophyllite, which usually has gray fibers

Chrysotile asbestos, with its curly fibers, is in the serpentine family of minerals. The other types of asbestos, which all have rod-like fibers, are known as amphiboles.

Asbestos fiber masses tend to break easily into a dust composed of tiny particles that can float in the air and stick to clothes. The fibers may be easily inhaled or swallowed and can cause serious health problems.

From "Asbestos Exposure: Questions and Answers," National Cancer Institute (http://www.cancer.gov), updated August 29, 2003.

How is asbestos used?

Asbestos was mined and used commercially in North America beginning in the late 1800s. Its use increased greatly during World War II. Since then, it has been used in many industries. For example, the building and construction industry has used it for strengthening cement and plastics as well as for insulation, fireproofing, and sound absorption. The shipbuilding industry has used asbestos to insulate boilers, steam pipes, and hot water pipes. The automotive industry uses asbestos in vehicle brakeshoes and clutch pads. More than 5,000 products contain or have contained asbestos. Some of them are listed below:

- Asbestos cement sheet and pipe products used for water supply and sewage piping, roofing and siding, casings for electrical wires, fire protection material, electrical switchboards and components, and residential and industrial building materials

- Friction products, such as clutch facings, brake linings for automobiles, gaskets, and industrial friction materials

- Products containing asbestos paper, such as table pads and heat-protective mats, heat and electrical wire insulation, industrial filters for beverages, and underlying material for sheet flooring

- Asbestos textile products, such as packing components, roofing materials, and heat-and-fire-resistant fabrics (including blankets and curtains)

- Other products, including ceiling and floor tile; gaskets and packings; paints, coatings, and adhesives; caulking and patching tape; artificial ashes and embers for use in gas-fired fireplaces; plastics; vermiculite-containing consumer garden products; and some talc-containing crayons

In the late 1970s, the U.S. Consumer Product Safety Commission (CPSC) banned the use of asbestos in wallboard patching compounds and gas fireplaces because the asbestos fibers in these products could be released into the environment during use. Additionally, asbestos was voluntarily withdrawn by manufacturers of electric hair dryers. In 1989, the U.S. Environmental Protection Agency (EPA) banned all new uses of asbestos; uses established prior to 1989 are still allowed. The EPA has established regulations that require school systems to inspect for damaged asbestos and to eliminate or reduce the exposure to occupants by removing the asbestos or encasing it. In June 2000, the CPSC concluded that the risk of children's exposure to asbestos fibers in crayons was extremely low. However, the U.S. manufacturers of these crayons agreed to reformulate their products within a year. In August 2000, the EPA recommended that consumers reduce possible asbestos exposure from vermiculite-containing garden products by limiting the amount of dust produced during use. The EPA suggested that consumers use vermiculite outdoors or in a well-ventilated area; keep vermiculite damp while using it; avoid bringing dust from vermiculite use into the home on clothing; and use premixed potting soil, which is less likely to generate dust.

The regulations described above and other actions, coupled with widespread public concern about the hazards of asbestos, have resulted in a significant annual decline in U.S. use of asbestos: Domestic consumption of asbestos amounted to about 719,000 metric tons in 1973, but it had dropped to about 9,000 metric tons by 2002. Asbestos is currently used most frequently in gaskets and in roofing and friction products.

What are the health hazards of exposure to asbestos?

Exposure to asbestos may increase the risk of several serious diseases:

- Asbestosis, a chronic lung ailment that can produce shortness of breath, coughing, and permanent lung damage

- Lung cancer

- Mesothelioma, a relatively rare cancer of the thin membranes that line the chest and abdomen

- Other cancers, such as those of the larynx, oropharynx, gastrointestinal tract, and kidney

Who is at risk?

Nearly everyone is exposed to asbestos at some time during their life. However, most people do not become ill from their exposure. People who become ill from asbestos are usually those who are exposed to it on a regular basis, most often in a job where they work directly with the material or through substantial environmental contact.

Since the early 1940s, millions of American workers have been exposed to asbestos. Health hazards from asbestos fibers have been recognized in workers exposed in shipbuilding trades, asbestos mining and milling, manufacturing of asbestos textiles and other asbestos products, insulation work in the construction and building trades, brake repair, and a variety of other trades. Demolition workers, drywall removers, and firefighters also may be exposed to asbestos fibers. As a result of government regulations and improved work practices, today's workers (those without previous exposure) are likely to face smaller risks than did those exposed in the past.

Although it is known that the risk to workers increases with heavier exposure and longer exposure time, investigators have found asbestos-related diseases in individuals with only brief exposures. Generally, those who develop asbestos-related diseases show no signs of illness for a long time after their first exposure. It can take from 10 to 40 years for symptoms of an asbestos-related condition to appear.

There is some evidence that family members of workers heavily exposed to asbestos face an increased risk of developing mesothelioma. This risk is thought to result from exposure to asbestos fibers brought into the home on the shoes, clothing, skin, and hair of workers. This type of exposure is called paraoccupational exposure. To decrease these exposures, people exposed to asbestos at work are required to shower and change their clothing before leaving the workplace.

How great is the risk?

Not all workers exposed to asbestos will develop diseases related to their exposure. The risk of developing asbestos-related diseases varies with the type of industry in which the exposure occurred and with the extent of the exposure. Asbestos that is bonded into finished products such as walls and tiles poses no risk to health as long as it is not damaged or disturbed (for example, by sawing or drilling) in such a way as to release fibers into the air. When asbestos fibers are set free and inhaled, however, exposed individuals are at risk of developing an asbestos-related disease.

In addition, different types of asbestos fibers may be associated with different health risks. For example, results of several studies suggest that amphibole forms of asbestos may be more harmful than chrysotile, particularly for mesothelioma. Even so, no fiber type can be considered harmless, and people working with asbestos should always take proper safety precautions to limit exposure.

170

How does smoking affect risk?

Many studies have shown that the combination of smoking and asbestos exposure is particularly hazardous. Smokers who are also exposed to asbestos have a greatly increased risk of lung cancer. However, smoking combined with asbestos exposure does not appear to increase the risk of mesothelioma.

There is evidence that quitting smoking will reduce the risk of lung cancer among asbestos-exposed workers. People who were exposed to asbestos on the job at any time during their life or who suspect they may have been exposed should not smoke. If they smoke, they should stop.

Who needs to be examined?

Individuals who have been exposed (or suspect they have been exposed) to asbestos fibers on the job or at home via a family contact should inform their physician of their exposure history and any symptoms. Asbestos fibers can be measured in urine, feces, mucus, or material rinsed out of the lungs. A thorough physical examination, including a chest x-ray and lung function tests, may be recommended. It is important to note that chest x-rays cannot detect asbestos fibers in the lungs, but they can help identify any lung changes resulting from asbestos exposure. Interpretation of the chest x-ray may require the help of a specialist who is experienced in reading x-rays for asbestos-related diseases. Other tests also may be necessary.

As noted earlier, the symptoms of asbestos-related diseases may not become apparent for many decades after exposure. If any of the following symptoms develop, a physical examination should be scheduled without delay:

- Shortness of breath
- A cough or a change in cough pattern
- Blood in the sputum (fluid) coughed up from the lungs
- Pain in the chest or abdomen
- Difficulty in swallowing or prolonged hoarseness
- Significant weight loss

How can workers protect themselves?

Employers are required to follow regulations dealing with asbestos exposure on the job that have been issued by the Occupational

Safety and Health Administration (OSHA), the federal agency responsible for health and safety regulations in maritime, construction, manufacturing, and service workplaces. The Mine Safety and Health Administration (MSHA) enforces regulations related to mine safety. Workers should use all protective equipment provided by their employers and follow recommended work practices and safety procedures. For example, National Institute of Occupational Safety and Health (NIOSH)-approved respirators that fit properly should be worn by workers when required.

Workers who are concerned about asbestos exposure in the workplace should discuss the situation with other employees, their employee health and safety representative, and their employers. If necessary, OSHA can provide more information or make an inspection. Regional offices of OSHA are listed in the "United States Government" section of telephone directories' blue pages (under "Department of Labor"). Regional offices can also be located at http://www.osha-slc.gov/html/RAmap.html on the internet, or by contacting OSHA's national office at:

Office of Public Affairs
Occupational Safety and Health Administration
U.S. Department of Labor
Room N-3647
200 Constitution Avenue, NW
Washington, DC 20210
Toll-Free: 800-321-6742
Phone: 202-693-1999
TTY (for deaf or hard of hearing callers): 877-889-5627
Website: http://www.osha.gov/as/opa/worker/index.html (Worker's Page)

Mine workers may contact:

Office of Information and Public Affairs
Mine Safety and Health Administration (MSHA)
U.S. Department of Labor
23rd Floor
1100 Wilson Boulevard
Arlington, VA 22209-3939
Phone: 202-693-9400
Website: http://www.msha.gov

The National Institute for Occupational Safety and Health (NIOSH) is another federal agency that is concerned with asbestos exposure in the workplace. The Institute conducts asbestos-related research, evaluates work sites for possible health hazards, and makes exposure control recommendations. In addition, NIOSH distributes publications on the health effects of asbestos exposure and can suggest additional sources of information. NIOSH can be contacted at:

Information Resources Branch
National Institute for Occupational Safety and Health (NIOSH)
Robert A. Taft Laboratories
Mail Stop C-19
4676 Columbia Parkway
Cincinnati, OH 45226-1998
Toll-Free: 800-356-4674
Website: http://www.cdc.gov/niosh
E-mail: eidtechinfo@cdc.gov

Will the government provide examinations and treatment for asbestos-related conditions? What about insurance coverage?

Medical services related to asbestos exposure are available through the government for certain groups of eligible individuals. In general, individuals must pay for their own medical services unless they are covered by private or government health insurance. Some people with symptoms of asbestos-related illness may be eligible for Medicare coverage. Information about benefits is available from the Medicare office serving each state. For the telephone number of the nearest office, call toll-free 800-633-4227 or visit http://www.medicare.gov.

People with asbestos-related diseases also may qualify for financial help, including medical payments, under state workers' compensation laws. Because eligibility requirements vary from state to state, workers should contact the workers' compensation program in their state. Contact information for the workers' compensation program in each state may be found in the blue pages of a local telephone directory or at http://www.dol.gov/esa/regs/compliance/owcp/wc.htm.

If exposure occurred during employment with a federal agency (military or civilian), medical expenses and other compensation may be covered by the Federal Employees' Compensation Program. Workers who are or were employed in a shipyard by a private employer may be covered under the Longshoremen and Harbor Workers' Compensation Act. Information about eligibility and how to file a claim is available from:

Office of Worker's Compensation Programs
Employment Standards Administration
U.S. Department of Labor
Room S-3229
200 Constitution Avenue, NW
Washington, DC 20210
Telephone: 202-693-0040
Website: http://www.dol.gov/esa/owcp_org.htm
E-mail: OWCP-Mail@dol-esa.gov

Workers also may wish to contact their international union for information on other sources of medical help and insurance matters.

Eligible veterans and their dependents may receive health care at a Department of Veterans Affairs (VA) Medical Center. Treatment for service-connected and nonservice-connected conditions is provided. If the VA cannot provide the necessary medical care, they will arrange for enrolled veterans to receive care in their community. Information about eligibility and benefits is available from the VA Health Benefits Service Center at 877-222-8387 or on the VA website at http://www.va .gov/health_benefits.

Is there a danger of nonoccupational exposure from the environment and products contaminated with asbestos fibers?

Asbestos is so widely used that the entire population has been exposed to some degree. Air, drinking water, and a variety of consumer products all may contain small amounts of asbestos. In addition, asbestos fibers are released into the environment from natural deposits in the earth and as a result of wear and deterioration of asbestos products. Disease is unlikely to result from a single, high-level exposure, or from a short period of exposure to lower levels of asbestos.

What other organizations offer information related to asbestos exposure?

The organizations listed below can provide more information about asbestos exposure.

The Agency for Toxic Substances and Disease Registry (ATSDR) is responsible for preventing exposure, adverse human health effects, and diminished quality of life associated with exposure to hazardous substances from waste sites, unplanned releases, and other sources of pollution present in the environment. The ATSDR provides information about asbestos and where to find occupational and environmental health clinics. The ATSDR Information Center can be reached at:

Agency for Toxic Substances and Disease Registry
Toll-Free: 800-CDC-INFO
Website: http://www.atsdr.cdc.gov
E-mail: cdcinfo@cdc.gov

The U.S. Environmental Protection Agency (EPA) regulates the general public's exposure to asbestos in buildings, drinking water, and the environment. The EPA's Toxic Substances Control Act (TSCA) Assistance Information Service, or TSCA Hotline, can answer questions about toxic substances, including asbestos. Printed material is available on a number of topics, particularly on controlling asbestos exposure in schools and other buildings. The EPA's Asbestos and Vermiculite Home Page has suggestions for homeowners who suspect asbestos in their homes, lists laws and regulations applicable to asbestos, and links to the Agency's findings on asbestos exposure at the World Trade Center and the Pentagon. Questions may be directed to:

TSCA Assistance Information Service
U.S. Environmental Protection Agency
Mailcode 74080
1200 Pennsylvania ave NW
Washington, DC 20460
Phone: 202-554-1404
Website: http://www.epa.gov/asbestos
E-mail: tsca-hotline@epa.gov

The U.S. Consumer Product Safety Commission (CPSC) is responsible for the regulation of asbestos in consumer products. The CPSC maintains a toll-free information line on the potential hazards of commercial products; the telephone number is 800-638-2772. In addition, CPSC provides information about laboratories for asbestos testing, guidelines for repairing and removing asbestos, and general information about asbestos in the home. Publications are available from:

Office of Information and Public Affairs
U.S. Consumer Product Safety Commission
4330 East-West Highway
Bethesda, MD 20814-4408
Phone: 800-638-2772

TTY (for deaf or hard of hearing callers): 800-638-8270
Website: http://www.cpsc.gov
E-mail: info@cpsc.gov

Information about asbestos is also available from the U.S. Department
of Health and Human Services website at http://www.hhs.gov/news/
press/2001pres/20010916a.html. In addition, people can contact their
local community or state health or environmental quality department
with questions or concerns about asbestos.

References

Agency for Toxic Substances and Disease Registry (September 2001).
Asbestos. Retrieved March 5, 2003, from: http://www.atsdr.cdc.gov/
toxprofiles/tp61.html.

Agency for Toxic Substances and Disease Registry (November 25, 2002).
Asbestos: Health Effects of Exposure to Asbestos. Retrieved March 5,
2003, from: http://www.atsdr.cdc.gov/asbestos/asbestos_effects .html.

Agency for Toxic Substances and Disease Registry (November 2000).
Case Studies in Environmental Medicine: Asbestos Toxicity. Retrieved
August 21, 2003, from: http://www.atsdr.cdc.gov/HEC/CSEM/asbestos/
index.html.

Agency for Toxic Substances and Disease Registry (September 11,
2001). *ToxFAQ's for Asbestos.* Retrieved March 5, 2003, from: http://
www.atsdr.cdc.gov/tfacts61.html.

Dollinger M, Jahan T, Rosenbaum EH, Jablons D. Mesothelioma. In:
Dollinger M, Rosenbaum EH, Tempero M, Mulvilhill SJ. *Everyone's
Guide to Cancer Therapy: How Cancer is Diagnosed, Treated, and
Managed Day to Day.* 4th ed. Kansas City, MO: Andrews McMeel Pub-
lishing, 2002.

Hillerdal G. Mesothelioma: Cases associated with non-occupational
and low dose exposures. *Occupational and Environmental Medicine.*
1999;56(8):505–13.

National Cancer Institute. *Cancer Rates and Risks, 4th ed.* NIH Publication No. 96–691, 1996.

National Cancer Institute. *What You Need To Know About™ Cancer
of the Larynx.* NIH Publication No. 95–1568, 1995.

National Cancer Institute. *What You Need To Know About™ Kidney Cancer.* NIH Publication No. 96–1569, 1996.

National Cancer Institute. *What You Need To Know About™ Lung Cancer.* Publication No. 99–1553, 1999.

National Institute of Environmental Health Sciences (August 14, 2000). *"Second-hand" Asbestos.* Retrieved March 5, 2003, from: http://www.niehs.nih.gov/external/faq/asbestos.htm.

National Toxicology Program. *10th Report on Carcinogens.* Research Triangle Park (NC): National Institute of Environmental Health Sciences, Public Health Service, U.S. Department of Health and Human Services, 2002. Available online at http://ehp.niehs.nih.gov/roc/toc10.html.

Ullrich RL. Etiology of cancer: Physical factors. In: DeVita VT Jr., Hellman S, Rosenberg SA. *Cancer: Principles and Practice of Oncology.* Vol. 1 and 2. 6th ed. Philadelphia: Lippincott Williams & Wilkins, 2001.

U.S. Consumer Product Safety Commission (June 13, 2000). *CPSC Releases Test Results on Crayons.* Retrieved March 5, 2003, from: http://www.cpsc.gov/CPSCPUB/PREREL/prhtml00/00123.html.

U.S. Environmental Protection Agency (January 6, 2000). *Asbestos Containing Materials.* Retrieved March 5, 2003, from: http://www.epa.gov/earth1r6/6pd/asbestos/asbmatl.htm.

U.S. Environmental Protection Agency (November 8, 2000). *Asbestos in Your Home.* Retrieved March 5, 2003, from: http://www.epa.gov/asbestos/ashome.html.

U.S. Environmental Protection Agency (June 14, 2001). *The Asbestos Informer.* Retrieved March 5, 2003, from: http://www.epa.gov/region04/air/asbestos/inform.htm.

U.S. Environmental Protection Agency (August 2000). *Sampling and Analysis of Consumer Garden Products That Contain Vermiculite.* Retrieved March 5, 2003, from: http://www.epa.gov/asbestos/vermiculite.pdf.

U.S. Environmental Protection Agency (August 2000). *Fact Sheet: Asbestos-Contaminated Vermiculite.* Retrieved June 25, 2003, from http://www.epa.gov/asbestos/vermfacts.pdf.

U.S. Geological Survey (March 2001). *Some Facts About Asbestos.* Retrieved March 5, 2003 from: http://pubs.usgs.gov/fs/fs012-01/.

Virta, RL. *Asbestos. Mineral Commodity Summaries.* U.S. Geological Survey Minerals Information. Retrieved March 5, 2003, from: http://minerals.usgs.gov/minerals/pubs/commodity/asbestos/070303.pdf.

Chapter 16

Questions and Answers about Formaldehyde and Cancer Risk

What is formaldehyde?

Formaldehyde is a colorless, flammable, strong-smelling gas. It is an important industrial chemical used to manufacture building materials and to produce many household products. It is used in pressed wood products such as particleboard, plywood, and fiberboard, glues and adhesives, permanent press fabrics, paper product coatings, and certain insulation materials. In addition, formaldehyde is commonly used as an industrial fungicide, germicide, and disinfectant, and as a preservative in mortuaries and medical laboratories.

How is the general population exposed to formaldehyde?

According to a 1997 report by the U.S. Consumer Product Safety Commission, formaldehyde is normally present in both indoor and outdoor air at low levels, usually less than 0.03 parts of formaldehyde per million parts of air (ppm). Materials containing formaldehyde can release formaldehyde gas or vapor into the air. Formaldehyde can also be released by burning wood, kerosene, natural gas, or cigarettes; through automobile emissions; or from natural processes.

During the 1970s, urea-formaldehyde foam insulation (UFFI) was used in many homes. However, few homes are now insulated with UFFI. Homes in which UFFI was installed many years ago are not likely to

From "Formaldehyde and Cancer: Questions and Answers," National Cancer Institute, July 30, 2004.

have high formaldehyde levels now. Pressed wood products containing formaldehyde resins are often a significant source of formaldehyde in homes. Other potential indoor sources of formaldehyde include cigarette smoke and the use of un-vented, fuel-burning appliances such as gas stoves, wood-burning stoves, and kerosene heaters.

Industrial workers who produce formaldehyde or formaldehyde-containing products, laboratory technicians, health care professionals, and mortuary employees may be exposed to higher levels of formaldehyde than the general public. Exposure occurs primarily by inhaling formaldehyde gas or vapor from the air or by absorbing liquids containing formaldehyde through the skin.

What are the short-term health effects of formaldehyde exposure?

When formaldehyde is present in the air at levels exceeding 0.1 ppm, some individuals may experience health effects such as watery eyes; burning sensations of the eyes, nose, and throat; coughing; wheezing; nausea; and skin irritation. Some people are very sensitive to formaldehyde, while others have no reaction to the same level of exposure.

Can formaldehyde cause cancer?

Although the short-term health effects of formaldehyde exposure are well known, less is known about its potential long-term health effects. In 1980, laboratory studies showed that exposure to formaldehyde could cause nasal cancer in rats. This finding raised the question of whether formaldehyde exposure could also cause cancer in humans. In 1987, the U.S. Environmental Protection Agency (EPA) classified formaldehyde as a probable human carcinogen under conditions of unusually high or prolonged exposure.[1] Since that time, some studies of industrial workers have suggested that formaldehyde exposure is associated with nasal cancer and nasopharyngeal cancer, and possibly with leukemia. In 1995, the International Agency for Research on Cancer (IARC) concluded that formaldehyde is a probable human carcinogen. However, in a reevaluation of existing data in June 2004, the IARC reclassified formaldehyde as a known human carcinogen.[2]

What have scientists learned about the relationship between formaldehyde and cancer?

Since 1980, the National Cancer Institute (NCI) has conducted studies to determine whether there is an association between occupational exposure to formaldehyde and an increase in the risk of cancer. The results of this research have provided the EPA and the Occupational Safety and Health Administration (OSHA) with information to evaluate the potential health effects of workplace exposure to formaldehyde.

Long-term effects of formaldehyde have been evaluated in epidemiological studies (studies that attempt to uncover the patterns and causes of disease in groups of people). One type of study, called a cohort study, looks at populations that have different exposures to a particular factor, such as formaldehyde. A cohort is a group of people who are followed over time to see whether a disease develops. Another kind of study, a case-control study, begins with people diagnosed as having a disease (cases) and compares them to people without the disease (controls).

Several NCI studies have found that anatomists and embalmers, professions with potential exposure to formaldehyde, are at an increased risk for leukemia and brain cancer compared with the general population. In 2003, a number of cohort studies were completed among workers exposed to formaldehyde. One study, conducted by the NCI, analyzed 25,619 workers in formaldehyde industries and estimated each worker's exposure to formaldehyde while at work.[3] The analysis found an increased risk of death due to leukemia, particularly myeloid leukemia, among the workers exposed to formaldehyde. This risk was associated with increasing peak and average levels of exposure and the duration of exposure, but not cumulative exposure. Another study of 14,014 textile workers performed by the National Institute for Occupational Safety and Health (NIOSH) also found an association between the duration of exposure to formaldehyde and leukemia deaths. However, an additional cohort study of 11,039 British industry workers found no association between cumulative formaldehyde exposure and leukemia deaths.

Formaldehyde undergoes rapid chemical changes immediately after absorption. Therefore, some scientists think effects of formaldehyde at sites other than the upper respiratory tract are unlikely. However, some laboratory studies suggest that formaldehyde may affect the lymphatic and blood systems. Based on both the epidemiologic data from cohort studies and the experimental data from laboratory research, NCI investigators have concluded that exposure to formaldehyde may cause leukemia, particularly myeloid leukemia, in humans. However, inconsistent results from other studies suggest that further research is needed before definite conclusions are drawn.

Several case-control studies and cohort studies, including analysis of the large NCI cohort, have reported an association between formaldehyde exposure and nasopharyngeal cancer, although others have not. Data from extended follow-up of the NCI study found that the excess of nasopharyngeal cancer observed in the earlier report persisted.[4]

Earlier analysis of the NCI cohort found increased lung cancer deaths among industrial workers compared with the general U.S. population. However, the rate of lung cancer deaths did not increase with higher levels of formaldehyde exposure. This observation led the researchers to conclude that factors other than formaldehyde exposure might have caused the increased deaths. New data on lung cancer from the extended follow-up did not find any relationship between formaldehyde exposure and lung cancer mortality.

What has been done to protect workers from formaldehyde?

In 1987, OSHA passed a law that reduced the amount of formaldehyde to which workers can be exposed over an 8-hour work day from 3 ppm to 1 ppm. In May 1992, the law was amended, and the formaldehyde exposure limit was further reduced to 0.75 ppm.

How can people limit formaldehyde exposure in their homes?

The EPA recommends the use of "exterior-grade" pressed wood products to limit formaldehyde exposure in the home. Before purchasing pressed wood products, including building materials, cabinetry, and furniture, buyers should ask about the formaldehyde content of these products. Formaldehyde levels in homes can also be reduced by ensuring adequate ventilation, moderate temperatures, and reduced humidity levels through the use of air conditioners and dehumidifiers.

Where can people find more information about formaldehyde?

The following organizations can provide additional resources that readers may find helpful:

The U.S. Consumer Product Safety Commission (CPSC) has information about household products that contain formaldehyde. The CPSC can be contacted at:

U.S. Consumer Product Safety Commission
4330 East-West Highway
Bethesda, MD 20814-4408
Toll-Free: 800-638- 2772

TTY: 800-638-8270
Website: http://www.cpsc.gov
E-mail: info@cpsc.gov

The U.S. Food and Drug Administration (FDA) maintains information about cosmetics and drugs that contain formaldehyde. The FDA can be contacted at:

U.S. Food and Drug Administration
5600 Fishers Lane
Rockville, MD 20857-0001
Toll-Free: 888-463-6332
Website: http://www.fda.gov

The Occupational Safety and Health Administration (OSHA) has information about occupational exposure limits for formaldehyde. OSHA can be contacted at:

U.S. Department of Labor
Occupational Safety and Health Administration
200 Constitution Avenue
Washington, DC 20210
Toll-Free: 800-321-6742
Website: http://www.osha.gov

Selected References

U.S. Environmental Protection Agency, Office of Air and Radiation. *Report to Congress on Indoor Air Quality, Volume II: Assessment and Control of Indoor Air Pollution*, 1989.

International Agency for Research on Cancer (June 2004). *IARC Classifies Formaldehyde as Carcinogenic to Humans*. Retrieved June 30, 2004, from: http://www.iarc.fr/ENG/Press_Releases/archives/pr153a.html.

Hauptmann M, Lubin JH, Stewart PA, Hayes RB, Blair A. Mortality from lymphohematopoietic malignancies among workers in formaldehyde industries. *Journal of the National Cancer Institute* 2003; 95(21): 1615–1623.

Hauptmann M, Lubin JH, Stewart PA, Hayes RB, Blair A. Mortality from solid cancers among workers in formaldehyde industries. *American Journal of Epidemiology* 2004; 159(12): 1117–1130.

Part Two

Types of Cancer

Chapter 17

Cancer Statistics

The Risk of Dying of Cancer

The risk of being diagnosed with cancer and the risk of dying of cancer have decreased since the early 1990s. Fewer than half the people diagnosed with cancer today will die of the disease. Some are completely cured, and many more people survive for years with a good quality of life, thanks to treatments that control many types of cancer.

Cancer is not one disease, but many different diseases with different causes. For that reason, one breakthrough "cure for cancer" is probably not likely to come along.

There probably won't be one date in history when people remember that the cure for cancer was announced—just as infectious diseases weren't conquered on one particular day. Instead, every year will bring more and more cures for more and more types of cancer.

Statistics for Specific Cancer Sites

Unless otherwise specified, statistical information in this chapter is for the United States and is based on the National Cancer Institute

This chapter begins with "The Risk of Dying of Cancer," reprinted by permission of the American Cancer Society, Inc. from www.cancer.org. All rights reserved. © 2005 American Cancer Society. The statistics that follow are from "Cancer Stat Fact Sheets," produced by Surveillance, Epidemiology, and End Results (SEER), National Cancer Institute, 2006. For additional statistical information about cancer, visit http://seer.cancer.gov.

(NCI)'s Surveillance Epidemiology and End Results (SEER) Cancer Statistics Review and other statistics from NCI's analysis of SEER incidence data and National Center for Health Statistics (NCHS) mortality data.

Survival rates can be calculated by different methods for different purposes. The survival rates presented here are based on the relative survival rate, which measures the survival of the cancer patients in comparison to the general population, to estimate the effect of cancer.

Statistical information on cancer prevalence includes any person alive on January 1, 2003 who had been diagnosed with cancer of the site specified at any point prior to January 1, 2003 and includes persons with active disease and those who are cured of their disease.

Cancer of All Sites

The American Cancer Society estimates that 1,399,790 men and women (720,280 men and 679,510 women) will be diagnosed with and 564,830 men and women will die of cancer of all sites in 2006.

Incidence and Mortality: From 2000–2003, the median age at diagnosis for cancer of all sites was 67 years of age. Approximately 1.1% were diagnosed under age 20; 2.7% between 20 and 34; 6.0% between 35 and 44; 13.5% between 45 and 54; 20.8% between 55 and 64; 26.0% between 65 and 74; 22.6% between 75 and 84; and 7.3% 85+ years of age. The age-adjusted incidence rate was 471.3 per 100,000 men and women per year. These rates are based on cases diagnosed in 2000–2003 from 17 SEER geographic areas.

From 2000–2003, the median age at death for cancer of all sites was 73 years of age. Approximately 0.4% died under age 20; 0.9% between 20 and 34; 2.9% between 35 and 44; 8.9% between 45 and 54; 16.6%

Table 17.1: Cancer Incidence Rates of All Sites by Race and Sex

Race/Ethnicity	Men	Women
All Races	558.1 per 100,000	412.0 per 100,000
White	558.3 per 100,000	424.6 per 100,000
Black	666.4 per 100,000	395.4 per 100,000
Asian/Pacific Islander	361.8 per 100,000	285.4 per 100,000
American Indian/Alaska Native	359.9 per 100,000	305.0 per 100,000
Hispanic	419.1 per 100,000	310.9 per 100,000

between 55 and 64; 26.3% between 65 and 74; 30.0% between 75 and 84; and 14.1% 85+ years of age. The age-adjusted death rate was 194.5 per 100,000 men and women per year. These rates are based on patients who died in 2000–2003 in the U.S.

Survival: The overall 5-year relative survival rate for 1996–2002 from 17 SEER geographic areas was 65.0%. Five-year relative survival rates by race and sex were: 66.8% for white men; 65.9% for white women; 59.7% for black men; 53.4% for black women.

Lifetime Risk: Based on rates from 2001–2003, 41.28% of men and women born today will be diagnosed with cancer of all sites at some time during their lifetime. This number can also be expressed as 1 in 2 men and women will be diagnosed with cancer of all sites during their lifetime. These statistics are called the lifetime risk of developing cancer. Sometimes it is more useful to look at the probability of developing cancer of all sites between two age groups. For example, 21.54% of men will develop cancer of all sites between their 50th and 70th birthdays compared to 15.87% for women.

Prevalence: On January 1, 2003, in the United States there were approximately 10,496,000 men and women alive who had a history of cancer of all sites—4,692,397 men and 5,803,603 women.

Cancer of the Anus, Anal Canal, and Anorectum

The American Cancer Society estimates that 4,660 men and women (1,910 men and 2,750 women) will be diagnosed with and 660 men and women will die of cancer of the anus, anal canal, and anorectum in 2006.

Table 17.2: Death Rates for Cancer of All Sites by Race and Sex

Race/Ethnicity	Men	Women
All Races	241.5 per 100,000	163.5 per 100,000
White	237.3 per 100,000	162.8 per 100,000
Black	326.8 per 100,000	191.1 per 100,000
Asian/Pacific Islander	143.3 per 100,000	98.0 per 100,000
American Indian/Alaska Native	150.0 per 100,000	111.1 per 100,000
Hispanic	165.1 per 100,000	108.1 per 100,000

Incidence and Mortality: From 2000–2003, the median age at diagnosis for cancer of the anus, anal canal, and anorectum was 61 years of age. The age-adjusted incidence rate was 1.5 per 100,000 men and women per year. The median age at death for cancer of the anus, anal canal, and anorectum was 66 years of age. The age-adjusted death rate was 0.2 per 100,000 men and women per year.

Survival and Stage: The overall 5-year relative survival rate for 1996–2002 from 17 SEER geographic areas was 66.7%. Five-year relative survival rates by race and sex were: 61.6% for white men; 72.6% for white women; 52.9% for black men; 65.8% for black women.

The stage distribution based on historic stage shows that 49% of anus cancer cases are diagnosed while the cancer is still confined to the primary site (localized stage); 32% are diagnosed after the cancer has spread to regional lymph nodes or directly beyond the primary site; 10% are diagnosed after the cancer has already metastasized (distant stage) and for the remaining 10% the staging information was unknown. The corresponding 5-year relative survival rates were: 82.4% for localized; 59.6% for regional; 19.4% for distant; and 55.7% for unstaged.

Cancer of the Bones and Joints

The American Cancer Society estimates that 2,760 men and women (1,500 men and 1,260 women) will be diagnosed with and 1,260 men and women will die of cancer of the bones and joints in 2006.

Incidence and Mortality: From 2000–2003, the median age at diagnosis for cancer of the bones and joints was 39 years of age. The age-adjusted incidence rate was 0.9 per 100,000 men and women per year. The median age at death for cancer of the bones and joints was 59 years of age. The age-adjusted death rate was 0.4 per 100,000 men and women per year.

Survival and Stage: The overall 5-year relative survival rate for 1996–2002 from 17 SEER geographic areas was 67.9%. Five-year relative survival rates by race and sex were: 64.4% for white men; 72.1% for white women; 65.5% for black men; 67.5% for black women.

The stage distribution based on historic stage shows that 37% of bone and joint cancer cases are diagnosed while the cancer is still confined to the primary site (localized stage); 38% are diagnosed after the cancer has spread to regional lymph nodes or directly beyond the primary site; 17% are diagnosed after the cancer has already metastasized (distant stage) and for the remaining 9% the staging information was unknown. The corresponding 5-year relative survival rates were: 85.8% for localized; 68.4% for regional; 28.4% for distant; and 62.1% for unstaged.

Cancer of the Brain and Other Nervous System

The American Cancer Society estimates that 18,820 men and women (10,730 men and 8,090 women) will be diagnosed with and 12,820 men and women will die of cancer of the brain and other nervous system in 2006.

Incidence and Mortality: From 2000–2003, the median age at diagnosis for cancer of the brain and other nervous system was 55 years of age. The age-adjusted incidence rate was 6.4 per 100,000 men and women per year. The median age at death for cancer of the brain and other nervous system was 64 years of age. The age-adjusted death rate was 4.5 per 100,000 men and women per year.

Survival: The overall 5-year relative survival rate for 1996–2002 from 17 SEER geographic areas was 33.5%. Five-year relative survival rates by race and sex were: 31.5% for white men; 34.3% for white women; 32.8% for black men; 38.1% for black women.

Cancer of the Breast

The American Cancer Society estimates that 212,920 women will be diagnosed with and 40,970 women will die of cancer of the breast in 2006.

Incidence and Mortality: From 2000–2003, the median age at diagnosis for cancer of the breast was 61 years of age. The age-adjusted incidence rate was 129.1 per 100,000 women per year. The median age at death for cancer of the breast was 69 years of age. The age-adjusted death rate was 25.8 per 100,000 women per year.

Survival and Stage: The overall 5-year relative survival rate for 1996–2002 from 17 SEER geographic areas was 88.5%. Five-year relative survival rates by race were: 89.7% for white women; 77.3% for black women.

The stage distribution based on historic stage shows that 61% of breast cancer cases are diagnosed while the cancer is still confined to the primary site (localized stage); 31% are diagnosed after the cancer

191

has spread to regional lymph nodes or directly beyond the primary site; 6% are diagnosed after the cancer has already metastasized (distant stage) and for the remaining 2% the staging information was unknown. The corresponding 5-year relative survival rates were: 98.1% for localized; 83.1% for regional; 26.0% for distant; and 54.1% for unstaged.

Lifetime Risk: Based on rates from 2001–2003, 12.67% of women born today will be diagnosed with cancer of the breast at some time during their lifetime. This number can also be expressed as 1 in 8 women will be diagnosed with cancer of the breast during their lifetime; 6.03% of women will develop cancer of the breast between their 50th and 70th birthdays.

Prevalence: On January 1, 2003, in the United States there were approximately 2,356,795 women alive who had a history of cancer of the breast.

Cancer of the Cervix Uteri

The American Cancer Society estimates that 9,710 women will be diagnosed with and 3,700 women will die of cancer of the cervix uteri in 2006.

Incidence and Mortality: From 2000–2003, the median age at diagnosis for cancer of the cervix uteri was 48 years of age. The age-adjusted incidence rate was 8.8 per 100,000 women per year. The median age at death for cancer of the cervix uteri was 57 years of age. The age-adjusted death rate was 2.6 per 100,000 women per year.

Survival and Stage: The overall 5-year relative survival rate for 1996–2002 from 17 SEER geographic areas was 71.6%. Five-year relative survival rates by race were: 72.8% for white women; 62.6% for black women.

The stage distribution based on historic stage shows that 52% of cervix uteri cancer cases are diagnosed while the cancer is still confined to the primary site (localized stage); 34% are diagnosed after the cancer has spread to regional lymph nodes or directly beyond the primary site; 9% are diagnosed after the cancer has already metastasized (distant stage) and for the remaining 5% the staging information was unknown. The corresponding 5-year relative survival rates were: 92.0% for localized; 55.5% for regional; 14.6% for distant; and 59.1% for unstaged.

Cancer of the Colon and Rectum

The American Cancer Society estimates that 148,610 men and women (72,800 men and 75,810 women) will be diagnosed with and 55,170 men and women will die of cancer of the colon and rectum in 2006.

Incidence and Mortality: From 2000-2003, the median age at diagnosis for cancer of the colon and rectum was 71 years of age. Approximately 0.0% were diagnosed under age 20; 0.9% between 20 and 34; 3.5% between 35 and 44; 10.9% between 45 and 54; 17.6% between 55 and 64; 25.9% between 65 and 74; 28.8% between 75 and 84; and 12.3% 85+ years of age. The age-adjusted incidence rate was 52.4 per 100,000 men and women per year.

From 2000-2003, the median age at death for cancer of the colon and rectum was 75 years of age. Approximately 0.0% died under age 20; 0.6% between 20 and 34; 2.4% between 35 and 44; 7.7% between 45 and 54; 14.3% between 55 and 64; 23.9% between 65 and 74; 31.1% between 75 and 84; and 20.0% 85+ years of age. The age-adjusted death rate was 19.8 per 100,000 men and women per year.

Survival and Stage: The overall 5-year relative survival rate for 1996–2002 from 17 SEER geographic areas was 64.1%. Five-year relative survival rates by race and sex were: 66.0% for white men; 64.2% for white women; 55.6% for black men; 53.9% for black women.

The stage distribution based on historic stage shows that 39% of colon and rectum cancer cases are diagnosed while the cancer is still confined to the primary site (localized stage); 37% are diagnosed after the cancer has spread to regional lymph nodes or directly beyond the primary site; 19% are diagnosed after the cancer has already metastasized (distant stage) and for the remaining 5% the staging information was unknown. The corresponding 5-year relative survival rates were: 90.4% for localized; 68.1% for regional; 9.8% for distant; and 34.6% for unstaged.

Lifetime Risk: Based on rates from 2001–2003, 5.56% of men and women born today will be diagnosed with cancer of the colon and rectum at some time during their lifetime. This number can also be expressed as 1 in 18 men and women will be diagnosed with cancer of the colon and rectum during their lifetime; 2.27% of men will develop cancer of the colon and rectum between their 50th and 70th birthdays compared to 1.64% for women.

Prevalence: On January 1, 2003, in the United States there were approximately 1,068,203 men and women alive who had a history of cancer of the colon and rectum—514,794 men and 553,409 women. This includes any person alive on January 1, 2003 who had been diagnosed with cancer of the colon and rectum at any point prior to January 1, 2003 and includes persons with active disease and those who are cured of their disease.

Cancer of the Corpus and Uterus, Not Otherwise Specified (NOS)

The American Cancer Society estimates that 41,200 women will be diagnosed with and 7,350 women will die of cancer of the corpus and uterus, nos in 2006.

Incidence and Mortality: From 2000–2003, the median age at diagnosis for cancer of the corpus and uterus, nos was 63 years of age. Approximately 0.0% were diagnosed under age 20; 1.4% between 20 and 34; 6.5% between 35 and 44; 18.5% between 45 and 54; 27.3% between 55 and 64; 23.6% between 65 and 74; 17.5% between 75 and 84; and 5.2% 85+ years of age. The age-adjusted incidence rate was 23.3 per 100,000 women per year. The median age at death for cancer of the corpus and uterus, nos was 73 years of age. The age-adjusted death rate was 4.1 per 100,000 women per year.

Survival and Stage: The overall 5-year relative survival rate for 1996–2002 from 17 SEER geographic areas was 83.2%. Five-year relative survival rates by race were: 85.0% for white women; 60.2% for black women.

The stage distribution based on historic stage shows that 70% of corpus and uterus, nos cancer cases are diagnosed while the cancer is still confined to the primary site (localized stage); 17% are diagnosed after the cancer has spread to regional lymph nodes or directly beyond the primary site; 9% are diagnosed after the cancer has already metastasized (distant stage) and for the remaining 4% the staging information was unknown. The corresponding 5-year relative survival rates were: 95.7% for localized; 66.9% for regional; 23.1% for distant; and 54.8% for unstaged.

Lifetime Risk: Based on rates from 2001–2003, 2.49% of women born today will be diagnosed with cancer of the corpus and uterus, nos at some time during their lifetime. This number can also be expressed as 1 in 40 women will be diagnosed with cancer of the corpus and uterus, nos during their lifetime; 1.30% of women will develop cancer of the corpus and uterus, nos between their 50th and 70th birthdays.

Prevalence: On January 1, 2003, in the United States there were approximately 570,806 women alive who had a history of cancer of the corpus and uterus, nos.

Cancer of the Esophagus

The American Cancer Society estimates that 14,550 men and women (11,260 men and 3,290 women) will be diagnosed with and 13,770 men and women will die of cancer of the esophagus in 2006.

Incidence and Mortality: From 2000–2003, the median age at diagnosis for cancer of the esophagus was 69 years of age. The age-adjusted incidence rate was 4.5 per 100,000 men and women per year. The median age at death for cancer of the esophagus was 70 years of age. The age-adjusted death rate was 4.4 per 100,000 men and women per year.

Survival and Stage: The overall 5-year relative survival rate for 1996–2002 from 17 SEER geographic areas was 15.6%. Five-year relative survival rates by race and sex were: 16.2% for white men; 16.8% for white women; 10.8% for black men; 11.8% for black women.

The stage distribution based on historic stage shows that 24% of esophagus cancer cases are diagnosed while the cancer is still confined to the primary site (localized stage); 29% are diagnosed after the cancer has spread to regional lymph nodes or directly beyond the primary site; 30% are diagnosed after the cancer has already metastasized (distant stage) and for the remaining 17% the staging information was unknown. The corresponding 5-year relative survival rates were: 33.6% for localized; 16.8% for regional; 2.6% for distant; and 10.8% for unstaged.

Cancer of the Eye and Orbit

The American Cancer Society estimates that 2,360 men and women (1,230 men and 1,130 women) will be diagnosed with and 230 men and women will die of cancer of the eye and orbit in 2006.

Incidence and Mortality: From 2000–2003, the median age at diagnosis for cancer of the eye and orbit was 60 years of age. The age-adjusted incidence rate was 0.8 per 100,000 men and women per year.

The median age at death for cancer of the eye and orbit was 69 years of age. The age-adjusted death rate was 0.1 per 100,000 men and women per year.

Survival and Stage: The overall 5-year relative survival rate for 1996–2002 from 17 SEER geographic areas was 84.3%. Five-year relative survival rates by race and sex were: 86.1% for white men; 81.8% for white women; 79.3% for black men; 87.7% for black women.

The stage distribution based on historic stage shows that 76% of eye and orbit cancer cases are diagnosed while the cancer is still confined to the primary site (localized stage); 8% are diagnosed after the cancer has spread to regional lymph nodes or directly beyond the primary site; 4% are diagnosed after the cancer has already metastasized (distant stage) and for the remaining 12% the staging information was unknown. The corresponding 5-year relative survival rates were: 87.3% for localized; 68.6% for regional; 70.1% for distant; and 77.9% for unstaged.

Cancer of the Kidney and Renal Pelvis

The American Cancer Society estimates that 38,890 men and women (24,650 men and 14,240 women) will be diagnosed with and 12,840 men and women will die of cancer of the kidney and renal pelvis in 2006.

Incidence and Mortality: From 2000–2003, the median age at diagnosis for cancer of the kidney and renal pelvis was 65 years of age. The age-adjusted incidence rate was 12.6 per 100,000 men and women per year. The median age at death for cancer of the kidney and renal pelvis was 71 years of age. The age-adjusted death rate was 4.2 per 100,000 men and women per year.

Survival and Stage: The overall 5-year relative survival rate for 1996–2002 from 17 SEER geographic areas was 65.6%. Five-year relative survival rates by race and sex were: 66.1% for white men; 65.1% for white women; 62.4% for black men; 66.3% for black women.

The stage distribution based on historic stage shows that 54% of kidney and renal pelvis cancer cases are diagnosed while the cancer is still confined to the primary site (localized stage); 20% are diagnosed after the cancer has spread to regional lymph nodes or directly beyond the primary site; 21% are diagnosed after the cancer has already metastasized (distant stage) and for the remaining 5% the staging information was unknown. The corresponding 5-year relative survival rates were: 90.4% for localized; 61.7% for regional; 9.5% for distant; and 33.1% for unstaged.

Lifetime Risk: Based on rates from 2001–2003, 1.30% of men and women born today will be diagnosed with cancer of the kidney and renal pelvis at some time during their lifetime. This number can also be expressed as 1 in 77 men and women will be diagnosed with cancer of the kidney and renal pelvis during their lifetime; 0.80% of men will develop cancer of the kidney and renal pelvis between their 50th and 70th birthdays compared to 0.41% for women.

Prevalence: On January 1, 2003, in the United States there were approximately 230,148 men and women alive who had a history of cancer of the kidney and renal pelvis—136,080 men and 94,068 women.

Cancer of the Larynx

The American Cancer Society estimates that 9,510 men and women (7,700 men and 1,810 women) will be diagnosed with and 3,740 men and women will die of cancer of the larynx in 2006.

Incidence and Mortality: From 2000–2003, the median age at diagnosis for cancer of the larynx was 65 years of age. The age-adjusted incidence rate was 3.8 per 100,000 men and women per year. The median age at death for cancer of the larynx was 69 years of age. The age-adjusted death rate was 1.3 per 100,000 men and women per year.

Survival and Stage: The overall 5-year relative survival rate for 1996–2002 from 17 SEER geographic areas was 64.1%. Five-year relative survival rates by race and sex were: 67.3% for white men; 60.3% for white women; 56.4% for black men; 44.4% for black women.

The stage distribution based on historic stage shows that 45% of larynx cancer cases are diagnosed while the cancer is still confined to the primary site (localized stage); 47% are diagnosed after the cancer has spread to regional lymph nodes or directly beyond the primary site; 4% are diagnosed after the cancer has already metastasized (distant stage) and for the remaining 3% the staging information was unknown. The corresponding 5-year relative survival rates were: 83.5% for localized; 50.4% for regional; 13.7% for distant; and 48.9% for unstaged.

Leukemia

The American Cancer Society estimates that 35,070 men and women (20,000 men and 15,070 women) will be diagnosed with and 22,280 men and women will die of leukemia in 2006.

Incidence and Mortality: From 2000–2003, the median age at diagnosis for leukemia was 67 years of age. The age-adjusted incidence rate was 12.2 per 100,000 men and women per year. The median age at death for leukemia was 74 years of age. The age-adjusted death rate was 7.5 per 100,000 men and women per year.

Survival: The overall 5-year relative survival rate for 1996–2002 from 17 SEER geographic areas was 48.2%. Five-year relative survival rates by race and sex were: 49.7% for white men; 49.0% for white women; 40.6% for black men; 39.6% for black women.

Lifetime Risk: Based on rates from 2001–2003, 1.26% of men and women born today will be diagnosed with leukemia at some time during their lifetime. This number can also be expressed as 1 in 79 men and women will be diagnosed with leukemia during their lifetime; 0.48% of men will develop leukemia between their 50th and 70th birthdays compared to 0.29% for women.

Prevalence: On January 1, 2003, in the United States there were approximately 199,013 men and women alive who had a history of leukemia—112,324 men and 86,689 women.

Acute Lymphocytic Leukemia

The American Cancer Society estimates that 3,930 men and women (2,150 men and 1,780 women) will be diagnosed with and 1,490 men and women will die of acute lymphocytic leukemia in 2006.

Incidence and Mortality: From 2000–2003, the median age at diagnosis for acute lymphocytic leukemia was 13 years of age. The age-adjusted incidence rate was 1.5 per 100,000 men and women per year. The median age at death for acute lymphocytic leukemia was 46 years of age. The age-adjusted death rate was 0.5 per 100,000 men and women per year.

Survival: The overall 5-year relative survival rate for 1996–2002 from 17 SEER geographic areas was 63.7%. Five-year relative survival rates by race and sex were: 63.2% for white men; 65.9% for white women; 52.7% for black men; 56.1% for black women.

Chronic Lymphocytic Leukemia

The American Cancer Society estimates that 10,020 men and women (6,280 men and 3,740 women) will be diagnosed with and 4,660 men and women will die of chronic lymphocytic leukemia in 2006.

Incidence and Mortality: From 2000–2003, the median age at diagnosis for chronic lymphocytic leukemia was 72 years of age. The age-adjusted incidence rate was 3.8 per 100,000 men and women per year. The median age at death for chronic lymphocytic leukemia was 78 years of age. The age-adjusted death rate was 1.5 per 100,000 men and women per year.

Survival: The overall 5-year relative survival rate for 1996–2002 from 17 SEER geographic areas was 73.7%. Five-year relative survival rates by race and sex were: 74.3% for white men; 75.8% for white women; 52.7% for black men; 67.7% for black women.

Acute Myeloid Leukemia

The American Cancer Society estimates that 11,930 men and women (6,350 men and 5,580 women) will be diagnosed with and 9,040 men and women will die of acute myeloid leukemia in 2006.

Incidence and Mortality: From 2000–2003, the median age at diagnosis for acute myeloid leukemia was 67 years of age. The age-adjusted incidence rate was 3.7 per 100,000 men and women per year. The median age at death for acute myeloid leukemia was 72 years of age. The age-adjusted death rate was 2.7 per 100,000 men and women per year.

Survival: The overall 5-year relative survival rate for 1996–2002 from 17 SEER geographic areas was 20.9%. Five-year relative survival rates by race and sex were: 19.1% for white men; 21.7% for white women; 24.6% for black men; 19.5% for black women.

Chronic Myeloid Leukemia

The American Cancer Society estimates that 4,500 men and women (2,550 men and 1,950 women) will be diagnosed with and 600 men and women will die of chronic myeloid leukemia in 2006.

Incidence and Mortality: From 2000–2003, the median age at diagnosis for chronic myeloid leukemia was 67 years of age. The age-adjusted incidence rate was 1.5 per 100,000 men and women per year. The median age at death for chronic myeloid leukemia was 71 years of age. The age-adjusted death rate was 0.5 per 100,000 men and women per year.

Survival: The overall 5-year relative survival rate for 1996–2002 from 17 SEER geographic areas was 43.8%. Five-year relative survival rates by race and sex were: 42.2% for white men; 45.6% for white women; 43.3% for black men; 39.1% for black women.

Cancer of the Liver and Intrahepatic Bile Duct

The American Cancer Society estimates that 18,510 men and women (12,600 men and 5,910 women) will be diagnosed with and 16,200 men and women will die of cancer of the liver and intrahepatic bile duct in 2006.

Incidence and Mortality: From 2000–2003, the median age at diagnosis for cancer of the liver and intrahepatic bile duct was 66 years of age. The age-adjusted incidence rate was 6.0 per 100,000 men and women per year. The median age at death for cancer of the liver and intrahepatic bile duct was 70 years of age. The age-adjusted death rate was 4.8 per 100,000 men and women per year.

Survival and Stage: The overall 5-year relative survival rate for 1996–2002 from 17 SEER geographic areas was 10.5%. Five-year relative survival rates by race and sex were: 9.5% for white men; 11.6% for white women; 7.3% for black men; 5.4% for black women.

The stage distribution based on historic stage shows that 33% of liver and intrahepatic bile duct cancer cases are diagnosed while the cancer is still confined to the primary site (localized stage); 25% are diagnosed after the cancer has spread to regional lymph nodes or directly beyond the primary site; 21% are diagnosed after the cancer has already metastasized (distant stage) and for the remaining 21% the staging information was unknown. The corresponding 5-year relative survival rates were: 21.9% for localized; 7.2% for regional; 3.3% for distant; and 4.1% for unstaged.

Cancer of the Lung and Bronchus

The American Cancer Society estimates that 174,470 men and women

(92,700 men and 81,770 women) will be diagnosed with and 162,460 men and women will die of cancer of the lung and bronchus in 2006.

Incidence and Mortality: From 2000–2003, the median age at diagnosis for cancer of the lung and bronchus was 70 years of age. The age-adjusted incidence rate was 64.8 per 100,000 men and women per year. The median age at death for cancer of the lung and bronchus was 71 years of age. The age-adjusted death rate was 55.1 per 100,000 men and women per year.

Survival and Stage: The overall 5-year relative survival rate for 1996–2002 from 17 SEER geographic areas was 15.0%. Five-year relative survival rates by race and sex were: 13.4% for white men; 17.4% for white women; 10.5% for black men; 14.5% for black women.

The stage distribution based on historic stage shows that 16% of lung and bronchus cancer cases are diagnosed while the cancer is still confined to the primary site (localized stage); 37% are diagnosed after the cancer has spread to regional lymph nodes or directly beyond the primary site; 39% are diagnosed after the cancer has already metastasized (distant stage) and for the remaining 8% the staging information was unknown. The corresponding 5-year relative survival rates were: 49.3% for localized; 15.5% for regional; 2.1% for distant; and 7.9% for unstaged.

Lifetime Risk: Based on rates from 2001–2003, 7.01% of men and women born today will be diagnosed with cancer of the lung and bronchus at some time during their lifetime. This number can also be expressed as 1 in 14 men and women will be diagnosed with cancer of the lung and bronchus during their lifetime; 3.32% of men will develop cancer of the lung and bronchus between their 50th and 70th birthdays compared to 2.44% for women.

Prevalence: On January 1, 2003, in the United States there were approximately 354,989 men and women alive who had a history of cancer of the lung and bronchus—173,431 men and 181,558 women.

Lymphoma

The American Cancer Society estimates that 66,670 men and women (34,870 men and 31,800 women) will be diagnosed with and 20,330 men and women will die of lymphoma in 2006.

Incidence and Mortality: From 2000–2003, the median age at diagnosis for lymphoma was 64 years of age. The age-adjusted incidence rate was 21.8 per 100,000 men and women per year. The median age at death for lymphoma was 74 years of age. The age-adjusted death rate was 8.2 per 100,000 men and women per year.

Survival: Survival rates can be calculated by different methods for different purposes. The survival rates presented here are based on the relative survival rate, which measures the survival of the cancer patients in comparison to the general population to estimate the effect of cancer. The overall 5-year relative survival rate for 1996–2002 from 17 SEER geographic areas was 66.1%. Five-year relative survival rates by race and sex were: 65.3% for white men; 69.2% for white women; 56.0% for black men; 64.0% for black women.

Hodgkin Lymphoma

The American Cancer Society estimates that 7,800 men and women (4,190 men and 3,610 women) will be diagnosed with and 1,490 men and women will die of Hodgkin lymphoma in 2006.

Incidence and Mortality: From 2000–2003, the median age at diagnosis for Hodgkin lymphoma was 37 years of age. The age-adjusted incidence rate was 2.7 per 100,000 men and women per year. The median age at death for Hodgkin lymphoma was 61 years of age. The age-adjusted death rate was 0.5 per 100,000 men and women per year.

Survival: The overall 5-year relative survival rate for 1996–2002 from 17 SEER geographic areas was 84.9%. Five-year relative survival rates by race and sex were: 84.0% for white men; 86.7% for white women; 78.5% for black men; 87.1% for black women.

Non-Hodgkin Lymphoma

The American Cancer Society estimates that 58,870 men and women (30,680 men and 28,190 women) will be diagnosed with and 18,840 men and women will die of non-Hodgkin lymphoma in 2006.

Incidence and Mortality: From 2000–2003, the median age at diagnosis for non-Hodgkin lymphoma was 67 years of age. The age-adjusted incidence rate was 19.1 per 100,000 men and women per year. The median age at death for non-Hodgkin lymphoma was 74 years of age. The age-adjusted death rate was 7.7 per 100,000 men and women per year.

Survival: The overall 5-year relative survival rate for 1996–2002 from 17 SEER geographic areas was 62.5%. Five-year relative survival rates by race and sex were: 61.6% for white men; 65.8% for white women; 50.6% for black men; 58.0% for black women.

Lifetime Risk: Based on rates from 2001–2003, 1.98% of men and women born today will be diagnosed with non-Hodgkin lymphoma at some time during their lifetime. This number can also be expressed as 1 in 51 men and women will be diagnosed with non-Hodgkin lymphoma during their lifetime; 0.83% of men will develop non-Hodgkin lymphoma between their 50th and 70th birthdays compared to 0.64% for women.

Prevalence: On January 1, 2003, in the United States there were approximately 364,485 men and women alive who had a history of non-Hodgkin lymphoma—189,637 men and 174,848 women.

Myeloma

The American Cancer Society estimates that 16,570 men and women (9,250 men and 7,320 women) will be diagnosed with and 11,310 men and women will die of myeloma in 2006.

Incidence and Mortality: From 2000–2003, the median age at diagnosis for myeloma was 70 years of age. The age-adjusted incidence rate was 5.5 per 100,000 men and women per year. The median age at death for myeloma was 74 years of age. The age-adjusted death rate was 3.8 per 100,000 men and women per year.

Survival: The overall 5-year relative survival rate for 1996–2002 from 17 SEER geographic areas was 32.9%. Five-year relative survival rates by race and sex were: 35.4% for white men; 30.0% for white women; 35.1% for black men; 31.5% for black women.

Cancer of the Oral Cavity and Pharynx

The American Cancer Society estimates that 30,990 men and women (20,180 men and 10,810 women) will be diagnosed with and 7,430 men and women will die of cancer of the oral cavity and pharynx in 2006.

Incidence and Mortality: From 2000–2003, the median age at diagnosis for cancer of the oral cavity and pharynx was 62 years of age. The age-adjusted incidence rate was 10.5 per 100,000 men and women per year. The median age at death for cancer of the oral cavity and pharynx was 68 years of age. The age-adjusted death rate was 2.7 per 100,000 men and women per year.

Survival and Stage: The overall 5-year relative survival rate for 1996–2002 from 17 SEER geographic areas was 58.8%. Five-year relative survival rates by race and sex were: 60.6% for white men; 61.6% for white women; 35.6% for black men; 49.1% for black women.

The stage distribution based on historic stage shows that 33% of oral cavity and pharynx cancer cases are diagnosed while the cancer is still confined to the primary site (localized stage); 52% are diagnosed after the cancer has spread to regional lymph nodes or directly beyond the primary site; 10% are diagnosed after the cancer has already metastasized (distant stage) and for the remaining 5% the staging information was unknown. The corresponding 5-year relative survival rates were: 81.3% for localized; 51.7% for regional; 26.4% for distant; and 45.0% for unstaged.

Lifetime Risk: Based on rates from 2001–2003, 1.01% of men and women born today will be diagnosed with cancer of the oral cavity and pharynx at some time during their lifetime. This number can also be expressed as 1 in 99 men and women will be diagnosed with cancer of the oral cavity and pharynx during their lifetime; 0.73% of men will develop cancer of the oral cavity and pharynx between their 50th and 70th birthdays compared to 0.25% for women.

Prevalence: On January 1, 2003, in the United States there were approximately 235,633 men and women alive who had a history of cancer of the oral cavity and pharynx—150,051 men and 85,582 women.

Cancer of the Tongue

The American Cancer Society estimates that 9,040 men and women (5,870 men and 3,170 women) will be diagnosed with and 1,780 men and women will die of cancer of the tongue in 2006.

Incidence and Mortality: From 2000–2003, the median age at diagnosis for cancer of the tongue was 61 years of age. The age-adjusted incidence rate was 2.7 per 100,000 men and women per year. The median age at death for cancer of the tongue was 67 years of age.

The age-adjusted death rate was 0.6 per 100,000 men and women per year.

Survival and Stage: The overall 5-year relative survival rate for 1996–2002 from 17 SEER geographic areas was 56.1%. Five-year relative survival rates by race and sex were: 58.4% for white men; 57.6% for white women; 37.1% for black men; 40.7% for black women.

The stage distribution based on historic stage shows that 37% of tongue cancer cases are diagnosed while the cancer is still confined to the primary site (localized stage); 48% are diagnosed after the cancer has spread to regional lymph nodes or directly beyond the primary site; 11% are diagnosed after the cancer has already metastasized (distant stage) and for the remaining 4% the staging information was unknown. The corresponding 5-year relative survival rates were: 74.5% for localized; 50.1% for regional; 27.9% for distant; and 40.1% for unstaged.

Cancer of the Ovary

The American Cancer Society estimates that 20,180 women will be diagnosed with and 15,310 women will die of cancer of the ovary in 2006.

Incidence and Mortality: From 2000–2003, the median age at diagnosis for cancer of the ovary was 63 years of age. The age-adjusted incidence rate was 13.7 per 100,000 women per year. The median age at death for cancer of the ovary was 71 years of age. The age-adjusted death rate was 8.9 per 100,000 women per year.

Survival and Stage: The overall 5-year relative survival rate for 1996–2002 from 17 SEER geographic areas was 44.7%. Five-year relative survival rates by race were: 44.2% for white women; 39.5% for black women.

The stage distribution based on historic stage shows that 19% of ovary cancer cases are diagnosed while the cancer is still confined to the primary site (localized stage); 7% are diagnosed after the cancer has spread to regional lymph nodes or directly beyond the primary site; 68% are diagnosed after the cancer has already metastasized (distant stage) and for the remaining 7% the staging information was unknown. The corresponding 5-year relative survival rates were: 93.1% for localized; 69.0% for regional; 29.6% for distant; and 23.3% for unstaged.

Lifetime Risk: Based on rates from 2001–2003, 1.44% of women born today will be diagnosed with cancer of the ovary at some time during their lifetime. This number can also be expressed as 1 in 69 women will be diagnosed with cancer of the ovary during their lifetime; 0.62% of women will develop cancer of the ovary between their 50th and 70th birthdays.

Prevalence: On January 1, 2003, in the United States there were approximately 171,840 women alive who had a history of cancer of the ovary.

Cancer of the Pancreas

The American Cancer Society estimates that 33,730 men and women (17,150 men and 16,580 women) will be diagnosed with and 32,300 men and women will die of cancer of the pancreas in 2006.

Incidence and Mortality: From 2000–2003, the median age at diagnosis for cancer of the pancreas was 72 years of age. The age-adjusted incidence rate was 11.3 per 100,000 men and women per year. The median age at death for cancer of the pancreas was 73 years of age. The age-adjusted death rate was 10.5 per 100,000 men and women per year.

Survival and Stage: The overall 5-year relative survival rate for 1996–2002 from 17 SEER geographic areas was 5.0%. Five-year relative survival rates by race and sex were: 5.3% for white men; 4.6% for white women; 3.4% for black men; 5.5% for black women.

The stage distribution based on historic stage shows that 7% of pancreas cancer cases are diagnosed while the cancer is still confined to the primary site (localized stage); 26% are diagnosed after the cancer has spread to regional lymph nodes or directly beyond the primary site; 52% are diagnosed after the cancer has already metastasized (distant stage) and for the remaining 15% the staging information was unknown. The corresponding 5-year relative survival rates were: 19.6% for localized; 8.2% for regional; 1.9% for distant; and 3.7% for unstaged.

Lifetime Risk: Based on rates from 2001–2003, 1.27% of men and women born today will be diagnosed with cancer of the pancreas at some time during their lifetime. This number can also be expressed as 1 in 78 men and women will be diagnosed with cancer of the pancreas during their lifetime 0.50% of men will develop cancer of the pancreas between their 50th and 70th birthdays compared to 0.38% for women.

Cancer of the Prostate

The American Cancer Society estimates that 234,460 men will be diagnosed with and 27,350 men will die of cancer of the prostate in 2006.

Incidence and Mortality: From 2000–2003, the median age at diagnosis for cancer of the prostate was 68 years of age. The age-adjusted incidence rate was 170.3 per 100,000 men per year. The median age at death for cancer of the prostate was 80 years of age. The age-adjusted death rate was 28.5 per 100,000 men per year.

Survival and Stage: The overall 5-year relative survival rate for 1996–2002 from 17 SEER geographic areas was 99.9%. Five-year relative survival rates by race were: 99.9% for white men; 97.6% for black men.
The stage distribution based on historic stage shows that 91% of prostate cancer cases are diagnosed while the cancer is still confined to the primary site or after the cancer has spread to regional lymph nodes (localized or regional stage); 5% are diagnosed after the cancer has already metastasized (distant stage) and for the remaining 4% the staging information was unknown. The corresponding 5-year relative survival rates were: 100.0% for localized/regional; 33.3% for distant; and 79.5% for unstaged.

Lifetime Risk: Based on rates from 2001–2003, 17.12% of men born today will be diagnosed with cancer of the prostate at some time during their lifetime. This number can also be expressed as 1 in 6 men will be diagnosed with cancer of the prostate during their lifetime; 8.74% of men will develop cancer of the prostate between their 50th and 70th birthdays.

Prevalence: On January 1, 2003, in the United States there were approximately 1,937,807 men alive who had a history of cancer of the prostate.

Cancer of the Skin (Excluding Basal and Squamous)

The American Cancer Society estimates that 68,780 men and women (38,360 men and 30,420 women) will be diagnosed with and 10,710 men and women will die of cancer of the skin (excluding basal and squamous) in 2006.

Incidence and Mortality: From 2000–2003, the median age at diagnosis for cancer of the skin (excluding basal and squamous) was 59 years of age. The age-adjusted incidence rate was 20.0 per 100,000 men and women per year. The median age at death for cancer of the skin (excluding basal and squamous) was 70 years of age. The age-adjusted death rate was 3.5 per 100,000 men and women per year.

Survival and Stage: The overall 5-year relative survival rate for 1996–2002 from 17 SEER geographic areas was 91.2%. Five-year relative survival rates by race and sex were: 89.9% for white men; 93.1% for white women; 84.5% for black men; 88.2% for black women.

The stage distribution based on historic stage shows that 79% of skin cancer (excluding basal and squamous) cases are diagnosed while the cancer is still confined to the primary site (localized stage); 14% are diagnosed after the cancer has spread to regional lymph nodes or directly beyond the primary site; 4% are diagnosed after the cancer has already metastasized (distant stage) and for the remaining 4% the staging information was unknown. The corresponding 5-year relative survival rates were: 98.7% for localized; 68.8% for regional; 16.3% for distant; and 77.6% for unstaged.

Melanoma of the Skin

The American Cancer Society estimates that 62,190 men and women (34,260 men and 27,930 women) will be diagnosed with and 7,910 men and women will die of melanoma of the skin in 2006.

Incidence and Mortality: From 2000–2003, the median age at diagnosis for melanoma of the skin was 58 years of age. The age-adjusted incidence rate was 18.2 per 100,000 men and women per year. The median age at death for melanoma of the skin was 67 years of age. The age-adjusted death rate was 2.6 per 100,000 men and women per year.

Survival and Stage: The overall 5-year relative survival rate for 1996–2002 from 17 SEER geographic areas was 91.5%. Five-year relative survival rates by race and sex were: 90.3% for white men; 93.4% for white women; 67.4% for black men; 74.5% for black women.

The stage distribution based on historic stage shows that 80% of melanoma of the skin cases are diagnosed while the cancer is still confined to the primary site (localized stage); 12% are diagnosed after the cancer has spread to regional lymph nodes or directly beyond the primary site; 4% are diagnosed after the cancer has already metastasized (distant stage) and for the remaining 4% the staging information was unknown. The corresponding 5-year relative survival rates were: 99.0% for localized; 64.9% for regional; 15.3% for distant; and 76.8% for unstaged.

Lifetime Risk: Based on rates from 2001–2003, 1.68% of men and women born today will be diagnosed with melanoma of the skin at some time during their lifetime. This number can also be expressed as 1 in 59 men and women will be diagnosed with melanoma of the skin during their lifetime; 0.88% of men will develop melanoma of the skin between their 50th and 70th birthdays compared to 0.51% for women.

Prevalence: On January 1, 2003, in the United States there were approximately 662,433 men and women alive who had a history of melanoma of the skin—320,178 men and 342,255 women.

Cancer of Other Non-Epithelial Skin

The American Cancer Society estimates that 6,590 men and women (4,100 men and 2,490 women) will be diagnosed with and 2,800 men and women will die of cancer of other non-epithelial skin in 2006.

Incidence and Mortality: From 2000–2003, the median age at diagnosis for cancer of other non-epithelial skin was 69 years of age. The age-adjusted incidence rate was 1.8 per 100,000 men and women per year. The median age at death for cancer of other non-epithelial skin was 75 years of age. The age-adjusted death rate was 0.8 per 100,000 men and women per year.

Survival and Stage: The overall 5-year relative survival rate for 1996–2002 from 17 SEER geographic areas was 88.1%. Five-year relative survival rates by race and sex were: 85.2% for white men; 89.0% for white women; 95.7% for black men; 96.6% for black women.

The stage distribution based on historic stage shows that 59% of other non-epithelial skin cancer cases are diagnosed while the cancer is still confined to the primary site (localized stage); 27% are diagnosed after the cancer has spread to regional lymph nodes or directly beyond the primary site; 3% are diagnosed after the cancer has already metastasized (distant stage) and for the remaining 11%

the staging information was unknown. The corresponding 5-year relative survival rates were: 93.0% for localized; 85.8% for regional; 29.2% for distant; and 79.2% for unstaged.

Cancer of the Small Intestine

The American Cancer Society estimates that 6,170 men and women (3,160 men and 3,010 women) will be diagnosed with and 1,070 men and women will die of cancer of the small intestine in 2006.

Incidence and Mortality: From 2000–2003, the median age at diagnosis for cancer of the small intestine was 67 years of age. The age-adjusted incidence rate was 1.8 per 100,000 men and women per year. The median age at death for cancer of the small intestine was 72 years of age. The age-adjusted death rate was 0.4 per 100,000 men and women per year.

Survival and Stage: The overall 5-year relative survival rate for 1996–2002 from 17 SEER geographic areas was 56.2%. Five-year relative survival rates by race and sex were: 57.3% for white men; 58.6% for white women; 48.3% for black men; 52.3% for black women.

The stage distribution based on historic stage shows that 30% of small intestine cancer cases are diagnosed while the cancer is still confined to the primary site (localized stage); 33% are diagnosed after the cancer has spread to regional lymph nodes or directly beyond the primary site; 29% are diagnosed after the cancer has already metastasized (distant stage) and for the remaining 7% the staging information was unknown. The corresponding 5-year relative survival rates were: 77.2% for localized; 61.3% for regional; 33.1% for distant; and 35.5% for unstaged.

Cancer of the Soft Tissue including Heart

The American Cancer Society estimates that 9,530 men and women (5,720 men and 3,810 women) will be diagnosed with and 3,500 men and women will die of cancer of the soft tissue including heart in 2006.

Incidence and Mortality: From 2000–2003, the median age at diagnosis for cancer of the soft tissue including heart was 56 years of age. The age-adjusted incidence rate was 3.0 per 100,000 men and women per year. The median age at death for cancer of the soft tissue including heart was 65 years of age. The age-adjusted death rate was 1.3 per 100,000 men and women per year.

Survival and Stage: The overall 5-year relative survival rate for 1996–2002 from 17 SEER geographic areas was 66.4%. Five-year relative survival rates by race and sex were: 68.0% for white men; 66.2% for white women; 59.4% for black men; 60.6% for black women.

The stage distribution based on historic stage shows that 53% of soft tissue including heart cancer cases are diagnosed while the cancer is still confined to the primary site (localized stage); 25% are diagnosed after the cancer has spread to regional lymph nodes or directly beyond the primary site; 15% are diagnosed after the cancer has already metastasized (distant stage) and for the remaining 7% the staging information was unknown. The corresponding 5-year relative survival rates were: 84.1% for localized; 61.5% for regional; 16.3% for distant; and 54.3% for unstaged.

Cancer of the Stomach

The American Cancer Society estimates that 22,280 men and women (13,400 men and 8,880 women) will be diagnosed with and 11,430 men and women will die of cancer of the stomach in 2006.

Incidence and Mortality: From 2000–2003, the median age at diagnosis for cancer of the stomach was 71 years of age. The age-adjusted incidence rate was 8.1 per 100,000 men and women per year. The median age at death for cancer of the stomach was 74 years of age. The age-adjusted death rate was 4.3 per 100,000 men and women per year.

Survival and Stage: The overall 5-year relative survival rate for 1996–2002 from 17 SEER geographic areas was 23.9%. Five-year relative survival rates by race and sex were: 20.9% for white men; 23.9% for white women; 20.5% for black men; 26.4% for black women.

The stage distribution based on historic stage shows that 23% of stomach cancer cases are diagnosed while the cancer is still confined to the primary site (localized stage); 31% are diagnosed after the cancer has spread to regional lymph nodes or directly beyond the primary site; 33% are diagnosed after the cancer has already metastasized (distant stage) and for the remaining 12% the staging information was unknown. The corresponding 5-year relative survival rates were: 61.9% for localized; 22.2% for regional; 3.4% for distant; and 13.0% for unstaged.

Cancer of the Testis

The American Cancer Society estimates that 8,250 men will be diagnosed with and 370 men will die of cancer of the testis in 2006.

Incidence and Mortality: From 2000–2003, the median age at diagnosis for cancer of the testis was 34 years of age. The age-adjusted incidence rate was 5.3 per 100,000 men per year. The median age at death for cancer of the testis was 40 years of age. The age-adjusted death rate was 0.3 per 100,000 men per year.

Survival and Stage: The overall 5-year relative survival rate for 1996–2002 from 17 SEER geographic areas was 95.7%. Five-year relative survival rates by race were: 95.9% for white men; 90.0% for black men.

The stage distribution based on historic stage shows that 70% of testis cancer cases are diagnosed while the cancer is still confined to the primary site (localized stage); 18% are diagnosed after the cancer has spread to regional lymph nodes or directly beyond the primary site; 11% are diagnosed after the cancer has already metastasized (distant stage) and for the remaining 1% the staging information was unknown. The corresponding 5-year relative survival rates were: 99.5% for localized; 96.3% for regional; 70.1% for distant; and 87.5% for unstaged.

Cancer of the Thyroid

The American Cancer Society estimates that 30,180 men and women (7,590 men and 22,590 women) will be diagnosed with and 1,500 men and women will die of cancer of the thyroid in 2006.

Incidence and Mortality: From 2000–2003, the median age at diagnosis for cancer of the thyroid was 47 years of age. The age-adjusted incidence rate was 8.2 per 100,000 men and women per year. The median age at death for cancer of the thyroid was 73 years of age. The age-adjusted death rate was 0.5 per 100,000 men and women per year.

Survival and Stage: The overall 5-year relative survival rate for 1996–2002 from 17 SEER geographic areas was 96.7%. Five-year relative survival rates by race and sex were: 94.8% for white men; 97.6% for white women; 89.1% for black men; 95.3% for black women.

The stage distribution based on historic stage shows that 58% of thyroid cancer cases are diagnosed while the cancer is still confined to the primary site (localized stage); 34% are diagnosed after the cancer has spread to regional lymph nodes or directly beyond the primary site; 5% are diagnosed after the cancer has already metastasized (distant stage) and for the remaining 3% the staging information was unknown. The corresponding 5-year relative survival rates were:

99.7% for localized; 96.9% for regional; 56.4% for distant; and 87.0% for unstaged.

Cancer of the Urinary Bladder

The American Cancer Society estimates that 61,420 men and women (44,690 men and 16,730 women) will be diagnosed with and 13,060 men and women will die of cancer of the urinary bladder in 2006.

Incidence and Mortality: From 2000–2003, the median age at diagnosis for cancer of the urinary bladder was 73 years of age. The age-adjusted incidence rate was 20.9 per 100,000 men and women per year. The median age at death for cancer of the urinary bladder was 78 years of age. The age-adjusted death rate was 4.3 per 100,000 men and women per year.

Survival and Stage: The overall 5-year relative survival rate for 1996–2002 from 17 SEER geographic areas was 80.8%. Five-year relative survival rates by race and sex were: 83.6% for white men; 76.8% for white women; 68.9% for black men; 53.9% for black women.

The stage distribution based on historic stage shows that 74% of urinary bladder cancer cases are diagnosed while the cancer is still confined to the primary site (localized stage); 19% are diagnosed after the cancer has spread to regional lymph nodes or directly beyond the primary site; 4% are diagnosed after the cancer has already metastasized (distant stage) and for the remaining 3% the staging information was unknown. The corresponding 5-year relative survival rates were: 93.7% for localized; 46.0% for regional; 6.2% for distant; and 60.4% for unstaged.

Lifetime Risk: Based on rates from 2001–2003, 2.30% of men and women born today will be diagnosed with cancer of the urinary bladder at some time during their lifetime. This number can also be expressed as 1 in 43 men and women will be diagnosed with cancer of the urinary bladder during their lifetime; 1.22% of men will develop cancer of the urinary bladder between their 50th and 70th birthdays compared to 0.35% for women.

Prevalence: On January 1, 2003, in the United States there were approximately 505,765 men and women alive who had a history of cancer of the urinary bladder—372,313 men and 133,452 women.

Cancer of the Vulva

The American Cancer Society estimates that 3,740 women will be diagnosed with and 880 women will die of cancer of the vulva in 2006.

Incidence and Mortality: From 2000–2003, the median age at diagnosis for cancer of the vulva was 69 years of age. The age-adjusted incidence rate was 2.2 per 100,000 women per year. The median age at death for cancer of the vulva was 79 years of age. The age-adjusted death rate was 0.4 per 100,000 women per year.

Survival and Stage: The overall 5-year relative survival rate for 1996–2002 from 17 SEER geographic areas was 78.1%. Five-year relative survival rates by race were: 78.1% for white women; 76.3% for black women.

The stage distribution based on historic stage shows that 61% of vulva cancer cases are diagnosed while the cancer is still confined to the primary site (localized stage); 28% are diagnosed after the cancer has spread to regional lymph nodes or directly beyond the primary site; 4% are diagnosed after the cancer has already metastasized (distant stage) and for the remaining 6% the staging information was unknown. The corresponding 5-year relative survival rates were: 93.2% for localized; 55.1% for regional; 18.0% for distant; and 59.8% for unstaged.

Chapter 18

Cancer of the Lip and Oral Cavity

Lip and oral cavity cancer is a disease in which malignant (cancer) cells form in the lips or mouth. The oral cavity includes the following:

- The front two thirds of the tongue
- The gingiva (gums)
- The buccal mucosa (the lining of the inside of the cheeks)
- The floor (bottom) of the mouth under the tongue
- The hard palate (the roof of the mouth)
- The retromolar trigone (the small area behind the wisdom teeth)

Most lip and oral cavity cancers start in squamous cells, the thin, flat cells that line the lips and oral cavity. These are called squamous cell carcinomas. Cancer cells may spread into deeper tissue as the cancer grows. Squamous cell carcinoma usually develops in areas of leukoplakia (white patches of cells that do not rub off).

Tobacco and alcohol use can affect the risk of developing lip and oral cavity cancer. Risk factors for lip and oral cavity cancer include the following:

- Using tobacco products
- Heavy alcohol use

PDQ® Cancer Information Summary. National Cancer Institute; Bethesda, MD. Lip and Oral Cavity Cancer (PDQ®): Treatment - Patient. Updated 07/2005. Available at: http://cancer.gov. Accessed July 14, 2006.

- Being exposed to sunlight
- Being male
- Being infected with human papillomavirus (HPV)

Possible signs of lip and oral cavity cancer include a sore or lump on the lips or in the mouth. These and other symptoms may be caused by lip and oral cavity cancer. Other conditions may cause the same symptoms. A doctor should be consulted if any of the following problems occur:

- A sore on the lip or in the mouth that does not heal
- A lump or thickening on the lips or gums or in the mouth
- A white or red patch on the gums, tongue, tonsils, or lining of the mouth
- Bleeding, pain, or numbness in the lip or mouth

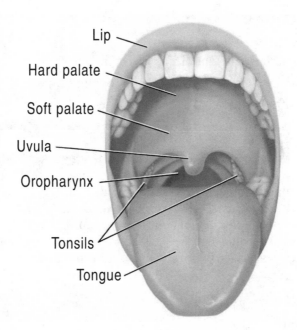

Figure 18.1. *This picture shows the parts of the mouth and throat (Source: From "What You Need to Know about™ Oral Cancer," National Cancer Institute, July 2005).*

- Change in voice
- Loose teeth or dentures that no longer fit well
- Trouble chewing or swallowing or moving the tongue or jaw
- Swelling of jaw
- Sore throat or feeling that something is caught in the throat

Lip and oral cavity cancer may not have any symptoms and is sometimes found during a regular dental exam.

Tests that examine the mouth and throat are used to detect (find), diagnose, and stage lip and oral cavity cancer. In addition to a physical exam of the lips and oral cavity, the following tests and procedures may be used:

- **Endoscopy:** A procedure to look at organs and tissues inside the body to check for abnormal areas. An endoscope (a thin, lighted

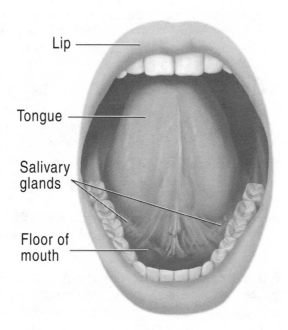

Figure 18.2. This picture shows the area under the tongue (Source: From "What You Need to Know about™ Oral Cancer," National Cancer Institute, July 2005).

tube) is inserted through an incision (cut) in the skin or opening in the body, such as the mouth. Tissue samples and lymph nodes may be taken for biopsy.

- **X-rays of the head, neck, and chest:** An x-ray is a type of energy beam that can go through the body and onto film, making a picture of areas inside the body.

- **Biopsy:** The removal of cells or tissues so they can be viewed under a microscope by a pathologist. If leukoplakia is found, cells taken from the patches are also checked under the microscope for signs of cancer.

- **MRI (magnetic resonance imaging):** A procedure that uses a magnet, radio waves, and a computer to make a series of detailed pictures of areas inside the body. This procedure is also called nuclear magnetic resonance imaging (NMRI).

- **CT scan (CAT scan):** A procedure that makes a series of detailed pictures of areas inside the body, taken from different angles. The pictures are made by a computer linked to an x-ray machine. A dye may be injected into a vein or swallowed to help the organs or tissues show up more clearly. This procedure is also called computed tomography, computerized tomography, or computerized axial tomography.

- **Exfoliative cytology:** A procedure to collect cells from the lip or oral cavity. A piece of cotton, a brush, or a small wooden stick is used to gently scrape cells from the lips, tongue, mouth, or throat. The cells are viewed under a microscope to find out if they are abnormal.

- **Barium swallow:** A series of x-rays of the esophagus and stomach. The patient drinks a liquid that contains barium (a silver-white metallic compound). The liquid coats the esophagus and x-rays are taken. This procedure is also called an upper GI series.

- **PET scan (positron emission tomography scan):** A procedure to find malignant tumor cells in the body. A small amount of radionuclide glucose (sugar) is injected into a vein. The PET scanner rotates around the body and makes a picture of where glucose is being used in the body. Malignant tumor cells show up brighter in the picture because they are more active and take up more glucose than normal cells do.

Certain factors affect prognosis (chance of recovery) and treatment options. Prognosis (chance of recovery) depends on the following:

- The stage of the cancer

- Where the tumor is in the lip or oral cavity

- Whether the cancer has spread to blood vessels

For patients who smoke, the chance of recovery is better if they stop smoking before beginning radiation therapy.

Patients who have had lip and oral cavity cancer have an increased risk of developing a second cancer in the head or neck. Frequent and careful follow-up is important. Clinical trials are studying the use of retinoid drugs to reduce the risk of a second head and neck cancer. Information about ongoing clinical trials is available from the National Cancer Institute (NCI)'s website (http://www.cancer .gov).

Stages of Lip and Oral Cavity Cancer

After lip and oral cavity cancer has been diagnosed, tests are done to find out if cancer cells have spread within the lip and oral cavity or to other parts of the body. The process used to find out if cancer has spread within the lip and oral cavity or to other parts of the body is called staging. The information gathered from the staging process determines the stage of the disease. It is important to know the stage in order to plan treatment. The results of the tests used to diagnose lip and oral cavity cancer are also used to stage the disease.

The following stages are used for lip and oral cavity cancer:

Stage 0 (carcinoma in situ): In stage 0, cancer is found only in the layer of cells lining the lips and oral cavity. Stage 0 cancer is also called carcinoma in situ.

Stage I: In stage I, the tumor is two centimeters or smaller and cancer has not spread to the lymph nodes.

Stage II: In stage II, the tumor is larger than two centimeters but not larger than four centimeters and cancer has not spread to the lymph nodes.

Stage III: In stage III, the tumor:

219

- may be any size and has spread to a single lymph node that is three centimeters or smaller, on the same side of the neck as the cancer; or

- is larger than four centimeters.

Stage IV: Stage IV is divided into stages IVA, IVB, and IVC as follows:

- In stage IVA, the tumor:

  - has spread to nearby tissues in the lip and oral cavity; or

  - is any size and may have spread to nearby tissues in the lip and oral cavity. Cancer has spread to one or more lymph nodes on one or both sides of the neck, and the involved lymph nodes are six centimeters or smaller.

- In stage IVB, the tumor:

  - may be any size and has spread to one or more lymph nodes that are larger than six centimeters; or

  - has spread to the muscles or bones in the oral cavity, or to the base or the skull and/or the carotid artery. Cancer may have spread to one or more lymph nodes on one or both sides of the neck.

- In stage IVC, the tumor has spread beyond the lip and oral cavity to other parts of the body. The tumor may be any size and may have spread to the lymph nodes.

Recurrent lip and oral cavity cancer: Recurrent lip and oral cavity cancer is cancer that has recurred (come back) after it has been treated. The cancer may come back in the lip or mouth or in other parts of the body.

Treatment Option Overview

Different types of treatment are available for patients with lip and oral cavity cancer. Some treatments are standard (the currently used treatment), and some are being tested in clinical trials. Before starting treatment, patients may want to think about taking part in a clinical trial. A treatment clinical trial is a research study meant to help improve current treatments or obtain information on new treatments for patients with cancer. When clinical trials show that a new treatment is better than the standard treatment, the new treatment may become the standard treatment.

Clinical trials are taking place in many parts of the country. Information about ongoing clinical trials is available from the NCI website. Choosing the most appropriate cancer treatment is a decision that ideally involves the patient, family, and health care team.

Patients with lip and oral cavity cancer should have their treatment planned by a team of doctors who are expert in treating head and neck cancer. Treatment will be overseen by a medical oncologist, a doctor who specializes in treating people with cancer. Because the lips and oral cavity are important for breathing, eating, and talking, patients may need special help adjusting to the side effects of the cancer and its treatment. The medical oncologist may refer the patient to other health professionals with special training in the treatment of patients with head and neck cancer. These include the following:

- Head and neck surgeon
- Radiation oncologist
- Dentist
- Speech therapist
- Dietitian
- Psychologist
- Rehabilitation specialist
- Plastic surgeon

Standard Treatment

Surgery: Surgery (removing the cancer in an operation) is a common treatment for all stages of lip and oral cavity cancer. Surgery may include the following:

- **Wide local excision:** Removal of the cancer and some of the healthy tissue around it. If cancer has spread into bone, surgery may include removal of the involved bone tissue.

- **Neck dissection:** Removal of lymph nodes and other tissues in the neck. This is done when cancer may have spread from the lip and oral cavity.

- **Plastic surgery:** An operation that restores or improves the appearance of parts of the body. Dental implants, a skin graft, or other plastic surgery may be needed to repair parts of the mouth, throat, or neck after removal of large tumors.

Even if the doctor removes all the cancer that can be seen at the time of the surgery, some patients may be given chemotherapy or radiation therapy after surgery to kill any cancer cells that are left. Treatment given after the surgery, to increase the chances of a cure, is called adjuvant therapy.

Radiation therapy: Radiation therapy is a cancer treatment that uses high-energy x-rays or other types of radiation to kill cancer cells. There are two types of radiation therapy. External radiation therapy uses a machine outside the body to send radiation toward the cancer. Internal radiation therapy uses a radioactive substance sealed in needles, seeds, wires, or catheters that are placed directly into or near the cancer. The way the radiation therapy is given depends on the type and stage of the cancer being treated.

For patients who smoke, radiation therapy works better when smoking is stopped before beginning treatment. It is also important for patients to have a dental exam before radiation therapy begins, so that existing problems can be treated.

New Treatments

New types of treatment are being tested in clinical trials. This summary section refers to specific treatments under study in clinical trials, but it may not mention every new treatment being studied. Information about ongoing clinical trials is available from the NCI website. New treatments include the following:

- **Chemotherapy:** Chemotherapy is a cancer treatment that uses drugs to stop the growth of cancer cells, either by killing the cells or by stopping the cells from dividing. When chemotherapy is taken by mouth or injected into a vein or muscle, the drugs enter the bloodstream and can reach cancer cells throughout the body (systemic chemotherapy). When chemotherapy is placed directly into the spinal column, an organ, or a body cavity such as the abdomen, the drugs mainly affect cancer cells in those areas (regional chemo-therapy). The way the chemotherapy is given depends on the type and stage of the cancer being treated.

- **Hyperfractionated radiation therapy:** Hyperfractionated radiation therapy is radiation treatment in which each day's total dose of radiation is divided into two or more, smaller doses, usually given hours apart, instead of giving it all at once. This is also called superfractionated radiation therapy.

- **Hyperthermia therapy:** Hyperthermia therapy is a treatment in which body tissue is heated above normal temperature to damage and kill cancer cells or to make cancer cells more sensitive to the effects of radiation and certain anticancer drugs.

Treatment Options by Stage

Stage I lip and oral cavity cancer: Treatment of stage I lip and oral cavity cancer depends on where cancer is found in the lip and oral cavity.

If cancer is in the lip, treatment may include the following:

- Surgery (wide local excision)
- Internal radiation therapy with or without external radiation therapy

If cancer is in the front of the tongue, treatment may include the following:

- Surgery (wide local excision)
- Internal radiation therapy with or without external radiation therapy
- Radiation therapy to lymph nodes in the neck

If cancer is in the buccal mucosa (the lining of the inside of the cheeks), treatment may include the following:

- Surgery (wide local excision) for tumors smaller than one centimeter, with or without internal and/or external radiation therapy
- Surgery (wide local excision with skin graft) or radiation therapy for larger tumors

If cancer is in the floor (bottom) of the mouth, treatment may include the following:

- Surgery (wide local excision) for tumors smaller than one half centimeter
- Surgery (wide local excision) or radiation therapy for larger tumors

If cancer is in the lower gingiva (gums), treatment may include the following:

- Surgery (wide local excision, which may include removing part of the jawbone, and skin graft)
- Radiation therapy with or without surgery

If cancer is in the retromolar trigone (the small area behind the wisdom teeth), treatment may include the following:

- Surgery (wide local excision, which may include removing part of the jawbone)
- Radiation therapy with or without surgery

If cancer is in the upper gingiva (gums) or the hard palate (the roof of the mouth), treatment is usually surgery (wide local excision) with or without radiation therapy.

Stage II lip and oral cavity cancer: Treatment of stage II lip and oral cavity cancer depends on where cancer is found in the lip and oral cavity.

If cancer is in the lip, treatment may include the following:

- Surgery (wide local excision)
- External radiation therapy and/or internal radiation therapy

If cancer is in the front of the tongue, treatment may include the following:

- Radiation therapy and/or surgery (wide local excision)
- Internal radiation therapy with surgery (neck dissection)

If cancer is in the buccal mucosa (the lining of the inside of the cheeks), treatment may include the following:

- Radiation therapy for tumors that are three centimeters or smaller
- Surgery (wide local excision) and/or radiation therapy for larger tumors

If cancer is in the floor (bottom) of the mouth, treatment may include the following:

- Surgery (wide local excision)
- Radiation therapy
- Surgery (wide local excision) followed by external radiation therapy, with or without internal radiation therapy, for large tumors

If cancer is in the lower gingiva (gums), treatment may include the following:

- Surgery (wide local excision, which may include removing part of the jawbone, and a skin graft)
- Radiation therapy alone or after surgery

If cancer is in the retromolar trigone (the small area behind the wisdom teeth), treatment may include the following:

- Surgery (wide local excision, which includes removing part of the jawbone)
- Radiation therapy with or without surgery

If cancer is in the upper gingiva (gums) or the hard palate (the roof of the mouth), treatment may include the following:

- Surgery (wide local excision) with or without radiation therapy
- Radiation therapy alone

Stage III lip and oral cavity cancer: Treatment of stage III lip and oral cavity cancer depends on where cancer is found in the lip and oral cavity.

If cancer is in the lip, treatment may include the following:

- Surgery and external radiation therapy with or without internal radiation therapy
- A clinical trial of chemotherapy before or after surgery
- A clinical trial of chemotherapy and radiation therapy
- A clinical trial of hyperfractionated radiation therapy

If cancer is in the front of the tongue, treatment may include the following:

- External radiation therapy with or without internal radiation therapy

- Surgery (wide local excision) followed by radiation therapy
- A clinical trial of chemotherapy and radiation therapy
- A clinical trial of hyperfractionated radiation therapy

If cancer is in the buccal mucosa (the lining of the inside of the cheeks), treatment may include the following:

- Surgery (wide local excision) with or without radiation therapy
- Radiation therapy
- A clinical trial of chemotherapy before or after surgery
- A clinical trial of chemotherapy and radiation therapy
- A clinical trial of hyperfractionated radiation therapy

If cancer is in the floor (bottom) of the mouth, treatment may include the following:

- Surgery (wide local excision, which may include removing part of the jawbone, with or without neck dissection)
- External radiation therapy with or without internal radiation therapy
- A clinical trial of chemotherapy before or after surgery
- A clinical trial of chemotherapy and radiation therapy
- A clinical trial of hyperfractionated radiation therapy

If cancer is in the lower gingiva (gums), treatment may include the following:

- Surgery (wide local excision) with or without radiation therapy. Radiation may be given before or after surgery
- A clinical trial of chemotherapy and radiation therapy
- A clinical trial of hyperfractionated radiation therapy

If cancer is in the retromolar trigone (the small area behind the wisdom teeth), treatment may include the following:

- Surgery to remove the tumor, lymph nodes, and part of the jawbone, with or without radiation therapy
- A clinical trial of chemotherapy before or after surgery

- A clinical trial of chemotherapy and radiation therapy
- A clinical trial of hyperfractionated radiation therapy

If cancer is in the upper gingiva (gums), treatment may include the following:

- Radiation therapy
- Surgery (wide local excision) and radiation therapy
- A clinical trial of chemotherapy and radiation therapy
- A clinical trial of hyperfractionated radiation therapy

If cancer is in the hard palate (the roof of the mouth), treatment may include the following:

- Radiation therapy
- Surgery (wide local excision) with or without radiation therapy
- A clinical trial of chemotherapy and radiation therapy
- A clinical trial of hyperfractionated radiation therapy

For cancer that may have spread to lymph nodes, treatment may include the following:

- Radiation therapy and/or surgery (neck dissection)
- A clinical trial of chemotherapy and radiation therapy
- A clinical trial of hyperfractionated radiation therapy

Stage IV lip and oral cavity cancer: Treatment of stage IV lip and oral cavity cancer depends on where cancer is found in the lip and oral cavity.

If cancer is in the lip, treatment may include the following:

- Surgery and external radiation therapy with or without internal radiation therapy
- A clinical trial of chemotherapy and radiation therapy
- A clinical trial of chemotherapy before or after surgery
- A clinical trial of hyperfractionated radiation therapy

If cancer is in the front of the tongue, treatment may include the following:

- Surgery to remove the tongue and sometimes the larynx (voice box) with or without radiation therapy
- Radiation therapy as palliative therapy to relieve symptoms and improve quality of life
- A clinical trial of chemotherapy and radiation therapy
- A clinical trial of chemotherapy before or after surgery
- A clinical trial of hyperfractionated radiation therapy

If cancer is in the buccal mucosa (the lining of the inside of the cheeks), treatment may include the following:

- Surgery (wide local excision) and/or radiation therapy
- A clinical trial of chemotherapy and radiation therapy
- A clinical trial of chemotherapy before or after surgery
- A clinical trial of hyperfractionated radiation therapy

If cancer is in the floor (bottom) of the mouth, treatment may include the following:

- Surgery before or after radiation therapy
- A clinical trial of chemotherapy and radiation therapy
- A clinical trial of chemotherapy before or after surgery
- A clinical trial of hyperfractionated radiation therapy

If cancer is in the lower gingiva (gums), treatment may include the following:

- Surgery and/or radiation therapy
- A clinical trial of chemotherapy and radiation therapy
- A clinical trial of chemotherapy before or after surgery
- A clinical trial of hyperfractionated radiation therapy

If cancer is in the retromolar trigone (the small area behind the wisdom teeth), treatment may include the following:

- Surgery to remove the tumor, lymph nodes, and part of the jawbone, followed by radiation therapy
- A clinical trial of chemotherapy and radiation therapy

- A clinical trial of chemotherapy before or after surgery
- A clinical trial of hyperfractionated radiation therapy

If cancer is in the upper gingiva (gums) or hard palate (the roof of the mouth), treatment may include the following:

- Surgery with radiation therapy
- A clinical trial of chemotherapy and radiation therapy
- A clinical trial of chemotherapy before or after surgery
- A clinical trial of hyperfractionated radiation therapy

For cancer that may have spread to lymph nodes, treatment may include the following:

- Radiation therapy and/or surgery (neck dissection)
- A clinical trial of chemotherapy and radiation therapy
- A clinical trial of chemotherapy before or after surgery
- A clinical trial of hyperfractionated radiation therapy

Treatment options for recurrent lip and oral cavity cancer: Treatment of recurrent lip and oral cavity cancer may include the following:

- Surgery, if radiation therapy was used before
- Surgery and/or radiation therapy, if surgery was used before
- A clinical trial of chemotherapy with or without radiation therapy
- A clinical trial of hyperthermia therapy

Chapter 19

Paranasal Sinus and Nasal Cavity Cancer

Cancer of the paranasal sinus and nasal cavity is a disease in which cancer (malignant) cells are found in the tissues of the paranasal sinuses or nasal cavity. The paranasal sinuses are small hollow spaces around the nose. The sinuses are lined with cells that make mucus, which keeps the nose from drying out; the sinuses are also a space through which the voice can echo to make sounds when a person talks or sings. The nasal cavity is the passageway just behind the nose through which air passes on the way to the throat during breathing. The area inside the nose is called the nasal vestibule.

There are several paranasal sinuses, including the frontal sinuses above the nose, the maxillary sinuses in the upper part of either side of the upper jawbone, the ethmoid sinuses just behind either side of the upper nose, and the sphenoid sinus behind the ethmoid sinus in the center of the skull.

Cancer of the paranasal sinus and nasal cavity most commonly starts in the cells that line the oropharynx. Much less often, cancer of the paranasal sinus and nasal cavity starts in the color-making cells called melanocytes, and is called a melanoma. If the cancer starts in the muscle or connecting tissue, it is called a sarcoma. Another type of cancer that can occur here, but grows more slowly, is called an inverting papilloma. Cancers called midline granulomas may also occur

PDQ® Cancer Information Summary. National Cancer Institute; Bethesda, MD. Paranasal Sinus and Nasal Cavity Cancer (PDQ®): Treatment - Patient. Updated 07/2005. Available at: http://cancer.gov. Accessed April 30, 2006.

in the paranasal sinuses or nasal cavity, and they cause the tissue around them to break down.

A doctor should be seen for any of the following problems:

- Blocked sinuses that do not clear
- A sinus infection
- Nosebleeds
- A lump or sore that doesn't heal inside the nose
- Frequent headaches or sinus pain
- Swelling or other trouble with the eyes
- Pain in the upper teeth
- Dentures that no longer fit well

If there are symptoms, a doctor will examine the nose using a mirror and lights. The doctor may order a CT scan (a special x-ray that uses a computer) or an MRI scan (an x-ray-like procedure that uses magnetic energy) to make a picture of the inside of parts of the body. A special instrument (called a rhinoscope or a nasoscope) may be put into the nose to see inside. If tissue that is not normal is found, the doctor will need to cut out a small piece and look at it under the microscope to see if there are any cancer cells. This is called a biopsy. Sometimes the doctor will need to cut into the sinus to do a biopsy.

The chance of recovery (prognosis) depends on where the cancer is in the sinuses, whether the cancer is just in the area where it started or has spread to other tissues (the stage), and the patient's general state of health.

Stage Explanation

Once cancer of the paranasal sinus and nasal cavity is found, more tests will be done to find out if cancer cells have spread to other parts of the body. This is called staging. It is important to know the stage of the disease to plan treatment. Staging systems have been established for the most common paranasal sinus cavity cancers.

Stages of Cancer of Maxillary Sinus

The following stages are used for maxillary sinus cancer:

Stage 0: In stage 0, cancer is found in the innermost lining of the maxillary sinus only. Stage 0 cancer is also called carcinoma in situ.

Stage I: In stage I, cancer is found in the mucous membranes of the maxillary sinus.

Stage II: In stage II, cancer has spread to bone around the maxillary sinus, including the roof of the mouth and the nose, but not to bones at the back of the maxillary sinus or the base of the skull.

Stage III: In stage III, cancer is found in any of the following places: bone at the back of the maxillary sinus; tissues under the skin; the eye socket; the base of the skull; the ethmoid sinuses.

Or, cancer is found in one lymph node on the same side of the neck as the cancer, and the lymph node is three centimeters or smaller; cancer also is found in any of the following places: the maxillary sinus; bones around the maxillary sinus; tissues under the skin; the eye socket; the base of the skull; the ethmoid sinuses.

Stage IV: Stage IV is divided into stages IVA, IVB, and IVC.

Stage IVA: In stage IVA, cancer has spread to either one lymph node on the same side of the neck as the cancer and the lymph node is larger than three centimeters but smaller than six centimeters; or, cancer has spread to more than one lymph node anywhere in the neck, and all are six centimeters or smaller; cancer is also found in any of the following areas: the maxillary sinus; bones around the maxillary sinus; tissues under the skin; the eye socket; the base of the skull; the ethmoid sinuses.

Or, cancer is found in one or more lymph nodes in the neck, none larger than six centimeters, and in any of the following areas: the front of the eye; the skin of the cheek; the base of the skull; behind the jaw; the bone between the eyes; the sphenoid or frontal sinuses.

Stage IVB: In stage IVB, cancer has spread to either:

- one or more lymph nodes larger than 6 centimeters; or
- the back of the eye, the brain, the base and middle parts of the skull, nerves in the head, and/or the upper part of the throat behind the nose; cancer may also be found in one or more lymph nodes.

Stage IVC: In stage IVC, cancer has spread to other parts of the body.

Stages of Cancer of Nasal Cavity and Ethmoid Sinus

The following stages are used for nasal cavity and ethmoid sinus cancer:

Stage 0: In stage 0, cancer is found in the innermost lining of the nasal cavity or ethmoid sinus only. Stage 0 cancer is also called carcinoma in situ.

Stage I: In stage 1, cancer is found in only one area (of either the nasal cavity or the ethmoid sinus) and may have spread into bone.

Stage II: In stage II, cancer is found in two areas (of either the nasal cavity or the ethmoid sinus) or has spread to a nearby area; the cancer may have spread into bone.

Stage III: In stage III, cancer is found in any of the following places: the eye socket; the maxillary sinus; the roof of the mouth; the bone between the eyes.

Or, cancer is found in a single lymph node on the same side of the neck as the cancer and the lymph node is three centimeters or smaller; cancer also is found in any of the following places: the nasal cavity or ethmoid sinus; the eye socket; the maxillary sinus; the roof of the mouth; the bone between the eyes.

Stage IV: Stage IV is divided into stages IVA, IVB, and IVC.

Stage IVA: In stage IVA, cancer has spread to either one lymph node on the same side of the neck as the cancer and the lymph node is larger than three centimeters but smaller than six centimeters; or, cancer has spread to more than one lymph node anywhere in the neck, and all are six centimeters or smaller; cancer is also found in any of the following places: the nasal cavity or ethmoid sinus; the eye socket; the maxillary sinus; the roof of the mouth; the bone between the eyes.

Or, cancer is found in one or more lymph nodes in the neck, and the lymph nodes are six centimeters or smaller; cancer is also found in any of the following areas: the front of the eye; the skin of the nose or cheek; front parts of the skull; the base of the skull; the sphenoid or frontal sinuses.

Stage IVB: In stage IVB, cancer is found in any of the following areas:

- The back of the eye
- The brain
- The middle parts of the skull
- Nerves in the head
- The upper part of the throat behind the nose
- The base of the skull

Cancer may also be found in one or more lymph nodes or in a lymph node that is larger than six centimeters.

Stage IVC: In stage IVC, cancer has spread to other parts of the body.

Recurrent: Recurrent disease means that the cancer has come back (recurred) after it has been treated. It may come back in the paranasal sinuses or nasal cavity or in another part of the body.

Treatment Option Overview

There are treatments for all patients with cancer of the paranasal sinus and nasal cavity. Three kinds of treatment are used:

- Surgery (taking out the cancer)
- Radiation therapy (using high-dose x-rays or other high-energy rays to kill cancer cells)
- Chemotherapy (using drugs to kill cancer cells)

Surgery is commonly used to remove cancers of the paranasal sinus or nasal cavity. Depending on where the cancer is and how far it has spread, a doctor may need to cut out bone or tissue around the cancer. If cancer has spread to lymph nodes in the neck, the lymph nodes may be removed (lymph node dissection).

Radiation therapy is also a common treatment of cancer of the paranasal sinus and nasal cavity. Radiation therapy uses high-energy x-rays to kill cancer cells and shrink tumors. Radiation may come from a machine outside the body (external radiation therapy) or from putting materials that produce radiation (radioisotopes) through thin plastic tubes in the area where the cancer cells are found (internal radiation therapy). External radiation to the thyroid or the pituitary gland may change the way the thyroid gland works. The doctor may wish to test the thyroid gland before and after therapy to make sure it is working properly.

Chemotherapy uses drugs to kill cancer cells. Chemotherapy may be taken by pill, or it may be put into the body by a needle in a vein or muscle. Chemotherapy is called a systemic treatment because the drug enters the bloodstream, travels through the body, and can kill cancer cells throughout the body.

Because the paranasal sinuses and nasal cavity help in talking and breathing, and are close to the face, patients may need special help adjusting to the side effects of the cancer and its treatment. A doctor will consult with several kinds of doctors who can help determine the best treatment. Trained medical staff can also help in recovery from treatment. Patients may need plastic surgery if a large amount of tissue or bone around the paranasal sinuses or nasal cavity is taken out.

Treatment by Stage

Treatment of cancer of the paranasal sinus and nasal cavity depends on where the cancer is, the stage of the disease, and the patient's age and overall health.

Standard treatment may be considered because of its effectiveness in patients in past studies, or participation in a clinical trial may be considered. Not all patients are cured with standard therapy, and some standard treatments may have more side effects than are desired. For these reasons, clinical trials are designed to find better ways to treat cancer patients and are based on the most up-to-date information. Clinical trials are ongoing in some parts of the country for patients with cancer of the paranasal sinus and nasal cavity. To learn more about clinical trials, call the Cancer Information Service at 800-4-CANCER (800-422-6237); TTY at 800-332-8615.

Stage I Paranasal Sinus and Nasal Cavity Cancer

Treatment depends on the type of cancer and where the cancer is found.

If cancer is in the maxillary sinus, treatment will probably be surgery to remove the cancer. Radiation therapy may be given after surgery.

If cancer is in the ethmoid sinus, treatment may be one of the following:

1. Radiation therapy, if the cancer cannot be removed with surgery

2. Surgery followed by radiation therapy

If cancer is in the sphenoid sinus, treatment is the same as for nasopharyngeal cancer and will probably be radiation therapy with or without chemotherapy.

If cancer is in the nasal cavity, treatment may be surgery, radiation therapy, or both.

If the cancer is an inverting papilloma, treatment will probably be surgery. If the cancer comes back after surgery, patients may receive more surgery or radiation therapy.

If the cancer is a melanoma or sarcoma, treatment will probably be surgery. For certain types of sarcoma, a combination of surgery, radiation therapy, and chemotherapy may be given.

If the cancer is a midline granuloma, treatment will probably be radiation therapy.

If cancer is in the nose (nasal vestibule), treatment may be surgery or radiation therapy.

Stage II Paranasal Sinus and Nasal Cavity Cancer

Treatment depends on the type of cancer and where the cancer is found.

If cancer is in the maxillary sinus, treatment will probably be surgery to remove the cancer. Radiation therapy is given before or after surgery.

If cancer is in the ethmoid sinus, treatment may be one of the following:

1. External-beam radiation therapy
2. Surgery followed by radiation therapy

If cancer is in the sphenoid sinus, treatment is the same as for nasopharyngeal cancer and will probably be radiation therapy with or without chemotherapy.

If cancer is in the nasal cavity, treatment may be one of the following:

1. Surgery and/or radiation therapy
2. Radiation with or without chemotherapy

If the cancer is an inverting papilloma, treatment will probably be surgery. If the cancer comes back after surgery, patients may receive more surgery or radiation therapy.

If the cancer is a melanoma or sarcoma, treatment will probably be surgery. For certain types of sarcoma, a combination of surgery, radiation therapy, and chemotherapy may be given.

If the cancer is a midline granuloma, treatment will probably be radiation therapy.

If the cancer is in the nose (nasal vestibule), treatment may be surgery or radiation therapy.

Stage III Paranasal Sinus and Nasal Cavity Cancer

Treatment depends on the type of cancer and where the cancer is found.

If cancer is in the maxillary sinus, treatment may be one of the following:

1. Surgery to remove the cancer. Radiation therapy is given before or after surgery.

2. A clinical trial of a special type of radiation therapy given before or after surgery

If cancer is in the ethmoid sinus, treatment may be one of the following:

1. Surgery followed by radiation therapy

2. A clinical trial of chemotherapy before surgery or radiation therapy

3. A clinical trial of chemotherapy after surgery or after a combination of treatments

If cancer is in the sphenoid sinus, treatment is the same as for nasopharyngeal cancer and will probably be radiation therapy with or without chemotherapy.

If cancer is in the nasal cavity, treatment may be one of the following:

1. Surgery

2. Radiation therapy with or without chemotherapy

3. Surgery plus radiation therapy

4. A clinical trial of chemotherapy before surgery or radiation therapy

5. A clinical trial of chemotherapy after surgery or after a combination of treatments

If the cancer is an inverting papilloma, treatment will probably be surgery. If the cancer comes back after surgery, patients may receive more surgery or radiation therapy.

If the cancer is a melanoma or sarcoma, treatment will probably be surgery. Radiation therapy may be given if the cancer cannot be removed with surgery. For certain types of sarcoma, a combination of surgery, radiation therapy, and chemotherapy may be given.

If the cancer is a midline granuloma, treatment will probably be radiation therapy.

If the cancer is in the nose (nasal vestibule), treatment may be one of the following:

1. External-beam and/or internal radiation therapy

2. Surgery if the cancer comes back following treatment

3. A clinical trial of chemotherapy before surgery or radiation therapy

4. A clinical trial of chemotherapy after surgery or after a combination of treatments

Stage IV Paranasal Sinus and Nasal Cavity Cancer

Treatment depends on the type of cancer and where the cancer is found.

If cancer is in the maxillary sinus, treatment will probably be one of the following:

1. Radiation therapy

2. A clinical trial of chemotherapy before surgery or radiation therapy

3. A clinical trial of radiation therapy

If cancer is in the ethmoid sinus, treatment may be one of the following:

1. Surgery followed by radiation therapy

2. Radiation therapy followed by surgery

3. Chemotherapy and radiation therapy given at the same time

4. A clinical trial of chemotherapy before surgery or radiation therapy

If cancer is in the sphenoid sinus, treatment is the same as for nasopharyngeal cancer and may be one of the following:

1. Radiation therapy with or without chemotherapy

2. A clinical trial of chemotherapy before surgery or radiation therapy

If cancer is in the nasal cavity, treatment may be one of the following:

1. Surgery

2. Radiation therapy with or without chemotherapy

3. Surgery plus radiation therapy

4. A clinical trial of chemotherapy before surgery or radiation therapy

If the cancer is an inverting papilloma, treatment may be one of the following:

1. Surgery. If the cancer comes back after surgery, patients may receive more surgery or radiation therapy.

2. A clinical trial of chemotherapy before surgery or radiation therapy

If the cancer is a melanoma or sarcoma, treatment may be one of the following:

1. Surgery

2. Radiation therapy

3. Chemotherapy

4. A clinical trial of chemotherapy before surgery or radiation therapy

If the cancer is a midline granuloma, treatment may be one of the following:

1. Radiation therapy

2. A clinical trial of chemotherapy before surgery or radiation therapy

If the cancer is in the nose (nasal vestibule), treatment may be one of the following:

1. External-beam and/or internal radiation therapy

2. Surgery if the cancer comes back following treatment

3. A clinical trial of chemotherapy before surgery or radiation therapy

Recurrent Paranasal Sinus and Nasal Cavity Cancer

Treatment depends on the type of cancer, where the cancer is found, and the type of treatment the patient received before.

If cancer is in the maxillary sinus, treatment will probably be one of the following:

1. Radiation therapy alone or after extensive surgery (if limited surgery was done for the original cancer)

2. Surgery (if radiation therapy was given for the original cancer)

3. Chemotherapy. Clinical trials are testing new chemotherapy drugs.

If cancer is in the ethmoid sinus, treatment may be one of the following:

1. Radiation therapy alone or after extensive surgery (if limited surgery was done for the original cancer)

2. Surgery (if radiation therapy was given for the original cancer)

3. Chemotherapy. Clinical trials are testing new chemotherapy drugs.

If cancer is in the sphenoid sinus, treatment will probably be radiation therapy. Chemotherapy is given if radiation therapy does not work.

If cancer is in the nasal cavity, treatment may be one of the following:

1. Radiation therapy alone or after extensive surgery (if limited surgery was done for the original cancer)

2. Surgery (if radiation therapy was given for the original cancer)

3. Chemotherapy. Clinical trials are testing new chemotherapy drugs.

If the cancer is an inverting papilloma, treatment will probably be surgery. If the cancer comes back after surgery, patients may receive more surgery or radiation therapy.

If the cancer is a melanoma or sarcoma, treatment may be surgery or chemotherapy.

If the cancer is a midline granuloma, treatment will probably be radiation therapy.

If the cancer is in the nose (nasal vestibule), treatment may be one of the following:

1. Surgery (if radiation therapy was given for the original cancer)

2. Radiation therapy alone or after extensive surgery (if limited surgery was done for the original cancer)

3. Chemotherapy. Clinical trials are testing new chemotherapy drugs.

Chapter 20

Oropharyngeal Cancer

Cancer of the oropharynx is a disease in which cancer cells are found in the tissues of the oropharynx. The oropharynx is the middle part of the throat (also called the pharynx). The pharynx is a hollow tube about five inches long that starts behind the nose and goes down to the neck to become part of the esophagus (tube that goes to the stomach). Air and food pass through the pharynx on the way to the windpipe (trachea) or the esophagus. The oropharynx includes the base of the tongue, the tonsils, the soft palate (the back of the mouth), and the walls of the pharynx. Cancer of the oropharynx most commonly starts in the cells that line the oropharynx.

A doctor should be seen if a person has a sore throat that does not go away, trouble swallowing, weight loss, a lump in the back of the mouth or throat, a change in the voice, or pain in the ear.

If there are symptoms, a doctor will examine the throat using a mirror and lights. The doctor will also feel the throat for lumps. If tissue that is not normal is found, the doctor will need to cut out a small piece and look at it under the microscope to see if there are any cancer cells. This is called a biopsy.

The chance of recovery (prognosis) depends on where the cancer is in the throat, whether the cancer is just in the throat or has spread to other tissues (the stage), and the patient's general state of health.

PDQ® Cancer Information Summary. National Cancer Institute; Bethesda, MD. Oropharyngeal Cancer (PDQ®): Treatment - Patient. Updated 06/2006. Available at: http://cancergov. Accessed August 7, 2006.

After the treatment, a doctor should be seen regularly because there is a chance of having a second primary cancer in the head or neck region. Smoking or drinking alcohol after treatment increases the chance of developing a second primary cancer.

Stage Explanation

Once cancer of the oropharynx is found, more tests will be done to find out if cancer cells have spread to other parts of the body. This is called staging. A doctor needs to know the stage of the disease to plan treatment. Imaging tests may be done, including special x-rays and an MRI (magnetic resonance imaging) scan, which uses a magnet, radio waves, and a computer to make a picture of the inside of the body. The following stages are used for cancer of the oropharynx.

Stage 0: Cancer is found only in cells lining the oropharynx. Stage 0 cancer is also called carcinoma in situ.

Stage I: The cancer is two centimeters (about three-quarters inch) or smaller and has not spread outside the oropharynx.

Stage II: The cancer is larger than two centimeters, but not larger than four centimeters (about one and a half inches), and has not spread outside the oropharynx.

Stage III: Stage III is either of the following:

- The cancer is larger than four centimeters and has not spread outside the oropharynx.

- The cancer is any size and has spread to only one lymph node on the same side of the neck as the cancer. (Lymph nodes are small, bean-shaped structures found throughout the body. They help fight infection and disease.) The lymph node that contains cancer is three centimeters (just over one inch) or smaller.

Stage IVA: Stage IVA is either of the following:

- The cancer has spread to tissues near the oropharynx, including the voice box, roof of the mouth, lower jaw, muscle of the tongue, or central muscles of the jaw. Cancer may have spread to one or more nearby lymph nodes, none larger than six centimeters (almost two and a half inches).

- The cancer is any size, is only in the oropharynx, and has spread to one lymph node that is larger than three centimeters but no larger than six centimeters, or to more than one lymph node, none larger than six centimeters.

Stage IVB: Stage IVB is either of the following:

- The cancer is found in a lymph node that is larger than six centimeters and may have spread to other tissues around the oropharynx.

- Cancer surrounds the main artery in the neck or has spread to bones in the jaw or skull, to muscle in the side of the jaw, or to the upper part of the throat behind the nose; the cancer may have spread to nearby lymph nodes.

Stage IVC: In stage IVC, cancer has spread to other parts of the body; the tumor may be any size and may have spread to lymph nodes.

Recurrent: Recurrent disease means that the cancer has come back (recurred) after it has been treated. It may come back in the oropharynx or in another part of the body.

Treatment Option Overview

There are treatments for all patients with cancer of the oropharynx. Three kinds of treatment are used:

- Surgery (taking out the cancer)
- Radiation therapy (using high-dose x-rays or other high-energy rays to kill cancer cells)
- Chemotherapy (using drugs to kill cancer cells)

Surgery is a common treatment of cancer of the oropharynx. A doctor may remove the cancer and some of the healthy tissue around the cancer. If cancer has spread to lymph nodes, the lymph nodes will be removed (lymph node dissection). A new type of surgery called micrographic surgery is being tested in clinical trials for early cancers of the oropharynx. Micrographic surgery removes the cancer and as little normal tissue as possible. During this surgery, the doctor removes the cancer and then uses a microscope to look at the cancerous area to make sure there are no cancer cells remaining.

Radiation therapy uses high-energy x-rays to kill cancer cells and shrink tumors. Radiation may come from a machine outside the body (external radiation therapy) or from putting materials that produce radiation (radioisotopes) through thin plastic tubes in the area where the cancer cells are found (internal radiation therapy). Fractionated radiation therapy is given in several smaller, equal doses over a period of several days. External radiation to the thyroid or the pituitary gland may change the way the thyroid gland works. The doctor may test the thyroid gland before and after therapy to make sure it is working properly. Giving drugs with the radiation therapy to make the cancer cells more sensitive to radiation (radiosensitization) is being tested in clinical trials. If smoking is stopped before radiation therapy is started, there is a better chance of surviving longer.

Chemotherapy uses drugs to kill cancer cells. Chemotherapy may be taken by pill, or it may be put into the body by a needle in the vein or muscle. Chemotherapy is called a systemic treatment because the drug enters the bloodstream, travels through the body, and can kill cancer cells throughout the body.

People with oropharyngeal cancer have a higher risk of getting other cancers in the head and neck area. Clinical trials of chemoprevention therapy are testing whether certain drugs can prevent second cancers from developing in the mouth, throat, windpipe, nose, or esophagus (the tube that connects the throat to the stomach).

Hyperthermia therapy (warming the body to kill cancer cells) is being tested in clinical trials. Hyperthermia therapy uses a special machine to heat the body for a certain period of time to kill cancer cells. Because cancer cells are often more sensitive to heat than normal cells, the cancer cells die and the cancer shrinks.

Because the oropharynx helps in breathing, eating, and talking, patients may need special help adjusting to the side effects of the cancer and its treatment. A doctor will consult with several kinds of doctors who can help determine the best treatment. Trained medical staff can also help patients recover from treatment and adjust to new ways of eating and talking. Plastic surgery, or help learning to eat and speak, may be needed if a large part of the oropharynx is taken out.

Treatment by Stage

Treatment of cancer of the oropharynx depends on where the cancer is in the oropharynx; the stage of the disease; the effect of treatment on the patient's ability to talk, eat, and breathe normally; and the patient's age and overall health.

246

Standard treatment may be considered because of its effectiveness in patients in past studies, or participation in a clinical trial may be considered. Not all patients are cured with standard therapy and some standard treatments may have more side effects than are desired. For these reasons, clinical trials are designed to find better ways to treat cancer patients and are based on the most up-to-date information. Clinical trials are ongoing in many parts of the country for patients with cancer of the oropharynx. To learn more about clinical trials, call the Cancer Information Service at 800-4-CANCER (800-422-6237); TTY at 800-332-8615.

Stage I oropharyngeal cancer: Treatment may be one of the following:

1. Radiation therapy or surgery

2. A clinical trial of fractionated radiation therapy

Stage II oropharyngeal cancer: Treatment will be surgery to remove the cancer or radiation therapy.

Stage III oropharyngeal cancer: Treatment may be one of the following:

1. Surgery to remove the cancer followed by radiation therapy with or without chemotherapy

2. Radiation therapy alone (which may be fractionated radiation therapy), for cancer in the tonsils or base of the tongue

3. Radiation therapy combined with chemotherapy

4. A clinical trial of chemotherapy followed by surgery or radiation therapy

5. A clinical trial of chemotherapy combined with radiation therapy for cancer that cannot be removed by surgery

6. A clinical trial of new ways of giving radiation therapy

Stage IV oropharyngeal cancer: If the cancer can be removed by surgery, treatment may be one of the following:

1. Surgery to remove the cancer followed by radiation therapy with or without chemotherapy

2. Radiation therapy

3. A clinical trial of chemotherapy combined with radiation therapy

4. A clinical trial of new ways of giving radiation therapy

If the cancer cannot be removed by surgery, treatment may be one of the following:

1. Radiation therapy with or without chemotherapy

2. A clinical trial of chemotherapy followed by surgery or radiation therapy

3. A clinical trial of chemotherapy with radiation therapy and drugs to make the cancer cells more sensitive to radiation therapy (radiosensitizers)

4. A clinical trial of chemotherapy and fractionated radiation therapy given at the same time

5. A clinical trial of new ways of giving radiation therapy

6. A clinical trial of hyperthermia therapy combined with radiation therapy

Following treatment, it is important to have careful head and neck examinations to look for recurrence. Check ups will be done monthly in the first year, every two months in the second year, every three months in the third year, and every six months thereafter.

Recurrent oropharyngeal cancer: Treatment may be one of the following:

1. Surgery to remove the cancer

2. Radiation therapy

3. A clinical trial of chemotherapy

4. A clinical trial of hyperthermia therapy plus radiation therapy

Following treatment, it is important to have careful head and neck examinations to look for recurrence. Check ups will be done monthly in the first year, every two months in the second year, every three months in the third year, and every six months thereafter.

Chapter 21

Laryngeal Cancer

Laryngeal cancer is a disease in which malignant (cancer) cells form in the tissues of the larynx (voice box), which is located just below the pharynx (throat) in the neck. The larynx contains the vocal cords, which vibrate and make sound when air is directed against them. The sound echoes through the pharynx, mouth, and nose to make a person's voice. Most laryngeal cancers form in squamous cells, the thin, flat cells lining the inside of the larynx.

There are three main parts of the larynx:

- **Supraglottis:** The upper part of the larynx above the vocal cords, including the epiglottis.

- **Glottis:** The middle part of the larynx where the vocal cords are located.

- **Subglottis:** The lower part of the larynx between the vocal cords and the trachea (windpipe).

Use of tobacco products and drinking too much alcohol can affect the risk of developing laryngeal cancer.

This chapter begins with PDQ® Cancer Information Summary. National Cancer Institute; Bethesda, MD. Laryngeal Cancer (PDQ®): Treatment - Patient. Updated 09/2004. Available at: http://cancer.gov. Accessed April 30, 2006. Text under the heading "Tips for People Who Have Had Laryngectomies" is excerpted from "What You Need to Know about™ Cancer of the Larynx," National Cancer Institute, May 2003.

Possible signs of laryngeal cancer include a sore throat and ear pain. These and other symptoms may be caused by laryngeal cancer or by other conditions. A doctor should be consulted if any of the following problems occur:

- A sore throat or cough that does not go away
- Trouble or pain when swallowing
- Ear pain
- A lump in the neck or throat
- A change or hoarseness in the voice

Diagnostic Procedures

Tests that examine the throat and neck are used to help detect (find), diagnose, and stage laryngeal cancer. The following tests and procedures may be used:

- **Physical exam of the throat and neck:** An examination in which the doctor feels for swollen lymph nodes in the neck and looks down the throat with a small, long-handled mirror to check for abnormal areas.

- **Laryngoscopy:** A procedure in which the doctor examines the larynx (voice box) with a mirror or with a laryngoscope (a thin, lighted tube).

- **Endoscopy:** A procedure to look at organs and tissues inside the body to check for abnormal areas. An endoscope (a thin, lighted tube) is inserted through an incision (cut) in the skin or opening in the body, such as the mouth. Tissue samples and lymph nodes may be taken for biopsy.

- **CT scan (CAT scan):** A procedure that makes a series of detailed pictures of areas inside the body, taken from different angles. The pictures are made by a computer linked to an x-ray machine. A dye may be injected into a vein or swallowed to help the organs or tissues show up more clearly. This procedure is also called computed tomography, computerized tomography, or computerized axial tomography.

- **MRI (magnetic resonance imaging):** A procedure that uses a magnet, radio waves, and a computer to make a series of detailed pictures of areas inside the body. This procedure is also called nuclear magnetic resonance imaging (NMRI).

- **Biopsy:** The removal of cells or tissues so they can be viewed under a microscope to check for signs of cancer.

- **Barium swallow:** A series of x-rays of the esophagus and stomach. The patient drinks a liquid that contains barium (a silver-white metallic compound). The liquid coats the esophagus and stomach, and x-rays are taken. This procedure is also called an upper GI series.

Prognosis

Certain factors affect prognosis (chance of recovery) and treatment options. Prognosis (chance of recovery) depends on the following:

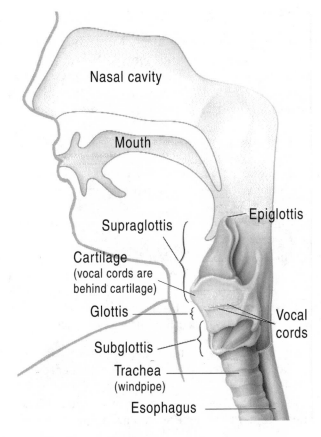

Figure 21.1. This picture shows the main parts of the larynx (Source: National Cancer Institute, May 2003).

- The stage of the disease
- The location and size of the tumor
- The grade of the tumor
- The patient's age, gender, and general health, including whether the patient is anemic

Treatment options depend on the following:

- The stage of the disease
- The location and size of the tumor
- Keeping the patient's ability to talk, eat, and breathe as normal as possible
- Whether the cancer has come back (recurred)

Smoking tobacco and drinking alcohol decrease the effectiveness of treatment for laryngeal cancer. Patients with laryngeal cancer who continue to smoke and drink are less likely to be cured and more likely to develop a second tumor. After treatment for laryngeal cancer, frequent and careful follow-up is important.

Stages of Laryngeal Cancer

After laryngeal cancer has been diagnosed, tests are done to find out if cancer cells have spread within the larynx or to other parts of the body.

The process used to find out if cancer has spread within the larynx or to other parts of the body is called staging. The information gathered from the staging process determines the stage of the disease. It is important to know the stage of the disease in order to plan treatment. The results of some of the tests used to diagnose laryngeal cancer are often also used to stage the disease.

The following stages are used for laryngeal cancer:

Stage 0 (carcinoma in situ): In stage 0, cancer is found only in the cells lining the larynx. Stage 0 cancer is also called carcinoma in situ.

Stage I: In stage I, cancer is in the area where it started. Stage I laryngeal cancer depends on where cancer is found in the larynx:

- **Supraglottis:** Cancer is in one area of the supraglottis only and the vocal cords can move normally.

- **Glottis:** Cancer is in one or both vocal cords and the vocal cords can move normally.

- **Subglottis:** Cancer is in the subglottis only.

Stage II: In stage II, cancer is in the larynx only. Stage II laryngeal cancer depends on where cancer is found in the larynx:

- **Supraglottis:** Cancer is in more than one area of the supraglottis or surrounding tissues.

- **Glottis:** Cancer has spread to the supraglottis and/or the subglottis and/or the vocal cords do not move normally.

- **Subglottis:** Cancer has spread to one or both vocal cords, which may not move normally.

Stage III: Stage III laryngeal cancer depends on whether cancer has spread from the supraglottis, glottis, or subglottis.

- **In stage III cancer of the supraglottis:** Cancer is in the larynx only and the vocal cords do not move normally, and/or cancer is in tissues next to the larynx; cancer may have spread to one lymph node on the same side of the neck as the original tumor and the lymph node is smaller than 3 centimeters; or cancer is in one area of the supraglottis only and in one lymph node on the same side of the neck as the original tumor; the lymph node is smaller than 3 centimeters and the vocal cords can move normally; or cancer is in more than one area of the supraglottis or surrounding tissues and in one lymph node on the same side of the neck as the original tumor; the lymph node is smaller than 3 centimeters and/or the vocal cords do not move normally.

- **In stage III cancer of the glottis:** Cancer is in the larynx only and the vocal cords do not move normally, and/or cancer is in tissues next to the larynx; cancer may have spread to one lymph node on the same side of the neck as the original tumor and the lymph node is smaller than 3 centimeters; or cancer is in one or both vocal cords and in one lymph node on the same side of the neck as the original tumor; the lymph node is smaller than 3 centimeters and the vocal cords can move normally; or cancer has spread to the supraglottis and/or the subglottis and/or the vocal cords do not move normally. The cancer has also spread to one lymph node on the same side of the neck as the original tumor and the lymph node is smaller than 3 centimeters.

- **In stage III cancer of the subglottis:** Cancer is in the larynx only and the vocal cords do not move normally; cancer may have spread to one lymph node on the same side of the neck as the original tumor and the lymph node is smaller than 3 centimeters; or cancer is in the subglottis only and in one lymph node on the same side of the neck as the original tumor; the lymph node is smaller than 3 centimeters; or cancer has spread to one or both vocal cords, which may not move normally, and to one lymph node on the same side of the neck as the original tumor; the lymph node is smaller than 3 centimeters.

Stage IV: Stage IV is divided into stage IVA, stage IVB, and stage IVC. Each substage is the same for cancer in the supraglottis, glottis, or subglottis.

- **In stage IVA:** Cancer has spread through the thyroid cartilage and/or has spread to tissues beyond the larynx such as the neck, trachea, thyroid, or esophagus, and may have spread to one lymph node on the same side of the neck as the original tumor; the lymph node is smaller than 3 centimeters; or cancer has spread to one or more lymph nodes anywhere in the neck and the lymph nodes are smaller than 6 centimeters; cancer may have spread to tissues beyond the larynx, such as the neck, trachea, thyroid, or esophagus. Vocal cords may not move normally.

- **In stage IVB:** Cancer has spread to the space in front of the spinal column and surrounds the carotid artery, or has spread to parts of the chest and may have spread to one or more lymph nodes anywhere in the neck (the lymph nodes may be any size); or cancer has spread to a lymph node that is larger than 6 centimeters and may have spread as far as the space in front of the spinal column, around the carotid artery or to parts of the chest. Vocal cords may not move normally.

- **In stage IVC:** Cancer has spread beyond the larynx to other parts of the body.

Recurrent laryngeal cancer: Recurrent laryngeal cancer is cancer that has recurred (come back) after it has been treated. The cancer is most likely to come back in the first 2 to 3 years. It may come back in the larynx or in other parts of the body.

Treatment Option Overview

Different types of treatment are available for patients with laryngeal cancer. Some treatments are standard (the currently used treatment), and some are being tested in clinical trials. Before starting treatment, patients may want to think about taking part in a clinical trial. A treatment clinical trial is a research study meant to help improve current treatments or obtain information on new treatments for patients with cancer. When clinical trials show that a new treatment is better than the standard treatment, the new treatment may become the standard treatment.

Clinical trials are taking place in many parts of the country. Information about ongoing clinical trials is available from the National Cancer Institute (NCI) website (http://www.cancer.gov). Choosing the most appropriate cancer treatment is a decision that ideally involves the patient, family, and health care team.

Three types of standard treatment are used:

Radiation therapy: Radiation therapy is a cancer treatment that uses high-energy x-rays or other types of radiation to kill cancer cells. There are two types of radiation therapy. External radiation therapy uses a machine outside the body to send radiation toward the cancer. Internal radiation therapy uses a radioactive substance sealed in needles, seeds, wires, or catheters that are placed directly into or near the cancer. The way the radiation therapy is given depends on the type and stage of the cancer being treated. Radiation therapy may work better in patients who have stopped smoking before beginning treatment.

Surgery: Surgery (removing the cancer in an operation) is a common treatment for all stages of laryngeal cancer. The following surgical procedures may be used:

- **Cordectomy:** Surgery to remove the vocal cords only.

- **Supraglottic laryngectomy:** Surgery to remove the supraglottis only.

- **Hemilaryngectomy:** Surgery to remove half of the larynx (voice box). A hemilaryngectomy saves the voice.

- **Partial laryngectomy:** Surgery to remove part of the larynx (voice box). A partial laryngectomy helps keep the patient's ability to talk.

- **Total laryngectomy:** Surgery to remove the whole larynx. During this operation, a hole is made in the front of the neck to allow the patient to breathe. This is called a tracheostomy.

- **Thyroidectomy:** The removal of all or part of the thyroid gland.

- **Laser surgery:** A surgical procedure that uses a laser beam (a narrow beam of intense light) as a knife to make bloodless cuts in tissue or to remove a surface lesion such as a tumor.

Even if the doctor removes all the cancer that can be seen at the time of the surgery, some patients may be given chemotherapy or radiation therapy after surgery to kill any cancer cells that are left. Treatment given after the surgery, to increase the chances of a cure, is called adjuvant therapy.

Chemotherapy: Chemotherapy is a cancer treatment that uses drugs to stop the growth of cancer cells, either by killing the cells or by stopping the cells from dividing. When chemotherapy is taken by mouth or injected into a vein or muscle, the drugs enter the bloodstream and can reach cancer cells throughout the body (systemic chemotherapy). When chemotherapy is placed directly into the spinal column, an organ, or a body cavity such as the abdomen, the drugs mainly affect cancer cells in those areas (regional chemotherapy). The way the chemotherapy is given depends on the type and stage of the cancer being treated.

New Treatments

Other types of treatment are being tested in clinical trials. These include the following:

- **Chemoprevention:** Chemoprevention is the use of drugs, vitamins, or other substances to reduce the risk of developing cancer or to reduce the risk cancer will recur (come back). The drug isotretinoin is being studied to prevent the development of a second cancer in patients who have had cancer of the head or neck.

- **Radiosensitizers:** Radiosensitizers are drugs that make tumor cells more sensitive to radiation therapy. Combining radiation therapy with radiosensitizers may kill more tumor cells.

Treatment Options by Stage

Stage I: Treatment of stage I laryngeal cancer depends on where cancer is found in the larynx. If cancer is in the supraglottis, treatment may include the following:

- Radiation therapy
- Supraglottic laryngectomy

If cancer is in the glottis, treatment may include the following:

- Radiation therapy
- Cordectomy
- Partial laryngectomy, hemilaryngectomy, or total laryngectomy
- Laser surgery

If cancer is in the subglottis, treatment may include the following:

- Radiation therapy with or without surgery
- Surgery alone

Stage II: Treatment of stage II laryngeal cancer depends on where cancer is found in the larynx. If cancer is in the supraglottis, treatment may include the following:

- Radiation therapy
- Supraglottic laryngectomy or total laryngectomy with or without radiation therapy
- A clinical trial of radiation therapy
- A clinical trial of chemoprevention

If cancer is in the glottis, treatment may include the following:

- Radiation therapy
- Partial laryngectomy, hemilaryngectomy, or total laryngectomy
- Laser surgery
- A clinical trial of radiation therapy
- A clinical trial of chemoprevention

257

If cancer is in the subglottis, treatment may include the following:

- Radiation therapy with or without surgery
- Surgery alone
- A clinical trial of radiation therapy
- A clinical trial of chemoprevention

Stage III: Treatment of stage III laryngeal cancer depends on where cancer is found in the larynx. If cancer is in the supraglottis or glottis, treatment may include the following:

- Surgery with or without radiation therapy
- Radiation therapy with or without surgery
- A clinical trial of radiation therapy
- A clinical trial of chemotherapy combined with radiation therapy, with or without laryngectomy
- A clinical trial of radiosensitizers
- A clinical trial of chemoprevention

If cancer is in the subglottis, treatment may include the following:

- Laryngectomy plus total thyroidectomy and removal of lymph nodes in the throat, usually followed by radiation therapy
- Radiation therapy with or without surgery
- A clinical trial of radiation therapy
- A clinical trial of chemotherapy
- A clinical trial of radiosensitizers
- A clinical trial of chemoprevention

Stage IV: Treatment of stage IV laryngeal cancer depends on where cancer is found in the larynx. If cancer is in the supraglottis or glottis, treatment may include the following:

- Total laryngectomy with radiation therapy
- Radiation therapy with or without surgery
- A clinical trial of radiation therapy
- A clinical trial of chemotherapy combined with radiation therapy, with or without laryngectomy

- A clinical trial of chemotherapy
- A clinical trial of radiosensitizers
- A clinical trial of chemoprevention

If cancer is in the subglottis, treatment may include the following:

- Laryngectomy plus total thyroidectomy and removal of lymph nodes in the throat, usually with radiation therapy
- Radiation therapy
- A clinical trial of radiation therapy
- A clinical trial of chemotherapy combined with radiation therapy
- A clinical trial of chemotherapy
- A clinical trial of radiosensitizers
- A clinical trial of chemoprevention

Recurrent laryngeal cancer: Treatment of recurrent laryngeal cancer may include the following:

- Surgery with or without radiation therapy
- Radiation therapy
- Chemotherapy
- A clinical trial of chemotherapy as palliative therapy to relieve symptoms caused by the cancer and improve quality of life

Tips for People Who Have Had Laryngectomies

Living with a Stoma

Learning to live with the changes brought about by cancer of the larynx is a special challenge. The medical team will make every effort to help you return to your normal routine as soon as possible. If you have a stoma, you will need to learn how to care for it:

- Before leaving the hospital, you will learn to remove and clean the trach tube, suction the trach, and care for the skin around the stoma.
- If the air is too dry, as it may be in heated buildings in the winter, the tissues of the windpipe and lungs may produce extra

mucus. Also, the skin around the stoma may get sore. Keeping the skin around the stoma clean and using a humidifier at home or at the office can lessen these problems.

• It is very dangerous for water to get into the windpipe and lungs through the stoma. Wearing a special plastic stoma shield or holding a washcloth over the stoma keeps water out when showering or shaving. Other types of stoma covers—such as scarves, neckties, and specially made covers—help keep moisture in and around the stoma. They help filter smoke and dust from the air before it enters the stoma. They also catch any fluids that come out of the windpipe when you cough or sneeze. Many people choose to wear something over their stoma even after the area heals. Stoma covers can be attractive as well as useful.

• When shaving, men should keep in mind that the neck may be numb for several months after surgery. To avoid nicks and cuts,

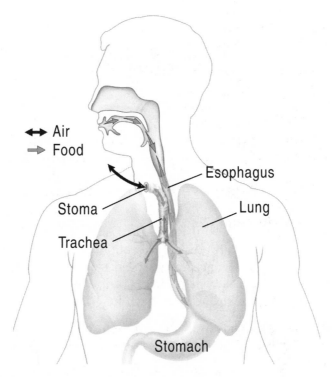

Figure 21.2. This picture shows the pathways for air and food after a total laryngectomy (Source: National Cancer Institute, May 2003.)

it may be best to use an electric shaver until the numbness goes away.

People with stomas work in almost every type of business and can do nearly all of the things they did before. However, they cannot hold their breath, so straining and heavy lifting may be difficult. Also, swimming and water skiing are not possible without special instruction and equipment to keep water from entering the stoma.

Some people may feel self-conscious about the way they look and speak. They may be concerned about how other people feel about them. They may be concerned about how their sexual relationships may be affected. Many people find that talking about these concerns helps them. Counseling or support groups may also be helpful.

Learning to Speak Again

Talking is part of nearly everything we do, so it's natural to be scared if your voice box must be removed. Losing the ability to talk—even for a short time—is hard. Patients and their families and friends need understanding and support during this time.

Within a week or so after a partial laryngectomy, you will be able to talk in the usual way. After a total laryngectomy, however, you must learn to speak in a new way. A speech pathologist usually meets with you before surgery to explain the methods that can be used. In many cases, speech lessons start before you leave the hospital.

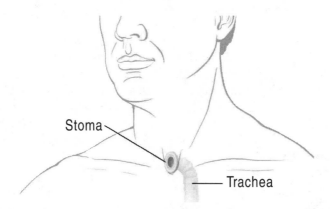

Figure 21.3. *The stoma is a new opening into the trachea (Source: National Cancer Institute, May 2003.)*

Until you begin to talk again, it is important to have other ways to communicate. Here are some ideas that you may find helpful:

- Keep pads of paper and pens or pencils in your pocket or purse.

- Use a typewriter, computer, or other electronic device. Your words can be printed on paper, displayed on a screen, or produced in a male or female voice.

- Carry a small dictionary or a picture book and point to the words you need.

- Write notes on a "magic slate" (a toy with a plastic sheet that covers black wax; lifting the plastic erases the sheet).

The health care team can help patients learn new ways to speak. It takes practice and patience to learn techniques such as esophageal speech or tracheoesophageal puncture speech, and not everyone is successful. How quickly a person learns, how understandable the speech is, and how natural the new voice sounds depend on the extent of the surgery on the larynx.

Esophageal speech: A speech pathologist can teach you how to force air into the top of your esophagus and then push it out again. The puff of air is like a burp. It vibrates the walls of the throat, making sound for the new voice. The tongue, lips, and teeth form words as the sound passes through the mouth. This type of speech sounds low pitched and gruff, but it usually sounds more like a natural voice than speech made by a mechanical larynx. There is also no device to carry around, so your hands are free.

Tracheoesophageal puncture: For tracheoesophageal puncture (TEP), the surgeon makes an opening between the trachea and the esophagus. The opening is made at the time of initial surgery or later. A small plastic or silicone valve fits into this opening. The valve keeps food out of the trachea. After TEP, patients can cover their stoma with a finger and force air into the esophagus through the valve. The air produces sound by making the walls of the throat vibrate. The sound is a lot like natural speech.

Mechanical speech: You may choose to use a mechanical larynx while you learn esophageal or TEP speech or if you are unable to use these methods. The device may be powered by batteries (electrolarynx) or by air (pneumatic larynx). Many different mechanical devices are available. The speech pathologist will help you choose the best device for your needs and abilities and will train you to use it.

One kind of electrolarynx looks like a small flashlight. It makes a humming sound. You hold the device against your neck, and the sound travels through your neck to your mouth. Another type of electrolarynx has a flexible plastic tube that carries sound into your mouth from a hand-held device. There are also devices that are built into a denture or retainer and can be worn inside your mouth and operated by a hand-held remote control.

A pneumatic larynx is held over the stoma and uses air from the lungs instead of batteries to make it vibrate. The sound it makes travels to the mouth through a plastic tube.

Chapter 22

Eye Cancers

Eye Tumors

Choroidal hemangioma: A hemangioma is a tumor comprised of blood vessels and can grow within the choroid, the blood vessel layer beneath the retina. Choroidal hemangiomas are not cancers and never metastasize. However, if the hemangioma is located in the area of central vision of the eye it can leak fluid that causes a retinal detachment and visual function may be affected.

Many choroidal hemangiomas can be safely monitored by your eye doctor without the need of further treatment. Photographs can be used to document evidence of growth or leakage and the need for treatment. Treatment options may include photodynamic therapy, laser photocoagulation to decrease the amount of fluid leakage, or low doses of external beam radiation therapy.

Choroidal melanoma: Choroidal melanoma is the most common primary intraocular (occurring inside the eye) tumor in adults. It arises from the pigmented cells of the choroid of the eye and is not a tumor that started somewhere else and spread to the eye.

A choroidal melanoma is malignant, meaning that the cancer may metastasize and eventually spread to other parts of the body. Because choroidal melanoma is intraocular and not usually visible, patients

This chapter includes "Eye Tumors," "Diagnosis," and "Treatment," undated fact sheets, accessed April 27, 2006. Reprinted with permission from www .eyecancermd.org. © Timothy G. Murray, M.D.

with this disease often do not recognize its presence until the tumor grows to a size that impairs vision by obstruction, retinal detachment, hemorrhage, or other complication. Pain is unusual, except with large tumors. Periodic retinal examination through a dilated pupil is the best means of early detection.

Cutting out the tumor and leaving the rest of the eye is not routinely advised for this type of cancer. Opening the eye during surgery would allow the tumor cells to float around into the spaces around the eye, which could spread cancer cells to other parts of the eye. In addition, some studies have shown that up to 50% of choroidal melanomas invade the sclera. Therefore if the tumor is removed from the eye there is a high possibility that cancer cells will remain within the sclera. Lastly, many eyes do not tolerate this procedure and severe complications may occur such as detachments of the retina, hemorrhages, and recurrence of the tumor which may result in having to remove the eye anyway.

Treatment recommendations for choroidal melanoma usually are based on the size of the tumor. Small suspicious melanomas usually are closely watched for evidence of growth before treatment is recommended. Medium-size tumors may be treated with either radioactive plaque therapy or enucleation (removal) of the eye. The Collaborative Ocular Melanoma Study (COMS), supported by the National Eye Institute of the National Institutes of Health, has documented equal success rates for plaque radiation therapy or enucleation for preventing the spread of cancer. Large-size tumors usually are best treated by enucleation. This is because the amount of radiation required to treat the tumor is too much for the eye to tolerate. The COMS study found no benefit to large-size tumor patients having radiation therapy prior to enucleation.

Choroidal metastasis: Malignant tumors from other parts of the body can spread in and around the eye. Metastatic cancers that appear in the eye usually come from a primary cancer of the breast in women and the lungs in men. Other, less common, sites of origin include the prostate, kidneys, thyroid, and the gastrointestinal tract. Blood cell tumors (lymphomas and leukemia) also can spread to the eye. The care of patients with metastasis to the eye should be coordinated between the eye cancer specialist, medical oncologist, and radiation oncologist. Treatment options may include chemotherapy, external beam radiation therapy, or, more rarely, enucleation.

Choroidal nevus: Like a raised freckle on the skin, a nevus can occur inside the eye. And, like a skin nevus, a choroidal freckle can become malignant, so should be closely monitored. A choroidal nevus should be examined by an ophthalmologist every four to six months to check if the pigmentation or size of the nevus has changed. In most cases, the only treatment recommended is close observation and monitoring by an ocular oncologist.

Conjunctival tumors: Conjunctival tumors are malignant cancers that grow on the outer surface of the eye. The most common types of conjunctival tumors are squamous cell carcinoma, malignant melanoma, and lymphoma. Squamous cell carcinomas rarely metastasize, but can invade the area around the eye into the orbit and sinuses. Malignant melanomas can start as a nevus (freckle) or can arise as newly formed pigmentation. Lymphoma of the eye can be a sign of systemic lymphoma or be confined to the conjunctiva.

Both squamous cell carcinomas and malignant conjunctival melanomas should be removed. Most small conjunctival tumors can be photographed and followed for evidence of growth prior to treatment. Small tumors can be completely removed surgically. In other instances cryotherapy (freezing therapy) may be necessary or chemotherapy eye drops may be used to treat the entire surface of the eye.

Eyelid tumors: Tumors of the eyelid may be benign cysts, inflammation, or malignant skin cancers. The most common type of eyelid cancer is basal cell carcinoma. Most basal cell carcinomas can be removed with surgery. If left untreated, these tumors can grow around the eye and into the orbit, sinuses, and brain. A simple biopsy can determine if an eyelid tumor is malignant. Malignant tumors are completely removed and the eyelid is repaired using plastic surgery techniques. Additional cryotherapy (freezing-therapy) and radiation therapy sometimes are required after surgery.

Iris tumors: Tumors can grow within and behind the iris. Though many iris tumors are cysts or a nevus, malignant melanomas can occur in this area. Most pigmented iris tumors do not grow. They are photographed and monitored with a special slit lamp and high frequency ultrasound to establish a baseline for future comparisons. When an iris tumor is documented to grow, treatment is recommended. Most small iris melanomas can be surgically removed. Radiation plaque therapy or enucleation may be considered for larger iris tumors.

Lymphoma/leukemia: Lymphoma tumors can appear in the eyelid tissue, tear ducts, and the eye itself. In most patients with large cell non-Hodgkin lymphoma, the disease is confined to the eye and central nervous system. In these patients, symptoms appear in the eye an average of two years before they are seen elsewhere. The disease itself as well as treatment, which may include external beam radiation, chemotherapy, or both (chemoradiation) to the central nervous system, can affect visual functioning.

Melanocytoma: This extremely slow-growing tumor usually is found on the surface of the optic disc. Almost all cases of melanocytoma are benign and malignant transformation is rare. It is probably present at birth and typically, there are no symptoms. Under clinical examination and fluorescein angiographic studies, melanocytoma appears as a deeply pigmented area located over the optic disc. In the majority of cases, close observation is recommended and no treatment is required. If malignant transformation does occur, enucleation, may be considered.

Orbital tumors: Tumors and inflammations can occur behind the eye. These tumors often push the eye forward causing a bulging of the eye called proptosis. The most common causes of proptosis are thyroid eye disease and lymphoid tumors. Other tumors include hemangiomas (blood vessel tumors), lachrymal (tear) gland tumors, and growths that extend from the sinuses into the orbit. Though CT (computed tomography) scans, MRIs (magnetic resonance imaging) and ultrasounds help in determining the probable diagnosis, most orbital tumors are diagnosed by a biopsy.

When possible, orbital tumors are totally removed. If they cannot be removed or if removal will cause too much damage to other important structures around the eye, a piece of tumor may be removed and sent for evaluation. If a tumor cannot be removed during surgery, most orbital tumors can be treated with external beam radiation therapy. Certain rare orbital tumors may require removal of the eye and orbital contents. In certain cases, orbital radiotherapy may be used to treat any residual tumor.

Diagnosis

A retinal oncologist (an eye cancer specialist) can determine if you have an eye cancer by performing a complete clinical examination. The examination may include asking questions about your medical history, examining both eyes, looking into the eye at the tumor, doing an ultrasound examination, and obtaining specialized photographs. Biopsy, which is often indicated to diagnose tumors in other parts of the body, is rarely needed with eye cancer. Though occasionally necessary, biopsies are usually avoided because they require opening the eye which risks spreading of the tumor cells.

Eye examination: Your ophthalmologist may be able to recognize an eye cancer by its appearance, including the degree of pigmentation of the tumor, its shape, and location, and by other features. Unlike tumors in other parts of the body, many eye cancers, including choroidal melanoma, may be directly visible through the "window" provided by the pupil.

Ultrasound (echography): During an ultrasound examination, sound waves are directed towards the tumor by a small probe placed on the eye. The patterns made by reflection of the sound waves helps to confirm that tumors are present. Ultrasound can determine if there is extraocular involvement (if the tumor has spread outside the eye) and helps to determine the thickness or height of the tumor. Black and white pictures of the ultrasound images may be taken for your physician to review.

Photography: There are two types of special photographs ophthalmologists use to assist in diagnosis: fluorescein angiography and fundus photographs.

- In fluorescein angiography, a special dye is injected into a vein in the arm. As the dye passes through the blood vessels in the back of the eye, this allows for a view of the circulation of the retina and the layers beneath the retina, highlighting any abnormalities. Although fluorescein angiography is not diagnostic, it is useful to exclude other possible disorders.

- The fundus of the eye includes the retina, macula, fovea, optic disc, and retinal vessels. In fundus photography, the inner lining of the eye is photographed with specially designed cameras through the dilated pupil. This is a non-invasive and painless procedure that produces a sharp view of the retina, the optic nerve and the retinal vessels.

Additional evaluations: Your doctor may request that you have a complete physical examination and specific tests depending upon what he sees inside your eye. Tests may include magnetic resonance imaging (MRI), a computerized tomography (CT) scan, chest x-ray, and complete blood count.

- A computerized tomography (CT) scan involves a series of x-ray images that provide a very clear picture of the eyes, the surrounding tissue, and the brain. Unlike an ordinary x-ray machine, which takes one picture at a time, the scanner takes a number of small pictures as it rotates around the patient.

- Magnetic resonance imaging (MRI) uses magnetic fields and radio waves linked to a computer to create pictures of areas inside the body. Because MRI can "see" through bone, it can provide clearer pictures of tumor located near bone and in the orbit.

Treatment

Your doctor will recommend treatment based on your medical history and the findings from the eye examination. It is not always necessary to treat all eye cancers immediately. If a tumor is very small or very slow growing, sometimes the doctor will closely monitor the tumor. If there are any concerns, then treatment can be started. Treatment usually is recommended when your physician determines that the tumor shows evidence of growth or if there is the possibility of spreading to other parts of the body if left untreated.

Chemotherapy: Although it is rarely used for eye cancer, chemotherapy is the most common type of treatment for many other types of cancer. Chemotherapy is the treatment of disease by means of drugs that have a specific toxic effect upon the cancer cells. Chemotherapy selectively destroys cancerous tissue.

There are many chemotherapeutic drugs available. Each type of drug has potential side effects such as skin problems, nausea, vomiting, and infections. Chemotherapy sometimes is recommended for choroidal metastasis, conjunctival tumors, and lymphoma.

Cryotherapy: Cryotherapy is the use of low temperatures to treat disease. Cryotherapy is applied under local anesthesia. The goal of cryotherapy is to freeze the malignant tissues in order to stimulate inflammation and scarring of this tissue. Cryotherapy may be recommended for conjunctival or eyelid tumors.

External beam radiation therapy: Radiation therapy uses high-energy radiation from x-rays and other sources to kill cancer cells and shrink tumors. Radiation that comes from a machine outside the body is called external-beam radiation therapy as opposed to radiation that is administered by placing a radiation plaque over or very near the tumor (internal radiation therapy or brachytherapy). External beam radiation therapy may be recommended for some choroidal metastasis, eyelid tumors, choroidal hemangiomas, lymphomas and orbital tumors.

Radiation plaque therapy (brachytherapy): Radiation plaque therapy is the most commonly used "eye-sparing" treatment for choroidal melanoma. A radioactive plaque is a small, gold covered, dish-shaped device that contains a radioactive source. Standard low-energy radioactive eye-plaques contain rice-sized radiation seeds that emit low energy photons. The gold coat of the plaque helps to aim the radiation photons directly at the tumor and decrease radiation damage to surrounding tissues. As the cells die, the tumor shrinks, although it usually does not disappear entirely. Radiation plaque therapy may be recommended for choroidal melanomas or iris melanomas.

Eye plaques are custom made to the dimensions of the tumor, usually ranging in size from about 12 to 22 mm. in diameter (about the size of a quarter). Careful calculations determine how long the plaque must remain in place to give the tumor the proper amount of radiation.

Surgical placement of the plaque lasts about an hour and usually is performed under local anesthesia. During surgery, an incision is made in the conjunctiva and the radioactive plaque is sutured to the sclera, outside of the eye, over the tumor. The conjunctiva is then sewn back over the plaque. Patients remain in the hospital for about three to five days at which time the plaque is surgically removed.

Most patients have no problems associated with plaque surgery. As with any ocular surgery, there can be secondary complications such as retinal detachments, hemorrhages, or infections. There are also risks associated with anesthesia.

The effects of radiation on the tumor typically are first evident three months after treatment. Eventually, eye melanomas shrink to about 40% of their pretreatment size. After successful treatment, although the tumors rarely completely disappear, they are considered to be inactive.

After radioactive plaque treatment, many patients note some dryness and irritation of the eye. In some instances, eyelashes may be permanently lost. In rare instances, the outside layer of the eye (sclera) may become very thin. Occasionally, prolonged redness, irritation, or infection may occur. Some patients may experience double vision, which can last a few days or several months. Radiation plaque therapy may cause eventual blurring, dimming, or rarely a total loss of vision in the treated eye. Plaque radiation does not affect the vision in the other eye. The amount of vision loss depends on what your vision was before treatment, how close the tumor is to the area of central vision of the eye, and how sensitive your tissues are to radiation. Most people maintain some central vision, and almost all retain peripheral vision.

Enucleation: The term enucleation may sound like an atomic bomb will be used to remove the eye, but the term simply means surgery for the removal of the eye. Enucleation is the surgical removal of the eye, leaving eye muscles and the contents of the eye socket intact. The eyelids, lashes, brow, and surrounding skin all remain.

This procedure is done when there is no other way to remove the cancer completely from the eye. Unfortunately, loss of vision for the eye removed is permanent because an eye cannot be transplanted. The eye is removed, and a spherical implant made of coral or hydroxyapatite is placed into the orbit. This allows the blood vessels to grow into the porous coral material. The muscles that help give movement to the eye are then sutured to the implant, which will allow for some movement of the prosthesis.

The eye is surrounded by bones; therefore, it is much easier to tolerate removal of an eye as compared to the loss of other organs. After a healing period, a temporary ocular prosthesis (plastic-eye) is inserted. The prosthesis is a plastic shell painted to match the other eye. It is inserted under the eyelid, much like a big contact lens. After a final prosthetic fitting most patients are happy with the way they look, and say others can't even tell they have vision in only one eye.

After enucleation, there is reduced visual field on the side of the body when looking straight ahead, and there is a loss of depth perception. Many of the skills of depth perception can be relearned and with time, almost all patients are able to do all the things they used to do before losing their eye. A few people who did very well with only one eye include: President Theodore Roosevelt, Israeli military leader Moshe Dayan, Congressman Morris Udall, entertainer Sammy Davis Jr., actor Peter Falk, painter Edgar Degas, aviator Wiley Post, inventor Guglielmo Marconi, and British naval hero Horatio Nelson.

Photodynamic therapy: Photodynamic therapy (also called PDT) is a treatment that can potentially destroy unwanted tissue and is sometimes used to treat choroidal hemangiomas. PDT destroys cancer cells with a fixed-frequency laser light in combination with a photosensitizing agent that is injected into the bloodstream. The photosensitizing agent alone is harmless and has no effect on either healthy or abnormal tissue. However, when laser is directed onto tissue containing the drug, the drug becomes activated and the tissue is rapidly destroyed. The laser light used in PDT is directed through a fiber-optic placed close to the hemangioma to deliver the proper amount of light and selectively target only the abnormal tissue.

An advantage of PDT is that it causes minimal damage to healthy tissue. However, PDT makes the skin and eyes sensitive to light for about six weeks after treatment. Patients are advised to avoid direct sunlight for at least six weeks after PDT treatment.

Chapter 23

Retinoblastoma

Retinoblastoma is a disease in which malignant (cancer) cells form in the tissues of the retina. The retina is the nerve tissue that lines the inside of the back of the eye. The retina senses light and sends images to the brain by way of the optic nerve.

Although retinoblastoma may occur at any age, it usually occurs in children younger than 5 years of age. The tumor may be in one eye or in both eyes. Retinoblastoma rarely spreads from the eye to nearby tissue or other parts of the body. Retinoblastoma is usually found in only one eye and can usually be cured.

Retinoblastoma is sometimes inherited (passed from the parent to the child). Retinoblastoma that is caused by an inherited gene mutation is called hereditary retinoblastoma. It usually occurs at a younger age than retinoblastoma that is not inherited. Retinoblastoma that occurs in only one eye is usually not inherited. Retinoblastoma that occurs in both eyes is always inherited. When hereditary retinoblastoma first occurs in only one eye, there is a chance it will develop later in the other eye. After diagnosis of retinoblastoma in one eye, regular follow-up exams of the healthy eye should be done every two to four months for at least 28 months. After treatment for retinoblastoma is finished, it is important that follow-up exams continue until the child is 7 years of age.

PDQ® Cancer Information Summary. National Cancer Institute; Bethesda, MD. Retinoblastoma (PDQ®): Treatment - Patient. Updated 12/2005. Available at: http://cancergov. Accessed April 30, 2006.

Treatment for both types of retinoblastoma should include genetic counseling (a discussion with a trained professional about inherited diseases). Brothers and sisters of a child who has retinoblastoma should also have regular check-ups and genetic counseling about the risk of developing the cancer.

A child who has hereditary retinoblastoma is at risk for developing pineal tumors in the brain. This is called trilateral retinoblastoma. Regular follow-up exams to check for this rare condition are important during treatment and for at least four years after the child is diagnosed with retinoblastoma. Hereditary retinoblastoma also increases the child's risk of developing other types of cancer in later years. Regular follow-up exams are important.

A doctor should be consulted if any of the following symptoms occur:

- Pupil of the eye appears white instead of red when light shines into it. This may be seen in flash photographs of the child.

- Eyes appear to be looking in different directions

- Pain or redness in the eye

In addition to a physical exam and history, the following tests and procedures may be used detect (find) and diagnose retinoblastoma:

- **Eye exam with dilated pupil:** An exam of the eye in which the pupil is dilated (opened wider) with medicated eye drops to allow the doctor to look through the lens and pupil to the retina. The inside of the eye, including the retina and the optic nerve, is examined with a light. Depending on the age of the child, this exam may be done under anesthesia.

- **Ultrasound exam:** A procedure in which high-energy sound waves (ultrasound) are bounced off internal tissues or organs and make echoes. The echoes form a picture of body tissues called a sonogram.

- **CT scan (CAT scan):** A procedure that makes a series of detailed pictures of areas inside the body, such as the eye, taken from different angles. The pictures are made by a computer linked to an x-ray machine. A dye may be injected into a vein or swallowed to help the organs or tissues show up more clearly. This procedure is also called computed tomography, computerized tomography, or computerized axial tomography.

- **MRI (magnetic resonance imaging):** A procedure that uses a magnet, radio waves, and a computer to make a series of detailed pictures of areas inside the body, such as the eye. This procedure is also called nuclear magnetic resonance imaging (NMRI).

- Retinoblastoma is usually diagnosed without a biopsy (removal of cells or tissues so they can be viewed under a microscope to check for signs of cancer).

Stages of Retinoblastoma

The following stages are used for retinoblastoma:

Intraocular retinoblastoma: Cancer is found in the eye but has not spread to tissues around the outside of the eye or to other parts of the body.

Extraocular retinoblastoma: The cancer has spread beyond the eye. It may be found in tissues around the eye or it may have spread to the central nervous system (brain and spinal cord) or to other parts of the body.

Recurrent retinoblastoma: Recurrent retinoblastoma is cancer that has recurred (come back) after it has been treated. The cancer may recur in the eye, in tissues around the eye, or in other places in the body. Tumors that were not treated with radiation therapy or surgery commonly recur, usually within six months.

Treatment Option Overview

Treatment will be overseen by a pediatric oncologist, a doctor who specializes in treating children with cancer. The pediatric oncologist works with other pediatric doctors who are experts in treating children with eye cancer and who specialize in certain areas of medicine.

Some cancer treatments cause side effects that continue or appear months or years after cancer treatment has ended. These are called late effects. Late effects of cancer treatment may include physical problems; changes in mood, feelings, thinking, learning or memory; and second cancers (new types of cancer.) Some late effects may be treated or controlled. It is important to talk with your child's doctors about the possible late effects caused by some treatments.

Children with the inherited form of retinoblastoma have an increased risk of developing second cancers. Children who have been treated for retinoblastoma with radiation therapy or certain chemotherapy agents also have a risk of developing second cancers. Regular follow-up by health professionals who are expert in finding and treating late effects is important.

Six types of standard treatment are used:

Enucleation: Enucleation is surgery to remove the eye and part of the optic nerve. The eye will be checked with a microscope to see if there are any signs that the cancer is likely to spread to other parts of the body. This is done if the tumor is large and there is little or no chance that vision can be saved. The patient will be fitted for an artificial eye after this surgery.

Radiation therapy: Radiation therapy is a cancer treatment that uses high-energy x-rays or other types of radiation to kill cancer cells. There are two types of radiation therapy. External radiation therapy uses a machine outside the body to send radiation toward the cancer. Internal radiation therapy uses a radioactive substance sealed in needles, seeds, wires, plaques, or catheters that are placed directly into or near the cancer. The way the radiation therapy is given depends on the type and stage of the cancer being treated. Methods of radiation therapy used to treat retinoblastoma include the following:

- **Intensity-modulated radiation therapy (IMRT):** A type of 3-dimensional (3-D) radiation therapy that uses a computer to make pictures of the size and shape of the tumor. Thin beams of radiation of different intensities (strengths) are aimed at the tumor from many angles. This type of radiation therapy causes less damage to healthy tissue near the tumor.

- **Stereotactic radiation therapy:** Radiation therapy that uses a rigid head frame attached to the skull to aim high-dose radiation beams directly at the tumors, causing less damage to nearby healthy tissue. It is also called stereotactic external-beam radiation, stereotactic radiosurgery, and stereotaxic radiosurgery. This procedure does not involve surgery.

- **Proton beam radiation therapy:** Radiation therapy that uses protons made by a special machine. A proton is a type of high-energy radiation that is different from an x-ray.

- **Plaque radiotherapy:** Radioactive seeds are attached to one side of a disk, called a plaque, and placed directly on the outside wall of the eye near the tumor. The side of the plaque with the seeds on it faces the eyeball, aiming radiation at the tumor. The plaque helps protect other nearby tissue from the radiation.

Cryotherapy: Cryotherapy is a treatment that uses an instrument to freeze and destroy abnormal tissue, such as carcinoma in situ. This type of treatment is also called cryosurgery.

Photocoagulation: Photocoagulation is a procedure that uses laser light to destroy blood vessels to the tumor, causing the tumor cells to die. Photocoagulation may be used to treat small tumors. This is also called light coagulation.

Thermotherapy: Thermotherapy is the use of heat to destroy cancer cells. Thermotherapy may be given using a laser beam aimed through the dilated pupil or onto the outside of the eyeball, or using ultrasound, microwaves, or infrared radiation (light that cannot be seen but can be felt as heat).

Chemotherapy: Chemotherapy is a cancer treatment that uses drugs to stop the growth of cancer cells, either by killing the cells or by stopping the cells from dividing. A form of chemotherapy called chemoreduction is used to treat retinoblastoma. Chemoreduction reduces the size of the tumor so it may be treated with local treatment (such as radiation therapy, cryotherapy, photocoagulation, or thermotherapy).

New Treatments

New types of treatment are being tested in clinical trials. These include the following:

Subtenon chemotherapy: Subtenon chemotherapy is the use of drugs injected through the membrane covering the muscles and nerves at the back of the eyeball. This is a type of regional chemotherapy. It is usually combined with systemic chemotherapy and local treatment (such as radiation therapy, cryotherapy, photocoagulation, or thermotherapy).

High-dose chemotherapy with stem cell transplant: High-dose chemotherapy with stem cell transplant is a method of giving high doses of chemotherapy and replacing blood-forming cells destroyed by the cancer treatment. Stem cells (immature blood cells) are removed from the blood or bone marrow of the patient or a donor and are frozen and stored. After the chemotherapy is completed, the stored stem cells are thawed and given back to the patient through an infusion. These reinfused stem cells grow into (and restore) the body's blood cells.

Treatment Options for Retinoblastoma

Intraocular retinoblastoma: If the cancer is in one eye and the tumor is large, treatment is usually enucleation. If the cancer is in one eye and it is expected that vision can be saved, treatment may include radiation therapy, photocoagulation, cryotherapy, thermotherapy, or chemotherapy (chemoreduction).

If the cancer is in both eyes, treatment may include the following:

- Enucleation of the eye with the most cancer and radiation therapy to the other eye

- Radiation therapy to both eyes or chemotherapy (chemoreduction) followed by local treatment. This may be done if there is a chance to save vision in both eyes

- Surgery only, when vision cannot be saved

- A clinical trial of subtenon chemotherapy combined with systemic chemotherapy and local treatment

Extraocular retinoblastoma: There is no standard treatment for extraocular retinoblastoma. Radiation therapy and chemotherapy have been used. Treatment may be a clinical trial of high-dose chemotherapy with stem cell transplant.

Recurrent retinoblastoma: If the cancer is small and in the eye only, treatment is usually local therapy (enucleation, radiation therapy, cryotherapy, photocoagulation, or thermotherapy).

If the cancer comes back outside of the eye, treatment will depend on many things and may be within a clinical trial. Information about ongoing clinical trials is available from the NCI website (http://www.cancer.gov).

Chapter 24

Brain Tumors

Types of Brain Tumors

A brain tumor is an abnormal mass of tissue in which cells grow and multiply uncontrollably, seemingly unchecked by the mechanisms that control normal cells. More than 150 different brain tumors have been documented, but to simplify matters, the two main brain tumor groups are primary and metastatic.

Primary brain tumors include tumors which originate from the tissues of the brain, or the brain's immediate surroundings. Primary tumors are categorized as glial or non-glial and benign or malignant.

Metastatic brain tumors include tumors which arise elsewhere in the body (such as the breast or lungs) and migrate to the brain, usually through the bloodstream. Metastatic tumors are considered cancer and are malignant.

Metastatic tumors to the brain affect nearly one in four patients with cancer—or an estimated 150,000 people a year. As many as 40 percent of people with lung cancer will develop metastatic brain tumors. In the past, the outcome for patients with these tumors was very poor, with typical survival rates just several weeks. More sophisticated diagnostic tools and innovative surgical and radiation approaches can now lead to longer survival and a better quality of life, measured in months to years.

Incidence in Adults

It is estimated that in 2005, there were a total of 18,500 new cases of brain and other nervous system tumors diagnosed—10,620 males and 7,880 females. The estimated number of deaths was 12,760, of which 7,280 were males and 5,480 were females.

From 1998–2002, the median age at diagnosis for cancer of the brain and central nervous system was age 55.

Types of Benign Brain Tumors

- Chordomas are benign, slowly growing tumors that are most prevalent in people ages 50 to 60. Their most common locations are the base of the skull and the lower portion of the spine. Although these tumors are benign, they may invade the adjacent bone and put pressure on nearby neural tissue. These are rare tumors, contributing to only 0.2 percent of all primary brain tumors.

- Craniopharyngiomas are typically benign but are difficult tumors to remove because of their location near critical structures deep in the brain. These tumors usually arise from a portion of the pituitary gland (the structure that regulates many hormones in the body), so nearly all patients will require some hormone replacement therapy.

- Gangliocytomas, gangliomas, and anaplastic gangliogliomas are rare tumors that include neoplastic nerve cells that are relatively well differentiated. They occur primarily in young adults.

- Glomus jugulare tumors are most frequently benign and are typically located just under the skull base at the top of the jugular vein. Glomus jugulare tumors are the most common form of glomus tumor. However, glomus tumors in general contribute to only 0.6 percent of neoplasms of the head and neck.

- Meningiomas are the most common benign intracranial tumors comprising 10 to 15 percent of all brain neoplasms, although a very small percentage are malignant. These tumors originate from the meninges, the membrane-like structures that surround the brain and spinal cord.

- Pineocytomas are generally benign lesions that arise from the pineal cells. They occur predominantly in adults. They are most often well-defined, noninvasive, homogeneous, and slow growing.

- Pituitary adenomas are the most common intracranial tumor after gliomas, meningiomas, and schwannomas. The large majority of pituitary adenomas are benign and fairly slow growing. Even malignant pituitary tumors rarely spread to other parts of the body. Adenomas are by far the most common disease affecting the pituitary. They more commonly affect people in their 30s or 40s, although they are diagnosed in children as well. Most of these tumors can be successfully treated.

- Schwannomas are common benign brain tumors in adults. They arise along nerves, comprised of cells that normally provide the "electrical insulation" for the nerve cells. Schwannomas often displace the remainder of the normal nerve instead of invading it. Acoustic neuromas are the most common schwannoma, arising from the eighth cranial nerve, or vestibular-cochlear nerve, which travels from the brain to the ear. Although these tumors are benign, they can cause serious complications and even death if they

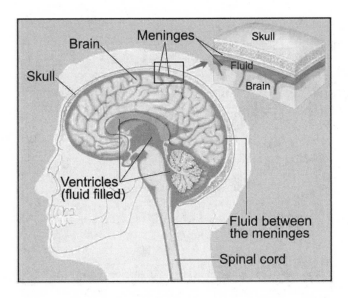

Figure 24.1. *The brain and nearby structures (Source: From "What You Need to Know about™ Brain Tumors," National Cancer Institute, March 2003).*

283

grow and exert pressure on nerves and eventually on the brain. Other locations include the spine, and, more rarely, along nerves that go to the limbs.

Types of Malignant Brain Tumors

Gliomas are the most prevalent type of adult brain tumor, accounting for 78 percent of malignant brain tumors. They arise from the supporting cells of the brain, called the glia. These cells are subdivided into astrocytes, ependymal cells, and oligodendroglial cells (or oligos). Glial tumors include the following:

- Astrocytomas are the most common glioma, accounting for about half of all primary brain and spinal cord tumors. Astrocytomas develop from star-shaped glial cells called astrocytes—part of the supportive tissue of the brain. They may occur in many parts of the brain, but most commonly occur in the cerebrum. People of all ages can develop astrocytomas, but they are more prevalent in adults, particularly middle-aged men. Astrocytomas in the base of the brain are more prevalent in children or younger people and account for the majority of children's brain tumors. In children,

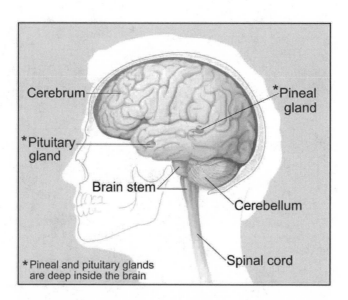

Figure 24.2. Major parts of the brain (Source: From "What You Need to Know about™ Brain Tumors," National Cancer Institute, March 2003).

most of these tumors are considered low-grade, while in adults most are high-grade.

- Ependymomas are derived from a neoplastic transformation of the ependymal cells lining the ventricular system. They account for 2 to 3 percent of all intracranial tumors. Most are well-defined, but some are not.

- Glioblastoma multiforme (GBM) is the most invasive type of glial tumor. These tumors tend to grow rapidly, spread to other tissue, and have a poor prognosis. They may be composed of several different kinds of cells, such as astrocytes and oligodendrocytes. GBM is more common in people ages 50 to 70 and more prevalent in men than women.

- Medulloblastomas usually arise in the cerebellum, most frequently in children. They are high-grade tumors, but they are usually responsive to radiation and chemotherapy.

- Oligodendrogliomas are derived from the cells which make myelin, which is the insulation for the wiring of the brain.

Other types of brain tumors include the following:

- Hemangioblastomas are slow growing tumors that are commonly located in the cerebellum. They originate from blood vessels, can be large in size, and are often accompanied by a cyst. These tumors are more common in people ages 40 to 60 and are more prevalent in men than women.

- Rhabdoid tumors are rare, highly aggressive tumors that tend to spread throughout the central nervous system. They often appear in multiple sites in the body, especially in the kidneys. They are more prevalent in young children but can also occur in adults.

Pediatric Brain Tumors

Brain tumors in children typically come from different tissues than those affecting adults. Treatments that are fairly well tolerated by the adult brain (like radiation therapy) may prevent normal development of a child's brain, especially in children younger than age 5.

It is estimated that in 2005, 3,410 new cases of childhood primary nonmalignant and malignant brain and central nervous system tumors were diagnosed. Of these cases, an estimated 2,590 were in children 15 and younger.

Some types of brain tumors are more common in children than in adults. The most common types of pediatric tumors are medulloblastomas, low-grade astrocytomas, ependymomas, craniopharyngiomas, and brain stem gliomas.

A grading system is used to indicate how benign or how malignant a tumor is, basically in terms of the tumor's histological features under a microscope. The World Health Organization (WHO) has developed the brain tumor grading system shown in Table 24.1.

Brain Tumor Causes

It is thought that brain tumors arise when certain genes on the chromosomes of a cell are damaged so that they no longer function properly. These genes normally regulate the rate at which the cell divides (if it divides at all). They also include repair genes that fix defects of

Table 24.1. World Health Organization (WHO) Brain Tumor Grades

Grade	Characteristics	Tumor Types
Low Grade		
WHO Grade I	• Least malignant (benign) • Possibly curable via surgery alone • Non-infiltrative • Long-term survival • Slow growing	Pilocytic astrocytoma Craniopharyngioma Gangliocytoma Ganglioglioma
WHO Grade II	• Relatively slow growing • Somewhat infiltrative • May recur as higher grade	"Diffuse" Astrocytoma Pineocytoma Pure oligodendroglioma
High Grade		
WHO Grade III	• Malignant • Infiltrative • Tend to recur as higher grade	Anaplastic astrocytoma Anaplastic ependymoma Anaplastic oligodendro-glioma
WHO Grade IV	• Most malignant • Rapid growth, aggressive • Widely infiltrative • Rapid recurrence • Necrosis prone	Glioblastoma Multiforme (GBM) Pineoblastoma Medulloblastoma Ependymoblastoma

other genes and genes that should cause the cell to self-destruct should the damage go beyond repair. In some cases, an individual may be born with partial defects in one or more of these genes. Environmental factors may then lead to further damage. In other cases the environmental injury to the genes may be the only cause. It is not known why some people in an "environment" develop brain tumors while others do not.

Once a cell is dividing too rapidly and internal mechanisms to check its growth are damaged, the cell can eventually grow into a tumor. Another line of defense may be the body's immune system, which optimally would detect the abnormal cell and kill it. Tumors may produce substances that block the immune system from recognizing the abnormal tumor cells and eventually overpower all internal and external checks to its growth.

A rapidly growing tumor may need more oxygen and nutrients than can be provided by the local blood supply intended for normal tissue. Tumors can produce substances which promote the growth of blood vessels, called angiogenesis factors. The new vessels that grow increase the supply of nutrients to the tumor, and eventually the tumor becomes dependent on these new vessels. Research is being done in this area, but more extensive research is necessary to translate this knowledge into potential therapies.

Symptoms

Symptoms vary depending on the location of the brain tumor, but the following are possible symptoms that may accompany different types of brain tumors.

- Headaches, which may be more severe in the morning
- Seizures or convulsions
- Difficulty thinking, speaking, or articulating
- Personality changes
- Weakness or paralysis in one part or one side of the body
- Loss of balance or dizziness
- Vision changes
- Hearing changes
- Facial numbness or tingling
- Nausea or vomiting
- Confusion and disorientation

Diagnosis

Sophisticated imaging techniques can pinpoint brain tumors. Diagnostic tools include computed tomography (CT or CAT scan) and magnetic resonance imaging (MRI). Intraoperative MRI is also used during surgery to guide tissue biopsies and tumor removal. Magnetic resonance spectroscopy (MRS) is used to examine the tumor's chemical profile and determine the nature of the lesions seen on the MRI. Positron emission tomography (PET scan) can help detect recurring brain tumors.

Sometimes, the only way to make a definitive diagnosis of a brain tumor is through a biopsy. The neurosurgeon performs the biopsy and the pathologist makes the final diagnosis, determining whether the tumor appears benign or malignant and grading it accordingly.

Brain Tumor Treatment

Brain tumors (whether primary or metastatic, benign or malignant) are usually treated with surgery, radiation, and/or chemotherapy—alone or in various combinations. While it is true that radiation and chemotherapy are more often used for malignant, residual, or recurrent tumors, decisions as to what treatment to use are made on a case-by-case basis and depend on a number of factors. There are risks and side effects associated with each type of therapy.

Surgery

It is generally accepted that complete or nearly complete surgical removal of a brain tumor is beneficial for a patient. The neurosurgeon's challenge is to remove as much tumor as possible—without injuring brain tissue important to the patient's neurological function (such as the ability to speak, walk, etc.). Traditionally, neurosurgeons open the skull through a craniotomy to insure that they can fully access the tumor and remove as much of it as possible.

Another procedure that is commonly done, sometimes before a craniotomy, is called a stereotactic biopsy. This is a smaller operation used to obtain tissue so that an accurate diagnosis can be made. Usually, a frame is attached to the patient's head, a scan is obtained, and then the patient is taken to the operating area where a small hole is drilled in the skull to allow access to the abnormal area. A small sample is obtained for examination under the microscope.

In the early 1990s, computerized devices called surgical navigation systems were first devised which eliminated the need for exploration. These systems assisted the neurosurgeon with guidance, localization, and orientation. This information reduced the risks and improved the extent of tumor removal. In many cases, this allowed previously inoperable tumors to be excised with acceptable risks. Some of these systems can also be used for biopsies without having to attach a frame to the skull. One limitation of these systems is that they utilize a scan (CT or MRI) obtained prior to surgery to guide the neurosurgeon. Thus, they cannot account for movements of the brain that may occur intraoperatively. Investigators are developing techniques using ultrasound and performing surgery in MRI scanners to help update the navigation system data during surgery.

Intraoperative language mapping is considered by some as a critically important technique for patients with tumors affecting language function, such as large, dominant-hemisphere gliomas. This procedure involves operating on an awake patient and mapping the anatomy of their language function during the operation prior to deciding which portions of the tumor are safe to resect. Recent studies have determined that cortical language mapping may be used as a safe and efficient adjunct to optimize glioma resection while preserving essential language sites.

Ventriculo-peritoneal shunting may be required for some patients with brain tumors. Everyone has cerebrospinal fluid (CSF) within the brain (and spine) that is slowly circulating or flowing all the time. If this flow becomes blocked, the sacs that contain the fluid (the ventricles) can become enlarged, creating increased pressure within the head, called hydrocephalus. If left untreated, hydrocephalus can cause brain damage and even death. The neurosurgeon may decide to use a shunt to divert the spinal fluid away from the brain, and therefore reduce the pressure. The body cavity in which the CSF is diverted is usually the peritoneal cavity (the area surrounding the abdominal organs). The shunt is usually permanent. If it becomes blocked, the symptoms are similar to that of the original condition of hydrocephalus and may include headaches, vomiting, visual problems, and/or confusion or lethargy, among others.

Radiation Therapy

Radiation therapy uses high-energy x-rays to kill cancer cells and abnormal brain cells and shrink tumors. Radiation therapy may be an option if the tumor cannot be treated effectively through medication or surgery.

- Standard external beam radiotherapy uses a radiation source that is nonselective and radiates all cells in the path of the beam. The radiation path beam may damage other portions of the brain in the general area of the tumor.

- Proton beam treatment employs a specific type of radiation in which "protons," a form of radioactivity, are directed specifically to the tumor. The advantage is that less tissue surrounding the tumor incurs damage.

- Stereotactic radiosurgery (like gamma knife, and Cyberknife) combines standard external beam radiotherapy with a technique that focuses the radiation through many different ports. This treatment tends to incur less damage to tissues adjacent to the tumor.

Chemotherapy

Chemotherapy is generally considered to be effective for specific pediatric tumors, lymphomas, and some oligodendrogliomas. While it has been proven that chemotherapy improves overall survival in patients with the most malignant primary brain tumors, it does so in only in about 20 percent of all patients, and physicians cannot readily predict which patients will benefit before treatment. As such, some physicians choose not to use chemotherapy because of the potential side effects (lung scarring, suppression of the immune system, nausea, etc.).

Chemotherapy works by inflicting cell damage that is better repaired by normal tissue than tumor tissue. Resistance to chemotherapy might involve survival of tumor tissue that cannot respond to the drug, or the inability of the drug to pass from the bloodstream into the brain. A special barrier exists between the bloodstream and the brain tissue called the blood-brain barrier. Some investigators have tried to improve the effect of chemotherapy by disrupting this barrier or injecting the drug into the tumor or brain. The goal of another class of drugs is not to kill the tumor cells but rather to block further tumor growth. In some cases, growth modifiers (such as tamoxifen) have been used to attempt to stop the growth of tumors resistant to other treatments.

In 1996, a new method of delivering chemotherapy directly into the area of the tumor was approved by the U.S. Food and Drug Administration. This allows patients to receive chemotherapy without the systemic side effects. Chemotherapy-impregnated wafers can be applied by the neurosurgeon at the time of surgery. The wafers slowly secrete the drug into the tumor.

Investigational Therapies

Many types of new therapies are currently being studied, especially for tumors for which the prognosis is generally poor through existing conventional therapies. It is unknown whether or not these therapies will work. Such therapies are given according to a protocol, and include various forms of immunotherapy, therapy using targeted toxins, anti-angiogenesis therapy, gene therapy, and differentiation therapy. Combinations of treatments may also be able to improve the outlook for patients, while lowering the adverse side effects.

Chapter 25

Brain Metastasis

Brain metastases are tumors that originate in tissues or organs outside the brain and spread secondarily to the brain. These tumors are a common complication of systemic cancer and an important cause of morbidity (rate of disease) and mortality (death) in cancer patients. They are the most common intracranial tumors (tumors inside the skull) and their incidence may be rising. Approximately 170,000 new cases of brain metastasis are diagnosed in the United States each year.

Risk Groups

Although virtually any malignancy can metastasize, or spread, to the brain, the incidence of brain metastasis varies dramatically from one type of cancer to another. Lung, breast, melanoma, renal, and colon cancers account for the greatest majority of all brain metastasis. Primary lung tumors rank first, accounting for 30 percent to 60 percent of all brain metastasis. Twenty percent to thirty percent of patients with breast cancer will develop brain metastasis.

The incidence of brain metastasis is based on age. It peaks in the fifth to seventh decades and tends to decline after that. There is a lower incidence of brain metastasis in children than in adults, with frequencies ranging from 6 percent to 13 percent in children.

Although brain metastasis occurs at a similar frequency among men and women some differences are seen in the types of primaries responsible for the brain metastasis in the two genders. Lung cancer is the most common source of brain metastasis in males, whereas breast cancer is the most common source in females.

Symptoms

Besides the following symptoms, many patients will have experienced symptoms caused by the original tumor and its related manifestations.

Increased intracranial pressure: In most of the patients, the symptoms of brain metastases are those of expanding (growing) mass lesions and increased intracranial pressure (ICP; the pressure within the skull). The most common symptoms, or "generalized manifestations" of increased ICP are headache, vomiting, and disturbance of consciousness.

Headache: Headache is the initial symptom in about half of brain tumor patients, and is eventually experienced by the majority of these patients at some point.

Vomiting: Vomiting is an occasional accompaniment to the headache. It is a far more common occurrence in children than in adults. In children, vomiting may be especially dramatic and forceful, so much so that it has been called "projectile" in nature.

Alteration in consciousness: Brain tumor patients at some points commonly experience alterations in consciousness, including both the level of consciousness and/or its quality. A brain tumor can induce a wide spectrum of changes in mental status ranging from subtle alterations in personality to states of profound and irretrievable coma.

Fits (epileptic seizures): Fits are associated with brain tumors in almost 35 percent of brain tumor patients. Age increases the risk of epilepsy being caused by a tumor especially in individuals beyond 45 years of age.

Focal (specific) neurological symptoms: Whereas headaches, altered mental status and seizures may be seen with tumors that occur in many parts of the brain, some symptoms are associated with tumors that occur in specific locations. These focal neurological symptoms affect the side of the body opposite from the side where the tumor resides and include different modalities of sensation, such as tingling, and motor changes, such as weakness (hemiparesis).

Radiological Diagnosis

Brain metastasis can be diagnosed by the following diagnostic tests:

- **CAT scan (computed axial tomography; also called a CT scan):** A CAT scan can be done with or without contrast (dye given to the patient intravenously before the study for better visualization of the tumor) with different views.

- **MRI (magnetic resonance imaging; also known as NMR):** It makes a clear picture of the brain using powerful magnets and radio waves. With the addition of a contrast agent given intravenously, this is the single best tool for radiographic evaluation of brain metastasis.

In addition to the above two diagnostic tests, the treating neuro-oncologist or neurosurgeon can ask for further sophisticated studies.

Treatment Modalities

Treatment varies with the size and type of the tumor, primary site of the tumor, and the general health of the person. Among the goals of treatment may be relief of symptoms, improved functioning, or comfort.

Drugs: Non-chemotherapeutic drugs: These drugs are given to relieve pain, such as headache pain, control epilepsy, and diminish swelling (edema) of the tumor. Examples of these drugs are analgesics, phenytoin and cortisone.

Chemotherapeutic drugs: These drugs are designed to attack and kill cells that divide rapidly, such as cancer cells. Chemotherapy can treat the whole brain. Additionally, multiple cancer sites can be treated at the same time.

Surgery: Surgery is an important part of the management for some patients with brain metastasis. During surgery, first tissue is obtained to confirm the diagnosis. Then the tumor, also called a lesion, is removed. Surgery is performed when the treating physician determines that it is likely to lead to greater relief of symptoms than might be achieved by other treatments and it possibly can extend survival.

Radiation: Another treatment approach uses radiation to destroy cancer cells. Like chemotherapy, radiotherapy can be given to the whole brain (WBRT, or whole brain radiotherapy) in fractionated (divided) doses. Stereotactic radiosurgery (SRS), a great advance in radiotherapy, uses a three-dimensional technique to target a single large dose of radiation with either a gamma knife or a linear accelerator. Its main advantage is its ability to treat lesions that are not easily treated by surgery. Also, it is not invasive, has fewer risks and results in shorter hospital stay.

Other types of treatment: New trials are being performed to use gene therapy for treatment of metastasis. However, gene therapy for brain metastasis is still in its infancy.

Prognosis

In general, the probable outcome is fairly poor. Many people with metastatic brain tumors have widespread tumor metastasis. Death often occurs within two years. The prognostic factors are complex and largely depend upon the status of systemic disease, extent of neurological deficit, length of time between first diagnosis of cancer and the diagnosis of brain metastasis, the type of primary (original) tumor, and the nature, size, and invasiveness of the metastatic lesion, among other factors.

—by Bahaa E. Hafez, MD, a post-doctoral fellow at the University of Texas in Houston and Instructor of Neurosurgery, Faculty of Medicine, Menofyia University, Shebin, El-kom, Egypt.

Chapter 26

Astrocytomas

Astrocytomas are the most common glioma, accounting for about half of all primary brain and spinal cord tumors. Astrocytomas develop from star-shaped glial cells called astrocytes, part of the supportive tissue of the brain. They may occur in many parts of the brain, but most commonly they occur in the cerebrum. They occur less commonly in the spinal cord. People of all ages can develop astrocytomas, but they are more prevalent in adults, particularly middle-aged men. Astrocytomas in the base of the brain are more prevalent in children or younger people and account for the majority of children's brain tumors. In children, most of these tumors are considered low-grade, while in adults most are high-grade.

There are different types of astrocytomas, and these lesions are classified into several categories according to their appearance under a microscope. This classification is important because the appearance of an astrocytoma will often predict its behavior and, therefore, a patient's prognosis.

Classification of Astrocytomas

Astrocytomas are generally classified (graded) into one of three types: low grade astrocytomas, anaplastic astrocytomas, and glioblastomas.

"Astrocytoma Tumors," August 2005, from NeurosurgeryToday.org, the public website for the American Association of Neurological Surgeons. Copyright © 2005. All rights reserved. Reproduced with permission from the American Association of Neurological Surgeons, 5550 Meadowbrook Dr., Rolling Meadows, IL 60008, http://www.aans.org.

Low grade astrocytomas account for 10 percent of astrocytomas. These tumors are typically slow growing and may not require specific treatment at the time of diagnosis. Many patients with low grade astrocytomas live for prolonged periods of time after their diagnosis. However, these tumors often advance into the higher grades and more rapidly growing forms of brain gliomas. Anaplastic astrocytomas and glioblastomas are the most aggressive and, unfortunately, the most common astrocytomas. Glioblastomas are fast growing astrocytomas that contain areas of dead tumor cells. In adults, glioblastoma occurs most often in the cerebrum, especially in the frontal and temporal lobes of the brain.

Symptoms

Symptoms vary depending on the location of the brain tumor but may include any of the following:

- Persistent headaches
- Double or blurred vision
- Vomiting
- Loss of appetite
- Changes in mood and personality
- Changes in ability to think and learn
- New seizures
- Speech difficulty of gradual onset

In early stages, children may experience headaches, nausea, vomiting, blurred or double vision, dizziness, and changes in coordination.

Diagnosis

Sophisticated imaging techniques can pinpoint brain tumors. Diagnostic tools include computed tomography (CT or CAT scan) and magnetic resonance imaging (MRI). Intraoperative MRI is also used during surgery to guide tissue biopsies and tumor removal. Magnetic resonance spectroscopy (MRS) is used to examine the tumor's chemical profile and determine the nature of the lesions seen on the MRI. Positron emission tomography (PET scan) can help detect recurring brain tumors.

Treatment Options

Treatment options include surgery, radiation, radiosurgery, and chemotherapy. The main goal of surgery is to remove as much of the tumor as possible without injuring brain tissue needed for neurological function (such as the ability to speak, walk, motor skills, etc.). However, high-grade tumors often have tentacle-like structures that invade surrounding tissues, making it more difficult to remove the entire tumor. If the tumor cannot be completely removed, surgery can still reduce or control tumor size. In most cases, surgeons open the skull through a craniotomy to best access the tumor site. The goal of radiation therapy is to selectively kill tumor cells while leaving normal brain tissue unharmed. In standard external beam radiation therapy, multiple treatments of standard-dose "fractions" of radiation are applied to the brain. Each treatment induces damage to both healthy and normal tissue. By the time the next treatment is given, most of the normal cells have repaired the damage, but the tumor tissue has not. This process is repeated for a total of 10 to 30 treatments, depending on the type of tumor. This additional treatment provides some patients with improved outcomes and longer survival rates.

Radiosurgery is a treatment method that uses computerized calculations to focus radiation at the site of the tumor while minimizing the radiation dose to the surrounding brain. Radiosurgery may be an adjunct to other treatments, or it may represent the primary treatment technique for some tumors.

Patients undergoing chemotherapy are administered special drugs designed to kill tumor cells. Although chemotherapy may improve overall survival in patients with the most malignant primary brain tumors, it does so in only about 20 percent of patients. Chemotherapy is often used in young children instead of radiation because radiation may have negative effects on the developing brain. The decision to prescribe this treatment is based on a patient's overall health, type of tumor, and extent of the cancer. Before considering chemotherapy, you should discuss it with your doctor because there are many side effects.

Because traditional treatment modalities are unlikely to result in a prolonged remission of malignant astrocytomas, researchers are presently investigating a number of promising new treatments including gene therapy, highly focused radiation therapy, immunotherapy, and novel chemotherapies. A number of new treatments are being made available on an investigational basis at centers specializing in brain tumor therapies.

Chapter 27

Neuroblastoma

What is neuroblastoma?

Neuroblastoma is the most common malignant (cancerous) abdominal tumor of childhood. It develops from the tissues that form the sympathetic nervous system, which is the part of the nervous system that regulates involuntary body functions.

The tumor usually begins in the nerve tissues of the adrenal gland (above the kidney), but may also begin in nerve tissues of the neck, chest or pelvis.

Although neuroblastoma often is present at birth, it generally is not detected until the tumor begins to grow and compress the surrounding organs.

Cancer cells can metastasize (spread) quickly to other areas of the body, such as lymph nodes, liver, lungs, bones, the central nervous system, and bone marrow. Close to 70 percent of children diagnosed with neuroblastoma will have metastatic disease.

Approximately 650 children in the United States are diagnosed with this tumor each year, and most children affected by the disease are diagnosed before age five. Neuroblastoma occurs with slightly more frequency in males than in females.

What causes neuroblastoma?

Most neuroblastoma cells have abnormalities involving a particular chromosome (chromosome #1), and the more malignant tumors often have multiple copies of the oncogene MYCN in the tumor cells, but a number of other genetic abnormalities may also be present. The likelihood of the disease being present in a future sibling of a child with neuroblastoma is about 1 percent.

Research is currently underway to determine if maternal exposure during pregnancy to toxic substances, environmental pollutants or radiation could be linked to development of the disease.

What are the symptoms of neuroblastoma?

The symptoms of neuroblastoma vary greatly depending on size, location and spread of the tumor; however, the most common symptoms include the following:

- An abdominal mass, either felt during an examination or seen as a swollen abdomen

- Uncontrolled eye movement caused by the tumor

- Swelling and bruising of the area around the eyes, caused by metastases (tumor spread)

- Compression of kidney or bladder by the tumor may cause changes in urination

- Pain, limping or weakness may be present from bone involvement

- Anemia or bruising may be present if there is bone marrow involvement

- Paralysis and weakness may be present if there is spinal cord involvement

- Diarrhea caused by a substance produced by the tumor (vasoactive intestinal peptide or VIP) may be present

- Fever

- High blood pressure and increased heart rate may occur depending on location of tumor and the organs the tumor compresses

How is neuroblastoma diagnosed?

In some cases, neuroblastoma can be detected before birth by a fetal ultrasound. For the most part, however, a complete medical and physical examination must be conducted, and a large number of diagnostic tests and procedures must be performed. These may include the following:

Blood tests: These should include a complete blood count, blood chemistries, and kidney and liver function tests.

Determination of urine catecholamine excretion levels: These levels are usually higher than normal due to tumor production.

Multiple imaging studies: These are done in order to evaluate the primary tumor and to determine the extent and location of any metastases:

- **Ultrasonography:** This imaging technique uses high-frequency sound waves and a computer to create images of blood vessels, tissues, and organs. It is used to view internal organs as they function, and to assess blood flow through various vessels. It is often the first test to screen for the presence of an abdominal tumor.

- **Computerized tomography scan (also called CT or CAT scan):** This is a diagnostic imaging procedure that uses a combination of x-rays and computer technology to produce cross-sectional images of the body. A CT scan shows detailed images of any part of the body, including bones, muscles, fat, and organs. CT scans are more detailed than standard x-rays.

- **Magnetic resonance imaging (MRI):** This procedure uses a combination of large magnets, radiofrequencies and a computer to produce detailed images of organs and structures within the body.

- **Bone scans:** These are x-rays of the bone that are taken after an injected dye is absorbed by bone tissue. Bone scans are used to detect tumors and bone abnormalities.

- **MIBG scans:** MIBG [metaiodobenzyl guanidine] is a substance selectively taken up by neuroblastoma cells. The MIBG is tagged with small amounts of radioactive iodine, which then can be localized in a patient's body by a nuclear medicine scan. This scan highlights the location of the tumors in a patient's body.

Bone marrow biopsy and/or aspiration: A small amount of bone marrow fluid and tissue is taken, usually from the hip bones, to further examine the number, size and maturity of blood cells and/or abnormal cells.

Biopsy: A biopsy is taken of the primary tumor and/or metastatic lesions.

What are the stages of the disease?

Diagnosing neuroblastoma involves staging and classifying the disease so treatment strategies can be determined and a prognosis can be made. The various stages, as classified by the International Neuroblastoma Staging System (INSS), are described below:

Stage 1 involves a tumor that does not cross the midline of the body. The tumor is completely resected (removed) and has not spread to other areas of the body. The lymph nodes on the same side of the body as the tumor do not have cancer cells present.

Stage 2A involves a tumor that does not cross the midline of the body. Though all visible tumor is removed, tumor removal is incomplete. This stage of tumor has not spread to other areas of the body, and lymph nodes on the same side as the tumor do not have tumor cells present.

Stage 2B involves a tumor that may or may not be completely resected, but has not spread to other areas of the body. Lymph nodes on the same side as the tumor have tumor cells present, while those on the opposite side do not.

Stage 3 involves a tumor that crosses the midline of the body and is not completely resected. Lymph nodes may or may not have tumor cells present. This stage also includes a tumor that does not cross the midline, but has lymph nodes on the opposite side of the body with tumor cells.

Stage 4 involves a tumor that has metastasized to distant lymph nodes, bone marrow, liver, skin, and/or other organs (except as defined in stage 4S).

Stage 4S involves a tumor that has metastasized to liver, skin, and/or bone marrow, but not to the bones. This stage generally occurs in children younger than one year of age.

How is neuroblastoma treated?

Decisions pertaining to treatment strategies should be jointly made by both parents and the child's physician(s). A number of factors must be considered:

- The child's age, medical history, and overall health
- Extent of the disease
- The child's tolerance for specific medications, procedures, or therapies

Treatment includes a wide range of approaches. Depending on individual circumstances, these approaches are used either alone or in combination:

- Surgery. This is done to remove the primary tumor and stage the patient in order to assess metastases.
- Chemotherapy
- Radiation therapy
- Blood and marrow transplant

Despite the benefits of these treatments, each treatment has certain associated side effects. Close attention is paid to these side effects and antibiotics to prevent or treat infections, as well as other supportive care, is given.

Also, new methods are continually being discovered to improve treatment approaches and to decrease side effects.

What is the outlook for a child with neuroblastoma?

As with any cancer, prognosis and long-term survival can vary greatly. While prompt medical attention and aggressive therapy are of utmost importance, prognosis depends upon a wide range of factors. These include the following:

- Extent of disease
- Size and location of the tumor
- Presence or absence of metastases
- Type of pathology (favorable or unfavorable)
- Biological factors, such as the number of copies per tumor cell of the N-myc oncogene, which is a tumor-specific protein

- Response of the tumor to therapy
- Child's tolerance of specific medications, procedures, and therapies

Depending on various prognostic factors, children are considered to be in low-, medium-, or high-risk categories, and different treatment protocols have been developed for each risk group.

With current therapies, low-risk patients (stages 1 and 2) carry more than a 90 percent long-term survival rate, regardless of age.

In higher-risk patients with more advanced stages of disease, survival rates diminish. Also, when the primary site of the tumor is in the chest, pelvic area, or the head and neck, the prognosis is better.

Treatment for children in the more advanced stages of neuroblastoma is much more aggressive, including chemotherapy, radiotherapy, and blood and marrow transplantation.

Despite treatment, however, the more advanced stages of neuroblastoma have a much less optimistic prognosis.

Is follow-up care necessary?

Continuous follow-up care is absolutely essential for the determination of response to treatment, recurrent disease and late effects of treatment.

Chapter 28

Primary Central Nervous System Lymphoma

Primary central nervous system (CNS) lymphoma is a disease in which malignant (cancer) cells form in the lymph tissue of the brain and/or spinal cord. Lymphoma is a disease in which malignant (cancer) cells form in the lymph system. The lymph system is part of the immune system and is made up of the lymph, lymph vessels, lymph nodes, spleen, thymus, tonsils, and bone marrow. Lymphocytes (carried in the lymph) travel in and out of the central nervous system (CNS). It is thought that some of these lymphocytes become malignant and cause lymphoma to form in the CNS. Primary CNS lymphoma can start in the brain, spinal cord, or meninges (the layers that form the outer covering of the brain). Because the eye is so close to the brain, primary CNS lymphoma can also start in the eye (called ocular lymphoma).

Having a weakened immune system may increase the risk of developing primary CNS lymphoma. Primary CNS lymphoma may occur in patients who have acquired immunodeficiency syndrome (AIDS) or other disorders of the immune system or who have had a kidney transplant.

Tests that examine the eyes, brain, and spinal cord are used to detect (find) and diagnose primary CNS lymphoma. The following tests and procedures may be used:

PDQ® Cancer Information Summary. National Cancer Institute; Bethesda, MD. Primary CNS Lymphoma (PDQ®): Treatment - Patient. Updated 02/2005. Available at: http://cancer.gov. Accessed April 30, 2006.

- **Physical exam and history:** An exam of the body to check general signs of health, including checking for signs of disease, such as lumps or anything else that seems unusual. A history of the patient's health habits and past illnesses and treatments will also be taken.

- **Neurological exam:** A series of questions and tests to check the brain, spinal cord, and nerve function. The exam checks a person's mental status, coordination, ability to walk normally, and how well the muscles, senses, and reflexes work. This may also be called a neuro exam or a neurologic exam.

- **Slit-lamp eye exam:** An exam that uses a special microscope with a bright, narrow slit of light to check the outside and inside of the eye.

- **Vitrectomy:** A surgical procedure to remove some or all of the vitreous humor (the gel-like fluid inside the eyeball). The fluid is removed through tiny incisions and then viewed under a microscope by a pathologist to check for cancer cells.

- **CT scan (CAT scan):** A procedure that makes a series of detailed pictures of areas inside the body, taken from different angles. The pictures are made by a computer linked to an x-ray machine. A dye may be injected into a vein or swallowed to help the organs or tissues show up more clearly. This procedure is also called computed tomography, computerized tomography, or computerized axial tomography. For primary CNS lymphoma, a CT scan is done of the chest, abdomen, and pelvis (the part of the body between the hips).

- **MRI (magnetic resonance imaging):** A procedure that uses a magnet, radio waves, and a computer to make a series of detailed pictures of areas inside the brain and spinal cord. A substance called gadolinium is injected into the patient through a vein. The gadolinium collects around the cancer cells so they show up brighter in the picture. This procedure is also called nuclear magnetic resonance imaging (NMRI).

- **Lumbar puncture:** A procedure used to collect cerebrospinal fluid (the fluid in the spaces around the brain and spinal cord) from the spinal column. This is done by placing a needle into the spinal column. This procedure is also called an LP or spinal tap. Laboratory tests to diagnose primary CNS lymphoma may include checking the protein level in the cerebrospinal fluid.

- **Stereotactic biopsy:** A biopsy procedure that uses a computer and a 3-dimensional (3-D) scanning device to find a tumor site and guide the removal of tissue so it can be viewed under a microscope to check for signs of cancer.

- **Complete blood count (CBC) with differential:** A procedure in which a sample of blood is drawn and checked for the following:
  - The number of red blood cells and platelets
  - The number and type of white blood cells
  - The amount of hemoglobin (the protein that carries oxygen) in the red blood cells
  - The portion of the blood sample made up of red blood cells

- **Blood chemistry studies:** A procedure in which a blood sample is checked to measure the amounts of certain substances released into the blood by organs and tissues in the body. An unusual (higher or lower than normal) amount of a substance can be a sign of disease in the organ or tissue that produces it.

Certain factors affect prognosis (chance of recovery) and treatment options. The prognosis (chance of recovery) depends on the following:

- The patient's age and general health
- The level of certain substances in the blood and cerebrospinal fluid (CSF)
- Where the tumor is in the central nervous system
- Whether the patient has AIDS

Treatment options depend on the following:

- The stage of the cancer
- Where the tumor is in the central nervous system
- The patient's age and general health
- Whether the cancer has just been diagnosed or has recurred (come back)

Treatment of primary CNS lymphoma works best when the tumor has not spread outside the cerebrum (the largest part of the brain) and the patient is younger than 60 years, able to carry out most daily activities, and does not have AIDS or other diseases that weaken the immune system.

Staging Primary CNS Lymphoma

After primary central nervous system (CNS) lymphoma has been diagnosed, tests are done to find out if cancer cells have spread within the brain and spinal cord or to other parts of the body. When primary CNS lymphoma continues to grow, it usually does not spread beyond the central nervous system or the eye. The process used to find out whether cancer has spread is called staging. The following tests and procedures may be used in the staging process:

- CT scan (CAT scan)
- Bone marrow biopsy
- Slit-lamp eye exam
- Vitrectomy

Recurrent Primary CNS Lymphoma

Recurrent primary central nervous system (CNS) lymphoma is cancer that has recurred (come back) after it has been treated. Primary CNS lymphoma commonly recurs in the brain or the eye.

Treatment Option Overview

Different types of treatment are available for patients with primary central nervous system (CNS) lymphoma. Some treatments are standard (the currently used treatment), and some are being tested in clinical trials. Before starting treatment, patients may want to think about taking part in a clinical trial. A treatment clinical trial is a research study meant to help improve current treatments or obtain information on new treatments for patients with cancer. When clinical trials show that a new treatment is better than the standard treatment, the new treatment may become the standard treatment.

Clinical trials are taking place in many parts of the country. Information about ongoing clinical trials is available from the National Cancer Institute (NCI) website. Choosing the most appropriate cancer treatment is a decision that ideally involves the patient, family, and health care team.

Surgery is not used to treat primary CNS lymphoma. Three standard treatments are used:

- **Radiation therapy:** Radiation therapy is a cancer treatment that uses high-energy x-rays or other types of radiation to kill cancer cells. There are two types of radiation therapy. External radiation therapy uses a machine outside the body to send radiation toward the cancer. Internal radiation therapy uses a radioactive substance sealed in needles, seeds, wires, or catheters that are placed directly into or near the cancer. The way the radiation therapy is given depends on the type of cancer being treated. High-dose radiation therapy to the brain can damage healthy tissue and cause disorders that can affect thinking, learning, problem solving, speech, reading, writing, and memory. Clinical trials have tested the use of chemotherapy alone or before radiation therapy to reduce the damage to healthy brain tissue that occurs with the use of radiation therapy.

- **Chemotherapy:** Chemotherapy is a cancer treatment that uses drugs to stop the growth of cancer cells, either by killing the cells or by stopping the cells from dividing. When chemotherapy is taken by mouth or injected into a vein or muscle, the drugs enter the bloodstream and can reach cancer cells throughout the body (systemic chemotherapy). When chemotherapy is placed directly into the spinal column (intrathecal chemotherapy), an organ, or a body cavity such as the abdomen, the drugs mainly affect cancer cells in those areas (regional chemotherapy). The way the chemotherapy is given depends on the type of cancer being treated. Primary CNS lymphoma may be treated with intrathecal chemotherapy and/or intraventricular chemotherapy, in which anticancer drugs are placed into the ventricles (fluid-filled cavities) of the brain. A network of blood vessels and tissue, called the blood-brain barrier, protects the brain from harmful substances. This barrier can also keep anticancer drugs from reaching the brain. In order to treat CNS lymphoma, certain drugs may be used to make openings between cells in the blood-brain barrier. This is called blood-brain barrier disruption. Anticancer drugs infused into the bloodstream may then reach the brain.

- **Steroid therapy:** Steroids are hormones made naturally in the body. They can also be made in a laboratory and used as drugs. Glucocorticoids are steroid drugs that have an anticancer effect in lymphomas.

Other types of treatment are being tested in clinical trials. These include the following:

- **High-dose chemotherapy with stem cell transplant:** High-dose chemotherapy with stem cell transplant is a method of giving high doses of chemotherapy and replacing blood-forming cells destroyed by the cancer treatment. Stem cells (immature blood cells) are removed from the blood or bone marrow of the patient or a donor and are frozen and stored. After the chemotherapy is completed, the stored stem cells are thawed and given back to the patient through an infusion. These re-infused stem cells grow into (and restore) the body's blood cells.

Treatment Options for Primary CNS Lymphoma

Primary CNS Lymphoma Not Related to AIDS

Treatment of primary central nervous system (CNS) lymphoma in patients who do not have AIDS may include the following:

- Chemotherapy
- Chemotherapy followed by radiation therapy
- Whole brain radiation therapy
- A clinical trial of high-dose chemotherapy with stem cell transplant

Primary CNS Lymphoma Related to AIDS

Treatment of primary central nervous system (CNS) lymphoma in patients who do have AIDS may include the following:

- Steroids with or without radiation therapy
- Radiation therapy alone
- Chemotherapy followed by radiation therapy

Treatment of primary CNS lymphoma is different in patients with AIDS because the treatment side effects may be more severe.

Recurrent Primary CNS Lymphoma

Treatment of recurrent primary central nervous system (CNS) lymphoma may include the following:

- Chemotherapy or radiation therapy (if not received in earlier treatment)
- A clinical trial of a new drug or treatment schedule

Chapter 29

Facts about Lung Cancer: An Overview

What is lung cancer?

Lung cancer is the leading cancer killer in both men and women. An estimated 173,700 new cases of lung cancer and an estimated 160,440 deaths from lung cancer will occur in the United States during 2004.

The rate of lung cancer cases appears to be dropping among white and African American men in the United States, while it continues to rise among both white and African American women.

There are two major types of lung cancer: non-small cell lung cancer and small cell lung cancer. Non-small cell lung cancer is much more common. It usually spreads to different parts of the body more slowly than small cell lung cancer. Squamous cell carcinoma, adenocarcinoma, and large cell carcinoma are three types of non-small cell lung cancer. Small cell lung cancer also called oat cell cancer, accounts for about 20% of all lung cancer.

What causes lung cancer?

Smoking is the number one cause of lung cancer. Lung cancer may also be the most tragic cancer because in most cases, it might have been prevented—87% of lung cancer cases are caused by smoking.

Cigarette smoke contains more than 4,000 different chemicals, many of which are proven cancer-causing substances, or carcinogens. Smoking cigars or pipes also increases the risk of lung cancer.

The more time and quantity you smoke, the greater your risk of lung cancer. But if you stop smoking, the risk of lung cancer decreases each year as normal cells replace abnormal cells. After ten years, the risk drops to a level that is one-third to one-half of the risk for people who continue to smoke. In addition, quitting smoking greatly reduces the risk of developing other smoking-related diseases, such as heart disease, stroke, emphysema, and chronic bronchitis.

Many of the chemicals in tobacco smoke also affect the nonsmoker inhaling the smoke, making "secondhand smoking" another important cause of lung cancer. It is responsible for approximately 3,000 lung cancer deaths annually.

Radon is considered to be the second leading cause of lung cancer in the U.S. today. Radon gas can come up through the soil under a home or building and enter through gaps and cracks in the foundation or insulation, as well as through pipes, drains, walls or other openings. Radon causes between 15,000 and 22,000 lung cancer deaths each year in the United States—12% of all lung cancer deaths are linked to radon.

Radon problems have been found in every state. The EPA estimates that nearly 1 out of every 15 homes in the U.S. has indoor radon levels at or above the level at which homeowners should take action—4 picocuries per liter of air (pCi/L) on a yearly average. Radon can be a problem in schools and workplaces, too.

Because you cannot see or smell radon, the only way to tell if you are being exposed to the gas is by measuring radon levels. Exposure to radon in combination with cigarette smoking greatly increases the risk of lung cancer. That means for smokers, exposure to radon is an even greater health risk.

Another leading cause of lung cancer is on-the-job exposure to cancer-causing substances or carcinogens. Asbestos is a well-known, work-related substance that can cause lung cancer, but there are many others, including uranium, arsenic, and certain petroleum products.

There are many different jobs that may involve exposure. Some examples are working with certain types of insulation, working in coke ovens, and repairing brakes. When exposure to job-related carcinogens is combined with smoking, the risk of getting lung cancer is sharply increased.

A study published in the *Journal of the American Medical Association* suggests that particulate matter pollution can cause lung cancer.

314

Lung cancer takes many years to develop. But changes in the lung can begin almost as soon as a person is exposed to cancer-causing substances. Soon after exposure begins, a few abnormal cells may appear in the lining of the bronchi (the main breathing tubes). If a person continues to be exposed to the cancer-causing substance, more abnormal cells will appear. These cells may be on their way to becoming cancerous and forming a tumor.

How is lung cancer detected?

In its early stages, lung cancer usually does not cause symptoms. When symptoms occur, the cancer is often advanced. Symptoms of lung cancer include the following:

- Chronic cough
- Hoarseness
- Coughing up blood
- Weight loss and loss of appetite
- Shortness of breath
- Fever without a known reason
- Wheezing
- Repeated bouts of bronchitis or pneumonia
- Chest pain

These conditions are also symptomatic of many other lung problems, so a person who has any of these symptoms should see a doctor to find out the cause. When a person goes for an exam, the doctor ask many questions about the person's medical history, including questions about the patient's exposure to hazardous substances. The doctor will also give the patient a physical exam. If the patient has a cough that produces a sputum (mucus), it may be examined for cancer cells. The doctor will order a chest x-ray or specialized x-ray such as the computed tomography (CT) scan, which help to locate any abnormal spots in the lungs. The doctor may insert a small tube called a bronchoscope through the nose or mouth and down the throat, to look inside the airways and lungs and take a sample, or biopsy, of the tumor. This is just one of several ways in which a doctor may take a biopsy sample.

A growing number of doctors are using a form of CT scan in smokers to spot small lung cancers, which are more likely than large tumors to be cured. The technique, called helical low-dose CT scan, is much more sensitive than a regular x-ray and can detect tumors when they are small.

More studies on this type of screening will show whether routine screening of smokers and others at risk for lung cancer will save lives.

If you are diagnosed with cancer, the doctor will do testing to find out whether the cancer has spread, and, if so, to which parts of the body. This information will help the doctor plan the most effective treatment. Tests to find out whether the cancer has spread can include a CT scan, magnetic resonance imaging (MRI), or a bone scan.

How is lung cancer treated?

The doctor will decide which treatment you will receive based on factors such as the type of lung cancer, the size, location and extent of the tumor (whether or not it has spread), and your general health. There are many treatments, which may be used alone or in combination. These include:

Surgery: Surgery may cure lung cancer. It is used in limited stages of the disease. The type of surgery depends on where the tumor is located in the lung. Some tumors cannot be removed because of their size or location.

Radiation therapy: Radiation therapy is a form of high energy x-ray that kills cancer cells. It is used:

- In combination with chemotherapy and sometimes with surgery.
- To offer relief from pain or blockage of the airways.

Chemotherapy: Chemotherapy is the use of drugs that are effective against cancer cells. Chemotherapy may be injected directly into a vein or given through a catheter, which is a thin tube that is placed into a large vein and kept there until it is no longer needed. Some chemotherapy drugs are taken by pill. Chemotherapy may be used:

- In conjunction with surgery.
- In more advanced stages of the disease to relieve symptoms.
- In all stages of small cell cancer.

Some patients may also be eligible to participate in clinical trials or research studies that look at new ways to treat lung cancer. For information, visit the National Cancer Institute website.

How can you prevent lung cancer?

- If you are a smoker, STOP SMOKING. Your local American Lung Association has books, videos, and group programs to help you quit for good.

- The Lung Association is also offering a new way to stop smoking through its Freedom From Smoking® online smoking cessation clinic. Find out more by visiting the American Lung Association website at www.ffsonline.org.

- If you are a nonsmoker, know your rights to a smoke-free environment at work and in public places. Make your home smoke-free.

- Test your home for radon.

- If you are exposed to dusts and fumes at work, ask questions about how you are being protected. Don't smoke—smoking increases your risk from many occupational exposures.

Chapter 30

Small Cell Lung Cancer

Small cell lung cancer is a disease in which malignant (cancer) cells form in the tissues of the lung. The lungs are a pair of cone-shaped breathing organs that are found within the chest. The lungs bring oxygen into the body when breathing in and take out carbon dioxide when breathing out. Each lung has sections called lobes. The left lung has two lobes. The right lung, which is slightly larger, has three. A thin membrane called the pleura surrounds the lungs. Two tubes called bronchi lead from the trachea (windpipe) to the right and left lungs. The bronchi are sometimes also involved in lung cancer. Small tubes called bronchioles and tiny air sacs called alveoli make up the inside of the lungs. There are two types of lung cancer: small cell lung cancer and non-small cell lung cancer.

There are three types of small cell lung cancer. These three types include many different types of cells. The cancer cells of each type grow and spread in different ways. The types of small cell lung cancer are named for the kinds of cells found in the cancer and how the cells look when viewed under a microscope:

- Small cell carcinoma (oat cell cancer)

- Mixed small cell/large cell carcinoma

- Combined small cell carcinoma

PDQ® Cancer Information Summary. National Cancer Institute; Bethesda, MD. Small Cell Lung Cancer (PDQ®): Treatment - Patient. Updated 08/2004. Available at: http://cancergov. Accessed April 30, 2006.

Smoking tobacco is the major risk factor for developing small cell lung cancer. Cigarette smoking is the most common cause of lung cancer. Risk factors for small cell lung cancer include the following:

- Smoking cigarettes, cigars, or pipes now or in the past
- Being exposed to second hand smoke
- Being exposed to asbestos or radon

A doctor should be consulted if any of the following symptoms occur:

- A cough that doesn't go away
- Shortness of breath
- Chest pain that doesn't go away
- Wheezing
- Coughing up blood
- Hoarseness
- Swelling of the face and neck
- Loss of appetite
- Unexplained weight loss
- Unusual tiredness

Tests and procedures that examine the lungs are used to detect (find) and diagnose small cell lung cancer. Chest x-rays, physical exam and history, and the following tests and procedures may be used:

- **Sputum cytology:** A microscope is used to check for cancer cells in the sputum (mucus coughed up from the lungs).
- **Laboratory tests:** Medical procedures that test samples of tissue, blood, urine, or other substances in the body. These tests help to diagnose disease, plan and check treatment, or monitor the disease over time.
- **Bronchoscopy:** A procedure to look inside the trachea and large airways in the lung for abnormal areas. A bronchoscope (a thin, lighted tube) is inserted through the nose or mouth into the trachea and lungs. Tissue samples may be taken for biopsy.
- **Fine needle aspiration biopsy:** The removal of part of a lump, suspicious tissue, or fluid, using a thin needle. A pathologist views

the tissue or fluid under a microscope to look for cancer cells. This procedure is also called a needle biopsy.

- **Thoracentesis:** Removal of fluid from the pleural cavity (the space between the lungs and chest wall) through a needle inserted between the ribs.

For most patients with small cell lung cancer, current treatments do not cure the cancer. If lung cancer is found, participation in one of the many clinical trials being done to improve treatment should be considered. Clinical trials are taking place in most parts of the country for patients with all stages of small cell lung cancer. Information about ongoing clinical trials is available from the National Cancer Institute (NCI)'s Cancer.gov website.

Stages of Small Cell Lung Cancer

After small cell lung cancer has been diagnosed, tests are done to find out if cancer cells have spread within the chest or to other parts of the body. The process used to find out if cancer has spread within the chest or to other parts of the body is called staging. The information gathered from the staging process determines the stage of the disease. It is important to know the stage in order to plan treatment. The following tests and procedures may be used in the staging process:

- **Bone marrow biopsy:** The removal of a small piece of bone and bone marrow by inserting a needle into the hipbone or breastbone. A pathologist views both the bone and the bone marrow samples under a microscope to look for signs of cancer.

- **CT scan (CAT scan) of brain, chest, and abdomen:** A procedure that makes a series of detailed pictures of areas inside the body, taken from different angles. The pictures are made by a computer linked to an x-ray machine. A dye may be injected into a vein or swallowed to help the organs or tissues show up more clearly. This procedure is also called computed tomography, computerized tomography, or computerized axial tomography.

- **MRI (magnetic resonance imaging):** A procedure that uses a magnet, radio waves, and a computer to make a series of detailed pictures of areas inside the body. This procedure is also called nuclear magnetic resonance imaging (NMRI).

- **Radionuclide bone scan:** A procedure to check if there are rapidly dividing cells, such as cancer cells, in the bone. A very small amount of radioactive material is injected into a vein and travels through the bloodstream. The radioactive material collects in the bones and is detected by a scanner.

- **PET scan (positron emission tomography scan):** A procedure to find malignant tumor cells in the body. A small amount of radionuclide glucose (sugar) is injected into a vein. The PET scanner rotates around the body and makes a picture of where glucose is being used in the body. Malignant tumor cells show up brighter in the picture because they are more active and take up more glucose than normal cells.

The following stages are used for small cell lung cancer:

- **Limited-stage small cell lung cancer:** In limited-stage, cancer is found in one lung, the tissues between the lungs, and nearby lymph nodes only.

- **Extensive-stage small cell lung cancer:** In extensive-stage, cancer has spread outside of the lung in which it began or to other parts of the body.

- **Recurrent small cell lung cancer:** Recurrent small cell lung cancer is cancer that has recurred (come back) after it has been treated. The cancer may come back in the chest, central nervous system, or in other parts of the body.

Treatment Option Overview

Different types of treatment are available for patients with small cell lung cancer. Some treatments are standard (the currently used treatment), and some are being tested in clinical trials. Before starting treatment, patients may want to think about taking part in a clinical trial. A treatment clinical trial is a research study meant to help improve current treatments or obtain information on new treatments for patients with cancer. When clinical trials show that a new treatment is better than the standard treatment, the new treatment may become the standard treatment.

Three types of standard treatment are used:

Surgery: Surgery may be used if the cancer is found in one lung and in nearby lymph nodes only. Because this type of lung cancer is usually found in both lungs, surgery alone is not often used. Occasionally, surgery may be used to help determine the patient's exact type of lung cancer. During surgery, the doctor will also remove lymph nodes to see if they contain cancer. Laser therapy (the use of an intensely powerful beam of light to kill cancer cells) may be used.

Even if the doctor removes all the cancer that can be seen at the time of the operation, some patients may be given chemotherapy or radiation therapy after surgery to kill any cancer cells that are left. Treatment given after the surgery, to increase the chances of a cure, is called adjuvant therapy.

Chemotherapy: Chemotherapy is a cancer treatment that uses drugs to stop the growth of cancer cells, either by killing the cells or by stopping the cells from dividing. When chemotherapy is taken by mouth or injected into a vein or muscle, the drugs enter the bloodstream and can reach cancer cells throughout the body (systemic chemotherapy). When chemotherapy is placed directly into the spinal column, an organ, or a body cavity such as the abdomen, the drugs mainly affect cancer cells in those areas (regional chemotherapy). The way the chemotherapy is given depends on the type and stage of the cancer being treated.

Radiation therapy: Radiation therapy is a cancer treatment that uses high-energy x-rays or other types of radiation to kill cancer cells. There are two types of radiation therapy. External radiation therapy uses a machine outside the body to send radiation toward the cancer. Internal radiation therapy uses a radioactive substance sealed in needles, seeds, wires, or catheters that are placed directly into or near the cancer. Prophylactic cranial irradiation (radiation therapy to the brain to reduce the risk that cancer will spread to the brain) may also be given. The way the radiation therapy is given depends on the type and stage of the cancer being treated.

Treatment Options by Stage

Limited-stage small cell lung cancer: Treatment of limited-stage small cell lung cancer may include the following:

- Combination chemotherapy and radiation therapy to the chest, with or without radiation therapy to the brain.

- Combination chemotherapy with or without radiation therapy to the brain in patients with complete response.

- Combination chemotherapy with or without radiation therapy to the chest.

- Surgery followed by chemotherapy or chemotherapy plus radiation therapy to the chest, with or without radiation therapy to the brain.

- Clinical trials of new chemotherapy, surgery, and radiation treatments.

Extensive-stage small cell lung cancer: Treatment of extensive-stage small cell lung cancer may include the following:

- Chemotherapy

- Combination chemotherapy

- Combination chemotherapy with or without radiation therapy to the brain for patients with complete response

- Radiation therapy to the brain, spine, bone, or other parts of the body where the cancer has spread, as palliative therapy to relieve symptoms and improve quality of life

- Clinical trials of new chemotherapy treatments

Recurrent small cell lung cancer: Treatment of recurrent small cell lung cancer may include the following:

- Radiation therapy as palliative therapy to relieve symptoms and improve quality of life

- Chemotherapy as palliative therapy to relieve symptoms and improve quality of life

- Laser therapy, surgical placement of devices to keep the airways open, and/or internal radiation therapy, as palliative therapy to relieve symptoms and improve quality of life

- Clinical trials of chemotherapy

Chapter 31

Non-Small Cell Lung Cancer

There are two main types of lung cancer: non-small cell lung cancer and small cell lung cancer. There are several types of non-small cell lung cancer. Each type of non-small cell lung cancer has different kinds of cancer cells. The cancer cells of each type grow and spread in different ways. The types of non-small cell lung cancer are named for the kinds of cells found in the cancer and how the cells look under a microscope:

- **Squamous cell carcinoma:** Cancer that begins in squamous cells, which are thin, flat cells that look like fish scales. This is also called epidermoid carcinoma.

- **Large cell carcinoma:** Cancer that may begin in several types of large cells.

- **Adenocarcinoma:** Cancer that begins in the cells that line the alveoli and make substances such as mucus.

Other less common types of non-small cell lung cancer are: pleomorphic, carcinoid tumor, salivary gland carcinoma, and unclassified carcinoma.

Smoking can increase the risk of developing non-small cell lung cancer. Smoking cigarettes or cigars is the most common cause of lung

Excerpted from PDQ® Cancer Information Summary. National Cancer Institute; Bethesda, MD. Non-Small Cell Lung Cancer (PDQ®): Treatment - Patient. Updated 03/2006. Available at: http://cancer.gov. Accessed April 30, 2006.

cancer. The more years a person smokes, the greater the risk. If a person has stopped smoking, the risk becomes lower as the years pass, but is never completely gone. Risk factors for lung cancer include the following:

- Smoking cigarettes or cigars, now or in the past
- Being exposed to second-hand smoke
- Being treated with radiation therapy to the breast or chest
- Being exposed to asbestos, radon, chromium, arsenic, soot, or tar
- Living where there is air pollution

When smoking is combined with other risk factors, the risk of developing lung cancer is increased.

Possible signs of non-small cell lung cancer include a cough that doesn't go away and shortness of breath. Sometimes lung cancer does not cause any symptoms and is found during a routine chest x-ray. Symptoms may be caused by lung cancer or by other conditions. A doctor should be consulted if any of the following problems occur:

- A cough that doesn't go away
- Trouble breathing
- Chest discomfort
- Wheezing
- Streaks of blood in sputum (mucus coughed up from the lungs)
- Hoarseness
- Loss of appetite
- Weight loss for no known reason
- Feeling very tired

Tests that examine the lungs are used to detect (find), diagnose, and stage non-small cell lung cancer. Tests and procedures to detect, diagnose, and stage non-small cell lung cancer are often done at the same time. In addition to a physical exam and history and chest x-ray, the following tests and procedures may be used:

- **CT scan (CAT scan):** A procedure that makes a series of detailed pictures of areas inside the body, such as the chest, taken from different angles. The pictures are made by a computer linked to an x-ray machine. A dye may be injected into a vein or swallowed to help the organs or tissues show up more clearly. This procedure is also called computed tomography, computerized tomography, or computerized axial tomography.

- **PET scan (positron emission tomography scan):** A procedure to find malignant tumor cells in the body. A small amount of radionuclide glucose (sugar) is injected into a vein. The PET scanner rotates around the body and makes a picture of where glucose is being used in the body. Malignant tumor cells show up brighter in the picture because they are more active and take up more glucose than normal cells do.

- **Sputum cytology:** A procedure in which a pathologist views a sample of sputum (mucus coughed up from the lungs) under a microscope, to check for cancer cells.

- **Fine-needle aspiration biopsy of the lung:** The removal of part of a lump, suspicious tissue, or fluid from the lung, using a thin needle. This procedure is also called needle biopsy. Ultrasound or another imaging procedure is used to locate the abnormal tissue or fluid in the lung. A small incision may be made in the skin where the biopsy needle is inserted into the abnormal tissue or fluid. A sample is removed with the needle and sent to the laboratory. A pathologist then views the sample under a microscope to look for cancer cells. A chest x-ray is done after the procedure to make sure no air is leaking from the lung.

- **Bronchoscopy:** A procedure to look inside the trachea and large airways in the lung for abnormal areas. A bronchoscope (a thin, lighted tube) is inserted through the nose or mouth into the trachea and lungs. Tissue samples may be taken for biopsy.

- **Thoracoscopy:** A surgical procedure to look at the organs inside the chest to check for abnormal areas. An incision (cut) is made between two ribs, and a thoracoscope (a thin, lighted tube) is inserted into the chest. Tissue samples and lymph nodes may be removed for biopsy. This procedure may be used to remove parts of the esophagus or lung. If certain tissues, organs, or lymph nodes can't be reached, a thoracotomy may be done. In this procedure, a larger incision is made between the ribs and the chest is opened.

- **Thoracentesis:** The removal of fluid from the space between the lining of the chest and the lung, using a needle. A pathologist views the fluid under a microscope to look for cancer cells.

For most patients with non-small cell lung cancer, current treatments do not cure the cancer. If lung cancer is found, taking part in one of the many clinical trials being done to improve treatment should be considered. Clinical trials are taking place in most parts of the country for patients with all stages of non-small cell lung cancer. Information about ongoing clinical trials is available from the National Cancer Institute (NCI)'s website at http://www.cancer.gov.

Stages of Non-Small Cell Lung Cancer

After lung cancer has been diagnosed, tests are done to find out if cancer cells have spread within the lungs or to other parts of the body. The process used to find out if cancer has spread within the lungs or to other parts of the body is called staging. The information gathered from the staging process determines the stage of the disease. It is important to know the stage in order to plan treatment. Some of the tests used to diagnose non-small cell lung cancer are also used to stage the disease. Laboratory tests, chest x-rays, and procedures, including the following, may be used in the staging process:

- **MRI (magnetic resonance imaging):** A procedure that uses a magnet, radio waves, and a computer to make a series of detailed pictures of areas inside the body, such as the brain. This procedure is also called nuclear magnetic resonance imaging (NMRI).

- **Endoscopic ultrasound (EUS):** A procedure in which an endoscope (a thin, lighted tube) is inserted into the body. The endoscope is used to bounce high-energy sound waves (ultrasound) off internal tissues or organs and make echoes. The echoes form a picture of body tissues called a sonogram. This procedure is also called endosonography. EUS may be used to guide fine needle aspiration biopsy of the lung, lymph nodes, or other areas.

- **Lymph node biopsy:** The removal of all or part of a lymph node. A pathologist views the tissue under a microscope to look for cancer cells.

- **Mediastinoscopy:** A surgical procedure to look at the organs, tissues, and lymph nodes between the lungs for abnormal areas. An incision (cut) is made at the top of the breastbone and an endoscope (a thin, lighted tube) is inserted into the chest. Tissue and lymph node samples may be taken for biopsy.

- **Anterior mediastinotomy:** A surgical procedure to look at the organs and tissues between the lungs and between the breastbone and spine for abnormal areas. An incision (cut) is made next to the breastbone and an endoscope (a thin, lighted tube) is inserted into the chest. Tissue and lymph node samples may be taken for biopsy. This is also called the Chamberlain procedure.

- **Bone scan:** A procedure to check if there are rapidly dividing cells, such as cancer cells, in the bone. A very small amount of radioactive material is injected into a vein and travels through the bloodstream. The radioactive material collects in the bones and is detected by a scanner.

The following stages are used for non-small cell lung cancer:

Occult (hidden) stage: In the occult (hidden) stage, cancer cells are found in sputum (mucus coughed up from the lungs), but no tumor can be found in the lung by imaging or bronchoscopy, or the primary tumor is too small to be checked.

Stage 0 (carcinoma in situ): In stage 0 (carcinoma in situ), cancer is in the lung only and has not spread beyond the innermost lining of the lung.

Stage I: Stage I is divided into stages IA and IB:

- Stage IA: The tumor is in the lung only and is three centimeters or smaller.
- Stage IB: One or more of the following is true:
  - The tumor is larger than three centimeters.
  - Cancer has spread to the main bronchus of the lung, and is at least two centimeters from the carina (where the trachea joins the bronchi).
  - Cancer has spread to the innermost layer of the membrane that covers the lungs.
  - The tumor partly blocks the bronchus or bronchioles and part of the lung has collapsed or developed pneumonitis (inflammation of the lung).

Stage II: Stage II is divided into stages IIA and IIB:

- Stage IIA: The tumor is three centimeters or smaller and cancer has spread to nearby lymph nodes on the same side of the chest as the tumor.

- Stage IIB: Cancer has spread to nearby lymph nodes on the same side of the chest as the tumor and one or more of the following is true: the tumor is larger than three centimeters; cancer has spread to the main bronchus of the lung and is two centimeters or more from the carina (where the trachea joins the bronchi); cancer has spread to the innermost layer of the membrane that covers the lungs; the tumor partly blocks the bronchus or bronchioles and part of the lung has collapsed or developed pneumonitis (inflammation of the lung). Or, cancer has not spread to lymph nodes and one or more of the following is true: the tumor may be any size and cancer has spread to the chest wall, or the diaphragm, or the pleura between the lungs, or membranes surrounding the heart; cancer has spread to the main bronchus of the lung and is no more than two centimeters from the carina (where the trachea meets the bronchi), but has not spread to the trachea; cancer blocks the bronchus or bronchioles and the whole lung has collapsed or developed pneumonitis (inflammation of the lung).

Stage IIIA: In stage IIIA, cancer has spread to lymph nodes on the same side of the chest as the tumor. Also:

- The tumor may be any size.
- Cancer may have spread to the main bronchus, the chest wall, the diaphragm, the pleura around the lungs, or the membrane around the heart, but has not spread to the trachea.
- Part or the entire lung may have collapsed or developed pneumonitis (inflammation of the lung).

Stage IIIB: In stage IIIB, the tumor may be any size and may have spread to any of the following:

- Heart
- Major blood vessels that lead to or from the heart
- Chest wall
- Diaphragm
- Trachea
- Esophagus
- Sternum (chest bone) or backbone
- More than one place in the same lobe of the lung

- The fluid of the pleural cavity surrounding the lung
- The lymph nodes on either side of the chest

Stage IV: In stage IV, cancer has spread to other parts of the body or to another lobe of the lungs and may have spread to lymph nodes.

Recurrent non-small cell lung cancer: Recurrent non-small cell lung cancer is cancer that has recurred (come back) after it has been treated. The cancer may come back in the brain, lung, or other parts of the body.

Treatment Option Overview

Six types of standard treatment are used:

Surgery: Four types of surgery are used:

- **Wedge resection:** Surgery to remove a triangle-shaped slice of tissue. Wedge resection is used to remove a tumor and a small amount of normal tissue around it. When a slightly larger amount of tissue is taken, it is called a segmental resection.

- **Lobectomy:** Surgery to remove a whole lobe (section) of the lung

- **Pneumonectomy:** Surgery to remove one whole lung

- **Sleeve resection:** Surgery to remove part of the bronchus

Radiation therapy: The way the radiation therapy is given depends on the type and stage of the cancer being treated. Radiation therapy is a cancer treatment that uses high-energy x-rays or other types of radiation to kill cancer cells. There are two types of radiation therapy. External radiation therapy uses a machine outside the body to send radiation toward the cancer. Internal radiation therapy uses a radioactive substance sealed in needles, seeds, wires, or catheters that are placed directly into or near the cancer.

Radiosurgery: Radiosurgery is a method of delivering radiation directly to the tumor with little damage to healthy tissue. It does not involve surgery and may be used to treat certain tumors in patients who cannot have surgery.

Chemotherapy: Chemotherapy is a cancer treatment that uses drugs to stop the growth of cancer cells, either by killing the cells or

331

by stopping the cells from dividing. When chemotherapy is taken by mouth or injected into a vein or muscle, the drugs enter the bloodstream and can reach cancer cells throughout the body (systemic chemotherapy). When chemotherapy is placed directly into the spinal column, an organ, or a body cavity such as the abdomen, the drugs mainly affect cancer cells in those areas (regional chemotherapy). The way the chemotherapy is given depends on the type and stage of the cancer being treated.

Laser therapy: Laser therapy is a cancer treatment that uses a laser beam (a narrow beam of intense light) to kill cancer cells.

Photodynamic therapy (PDT): Photodynamic therapy (PDT) is a cancer treatment that uses a drug and a certain type of laser light to kill cancer cells. A drug that is not active until it is exposed to light is injected into a vein. The drug collects more in cancer cells than in normal cells. Fiberoptic tubes are then used to deliver the laser light to the cancer cells, where the drug becomes active and kills the cells. Photodynamic therapy causes little damage to healthy tissue. It is used mainly to treat tumors on or just under the skin or in the lining of internal organs.

Watchful waiting: Watchful waiting is closely monitoring a patient's condition without giving any treatment until symptoms appear or change. This may be done in certain rare cases of non-small cell lung cancer.

New Treatments

New types of treatment and prevention are being tested in clinical trials. These include the following:

- **Chemoprevention:** Chemoprevention is the use of drugs, vitamins, or other substances to reduce the risk of developing cancer or to reduce the risk cancer will recur (come back).

- **Biologic therapy:** Biologic therapy is a treatment that uses the patient's immune system to fight cancer. Substances made by the body or made in a laboratory are used to boost, direct, or restore the body's natural defenses against cancer. This type of cancer treatment is also called biotherapy or immunotherapy.

- **New combinations:** New combinations of treatments are being studied in clinical trials.

Treatment Options by Stage

Occult non-small cell lung cancer: Treatment of occult non-small cell lung cancer depends on where the cancer has spread. It can usually be cured by surgery.

Stage 0 non-small cell lung cancer: Treatment of stage 0 non-small cell lung cancer may include the following:

- Surgery (wedge resection or segmental resection)
- Photodynamic therapy using an endoscope

Stage I non-small cell lung cancer: Treatment of stage I non-small cell lung cancer may include the following:

- Surgery (wedge resection, segmental resection, or lobectomy)
- External radiation therapy (for patients who cannot have surgery or choose not to have surgery)
- Surgery followed by chemotherapy
- A clinical trial of photodynamic therapy using an endoscope
- A clinical trial of surgery followed by chemoprevention

Stage II non-small cell lung cancer: Treatment of stage II non-small cell lung cancer may include the following:

- Surgery (wedge resection, segmental resection, lobectomy, or pneumonectomy)
- External radiation therapy (for patients who cannot have surgery or choose not to have surgery)
- Surgery followed by chemotherapy, with or without other treatments
- A clinical trial of external radiation therapy following surgery

Stage IIIA and stage IIIB non-small cell lung cancer: Treatment of stage IIIA non-small cell lung cancer may include the following:

- Surgery with or without radiation therapy
- External radiation therapy alone
- Chemotherapy combined with other treatments

- A clinical trial of new ways of giving radiation therapy and chemotherapy
- A clinical trial of new combinations of treatments

Treatment of stage IIIB non-small cell lung cancer may include the following:

- External radiation therapy alone
- Chemotherapy combined with external radiation therapy
- Chemotherapy combined with external radiation therapy, followed by surgery
- Chemotherapy alone
- A clinical trial of new ways of giving radiation therapy
- A clinical trial of new combinations of treatments

Stage IV non-small cell lung cancer: Treatment of stage IV non-small cell lung cancer may include the following:

- Watchful waiting
- External radiation therapy as palliative therapy, to relieve pain and other symptoms and improve the quality of life
- Chemotherapy
- Laser therapy and/or internal radiation therapy
- A clinical trial of chemotherapy with or without biologic therapy

Treatment options for recurrent non-small cell lung cancer: Treatment of recurrent non-small cell lung cancer may include the following:

- External radiation therapy as palliative therapy, to relieve pain and other symptoms and improve the quality of life
- Chemotherapy alone
- Surgery (for some patients who have a very small amount of cancer that has spread to the brain)
- Laser therapy or internal radiation therapy
- Radiosurgery (for certain patients who cannot have standard surgery)
- A clinical trial of biologic therapy or other new treatments

Chapter 32

Pleural and Other Forms of Mesothelioma

Malignant mesothelioma is a disease in which malignant (cancer) cells are found in the pleura (the thin layer of tissue that lines the chest cavity and covers the lungs) or the peritoneum (the thin layer of tissue that lines the abdomen and covers most of the organs in the abdomen). Being exposed to asbestos can affect the risk of developing malignant mesothelioma.

What is the mesothelium?

The mesothelium is a membrane that covers and protects most of the internal organs of the body. It is composed of two layers of cells: One layer immediately surrounds the organ; the other forms a sac around it. The mesothelium produces a lubricating fluid that is released between these layers, allowing moving organs (such as the beating heart and the expanding and contracting lungs) to glide easily against adjacent structures.

The mesothelium has different names, depending on its location in the body. The peritoneum is the mesothelial tissue that covers most

The introductory paragraph and text under the question "What types of surgical procedures are used to treat mesothelioma?" are excerpted from PDQ® Cancer Information Summary. National Cancer Institute; Bethesda, MD. Malignant Mesothelioma (PDQ®): Treatment - Patient. Updated 011/2005. Available at: http://cancer.gov. Accessed April 30, 2006. Other questions and answers are from "Mesothelioma: Questions and Answers," National Cancer Institute, May 2002.

of the organs in the abdominal cavity. The pleura is the membrane that surrounds the lungs and lines the wall of the chest cavity. The pericardium covers and protects the heart. The mesothelial tissue surrounding the male internal reproductive organs is called the tunica vaginalis testis. The tunica serosa uteri covers the internal reproductive organs in women.

What is mesothelioma?

Mesothelioma (cancer of the mesothelium) is a disease in which cells of the mesothelium become abnormal and divide without control or order. They can invade and damage nearby tissues and organs. Cancer cells can also metastasize (spread) from their original site to other parts of the body. Most cases of mesothelioma begin in the pleura or peritoneum.

How common is mesothelioma?

Although reported incidence rates have increased in the past 20 years, mesothelioma is still a relatively rare cancer. About 2,000 new cases of mesothelioma are diagnosed in the United States each year. Mesothelioma occurs more often in men than in women and risk increases with age, but this disease can appear in either men or women at any age.

What are the risk factors for mesothelioma?

Working with asbestos is the major risk factor for mesothelioma. A history of asbestos exposure at work is reported in about 70 percent to 80 percent of all cases. However, mesothelioma has been reported in some individuals without any known exposure to asbestos.

Asbestos is the name of a group of minerals that occur naturally as masses of strong, flexible fibers that can be separated into thin threads and woven. Asbestos has been widely used in many industrial products, including cement, brake linings, roof shingles, flooring products, textiles, and insulation. If tiny asbestos particles float in the air, especially during the manufacturing process, they may be inhaled or swallowed, and can cause serious health problems. In addition to mesothelioma, exposure to asbestos increases the risk of lung cancer, asbestosis (a noncancerous, chronic lung ailment), and other cancers, such as those of the larynx and kidney.

Smoking does not appear to increase the risk of mesothelioma. However, the combination of smoking and asbestos exposure significantly increases a person's risk of developing cancer of the air passageways in the lung.

What are the symptoms of mesothelioma?

Symptoms of mesothelioma may not appear until 30 to 50 years after exposure to asbestos. Shortness of breath and pain in the chest due to an accumulation of fluid in the pleura are often symptoms of pleural mesothelioma. Symptoms of peritoneal mesothelioma include weight loss and abdominal pain and swelling due to a buildup of fluid in the abdomen. Other symptoms of peritoneal mesothelioma may include bowel obstruction, blood clotting abnormalities, anemia, and fever. If the cancer has spread beyond the mesothelium to other parts of the body, symptoms may include pain, trouble swallowing, or swelling of the neck or face.

These symptoms may be caused by mesothelioma or by other, less serious conditions. It is important to see a doctor about any of these symptoms. Only a doctor can make a diagnosis.

How is mesothelioma diagnosed?

Diagnosing mesothelioma is often difficult, because the symptoms are similar to those of a number of other conditions. Diagnosis begins with a review of the patient's medical history, including any history of asbestos exposure. A complete physical examination may be performed, including x-rays of the chest or abdomen and lung function tests. A computed tomography (CT or CAT) scan or magnetic resonance imaging (MRI) may also be useful. A CT scan is a series of detailed pictures of areas inside the body created by a computer linked to an x-ray machine. In an MRI, a powerful magnet linked to a computer is used to make detailed pictures of areas inside the body. These pictures are viewed on a monitor and can also be printed.

A biopsy is needed to confirm a diagnosis of mesothelioma. In a biopsy, a surgeon or a medical oncologist (a doctor who specializes in diagnosing and treating cancer) removes a sample of tissue for examination under a microscope by a pathologist. A biopsy may be done in different ways, depending on where the abnormal area is located. If the cancer is in the chest, the doctor may perform a thoracoscopy. In this procedure, the doctor makes a small cut through the chest wall and puts a thin, lighted tube called a thoracoscope into the chest between two ribs. Thoracoscopy allows the doctor to look inside the chest and obtain tissue samples. If the cancer is in the abdomen, the doctor may perform a peritoneoscopy. To obtain tissue for examination, the doctor makes a small opening in the abdomen and inserts a special instrument called a peritoneoscope into the abdominal cavity. If these procedures do not yield enough tissue, more extensive diagnostic surgery may be necessary.

If the diagnosis is mesothelioma, the doctor will want to learn the stage (or extent) of the disease. Staging involves more tests in a careful attempt to find out whether the cancer has spread and, if so, to which parts of the body. Knowing the stage of the disease helps the doctor plan treatment.

Mesothelioma is described as localized if the cancer is found only on the membrane surface where it originated. It is classified as advanced if it has spread beyond the original membrane surface to other parts of the body, such as the lymph nodes, lungs, chest wall, or abdominal organs.

How is mesothelioma treated?

Treatment for mesothelioma depends on the location of the cancer, the stage of the disease, and the patient's age and general health. Standard treatment options include surgery, radiation therapy, and chemotherapy. Sometimes, these treatments are combined.

Surgery is a common treatment for mesothelioma. The doctor may remove part of the lining of the chest or abdomen and some of the tissue around it. For cancer of the pleura (pleural mesothelioma), a lung may be removed in an operation called a pneumonectomy. Sometimes part of the diaphragm, the muscle below the lungs that helps with breathing, is also removed.

Radiation therapy, also called radiotherapy, involves the use of high-energy rays to kill cancer cells and shrink tumors. Radiation therapy affects the cancer cells only in the treated area. The radiation may come from a machine (external radiation) or from putting materials that produce radiation through thin plastic tubes into the area where the cancer cells are found (internal radiation therapy).

Chemotherapy is the use of anticancer drugs to kill cancer cells throughout the body. Most drugs used to treat mesothelioma are given by injection into a vein (intravenous, or IV). Doctors are also studying the effectiveness of putting chemotherapy directly into the chest or abdomen (intracavitary chemotherapy).

To relieve symptoms and control pain, the doctor may use a needle or a thin tube to drain fluid that has built up in the chest or abdomen. The procedure for removing fluid from the chest is called thoracentesis.

Removal of fluid from the abdomen is called paracentesis. Drugs may be given through a tube in the chest to prevent more fluid from accumulating. Radiation therapy and surgery may also be helpful in relieving symptoms.

What types of surgical procedures are used to treat mesothelioma?

The following surgical treatments may be used for malignant mesothelioma:

- **Wide local excision:** Surgery to remove the cancer and some of the healthy tissue around it

- **Pleurectomy and decortication:** Surgery to remove part of the covering of the lungs and lining of the chest and part of the outside surface of the lungs

- **Extrapleural pneumonectomy:** Surgery to remove one whole lung and part of the lining of the chest, the diaphragm, and the lining of the sac around the heart

- **Pleurodesis:** A surgical procedure that uses chemicals or drugs to make a scar in the space between the layers of the pleura. Fluid is first drained from the space using a catheter or chest tube and the chemical or drug is put into the space. The scarring stops the build-up of fluid in the pleural cavity.

Even if the doctor removes all the cancer that can be seen at the time of the surgery, some patients may be given chemotherapy or radiation therapy after surgery to kill any cancer cells that are left. Treatment given after surgery, to increase the chances of a cure, is called adjuvant therapy.

Are new treatments for mesothelioma being studied?

Yes. Because mesothelioma is very hard to control, the National Cancer Institute (NCI) is sponsoring clinical trials (research studies with people) that are designed to find new treatments and better ways to use current treatments. Before any new treatment can be recommended for general use, doctors conduct clinical trials to find out whether the treatment is safe for patients and effective against the disease. Participation in clinical trials is an important treatment option for many patients with mesothelioma.

People interested in taking part in a clinical trial should talk with their doctor. Information about clinical trials is available from the Cancer Information Service (CIS) 800-4-CANCER. Information specialists at the CIS use PDQ®, NCI's cancer information database, to identify and provide detailed information about specific ongoing clinical trials. Patients also have the option of searching for clinical trials on their own. The clinical trials page on the NCI website, located at http://www.cancer.gov/clinical_trials, provides general information about clinical trials and links to PDQ.

Chapter 33

Esophageal Cancer

Esophageal cancer is a disease in which malignant (cancer) cells form in the tissues of the esophagus. The esophagus is the hollow, muscular tube that moves food and liquid from the throat to the stomach. The wall of the esophagus is made up of several layers of tissue, including mucous membrane, muscle, and connective tissue. Esophageal cancer starts at the inside lining of the esophagus and spreads outward through the other layers as it grows.

The two most common forms of esophageal cancer are named for the type of cells that become malignant (cancerous):

- **Squamous cell carcinoma:** Cancer that forms in squamous cells, the thin, flat cells lining the esophagus. This cancer is most often found in the upper and middle part of the esophagus, but can occur anywhere along the esophagus. This is also called epidermoid carcinoma.

- **Adenocarcinoma:** Cancer that begins in glandular (secretory) cells. Glandular cells in the lining of the esophagus produce and release fluids such as mucus. Adenocarcinomas usually form in the lower part of the esophagus, near the stomach.

Risk factors of esophageal cancer include the following:

PDQ® Cancer Information Summary. National Cancer Institute; Bethesda, MD. Esophageal Cancer (PDQ®): Treatment - Patient. Updated 08/2005. Available at: http://cancer.gov. Accessed June 22, 2006.

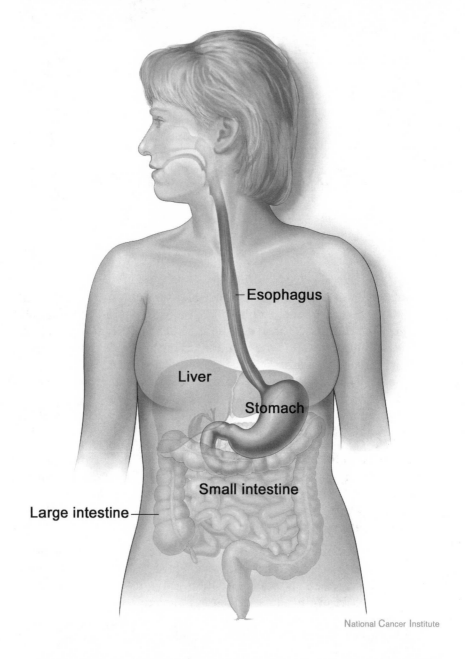

National Cancer Institute

Figure 33.1: *The stomach and esophagus are part of the upper digestive system (Source: Image by Therese Winslow, NCI Visuals Online, 2005).*

- Tobacco use
- Heavy alcohol use
- Barrett esophagus: A condition in which the cells lining the lower part of the esophagus have changed or been replaced with abnormal cells that could lead to cancer of the esophagus. Gastric reflux (the backing up of stomach contents into the lower section of the esophagus) may irritate the esophagus and, over time, cause Barrett esophagus.
- Older age
- Being male
- Being African-American

A doctor should be consulted if any of the following symptoms occur:

- Painful or difficult swallowing
- Weight loss
- Pain behind the breastbone
- Hoarseness and cough
- Indigestion and heartburn

The following tests and procedures may be used to detect (find) and diagnose esophageal cancer:

- **Chest x-ray:** An x-ray of the organs and bones inside the chest. An x-ray is a type of energy beam that can go through the body and onto film, making a picture of areas inside the body.
- **Barium swallow:** A series of x-rays of the esophagus and stomach. The patient drinks a liquid that contains barium (a silver-white metallic compound). The liquid coats the esophagus and x-rays are taken. This procedure is also called an upper GI series.
- **Esophagoscopy:** A procedure to look inside the esophagus to check for abnormal areas. An esophagoscope (a thin, lighted tube) is inserted through the mouth or nose and down the throat into the esophagus. Tissue samples may be taken for biopsy.
- **Biopsy:** The removal of cells or tissues so they can be viewed under a microscope to check for signs of cancer. The biopsy is usually done during an esophagoscopy. Sometimes a biopsy

shows changes in the esophagus that are not cancer but may lead to cancer.

The prognosis (chance of recovery) and treatment options depend on the following:

- The stage of the cancer (whether it affects part of the esophagus, involves the whole esophagus, or has spread to other places in the body)

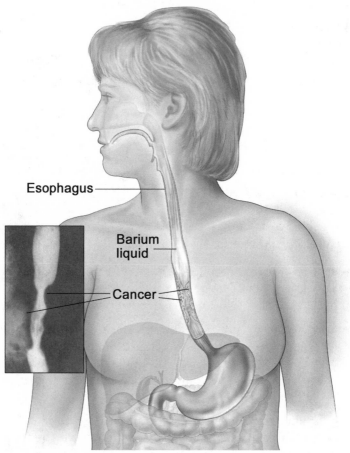

National Cancer Institute

Figure 33.2: Barium swallow. The patient swallows barium liquid and it flows through the esophagus and into the stomach. X-rays are taken to look for abnormal areas (Source: Image by Therese Winslow, NCI Visuals Online, 2005).

- The size of the tumor
- The patient's general health

When esophageal cancer is found very early, there is a better chance of recovery. Esophageal cancer is often in an advanced stage when it is diagnosed. At later stages, esophageal cancer can be treated but rarely can be cured. Taking part in one of the clinical trials being done to improve treatment should be considered. Information about ongoing clinical trials is available from the NCI (National Cancer Institute) website at http://www.cancer.gov.

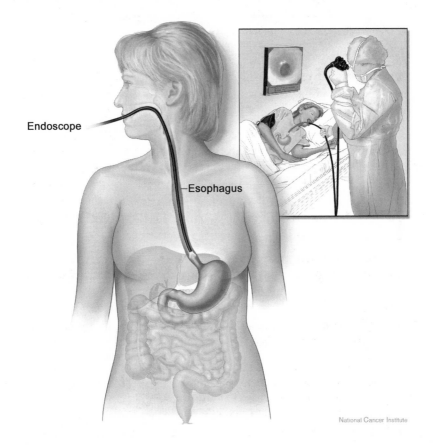

Endoscope

Esophagus

National Cancer Institute

Figure 33.3: *Esophagoscopy. A thin, lighted tube is inserted through the mouth and into the esophagus to look for abnormal areas (Source: Image by Therese Winslow, NCI Visuals Online, 2005).*

Stages of Esophageal Cancer

After esophageal cancer has been diagnosed, tests are done to find out if cancer cells have spread within the esophagus or to other parts of the body. The process used to find out if cancer cells have spread within the esophagus or to other parts of the body is called staging. The information gathered from the staging process determines the stage of the disease. It is important to know the stage in order to plan treatment. The following tests and procedures may be used in the staging process:

- **Bronchoscopy:** A procedure to look inside the trachea and large airways in the lung for abnormal areas. A bronchoscope (a thin, lighted tube) is inserted through the nose or mouth into the trachea and lungs. Tissue samples may be taken for biopsy.

- **Chest x-ray**

- **Laryngoscopy:** A procedure in which the doctor examines the larynx (voice box) with a mirror or with a laryngoscope (a thin, lighted tube).

- **CT scan (CAT scan):** A procedure that makes a series of detailed pictures of areas inside the body, taken from different angles. The pictures are made by a computer linked to an x-ray machine. A dye may be injected into a vein or swallowed to help the organs or tissues show up more clearly. This test is also called computed tomography, computerized tomography, or computerized axial tomography.

- **Endoscopic ultrasound (EUS):** A procedure in which an endoscope (a thin, lighted tube) is inserted into the body. The endoscope is used to bounce high-energy sound waves (ultrasound) off internal tissues or organs and make echoes. The echoes form a picture of body tissues called a sonogram. This procedure is also called endosonography.

- **Thoracoscopy:** A surgical procedure to look at the organs inside the chest to check for abnormal areas. An incision (cut) is made between two ribs and a thoracoscope (a thin, lighted tube) is inserted into the chest. Tissue samples and lymph nodes may be removed for biopsy. In some cases, this procedure may be used to remove portions of the esophagus or lung.

- **Laparoscopy:** A surgical procedure to look at the organs inside the abdomen to check for signs of disease. Small incisions (cuts) are made in the wall of the abdomen, and a laparoscope (a thin, lighted tube) is inserted into one of the incisions. Other instruments may be inserted through the same or other incisions to perform procedures such as removing organs or taking tissue samples for biopsy.

- **PET scan (positron emission tomography scan):** A procedure to find malignant tumor cells in the body. A small amount of radionuclide glucose (sugar) is injected into a vein. The PET scanner rotates around the body and makes a picture of where glucose is being used in the body. Malignant tumor cells show up brighter in the picture because they are more active and take up more glucose than normal cells. The use of PET for staging esophageal cancer is being studied in clinical trials.

The following stages are used for esophageal cancer:

Stage 0 (carcinoma in situ): In stage 0, cancer is found only in the innermost layer of cells lining the esophagus. Stage 0 is also called carcinoma in situ.

Stage I: In stage I, cancer has spread beyond the innermost layer of cells to the next layer of tissue in the wall of the esophagus.

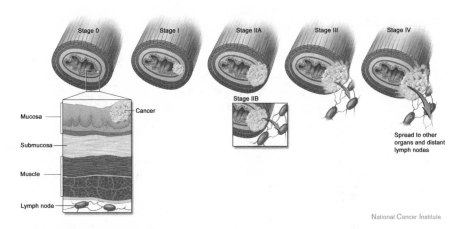

Figure 33.4: *As esophageal cancer progresses from Stage 0 to Stage IV, the cancer cells grow through the layers of the esophagus wall and spread to lymph nodes and other organs (Source: Image by Therese Winslow, NCI Visuals Online, 2005).*

347

Stage II: Stage II esophageal cancer is divided into stage IIA and stage IIB, depending on where the cancer has spread.

- **Stage IIA:** Cancer has spread to the layer of esophageal muscle or to the outer wall of the esophagus.
- **Stage IIB:** Cancer may have spread to any of the first three layers of the esophagus and to nearby lymph nodes.

Stage III: In stage III, cancer has spread to the outer wall of the esophagus and may have spread to tissues or lymph nodes near the esophagus.

Stage IV: Stage IV esophageal cancer is divided into stage IVA and stage IVB, depending on where the cancer has spread.

- **Stage IVA:** Cancer has spread to nearby or distant lymph nodes.
- **Stage IVB:** Cancer has spread to distant lymph nodes and/or organs in other parts of the body.

Recurrent esophageal cancer: Recurrent esophageal cancer is cancer that has recurred (come back) after it has been treated. The cancer may come back in the esophagus or in other parts of the body.

Treatment Option Overview

Different types of treatment are available for patients with esophageal cancer. Some treatments are standard (the currently used treatment), and some are being tested in clinical trials. Before starting treatment, patients may want to think about taking part in a clinical trial. A treatment clinical trial is a research study meant to help improve current treatments or obtain information on new treatments for patients with cancer. When clinical trials show that a new treatment is better than the standard treatment, the new treatment may become the standard treatment.

Clinical trials are taking place in many parts of the country. Information about ongoing clinical trials is available from the NCI website (http://www.cancer.gov). Choosing the most appropriate cancer treatment is a decision that ideally involves the patient, family, and health care team.

Five types of standard treatment are used:

Surgery: Surgery is the most common treatment for cancer of the esophagus. Part of the esophagus may be removed in an operation called an esophagectomy.

The doctor will connect the remaining healthy part of the esophagus to the stomach so the patient can still swallow. A plastic tube or part of the intestine may be used to make the connection. Lymph nodes near the esophagus may also be removed and viewed under a microscope to see if they contain cancer. If the esophagus is partly blocked by the tumor, an expandable metal stent (tube) may be placed inside the esophagus to help keep it open.

Radiation therapy: Radiation therapy is a cancer treatment that uses high-energy x-rays or other types of radiation to kill cancer cells. There are two types of radiation therapy. External radiation therapy uses a machine outside the body to send radiation toward the cancer. Internal radiation therapy uses a radioactive substance sealed in needles, seeds, wires, or catheters that are placed directly into or near the cancer. The way the radiation therapy is given depends on the type and stage of the cancer being treated.

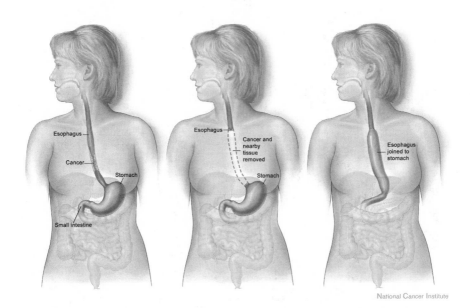

National Cancer Institute

Figure 33.5: Esophagectomy. A portion of the esophagus is removed and the stomach is pulled up and joined to the remaining esophagus (Source: Image by Therese Winslow, NCI Visuals Online, 2005).

A plastic tube may be inserted into the esophagus to keep it open during radiation therapy. This is called intraluminal intubation and dilation.

Chemotherapy: Chemotherapy is a cancer treatment that uses drugs to stop the growth of cancer cells, either by killing the cells or by stopping the cells from dividing. When chemotherapy is taken by mouth or injected into a vein or muscle, the drugs enter the bloodstream and can reach cancer cells throughout the body (systemic chemotherapy). When chemotherapy is placed directly into the spinal column, an organ, or a body cavity such as the abdomen, the drugs mainly affect cancer cells in those areas (regional chemotherapy). The way the chemotherapy is given depends on the type and stage of the cancer being treated.

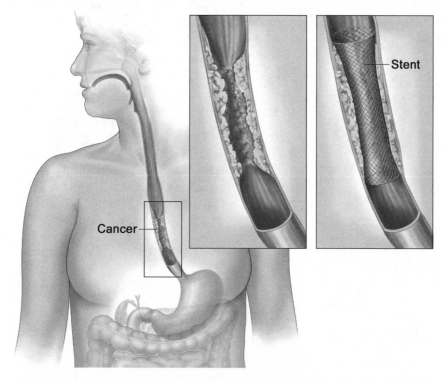

Figure 33.6: Esophageal stent. A device (stent) is placed in the esophagus to keep it open to allow food and liquids to pass through into the stomach (Source: Image by Therese Winslow, NCI Visuals Online, 2005).

Laser therapy: Laser therapy is a cancer treatment that uses a laser beam (a narrow beam of intense light) to kill cancer cells.

Electrocoagulation: Electrocoagulation is the use of an electric current to kill cancer cells.

Patients have special nutritional needs during treatment for esophageal cancer. Many people with esophageal cancer find it hard to eat because they have difficulty swallowing. The esophagus may be narrowed by the tumor or as a side effect of treatment. Some patients may receive nutrients directly into a vein. Others may need a feeding tube (a flexible plastic tube that is passed through the nose or mouth into the stomach) until they are able to eat on their own.

Treatment Options by Stage

Stage 0 esophageal cancer (carcinoma in situ): Treatment of stage 0 esophageal cancer (carcinoma in situ) is usually surgery.

Stage I esophageal cancer: Treatment of stage I esophageal cancer may include the following:

- Surgery
- Clinical trials of chemotherapy plus radiation therapy, with or without surgery
- Clinical trials of new therapies used before or after surgery

Stage II esophageal cancer: Treatment of stage II esophageal cancer may include the following:

- Surgery
- Clinical trials of chemotherapy plus radiation therapy, with or without surgery
- Clinical trials of new therapies used before or after surgery

Stage III esophageal cancer: Treatment of stage III esophageal cancer may include the following:

- Surgery
- Clinical trials of chemotherapy plus radiation therapy, with or without surgery
- Clinical trials of new therapies used before or after surgery

Stage IV esophageal cancer: Treatment of stage IV esophageal cancer may include the following:

- External or internal radiation therapy as palliative therapy to relieve symptoms and improve quality of life
- Laser surgery or electrocoagulation as palliative therapy to relieve symptoms and improve quality of life
- Chemotherapy
- Clinical trials of chemotherapy

Recurrent esophageal cancer: Treatment of recurrent esophageal cancer may include the following:

- Use of any standard treatments as palliative therapy to relieve symptoms and improve quality of life
- Clinical trials of new therapies used before or after surgery

Chapter 34

Stomach (Gastric) Cancer

The Stomach

The stomach is part of the digestive system. It is a hollow organ in the upper abdomen, under the ribs. The wall of the stomach has five layers:

- **Inner layer or lining (mucosa):** Juices made by glands in the inner layer help digest food. Most stomach cancers begin in this layer.

- **Submucosa:** This is the support tissue for the inner layer.

- **Muscle layer:** Muscles in this layer create a rippling motion that mixes and mashes food.

- **Subserosa:** This is the support tissue for the outer layer.

- **Outer layer (serosa):** The outer layer covers the stomach. It holds the stomach in place.

Food moves from the mouth through the esophagus to reach the stomach. In the stomach, the food becomes liquid. The liquid then moves into the small intestine, where it is digested even more.

Cancer Risk Factors

Studies have found the following risk factors for stomach cancer:

From "What You Need to Know about™ Stomach Cancer," National Cancer Institute, August 30, 2005.

- **Age:** Most people with this disease are 72 or older.

- **Sex:** Men are more likely than women to develop stomach cancer.

- **Race:** Stomach cancer is more common in Asian, Pacific Islander, Hispanic, and African Americans than in non-Hispanic white Americans.

- **Diet:** Studies suggest that people who eat a diet high in foods that are smoked, salted, or pickled may be at increased risk for stomach cancer. On the other hand, eating fresh fruits and vegetables may protect against this disease.

- *Helicobacter pylori* **infection:** *H. pylori* is a type of bacteria that commonly lives in the stomach. *H. pylori* infection increases the risk of stomach inflammation and stomach ulcers. It also

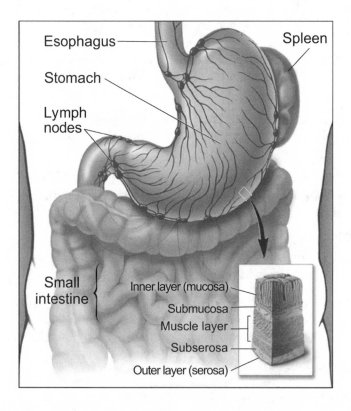

Figure 34.1. This picture shows the stomach and nearby organs (Source: NCI, August 2005).

increases the risk of stomach cancer, but only a small number of infected people develop stomach cancer. Although infection increases the risk, cancer is not contagious. You cannot catch stomach cancer from another person who has it.

- **Smoking:** People who smoke are more likely to develop stomach cancer than people who do not smoke.

- **Certain health problems:** Conditions that cause inflammation or other problems in the stomach may increase the risk of stomach cancer:

  - Stomach surgery

  - Chronic gastritis (long-term inflammation of the stomach lining)

  - Pernicious anemia (a blood disease that affects the stomach)

- **Family history:** A rare type of stomach cancer runs in some families.

Most people who have known risk factors do not develop stomach cancer. For example, many people have *H. pylori* in their stomach but never develop cancer. On the other hand, people who do develop the disease sometimes have no known risk factors.

If you think you may be at risk, you should talk with your doctor. Your doctor may be able to suggest ways to reduce your risk and can plan a schedule for checkups.

Symptoms

Early stomach cancer often does not cause clear symptoms. As the cancer grows, the most common symptoms are these:

- Discomfort in the stomach area
- Feeling full or bloated after a small meal
- Nausea and vomiting
- Weight loss

Most often, these symptoms are not due to cancer. Other health problems, such as an ulcer or infection, can cause the same symptoms. Anyone with these symptoms should tell the doctor so that problems can be found and treated as early as possible.

Stomach cancer can affect nearby organs and lymph nodes:

- A stomach tumor can grow through the stomach's outer layer into nearby organs, such as the pancreas, esophagus, or intestine.

- Stomach cancer cells can spread through the blood to the liver, lungs, and other organs.

- Cancer cells also can spread through the lymphatic system to lymph nodes all over the body.

When cancer spreads from its original place to another part of the body, the new tumor has the same kind of abnormal cells and the same name as the original tumor. For example, if stomach cancer spreads to the liver, the cancer cells in the liver are actually stomach cancer cells. The disease is metastatic stomach cancer, not liver cancer. For that reason, it is treated as stomach cancer, not liver cancer. Doctors call the new tumor "distant" or metastatic disease.

Diagnosis

If you have a symptom that suggests stomach cancer, your doctor must find out whether it is really due to cancer or to some other cause. Your doctor may refer you to a gastroenterologist, a doctor whose specialty is diagnosing and treating digestive problems.

The doctor asks about your personal and family health history. You may have blood or other lab tests. You also may have:

- **Physical exam:** The doctor checks your abdomen for fluid, swelling, or other changes. The doctor also feels for swollen lymph nodes. Your skin and eyes are checked to see if they seem yellow.

- **Upper GI (gastrointestinal) series:** The doctor orders x-rays of your esophagus and stomach. The x-rays are taken after you drink a barium solution. The solution makes your stomach show up more clearly on the x-rays.

- **Endoscopy:** The doctor uses a thin, lighted tube (endoscope) to look into your stomach. The doctor first numbs your throat with an anesthetic spray. You also may receive medicine to help you relax. The tube is passed through your mouth and esophagus to the stomach.

- **Biopsy:** The doctor uses an endoscope to remove tissue from the stomach. A pathologist checks the tissue under a microscope for cancer cells. A biopsy is the only sure way to know if cancer cells are present.

Staging

To plan the best treatment, your doctor needs to know the extent (stage) of the disease. The stage is based on whether the tumor has invaded nearby tissues, whether the cancer has spread, and if so, to what parts of the body. Stomach cancer can spread to the lymph nodes, liver, pancreas, and other organs. The doctor may order tests to check these areas:

- **Blood tests:** The lab does a complete blood count to check for anemia. Blood tests also show how well your liver is working.

- **Chest x-ray:** An x-ray machine takes pictures of your lungs. The doctor can then study these pictures on film. Tumors in your lungs can show up on the x-ray.

- **CT scan:** An x-ray machine linked to a computer takes a series of detailed pictures of your organs. You may receive an injection of dye. The dye makes abnormal areas easier to see. Tumors in your liver, pancreas, or elsewhere in the body can show up on a CT scan.

- **Endoscopic ultrasound:** The doctor passes a thin, lighted tube (endoscope) down your throat. A probe at the end of the tube sends out sound waves that you cannot hear. The waves bounce off tissues in your stomach and other organs.

- **Laparoscopy:** A surgeon makes small incisions (cuts) in your abdomen. The surgeon inserts a thin, lighted tube (laparoscope) into the abdomen. The surgeon may remove lymph nodes or take tissue samples for biopsy.

Sometimes staging is not complete until after surgery to remove the tumor and nearby lymph nodes.

These are the stages of stomach cancer:

Stage 0: The cancer is found only in the inner layer of the stomach. It is carcinoma in situ.

Stage I: Stage I is one of the following:

- The tumor has invaded only the submucosa. Cancer cells may be found in up to six lymph nodes.

- Or, the tumor has invaded the muscle layer or subserosa. Cancer cells have not spread to lymph nodes or other organs.

357

Stage II: Stage II is one of the following:

- The tumor has invaded only the submucosa. Cancer cells have spread to seven to 15 lymph nodes.

- Or, the tumor has invaded the muscle layer or subserosa. Cancer cells have spread to one to six lymph nodes.

- Or, the tumor has penetrated the outer layer of the stomach. Cancer cells have not spread to lymph nodes or other organs.

Stage III: Stage III is one of the following:

- The tumor has invaded the muscle layer or subserosa. Cancer cells have spread to seven to 15 lymph nodes.

- Or, the tumor has penetrated the outer layer. Cancer cells have spread to one to 15 lymph nodes.

- Or, the tumor has invaded nearby organs, such as the liver or spleen. Cancer cells have not spread to lymph nodes or to distant organs.

Stage IV: Stage IV is one of the following:

- Cancer cells have spread to more than 15 lymph nodes.

- Or, the tumor has invaded nearby organs and at least one lymph node.

- Or, cancer cells have spread to distant organs.

Recurrent cancer: The cancer has come back (recurred) after a period of time when it could not be detected. It may recur in the stomach or in another part of the body.

Treatment

The choice of treatment depends mainly on the size and place of the tumor, the stage of disease, and your general health. Treatment for stomach cancer may involve surgery, chemotherapy, or radiation therapy. Many people have more than one type of treatment.

Cancer treatment is either local therapy or systemic therapy:

- **Local therapy:** Surgery and radiation therapy are local therapies. They remove or destroy cancer in or near the stomach.

When stomach cancer has spread to other parts of the body, local therapy may be used to control the disease in those specific areas.

- **Systemic therapy:** Chemotherapy is systemic therapy. The drug enters the bloodstream and destroys or controls cancer throughout the body.

Because cancer treatments often damage healthy cells and tissues, side effects are common. Side effects depend mainly on the type and extent of the treatment. Side effects may not be the same for each person, and they may change from one treatment session to the next.

Before treatment starts, your health care team will explain possible side effects and suggest ways to help you manage them.

At any stage of disease, supportive care is available to relieve the side effects of treatment, to control pain and other symptoms, and to ease emotional concerns. Information about such care is available on NCI's website at http://www.cancer.gov/cancertopics/coping, and from Information Specialists at 800-4-CANCER or LiveHelp (http://cis.nci .nih.gov).

You may want to talk to your doctor about taking part in a clinical trial, a research study of new treatment methods.

Surgery: Surgery is the most common treatment for stomach cancer. The type of surgery depends on the extent of the cancer. There are two main types of stomach cancer surgery:

- **Partial (subtotal) gastrectomy:** The surgeon removes the part of the stomach with cancer. The surgeon also may remove part of the esophagus or part of the small intestine. Nearby lymph nodes and other tissues may be removed.

- **Total gastrectomy:** The doctor removes the entire stomach, nearby lymph nodes, parts of the esophagus and small intestine, and other tissues near the tumor. The spleen also may be removed. The surgeon then connects the esophagus directly to the small intestine. The surgeon makes a new "stomach" out of tissue from the intestine.

It is natural to be concerned about eating after surgery for stomach cancer. During surgery, the surgeon may place a feeding tube into your small intestine. This tube helps you get enough nutrition while you heal. Information about eating after surgery is in the "Nutrition" section.

The time it takes to heal after surgery is different for each person. You may be uncomfortable for the first few days. Medicine can help control your pain. Before surgery, you should discuss the plan for pain relief with your doctor or nurse. After surgery, your doctor can adjust the plan if you need more pain relief.

Many people who have stomach surgery feel tired or weak for a while. The surgery also can cause constipation or diarrhea. These symptoms usually can be controlled with diet changes and medicine. Your health care team will watch for signs of bleeding, infection, or other problems that may require treatment.

Chemotherapy: Chemotherapy uses anticancer drugs to kill cancer cells. The drugs enter the bloodstream and can affect cancer cells all over the body.

Most people who receive chemotherapy have it after surgery. Radiation therapy may be given along with chemotherapy.

Anticancer drugs for stomach cancer are usually injected into a blood vessel. But some drugs may be given by mouth. You may have your treatment in a clinic at the hospital, at the doctor's office, or at home. Some people may need to stay in the hospital during treatment.

The side effects of chemotherapy depend mainly on the specific drugs and the dose. The drugs affect cancer cells and other cells that divide rapidly:

- **Blood cells:** These cells fight infection, help blood to clot, and carry oxygen to all parts of your body. When drugs affect your blood cells, you are more likely to get infections, bruise or bleed easily, and feel very weak and tired.

- **Cells in hair roots:** Chemotherapy drugs can cause hair loss. Your hair will grow back, but it may be somewhat different in color and texture.

- **Cells that line the digestive tract:** Chemotherapy can cause poor appetite, nausea and vomiting, diarrhea, or mouth and lip sores.

The drugs used for stomach cancer also may cause a skin rash or itching. Your health care team can suggest ways to control many of these side effects.

Radiation therapy: Radiation therapy (also called radiotherapy) uses high-energy rays to kill cancer cells. It affects cells only in the treated area.

The radiation comes from a large machine outside the body. Most people go to a hospital or clinic for treatment. Treatments are usually five days a week for several weeks.

Side effects depend mainly on the dose of radiation and the part of your body that is treated. Radiation therapy to the abdomen may cause pain in the stomach or the intestine. You may have nausea and diarrhea. Also, your skin in the treated area may become red, dry, and tender.

You are likely to become very tired during radiation therapy, especially in the later weeks of treatment. Resting is important, but doctors usually advise patients to try to stay as active as they can.

Although the side effects of radiation therapy can be distressing, your doctor can usually treat or control them. Also, side effects usually go away after treatment ends.

Complementary and alternative medicine: Some people with cancer use complementary and alternative medicine (CAM):

- An approach is generally called complementary medicine when it is used along with standard treatment.

- An approach is called alternative medicine when it is used instead of standard treatment.

- Acupuncture, massage therapy, herbal products, vitamins or special diets, visualization, meditation, and spiritual healing are types of CAM.

Many people say that CAM helps them feel better. However, some types of CAM may change the way standard treatment works. These changes could be harmful. And some types of CAM could be harmful even if used alone. Before trying any type of CAM, you should discuss its possible benefits and risks with your doctor.

Some types of CAM are expensive. Health insurance may not cover the cost.

Nutrition

It is important to eat well during and after cancer treatment. You need the right amount of calories, protein, vitamins, and minerals. Eating well may help you feel better and have more energy.

Eating well can be hard. Sometimes, especially during or soon after treatment, you may not feel like eating. You may be uncomfortable or tired. You may find that foods do not taste as good as they used to. You also may have side effects of treatment such as poor appetite, nausea, vomiting, or diarrhea.

A registered dietitian can suggest ways to deal with these problems. Some people with stomach cancer are helped by receiving nutrition by a feeding tube or by injection into a blood vessel. Some are helped by nutritional beverage products.

Nutrition after Stomach Surgery

Weight loss after surgery for stomach cancer is common. You may need to change the types of food you eat. A registered dietitian can help you plan a diet that will give you the nutrition you need.

Another common problem after stomach surgery is dumping syndrome. This problem occurs when food or liquid enters the small intestine too fast. It can cause cramps, nausea, bloating, diarrhea, and dizziness. Eating smaller meals can help prevent dumping syndrome. Also, you may wish to cut down on very sweet foods and drinks, such as cookies, candy, soda, and juices. A registered dietitian can suggest foods to try. Also, your health care team may suggest medicine to control the symptoms.

You may need to take daily supplements of vitamins and minerals, such as calcium. You also may need injections of vitamin B_{12}.

You may want to ask a registered dietitian these questions about nutrition:

- What foods are best soon after surgery?
- How can I avoid dumping syndrome?
- Are there foods or drinks I should avoid?

Follow-up Care

Follow-up care after treatment for stomach cancer is important. Even when there are no longer any signs of cancer, the disease sometimes returns because undetected cancer cells remained somewhere in the body after treatment. Your doctor will monitor your recovery and check for recurrence of the cancer. Checkups help ensure that any changes in your health are noted and treated if needed. Checkups may include a physical exam, lab tests, x-rays, CT scans, endoscopy, or other tests. Between scheduled visits, you should contact the doctor if you have any health problems.

Chapter 35

Gallbladder Cancer

Gallbladder cancer is a rare disease in which malignant (cancer) cells are found in the tissues of the gallbladder. The gallbladder is a pear-shaped organ that lies just under the liver in the upper abdomen. The gallbladder stores bile, a fluid made by the liver to digest fat. When food is being broken down in the stomach and intestines, bile is released from the gallbladder through a tube called the common bile duct, which connects the gallbladder and liver to the first part of the small intestine.

The wall of the gallbladder has three main layers of tissue:

- Mucosal (innermost) layer
- Muscularis (middle, muscle) layer
- Serosal (outer) layer

Between these layers is supporting connective tissue. Primary gallbladder cancer starts in the innermost layer and spreads through the outer layers as it grows.

Anything that increases your chance of getting a disease is called a risk factor. Risk factors for gallbladder cancer include being female or being Native American.

A doctor should be consulted if any of the following symptoms occur:

Excerpted from PDQ® Cancer Information Summary. National Cancer Institute; Bethesda, MD. Gallbladder Cancer (PDQ®): Treatment - Patient. Updated 12/2005. Available at: http://cancer.gov. Accessed June 22, 2006.

- Jaundice (yellowing of the skin and whites of the eyes)
- Pain above the stomach
- Fever
- Nausea and vomiting
- Bloating
- Lumps in the abdomen

Gallbladder cancer is difficult to detect and diagnose for the following reasons:

- There aren't any noticeable signs or symptoms in the early stages of gallbladder cancer.
- The symptoms of gallbladder cancer, when present, are like the symptoms of many other illnesses.
- The gallbladder is hidden behind the liver.

Gallbladder cancer is sometimes found when the gallbladder is removed for other reasons. Patients with gallstones rarely develop gallbladder cancer.

Procedures that create pictures of the gallbladder and the area around it help diagnose gallbladder cancer and show how far the cancer has spread. The process used to find out if cancer cells have spread within and around the gallbladder is called staging.

In order to plan treatment, it is important to know if the gallbladder cancer can be removed by surgery. Tests and procedures to detect, diagnose, and stage gallbladder cancer are usually done at the same time. In addition to a physical exam and history, the following tests and procedures may be used:

- **Ultrasound exam:** A procedure in which high-energy sound waves (ultrasound) are bounced off internal tissues or organs and make echoes. The echoes form a picture of body tissues called a sonogram. An abdominal ultrasound is done to diagnose gallbladder cancer.

- **Liver function tests:** A procedure in which a blood sample is checked to measure the amounts of certain substances released into the blood by the liver. A higher than normal amount of a substance can be a sign of liver disease that may be caused by gallbladder cancer.

- **Carcinoembryonic antigen (CEA) assay:** A test that measures the level of CEA in the blood. CEA is released into the bloodstream from both cancer cells and normal cells. When found in higher than normal amounts, it can be a sign of gallbladder cancer or other conditions.

- **CA 19-9 assay:** A test that measures the level of CA 19-9 in the blood. CA 19-9 is released into the bloodstream from both cancer cells and normal cells. When found in higher than normal amounts, it can be a sign of gallbladder cancer or other conditions.

- **CT scan (CAT scan):** A procedure that makes a series of detailed pictures of areas inside the body, taken from different angles. The pictures are made by a computer linked to an x-ray machine. A dye may be injected into a vein or swallowed to help the organs or tissues show up more clearly. This procedure is also called computed tomography, computerized tomography, or computerized axial tomography.

- **Blood chemistry studies:** A procedure in which a blood sample is checked to measure the amounts of certain substances released into the blood by organs and tissues in the body. An unusual (higher or lower than normal) amount of a substance can be a sign of disease in the organ or tissue that produces it.

- **Chest x-ray:** An x-ray of the organs and bones inside the chest. An x-ray is a type of energy beam that can go through the body and onto film, making a picture of areas inside the body.

- **MRI (magnetic resonance imaging):** A procedure that uses a magnet, radio waves, and a computer to make a series of detailed pictures of areas inside the body. This procedure is also called nuclear magnetic resonance imaging (NMRI). A dye may be injected into the gallbladder area so the ducts (tubes) that carry bile from the liver to the gallbladder and from the gallbladder to the small intestine will show up better in the image. This procedure is called MRCP (magnetic resonance cholangiopancreatography). To create detailed pictures of blood vessels near the gallbladder, the dye is injected into a vein. This procedure is called MRA (magnetic resonance angiography).

- **ERCP (endoscopic retrograde cholangiopancreatography):** A procedure used to x-ray the ducts (tubes) that carry bile from the liver to the gallbladder and from the gallbladder to the small intestine. Sometimes gallbladder cancer causes these ducts to narrow and block or slow the flow of bile, causing jaundice. An endoscope (a thin, lighted tube) is passed through the mouth, esophagus, and stomach into the first part of the small intestine. A catheter (a smaller tube) is then inserted through the endoscope into the bile ducts. A dye is injected through the catheter into the ducts and an x-ray is taken. If the ducts are blocked by a tumor, a fine tube may be inserted into the duct to unblock it. This tube (or stent) may be left in place to keep the duct open. Tissue samples may also be taken.

- **Biopsy:** The removal of cells or tissues so they can be viewed under a microscope by a pathologist to check for signs of cancer. The biopsy may be done after surgery to remove the tumor. If the tumor clearly cannot be removed by surgery, the biopsy may be done using a fine needle to remove cells from the tumor.

- **Laparoscopy:** A surgical procedure to look at the organs inside the abdomen to check for signs of disease. Small incisions (cuts) are made in the wall of the abdomen and a laparoscope (a thin, lighted tube) is inserted into one of the incisions. Other instruments may be inserted through the same or other incisions to perform procedures such as removing organs or taking tissue samples for biopsy. The laparoscopy helps to determine if the cancer is within the gallbladder only or has spread to nearby tissues and if it can be removed by surgery.

- **PTC (percutaneous transhepatic cholangiography):** A procedure used to x-ray the liver and bile ducts. A thin needle is inserted through the skin below the ribs and into the liver. Dye is injected into the liver or bile ducts and an x-ray is taken. If a blockage is found, a thin, flexible tube called a stent is sometimes left in the liver to drain bile into the small intestine or a collection bag outside the body.

Gallbladder cancer can be cured only if it is found before it has spread, when it can be removed by surgery. If the cancer has spread, palliative treatment can improve the patient's quality of life by controlling the symptoms and complications of this disease.

Stages of Gallbladder Cancer

Tests and procedures to stage gallbladder cancer are usually done at the same time as diagnosis. The following stages are used for gallbladder cancer:

Stage 0 (carcinoma in situ): In stage 0, cancer is found only in the innermost (mucosal) layer of the gallbladder. Stage 0 cancer is also called carcinoma in situ.

Stage I: Stage I is divided into stage IA and stage IB.

- **Stage IA:** Cancer has spread beyond the innermost (mucosal) layer to the connective tissue or to the muscle (muscularis) layer.
- **Stage IB:** Cancer has spread beyond the muscle layer to the connective tissue around the muscle.

Stage II: Stage II is divided into stage IIA and stage IIB.

- **Stage IIA:** Cancer has spread beyond the visceral peritoneum (tissue that covers the gallbladder) and/or to the liver and/or one nearby organ (such as the stomach, small intestine, colon, pancreas, or bile ducts outside the liver).
- **Stage IIB:** Cancer has spread:
  - beyond the innermost layer to the connective tissue and to nearby lymph nodes; or
  - to the muscle layer and nearby lymph nodes; or
  - beyond the muscle layer to the connective tissue around the muscle and to nearby lymph nodes; or
  - through the visceral peritoneum (tissue that covers the gallbladder) and/or to the liver and/or to one nearby organ (such as the stomach, small intestine, colon, pancreas, or bile ducts outside the liver), and to nearby lymph nodes.

Stage III: In stage III, cancer has spread to a main blood vessel in the liver or to nearby organs and may have spread to nearby lymph nodes.

Stage IV: In stage IV, cancer has spread to nearby lymph nodes and/or to organs far away from the gallbladder.

For gallbladder cancer, stages are also grouped according to how the cancer may be treated. There are two treatment groups:

Localized (stage I): Cancer is found in the wall of the gallbladder and can be completely removed by surgery.

Unresectable (stage II, stage III, and stage IV): Cancer has spread through the wall of the gallbladder to surrounding tissues or organs or throughout the abdominal cavity. Except in patients whose cancer has spread only to lymph nodes, the cancer is unresectable (cannot be completely removed by surgery).

Recurrent gallbladder cancer: Recurrent gallbladder cancer is cancer that has recurred (come back) after it has been treated. The cancer may come back in the gallbladder or in other parts of the body.

Treatment Option Overview

Three types of standard treatment are used:

Surgery: Gallbladder cancer may be treated with a cholecystectomy, surgery to remove the gallbladder and some of the tissues around it. Nearby lymph nodes may be removed. A laparoscope is sometimes used to guide gallbladder surgery. The laparoscope is attached to a video camera and inserted through an incision (port) in the abdomen. Surgical instruments are inserted through other ports to perform the surgery. Because there is a risk that gallbladder cancer cells may spread to these ports, tissue surrounding the port sites may also be removed.

If the cancer has spread and cannot be removed, the following types of palliative surgery may relieve symptoms:

- **Surgical biliary bypass:** If the tumor is blocking the small intestine and bile is building up in the gallbladder, a biliary bypass may be done. During this operation, the gallbladder or bile duct will be cut and sewn to the small intestine to create a new pathway around the blocked area.

- **Endoscopic stent placement:** If the tumor is blocking the bile duct, surgery may be done to put in a stent (a thin, flexible tube) to drain bile that has built up in the area. The stent may be placed through a catheter that drains to the outside of the body or the stent may go around the blocked area and drain the bile into the small intestine.

- **Percutaneous transhepatic biliary drainage:** A procedure done to drain bile when there is a blockage and endoscopic stent placement is not possible. An x-ray of the liver and bile ducts is done to locate the blockage. Images made by ultrasound are used to guide placement of a stent, which is left in the liver to drain bile into the small intestine or a collection bag outside the body. This procedure may be done to relieve jaundice before surgery.

Radiation therapy: Radiation therapy is a cancer treatment that uses high-energy x-rays or other types of radiation to kill cancer cells. There are two types of radiation therapy. External radiation therapy uses a machine outside the body to send radiation toward the cancer. Internal radiation therapy uses a radioactive substance sealed in needles, seeds, wires, or catheters that are placed directly into or near the cancer. The way the radiation therapy is given depends on the type and stage of the cancer being treated.

Chemotherapy: Chemotherapy is a cancer treatment that uses drugs to stop the growth of cancer cells, either by killing the cells or by stopping the cells from dividing. When chemotherapy is taken by mouth or injected into a vein or muscle, the drugs enter the bloodstream and can reach cancer cells throughout the body (systemic chemotherapy). When chemotherapy is placed directly into the spinal column, an organ, or a body cavity such as the abdomen, the drugs mainly affect cancer cells in those areas (regional chemotherapy). The way the chemotherapy is given depends on the type and stage of the cancer being treated.

New Treatment

New types of treatment are being tested in clinical trials. These include the following:

Radiosensitizers: Radiosensitizers are drugs that make tumor cells more sensitive to radiation therapy. Combining radiation therapy with radiosensitizers may kill more tumor cells.

Treatment Options for Gallbladder Cancer

Localized gallbladder cancer: Treatment of localized gallbladder cancer may include the following:

- Surgery to remove the gallbladder and some of the tissue around it. The liver and nearby lymph nodes may also be removed. Radiation therapy with or without chemotherapy may follow surgery.

- Radiation therapy with or without chemotherapy

- A clinical trial of radiation therapy with radiosensitizers

Unresectable gallbladder cancer: Treatment of unresectable gallbladder cancer may include the following:

- Radiation therapy as palliative treatment, with or without surgery or the placement of stents, to relieve symptoms caused by blocked bile ducts

- Surgery as palliative treatment to relieve symptoms caused by blocked bile ducts

- Chemotherapy as palliative treatment to relieve symptoms caused by the cancer

- A clinical trial of internal radiation therapy or radiosensitizers

- A clinical trial of chemotherapy

Recurrent gallbladder cancer: Treatment of recurrent gallbladder cancer is usually done in a clinical trial.

Chapter 36

Extrahepatic Bile Duct Cancer

Extrahepatic bile duct cancer is a rare disease in which malignant (cancer) cells form in the part of bile duct that is outside the liver. A network of bile ducts (tubes) connects the liver and the gallbladder to the small intestine. This network begins in the liver where many small ducts collect bile, a fluid made by the liver to break down fats during digestion. The small ducts come together to form the right and left hepatic bile ducts, which lead out of the liver. The two ducts join outside the liver to become the common hepatic duct. The part of the common hepatic duct that is outside the liver is called the extrahepatic bile duct. The extrahepatic bile duct is joined by a duct from the gallbladder (which stores bile) to form the common bile duct. Bile is released from the gallbladder through the common bile duct into the small intestine when food is being digested.

Risk factors include having any of the following disorders:

- Primary sclerosing cholangitis
- Chronic ulcerative colitis
- Choledochal cysts
- Infection with a Chinese liver fluke parasite

A doctor should be consulted if any of the following symptoms occur:

PDQ® Cancer Information Summary. National Cancer Institute; Bethesda, MD. Extrahepatic Bile Duct Cancer (PDQ®): Treatment - Patient. Updated 05/2004. Available at: http://cancer.gov. Accessed June 22, 2006.

- Jaundice (yellowing of the skin or whites of the eyes)
- Pain in the abdomen
- Fever
- Itchy skin

Tests that examine the bile duct and liver are used to detect (find) and diagnose extrahepatic bile duct cancer. The following tests and procedures may be used:

Physical exam and history: An exam of the body to check general signs of health, including checking for signs of disease, such as lumps or anything else that seems unusual. A history of the patient's health habits and past illnesses and treatments will also be taken.

Ultrasound: A procedure in which high-energy sound waves (ultrasound) are bounced off internal tissues or organs and make echoes. The echoes form a picture of body tissues called a sonogram.

CT scan (CAT scan): A procedure that makes a series of detailed pictures of areas inside the body, taken from different angles. The pictures are made by a computer linked to an x-ray machine. A dye may be injected into a vein or swallowed to help the organs or tissues show up more clearly. This procedure is also called computed tomography, computerized tomography, or computerized axial tomography. A spiral or helical CT scan makes detailed pictures of areas inside the body using an x-ray machine that scans the body in a spiral path.

MRI (magnetic resonance imaging): A procedure that uses a magnet, radio waves, and a computer to make a series of detailed pictures of areas inside the body. This procedure is also called nuclear magnetic resonance imaging (NMRI).

ERCP (endoscopic retrograde cholangiopancreatography): A procedure used to x-ray the ducts (tubes) that carry bile from the liver to the gallbladder and from the gallbladder to the small intestine. Sometimes bile duct cancer causes these ducts to narrow and block or slow the flow of bile, causing jaundice. An endoscope (a thin, lighted tube) is passed through the mouth, esophagus, and stomach into the first part of the small intestine. A catheter (a smaller tube) is then inserted through the endoscope into the pancreatic ducts. A dye is injected through the catheter into the ducts and an x-ray is taken. If the ducts are blocked by a tumor, a fine tube may be inserted into the duct to unblock it. This tube (or stent) may be left in place to keep the duct open. Tissue samples may also be taken.

PTC (percutaneous transhepatic cholangiography): A procedure used to x-ray the liver and bile ducts. A thin needle is inserted through the skin below the ribs and into the liver. Dye is injected into the liver or bile ducts and an x-ray is taken. If a blockage is found, a thin, flexible tube called a stent is sometimes left in the liver to drain bile into the small intestine or a collection bag outside the body.

Biopsy: The removal of cells or tissues so they can be viewed under a microscope to check for signs of cancer. The sample may be taken using a fine needle inserted into the duct during an x-ray or ultrasound. This is called needle biopsy or fine-needle aspiration biopsy. The biopsy is usually done during PTC or ERCP. Tissue may also be removed during surgery.

Liver function tests: A procedure in which a blood sample is checked to measure the amounts of certain substances released into the blood by the liver. A higher than normal amount of a substance can be a sign of liver disease that may be caused by extrahepatic bile duct cancer.

The prognosis (chance of recovery) and treatment options depend on the following:

- The stage of the cancer (whether it affects only the bile duct or has spread to other places in the body)

- Whether the tumor can be completely removed by surgery

- Whether the tumor is in the upper or lower part of the duct

- Whether the cancer has just been diagnosed or has recurred (come back)

- Treatment options may also depend on the symptoms caused by the tumor. Extrahepatic bile duct cancer is usually found after it has spread and can rarely be removed completely by surgery. Palliative therapy may relieve symptoms and improve the patient's quality of life.

Stages of Extrahepatic Bile Duct Cancer

After extrahepatic bile duct cancer has been diagnosed, tests are done to find out if cancer cells have spread within the bile duct or to other parts of the body. The process used to find out if cancer has spread within the extrahepatic bile duct or to other parts of the body is called staging. The information gathered from the staging process determines the stage of the disease. It is important to know the stage in order to plan treatment.

Extrahepatic bile duct cancer is usually staged following a laparotomy. A surgical incision is made in the wall of the abdomen to check the inside of the abdomen for signs of disease and to remove tissue and fluid for examination under a microscope. The results of the diagnostic imaging tests, laparotomy, and biopsy are viewed together to determine the stage of the cancer. Sometimes, a laparoscopy will be done before the laparotomy to see if the cancer has spread. If the cancer has spread and cannot be removed by surgery, the surgeon may decide not to do a laparotomy.

The following stages are used for extrahepatic bile duct cancer:

Stage 0 (carcinoma in situ): In stage 0, cancer is found only in the innermost layer of cells lining the extrahepatic bile duct. Stage 0 cancer is also called carcinoma in situ.

Stage I: Stage I is divided into stage IA and stage IB.

- **Stage IA:** Cancer is found in the bile duct only.
- **Stage IB:** Cancer has spread through the wall of the bile duct.

Stage II: Stage II is divided into stage IIA and stage IIB.

- **Stage IIA:** Cancer has spread to the liver, gallbladder, pancreas, and/or to either the right or left branches of the hepatic artery or to right or left branches of the portal vein.
- **Stage IIB:** Cancer has spread to nearby lymph nodes and:
  - is found in the bile duct; or
  - has spread through the wall of the bile duct; or
  - has spread to the liver, gallbladder, pancreas, and/or the right or left branches of the hepatic artery or portal vein.

Stage III: In stage III, cancer has spread:

- to the portal vein or to both right and left branches of the portal vein; or
- to the hepatic artery; or

- to other nearby organs or tissues, such as the colon, stomach, small intestine, or abdominal wall; or

- to nearby lymph nodes.

Stage IV: In stage IV, cancer has spread to lymph nodes and/or organs far away from the extrahepatic bile duct.

Grouped by Treatment

Extrahepatic bile duct cancer can also be grouped according to how the cancer may be treated. There are two treatment groups:

Localized (and resectable): The cancer is in an area where it can be removed completely by surgery.

Unresectable: The cancer cannot be removed completely by surgery. The cancer may have spread to nearby blood vessels, the liver, the common bile duct, nearby lymph nodes, or other parts of the abdominal cavity.

Recurrent extrahepatic bile duct cancer: Recurrent extrahepatic bile duct cancer is cancer that has recurred (come back) after it has been treated. The cancer may come back in the bile duct or in other parts of the body.

Treatment Option Overview

Different types of treatment are available for patients with extrahepatic bile duct cancer. Some treatments are standard (the currently used treatment), and some are being tested in clinical trials. Before starting treatment, patients may want to think about taking part in a clinical trial. A treatment clinical trial is a research study meant to help improve current treatments or obtain information on new treatments for patients with cancer. When clinical trials show that a new treatment is better than the standard treatment, the new treatment may become the standard treatment.

Clinical trials are taking place in many parts of the country. Information about ongoing clinical trials is available from the NCI (National Cancer Institute) website (http://www.cancer.gov). Choosing the most appropriate cancer treatment is a decision that ideally involves the patient, family, and health care team.

Two types of standard treatment are used:

Surgery: The following types of surgery are used to treat extra-hepatic bile duct cancer:

- **Removal of the bile duct:** If the tumor is small and only in the bile duct, the entire bile duct may be removed. A new duct is made by connecting the duct openings in the liver to the intestine. Lymph nodes are removed and viewed under a microscope to see if they contain cancer.

- **Partial hepatectomy:** Removal of the part of the liver where cancer is found. The part removed may be a wedge of tissue, an entire lobe, or a larger part of the liver, along with some normal tissue around it.

- **Whipple procedure:** A surgical procedure in which the head of the pancreas, the gallbladder, part of the stomach, part of the small intestine, and the bile duct are removed. Enough of the pancreas is left to produce digestive juices and insulin.

- **Surgical biliary bypass:** If the tumor cannot be removed but is blocking the small intestine and causing bile to build up in the gallbladder, a biliary bypass may be done. During this operation, the gallbladder or bile duct will be cut and sewn to the small intestine to create a new pathway around the blocked area. This procedure helps to relieve jaundice caused by the build-up of bile.

- **Stent placement:** If the tumor is blocking the bile duct, a stent (a thin tube) may be placed in the duct to drain bile that has built up in the area. The stent may drain to the outside of the body or it may go around the blocked area and drain the bile into the small intestine. The doctor may place the stent during surgery or PTC, or with an endoscope.

Radiation therapy: Radiation therapy is a cancer treatment that uses high-energy x-rays or other types of radiation to kill cancer cells. There are two types of radiation therapy. External radiation therapy uses a machine outside the body to send radiation toward the cancer. Internal radiation therapy uses a radioactive substance sealed in needles, seeds, wires, or catheters that are placed directly into or near the cancer. The way the radiation therapy is given depends on the type and stage of the cancer being treated.

Other Treatments

Other types of treatment are being tested in clinical trials. These include the following:

Radiation sensitizers: Clinical trials are studying ways to improve the effect of radiation therapy on tumor cells, including the following:

- **Hyperthermia therapy:** A treatment in which body tissue is exposed to high temperatures to damage and kill cancer cells or to make cancer cells more sensitive to the effects of radiation therapy and certain anticancer drugs.

- **Radiosensitizers:** Drugs that make tumor cells more sensitive to radiation therapy. Combining radiation therapy with radiosensitizers may kill more tumor cells.

Chemotherapy: Chemotherapy is a cancer treatment that uses drugs to stop the growth of cancer cells, either by killing the cells or by stopping the cells from dividing. When chemotherapy is taken by mouth or injected into a vein or muscle, the drugs enter the bloodstream and can reach cancer cells throughout the body (systemic chemotherapy). When chemotherapy is placed directly into the spinal column, an organ, or a body cavity such as the abdomen, the drugs mainly affect cancer cells in those areas (regional chemotherapy). The way the chemotherapy is given depends on the type and stage of the cancer being treated.

Biologic therapy: Biologic therapy is a treatment that uses the patient's immune system to fight cancer. Substances made by the body or made in a laboratory are used to boost, direct, or restore the body's natural defenses against cancer. This type of cancer treatment is also called biotherapy or immunotherapy.

Treatment Options for Extrahepatic Bile Duct Cancer

Localized extrahepatic bile duct cancer: Treatment of localized extrahepatic bile duct cancer may include the following:

- Stent placement or biliary bypass to relieve blockage of the bile duct may be done before surgery to relieve jaundice

- Surgery, with or without external-beam radiation therapy

Unresectable extrahepatic bile duct cancer: Treatment of unresectable extrahepatic bile duct cancer may include the following:

- Stent placement or biliary bypass with or without internal or external radiation therapy, as palliative treatment to relieve symptoms and improve the quality of life

- A clinical trial of hyperthermia therapy, radiosensitizers, chemotherapy, or biologic therapy

Recurrent extrahepatic bile duct cancer: Treatment of recurrent extrahepatic bile duct cancer may include the following:

- Palliative treatment to relieve symptoms and improve quality of life

- A clinical trial

Chapter 37

Pancreatic Cancer

What is the pancreas?

The pancreas is an oblong flattened gland located deep in the abdomen. It is an integral part of the digestive system. It is about six inches long and is shaped like a flat pear. The widest part of the pancreas is the head, the middle section is the body, and the thinnest part is the tail.

What does the pancreas do?

The pancreas produces insulin and other hormones. These hormones help the body use or store the energy that comes from food. The pancreas also makes pancreatic juices which contain enzymes that help digest food. The pancreas releases the juices into a system of ducts leading to the common bile duct. The common bile duct empties into the duodenum, the first section of the small intestine.

What is cancer?

Cancer is the illness or condition that is caused when cells multiply uncontrollably forming a growth or tumor and destroying healthy tissue.

What is the difference between a benign and malignant tumor?

Benign tumors are not cancer and are usually not life threatening. In most cases, benign tumors can be removed and do not come back. Cells from benign tumors do not spread to tissues around them or to other parts of the body.

Malignant tumors are cancer. The term malignant is used to describe a tumor that invades the tissue around it and may spread to other parts of the body. Malignant tumors are more serious and may be life threatening.

How does cancer spread?

Cancer cells can break away from a malignant tumor and enter the bloodstream or lymphatic system. That is how cancer cells metastasize,

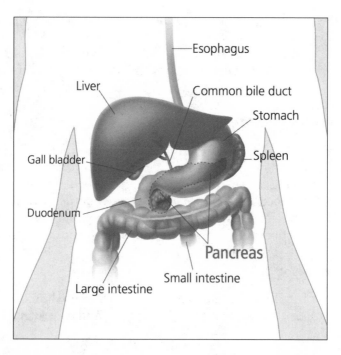

Figure 37.1: This picture shows the pancreas and nearby organs (Source: From "What You Need to Know about™ Cancer of the Pancreas," National Cancer Institute, September 2001).

or spread, from the original cancer (primary tumor) to form new tumors in other organs.

Where does pancreatic cancer begin?

Most pancreatic cancers begin in the ducts that carry pancreatic juices. Cancer of the pancreas may be called pancreatic cancer or carcinoma of the pancreas.

What is islet cell cancer?

A rare type of pancreatic cancer that begins in the cells that make insulin and other hormones.

What is metastatic pancreatic cancer?

When cancer spreads from its original place to another part of the body, the new tumor has the same kind of abnormal cells and the same name as the primary tumor. For example, if cancer of the pancreas spreads to the liver, the cancer cells in the liver are pancreatic cancer cells. The disease is metastatic pancreatic cancer, not liver cancer. It is treated as pancreatic cancer, not liver cancer.

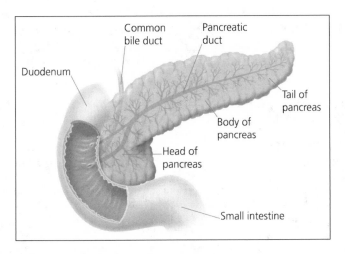

Figure 37.2: This picture shows the pancreas, common bile duct, and small intestine (Source: From "What You Need to Know about™ Cancer of the Pancreas," National Cancer Institute, September 2001).

Is pancreatic cancer contagious?

No. Cancer does not spread from person to person.

What causes pancreatic cancer?

No one knows the exact causes of pancreatic cancer though research has shown that people with certain risk factors are more likely to develop pancreatic cancer. Risk factors include the following:

- **Cigarette smoking:** Cigarette smoke contains a large number of carcinogens (cancer causing chemicals.) Therefore, it is not surprising that cigarette smoking is one of the biggest risk factors for developing pancreatic cancer. According to some reports smokers have a 2–3 fold increased risk of developing pancreatic cancer.

- **Age:** The risk of developing pancreatic cancer increases with age. Over 80% of the cases develop between the ages of 60 and 80.

- **Race:** Studies in the United States have shown that pancreatic cancer is more common in the African-American population than it is in the white population. Some of this increased risk may be due to socioeconomic factors and to cigarette smoking.

- **Gender:** Cancer of the pancreas is more common in men than in women. This may be, in part, because men are more likely to smoke than women.

- **Religious background:** Pancreatic cancer is proportionally more common in Jews than the rest of the population. This may be because of a particular inherited mutation in the breast cancer gene (BRCA2) which runs in some Jewish families.

- **Chronic pancreatitis:** Long-term inflammation of the pancreas (pancreatitis) has been linked to cancer of the pancreas.

- **Diabetes:** There have been a number of reports which suggest that diabetics have an increased risk of developing pancreatic cancer.

- **Peptic ulcer surgery:** Patients who have had a portion of their stomach removed (partial gastrectomy) appear to have an increased risk for developing pancreatic cancer.

- **Diet:** Diets high in meats, cholesterol, fried foods, and nitrosamines may increase the risk, while diets high in fruits and vegetables may reduce the risk of pancreatic cancer.

If I think I may be at risk, what should I do?

People who think they may be at risk for pancreatic cancer should discuss this concern with their doctor. The doctor may suggest ways to reduce the risk and can plan an appropriate schedule for checkups.

What are the symptoms?

In the early stages, pancreatic cancer is extremely difficult to detect because often there are no symptoms. But, as the cancer grows, symptoms may include the following:

- Pain in the upper abdomen or upper back
- Yellow skin and eyes, and dark urine from jaundice
- Weakness
- Loss of appetite
- Nausea and vomiting
- Weight loss

These symptoms are not sure signs of pancreatic cancer. An infection or other problem could also cause these symptoms. Only a doctor can diagnose the cause of a person's symptoms. Anyone with these symptoms should see a doctor so that the doctor can treat any problem as early as possible.

How is pancreatic cancer diagnosed?

Pancreatic cancer can be difficult to detect and diagnose. A variety of techniques can be used to establish a diagnosis. These techniques include lab tests, CT scan, endoscopic ultrasound (EUS), and endoscopic retrograde cholangiopancreatography (ERCP).

Although all of these techniques may reveal a suspicious mass in the pancreas, by far the best diagnostic method remains histopathology.

Lab tests: The doctor may take blood, urine, and stool samples to check for bilirubin and other substances. Bilirubin is a substance that passes from the liver to the gallbladder to the intestine. If the common bile duct is blocked by a tumor, the bilirubin cannot pass through normally. Blockage may cause the level of bilirubin in the blood, stool, or urine to become very high. High bilirubin levels can result from cancer or from noncancerous conditions.

CT scan (computed tomography): An x-ray machine linked to a computer takes a series of detailed pictures. The x-ray machine is shaped like a donut with a large hole. The patient lies on a bed that passes through the hole. As the bed moves slowly through the hole, the machine takes many x-rays. The computer puts the x-rays together to create pictures of the pancreas and other organs and blood vessels in the abdomen.

Ultrasonography: The ultrasound device uses sound waves to produce a pattern of echoes as they bounce off internal organs. The echoes create a picture of the pancreas and other organs inside the abdomen. The echoes from tumors are different from echoes made by healthy tissues. The ultrasound procedure may use an external or internal device, or both types:

- Transabdominal ultrasound: To make images of the pancreas, the doctor places the ultrasound device on the abdomen and slowly moves it around.

- EUS (endoscopic ultrasound): The doctor passes a thin, lighted tube (endoscope) through the patient's mouth and stomach, down into the first part of the small intestine. At the tip of the endoscope is an ultrasound device. The doctor slowly withdraws the endoscope from the intestine toward the stomach to make images of the pancreas and surrounding organs and tissues.

ERCP (endoscopic retrograde cholangiopancreatography): The doctor passes an endoscope through the patient's mouth and stomach, down into the first part of the small intestine. The doctor slips a smaller tube (catheter) through the endoscope into the bile ducts and pancreatic ducts. After injecting dye through the catheter into the ducts, the doctor takes x-ray pictures. The x-rays can show whether the ducts are narrowed or blocked by a tumor or other condition.

PTC (percutaneous transhepatic cholangiography): A dye is injected through a thin needle inserted through the skin into the liver. Unless there is a blockage, the dye should move freely through the bile ducts. The dye makes the bile ducts show up on x-ray pictures. From the pictures, the doctor can tell whether there is a blockage from a tumor or other condition.

Biopsy: In some cases, the doctor may remove tissue. A pathologist then uses a microscope to look for cancer cells in the tissue. The doctor may obtain tissue in several ways. One way is by inserting a needle into the pancreas to remove cells. This is called fine-needle aspiration. The doctor uses x-ray or ultrasound to guide the needle. Sometimes the doctor obtains a sample of tissue during EUS or ERCP. Another way is to open the abdomen during an operation.

The following are questions you may want to ask your doctor about you biopsy:

- What kind of biopsy will I have?
- How long will it take? Will I be awake? Will it hurt?
- Are there any risks?
- How soon will I know the results?
- If I do have cancer, who will talk to me about treatment? When?

What is staging?

When pancreatic cancer is diagnosed, the doctor needs to know the stage, or extent, of the disease to plan the best treatment. Staging is a careful attempt to find out the size of the tumor in the pancreas, whether the cancer has spread, and if so, to what parts of the body. The results of various diagnostic tests will indicate how far the cancer has progressed and determine the stage. Subsequent decisions about treatment will be based upon the stage assigned.

What kinds of question should I ask my doctor(s)?

The shock and stress that people may feel after a diagnosis of cancer can make it hard for them to think of everything they want to ask the doctor. Often it helps to make a list of questions before an appointment. To help remember what the doctor says, patients may take notes or ask whether they may use a tape recorder. Some patients also want to have a family member or friend with them when they talk to the doctor—to take part in the discussion, to take notes, or just to listen. Always remember that the doctor is there to answer your questions don't be afraid to voice your opinion or question any action or procedure.

If you are meeting with a surgeon or oncologist for the first time, you may want to ask questions like these:

- Have you ever treated a pancreatic cancer patient before?
- If this is a surgeon: How many surgeries have you performed on pancreatic cancer patients?

- What has the general outcome of those patients been?

- Where were you trained (medical school, residency)?

- Which surgeons did you study under?

At any point in the relationship with your physician, you have the right to ask these questions:

- What is the diagnosis?

- What treatments are recommended?

- Are there other treatment options available that you do not provide (protocol treatments, herbal therapy, touch therapy, other alternative therapies)?

- What are the benefits of each treatment?

- What are the side effects of each treatment?

- What are the medications being prescribed?

- What are they for?

- What are their side effects?

- Are there any clinical drug trials I can participate in?

- How should I expect to feel during the treatment(s)?

- What are the risks of the treatment(s)?

- Will my diet need to be changed or modified?

- Will I need to take enzymes or vitamins?

Do not forget to ask about the things that are most important to you:

- How will this affect my ability to work?

- Can this treatment be done as an outpatient so that I can spend more time at home with family?

- Will I have any physical limitations?

- How will my current lifestyle be changed?

Finally—and most importantly—ask these questions of yourself:

- Does my doctor appear interested in answering my questions?

- Or, does my doctor look annoyed when I ask questions, like I am doubting his or her expertise or holding him or her up?

- Do I feel that my doctor cares about my medical outcome?

If you are uncomfortable with the results of some of these questions, you may want to re-evaluate your choice of physician or get a second opinion.

Should I participate in a clinical trial?

Cancer of the pancreas is very hard to control with current treatments. For that reason, many doctors encourage patients with this disease to consider taking part in a clinical trial. Clinical trials are an important option for people with all stages of pancreatic cancer.

What is palliative therapy?

Palliative therapy aims to improve quality of life by controlling pain and other problems caused by pancreatic cancer.

What is an oncologist?

An oncologist is a doctor who specializes in treating cancer. Specialists who treat pancreatic cancer include surgeons, medical oncologists, and radiation oncologists.

Should I get a second opinion?

Yes. While some insurance companies require a second opinion, others may cover a second opinion if the patient requests it. Gathering medical records and arranging to see another doctor may take a little time. But in most cases, a brief delay to get another opinion will not make therapy less helpful.

There are a number of ways to find a doctor for a second opinion:

- The Cancer Information Service (800-4-CANCER) can tell callers about treatment facilities, including cancer centers and other programs supported by the National Cancer Institute, and can send printed information about finding a doctor.

- A local medical society, a nearby hospital, or a medical school can usually provide the name of specialists.

- The *Official ABMS Directory of Board Certified Medical Specialists* lists doctors' names along with their specialty and their educational background. This resource is available in most public libraries.

- The American Board of Medical Specialties (ABMS) also offers information by telephone and on the Internet. The public may use these services to check whether a doctor is board certified. The telephone number is 866-ASK-ABMS (866-275-2267). The internet address is http://www.abms.org/newsearch.asp.

What are the available treatment options?

People with pancreatic cancer may have several treatment options. Depending on the type and stage, pancreatic cancer may be treated with surgery, radiation therapy, or chemotherapy. Some patients have a combination of therapies.

When is surgery possible?

Generally if the cancer is localized, surgical treatment, through resection or removal of the tumor, can be pursued. This means that the cancer has not spread to any blood vessels, distant lymph nodes, or other organs, such as the liver or lung. These characteristics are determined through various diagnostic techniques.

What types of surgical procedures are performed to treat pancreatic cancer?

This depends where the tumor is located within the pancreas.

What are some questions I should ask my doctor before surgery?

- What kind of operation will I have?
- How will I feel after the operation?
- How will you treat my pain?
- What other treatment will I need?
- How long will I be in the hospital?
- Will I need a feeding tube after surgery? Will I need a special diet?
- What are the long-term effects?
- When can I get back to my normal activities?
- How often will I need checkups?

What is radiation therapy?

Radiation therapy (also referred to as radiotherapy) uses high-energy rays to kill cancer cells. Radiation therapy may be administered alone or in combination with surgery, chemotherapy, or both.

What are some questions I should ask my doctor before radiation therapy?

- Why do I need this treatment?
- When will the treatments begin? When will they end?
- How will I feel during therapy? Are there side effects?
- What can I do to take care of myself during therapy? Are there certain foods that I should eat or avoid?
- How will we know if the radiation is working?
- Will I be able to continue my normal activities during treatment?

What is chemotherapy?

Chemotherapy is the use of drugs to kill cancer cells. Doctors also give chemotherapy to help reduce pain and other problems caused by pancreatic cancer. It may be given alone, with radiation, or in combination with surgery and radiation.

Chemotherapy is systemic therapy and is most often delivered intravenously. Once in the bloodstream, the drugs travel throughout the body.

Usually chemotherapy is an outpatient treatment. However, depending on which drugs are given and the patient's general health, the patient may need to stay in the hospital.

What are some question I should ask my doctor before chemotherapy?

- Why do I need this treatment?
- What will it do?
- What drugs will I be taking? How will they be given? Will I need to stay in the hospital?
- Will the treatment cause side effects? What can I do about them?
- How long will I be on this treatment?

What are the possible side effects?

Because cancer treatment may damage healthy cells and tissues, unwanted side effects are common. These side effects depend on many factors, including the type and extent of the treatment. Side effects may not be the same for each person, and they may even change from one treatment session to the next. The health care team will explain possible side effects and how they will help the patient manage them.

Surgery: The side effects of surgery depend on the extent of the operation, the person's general health, and other factors. Most patients have pain for the first few days after surgery. Pain can be controlled with medicine, and patients should discuss pain relief with the doctor or nurse.

Removal of part, or all, of the pancreas may make it hard for a patient to digest foods. The health care team can suggest a diet plan and medicines to help relieve diarrhea, pain, cramping, or feelings of fullness. During the recovery from surgery, the doctor will carefully monitor the patient's diet and weight. At first, a patient may have only liquids and may receive extra nourishment intravenously or by feeding tube into the intestine. Solid foods are added to the diet gradually.

Patients may not have enough pancreatic enzymes or hormones after surgery. Those who do not have enough insulin may develop diabetes. The doctor can give the patient insulin, other hormones, and enzymes.

Radiation therapy: Radiation therapy may cause patients to become very tired as treatment continues. Rest is important, but doctors usually advise patients to try to stay as active as possible. In addition, when patients receive radiation therapy, the skin in the treated area may sometimes become red, dry, and tender.

Radiation therapy to the abdomen may cause nausea, vomiting, diarrhea, or other problems with digestion. The health care team can offer medicine or suggest diet changes to control these problems. For most patients, the side effects of radiation therapy go away when treatment is over.

Chemotherapy: The side effects of chemotherapy depend on the drugs and the doses the patient receives as well as how the drugs are administered. As with other types of treatment, side effects vary from patient to patient.

Patients who undergo chemotherapy may also be more likely to get infections, bruise or bleed easily, and may have less energy. Since systemic therapy affects rapidly dividing cells, patients may lose their hair and may have other side effects such as poor appetite, nausea and vomiting, diarrhea, or mouth sores. Usually, these side effects go away gradually during the recovery periods between treatments or after treatment is over. The health care team can suggest ways to relieve side effects.

How is pain controlled?

The management of pain for patients with pancreatic cancer is one of the most important aspects of their care. Pain is a common symptom that can be successfully controlled. The best management of pain is aggressive therapy with constant assessment. The patient with pancreatic cancer who is experiencing pain can maintain their quality of life. Pain can be relieved or reduced in several ways:

Medication: The use of opioids (or narcotics, the strongest pain relievers that are only available by prescription) is the main way to treat pain from pancreatic cancer. Other types of medicines used to relieve pain that are not opioids are: acetaminophen and non-steroidal anti-inflammatory drugs (NSAIDs). At times, medicines called adjuvant analgesics are also used. These are medicines used for purposes other than the treatment of pain but help in relieving pain in some situations. See Table 37.1 for a list of commonly used medications.

Radiation: High-energy rays can help relieve pain by shrinking the tumor.

Nerve block: The doctor may inject alcohol into the area around certain nerves in the abdomen to block the feeling of pain.

Surgery: The surgeon may cut certain nerves to block pain.

Other options: The doctor may suggest other ways to relieve or reduce pain. For example, massage, acupuncture, or acupressure may be used along with other approaches to help relieve pain. Also, the patient may learn relaxation techniques such as listening to slow music or breathing slowly and comfortably.

What are some questions I should ask my doctor about pain control?

- What can be done to relieve my pain?

Table 37.1. Pain Medications Used for Patients with Pain from Pancreatic Cancer

Types of Opioids Recommended for Pain of Pancreatic Cancer

Codeine

Hydrocodone (Vicodin, Vicoprofen)

Hydromorphone (Dilaudid)

Levorphanol (Levo-Dromoran)

Morphine (Kadian, MSIR, MS Contin, Oramorph-SR)

Oxycodone (Roxicodone, OxyIR, OxyContin, Percodan)

Fentanyl (Duragesic, Actiq)

Methadone (Dolophine)

Tramadol (Ultram)

MSIR (morphine sulfate immediate release)

MS Contin (morphine sulfate sustained release)

Oramorph-SR (morphine sulfate sustained release)

Roxicodone (oxycodone immediate release)

OxyIR (oxycodone immediate release)

OxyContin (oxycodone sustained release)

Percodan (oxycodone immediate release)

Non-Opioids Recommended for Pain of Pancreatic Cancer

NSAIDs	Antidepressants	Anticonvulsants
Aspirin	Amitriptyline	Carbamazepine
Bufferin	Elavil	Tegretol
Ecotrin	Nortriptyline	Phenytoin
Trilisate	Pamelor	Dilantin
Dolobid	Desipramine	Valproate
Ibuprofen	Norpramin	Depakote
Motrin, Advil	Doxepin	Clonazepam
Ansaid	Sinequan	Klonopin
Orudis	Imipramine	Gabapentin
Aleve, Anaprox	Tofranil	Neurontin
Daypro	Venlafaxine	Lamotrigine
Lodine	Effexor	Lamictal
Voltaren	Citalopram	
Arthrotec	Celexa	
Celebrex		

Acetaminophen
  Tylenol (classified as a non-opioid)

- What can we do if the medicine does not work?
- What other options do I have for pain control?
- Will the pain medicines have side effects?
- What can be done to manage the side effects?
- Will the treatment limit my activities (for example working or driving)?

Are there support groups for people with pancreatic cancer?

Living with a serious disease such as pancreatic cancer is not easy. Some people find they need help coping with the emotional and practical aspects of their disease. Support groups can help. In these groups, patients or their family members get together to share what they have learned about coping with their disease and the effects of treatment.

People living with pancreatic cancer may worry about the future. They may worry about caring for themselves or their families, keeping their jobs, or continuing daily activities. Concerns about treatments and managing side effects, hospital stays, and medical bills are also common. Doctors, nurses, and other members of the health care team can answer questions about treatment, diet, working, or other matters. Meeting with a social worker, counselor, or member of the clergy can be helpful to those who want to talk about their feelings or discuss their concerns. Often, a social worker can suggest resources for financial aid, transportation, home care, emotional support, or other services.

What are clinical trails?

Doctors in clinics and hospitals are searching for a cure. In their efforts, they often conduct clinical trials. These are research studies in which people take part voluntarily. In these trials, researchers are studying ways to treat pancreatic cancer. Research already has led to advances in treatment methods, and researchers continue to search for more effective approaches to treat this disease.

Patients who join clinical trials have the first chance to benefit from new treatments that have shown promise in earlier research. They also make an important contribution to medical science by helping doctors learn more about the disease.

Although clinical trials may pose some risks, researchers take very careful steps to protect their patients.

In trials with people who have pancreatic cancer, doctors are studying new drugs, new combinations of chemotherapy, and combinations of chemotherapy and radiation before and after surgery.

What about alternative treatments?

Biological therapy is also under investigation. Scientists are studying several cancer vaccines to help the immune system fight cancer. Other studies use monoclonal antibodies to slow or stop the growth of cancer.

Chapter 38

Islet Cell Carcinoma

Islet cell cancer, a rare cancer, is a disease in which cancer (malignant) cells are found in certain tissues of the pancreas. The pancreas is about six inches long and is shaped like a thin pear, wider at one end and narrower at the other. The pancreas lies behind the stomach, inside a loop formed by part of the small intestine. The broader right end of the pancreas is called the head, the middle section is called the body, and the narrow left end is the tail.

The pancreas has two basic jobs in the body. It produces digestive juices that help break down (digest) food and hormones (such as insulin) that regulate how the body stores and uses food. The area of the pancreas that produces digestive juices is called the exocrine pancreas. About 95% of pancreatic cancers begin in the exocrine pancreas. The hormone-producing area of the pancreas has special cells called islet cells and is called the endocrine pancreas. Only about 5% of pancreatic cancers start here.

The islet cells in the pancreas make many hormones, including insulin, which help the body store and use sugars. When islet cells in the pancreas become cancerous, they may make too many hormones. Islet cell cancers that make too many hormones are called functioning tumors. Other islet cell cancers may not make extra hormones and are called nonfunctioning tumors. Tumors that do not spread to other parts of the body can also be found in the islet cells. These are called

PDQ® Cancer Information Summary. National Cancer Institute; Bethesda, MD. Islet Cell Carcinoma (Endocrine Pancreas) (PDQ®): Treatment - Patient. Updated 07/2005. Available at: http://cancer.gov. Accessed April 30, 2006.

benign tumors and are not cancer. A doctor will need to determine whether the tumor is cancer or a benign tumor.

A doctor should be seen if there is pain in the abdomen, diarrhea, stomach pain, a tired feeling all the time, fainting, or weight gain without eating too much. If there are symptoms, the doctor will order blood and urine tests to see whether the amounts of hormones in the body are normal. Other tests, including x-rays and special scans, may also be done.

The chance of recovery (prognosis) depends on the type of islet cell cancer the patient has, how far the cancer has spread, and the patient's overall health.

Stages of Islet Cell Cancer

Once islet cell cancer is found, more tests will be done to find out if cancer cells have spread to other parts of the body. This is called staging. The staging system for islet cell cancer is still being developed. These tumors are most often divided into one of three groups:

1. Islet cell cancers occurring in one site within the pancreas

2. Islet cell cancers occurring in several sites within the pancreas

3. Islet cell cancers that have spread to lymph nodes near the pancreas or to distant sites

A doctor also needs to know the type of islet cell tumor to plan treatment. The following types of islet cell tumors are found:

- **Gastrinoma:** The tumor makes large amounts of a hormone called gastrin, which causes too much acid to be made in the stomach. Ulcers may develop as a result of too much stomach acid.

- **Insulinoma:** The tumor makes too much of the hormone insulin and causes the body to store sugar instead of burning the sugar for energy. This causes too little sugar in the blood, a condition called hypoglycemia.

- **Glucagonoma:** This tumor makes too much of the hormone glucagon and causes too much sugar in the blood, a condition called hyperglycemia.

- **Miscellaneous:** Other types of islet cell cancer can affect the pancreas and/or small intestine. Each type of tumor may affect different hormones in the body and cause different symptoms.

- **Recurrent:** Recurrent disease means that the cancer has come back (recurred) after it has been treated. It may come back in the pancreas or in another part of the body.

Treatment Option Overview

There are treatments for all patients with islet cell cancer. Three types of treatment are used:

- Surgery (taking out the cancer)
- Chemotherapy (using drugs to kill cancer cells)
- Hormone therapy (using hormones to stop cancer cells from growing)

Surgery is the most common treatment of islet cell cancer. The doctor may take out the cancer and most or part of the pancreas. Sometimes the stomach is taken out (gastrectomy) because of ulcers. Lymph nodes in the area may also be removed and looked at under a microscope to see if they contain cancer.

Chemotherapy uses drugs to kill cancer cells. Chemotherapy may be taken by pill, or it may be put into the body by a needle in the vein or muscle. Chemotherapy is called a systemic treatment because the drug enters the bloodstream, travels through the body, and can kill cancer cells throughout the body.

Hormone therapy uses hormones to stop the cancer cells from growing or to relieve symptoms caused by the tumor.

Treatment by Type

Treatment of islet cell cancer depends on the type of tumor, the stage, and the patient's overall health.

Standard treatment may be considered because of its effectiveness in patients in past studies, or participation in a clinical trial may be considered. Not all patients are cured with standard therapy and some standard treatments may have more side effects than are desired. For these reasons, clinical trials are designed to find better ways to treat cancer patients and are based on the most up-to-date information. Clinical trials are ongoing in many parts of the country for patients with islet cell cancer. To learn more about clinical trials, call the Cancer Information Service 800-4-CANCER or visit the National Cancer Institute's website at http://www.cancer.gov.

Gastrinoma: Treatment may be one of the following:

• Surgery to remove the cancer
• Surgery to remove the stomach (gastrectomy)
• Surgery to cut the nerve that stimulates the pancreas
• Chemotherapy
• Hormone therapy
• Hepatic arterial occlusion or embolization to kill cancer cells growing in the liver

Insulinoma: Treatment may be one of the following:

• Surgery to remove the cancer
• Chemotherapy
• Hormone therapy
• Drugs to relieve symptoms
• Hepatic arterial occlusion or embolization to kill cancer cells growing in the liver

Glucagonoma: Treatment may be one of the following:

• Surgery to remove the cancer
• Chemotherapy
• Hormone therapy
• Hepatic arterial occlusion or embolization to kill cancer cells growing in the liver

Miscellaneous islet cell cancer: Treatment may be one of the following:

• Surgery to remove the cancer
• Chemotherapy
• Hormone therapy
• Hepatic arterial occlusion or embolization to kill cancer cells growing in the liver

Recurrent islet cell carcinoma: Treatment depends on many factors, including what treatment the patient had before and where the cancer has come back. Treatment may be chemotherapy, or patients may want to consider taking part in a clinical trial.

Chapter 39

Gastrointestinal Carcinoid Tumors

A gastrointestinal carcinoid tumor is cancer that forms in the lining of the gastrointestinal tract. The gastrointestinal tract includes the stomach, small intestine, and large intestine. These organs are part of the digestive system, which processes nutrients (vitamins, minerals, carbohydrates, fats, proteins, and water) in foods that are eaten and helps pass waste material out of the body. Gastrointestinal carcinoid tumors develop from a certain type of hormone-making cell in the lining of the gastrointestinal tract. These cells produce hormones that help regulate digestive juices and the muscles used in moving food through the stomach and intestines. A gastrointestinal carcinoid tumor may also produce hormones. Carcinoid tumors that start in the rectum (the last several inches of the large intestine) usually do not produce hormones.

Gastrointestinal carcinoid tumors grow slowly. Most of them occur in the appendix (an organ attached to the large intestine), small intestine, and rectum. It is common for more than one tumor to develop in the small intestine. Having a carcinoid tumor increases a person's chance of getting other cancers in the digestive system, either at the same time or later.

Risk factors include the following:

- Having a family history of multiple endocrine neoplasia type 1 (MEN1) syndrome

PDQ® Cancer Information Summary. National Cancer Institute; Bethesda, MD. Gastrointestinal Carcinoid Tumors (PDQ®): Treatment - Patient. Updated 05/2004. Available at: http://cancer.gov. Accessed June 22, 2006.

- Having certain conditions that affect the stomach's ability to produce stomach acid, such as atrophic gastritis, pernicious anemia, or Zollinger-Ellison syndrome
- Smoking tobacco

A gastrointestinal carcinoid tumor often has no signs in its early stages. Carcinoid syndrome may occur if the tumor spreads to the liver or other parts of the body. The hormones produced by gastrointestinal carcinoid tumors are usually destroyed by blood and liver enzymes. If the tumor has spread to the liver, however, high amounts of these hormones may remain in the body and cause the following group of symptoms, called carcinoid syndrome:

- Redness or a feeling of warmth in the face and neck
- Diarrhea
- Shortness of breath, fast heartbeat, tiredness, or swelling of the feet and ankles
- Wheezing
- Pain or a feeling of fullness in the abdomen

These symptoms and others may be caused by gastrointestinal carcinoid tumors or by other conditions. A doctor should be consulted if any of these symptoms occur.

The following tests and procedures may be used to detect (find) and diagnose gastrointestinal carcinoid tumors:

Complete blood count: A procedure in which a sample of blood is drawn and checked for the following:

- The number of red blood cells, white blood cells, and platelets
- The amount of hemoglobin (the protein that carries oxygen) in the red blood cells
- The portion of the sample made up of red blood cells

Physical exam and history: An exam of the body to check general signs of health, including checking for signs of disease, such as lumps or anything else that seems unusual. A history of the patient's health habits and past illnesses and treatments will also be taken.

Blood chemistry studies: A procedure in which a blood sample is checked to measure the amounts of certain substances, such as hormones, released into the blood by organs and tissues in the body. An unusual (higher or lower than normal) amount of a substance can be a sign of disease in the organ or tissue that produces it. The blood sample is checked to see if it contains a hormone produced by carcinoid tumors. This test is used to help diagnose carcinoid syndrome.

Twenty-four-hour urine test: A test in which a urine sample is checked to measure the amounts of certain substances, such as hormones. An unusual (higher or lower than normal) amount of a substance can be a sign of disease in the organ or tissue that produces it. The urine sample is checked to see if it contains a hormone produced by carcinoid tumors. This test is used to help diagnose carcinoid syndrome.

Prognosis

The prognosis (chance of recovery) and treatment options depend on the following:

- Whether the cancer can be completely removed by surgery
- Whether the cancer has spread from the stomach and intestines to other parts of the body, such as the liver or lymph nodes
- The size of the tumor
- Where the tumor is in the gastrointestinal tract
- Whether the cancer is newly diagnosed or has recurred

Treatment options also depend on whether the cancer is causing symptoms. Most gastrointestinal carcinoid tumors are slow-growing and can be treated and often cured. Even when not cured, many patients may live for a long time.

Stages of Gastrointestinal Carcinoid Tumors

After a gastrointestinal carcinoid tumor has been diagnosed, tests are done to find out if cancer cells have spread within the stomach and intestines or to other parts of the body. Staging is the process used to find out how far the cancer has spread. The information gathered from the staging process determines the stage of the disease. There are no standard stages for gastrointestinal carcinoid tumors. In order to plan treatment, it is important to know the extent of the disease and whether the tumor can be removed by surgery. The following tests and procedures may be used:

Gastrointestinal endoscopy: A procedure to look inside the gastrointestinal tract for abnormal areas or cancer. An endoscope (a thin, lighted tube) is inserted through the mouth and esophagus into the stomach and first part of the small intestine. Also, a colonoscope (a thin, lighted tube) is inserted through the rectum into the colon (large intestine); this is called a colonoscopy.

CT scan (CAT scan): A procedure that makes a series of detailed pictures of areas inside the body, taken from different angles. The pictures are made by a computer linked to an x-ray machine. A dye may be injected into a vein or swallowed to help the organs or tissues show up more clearly. This procedure is also called computed tomography, computerized tomography, or computerized axial tomography.

Somatostatin receptor scintigraphy (SRS): A type of radionuclide scan used to find carcinoid tumors. In SRS, radioactive octreotide, a drug similar to somatostatin, is injected into a vein and travels through the bloodstream. The radioactive octreotide attaches to carcinoid tumor cells that have somatostatin receptors. A radiation-measuring device detects the radioactive material, showing where the carcinoid tumor cells are in the body. This procedure is also called an octreotide scan.

Biopsy: The removal of cells or tissues so they can be viewed under a microscope to check for signs of cancer. Tissue samples may be taken during endoscopy and colonoscopy.

Angiogram: A procedure to look at blood vessels and the flow of blood. A contrast dye is injected into the blood vessel. As the contrast dye moves through the blood vessel, x-rays are taken to see if there are any blockages.

PET scan (positron emission tomography scan): A procedure to find malignant tumor cells in the body. A small amount of radionuclide glucose (sugar) is injected into a vein. The PET scanner rotates around the body and makes a picture of where glucose is being used in the body. Malignant tumor cells show up brighter in the picture because they are more active and take up more glucose than normal cells.

X-ray of the abdomen: An x-ray of the organs and tissues inside the abdomen. An x-ray is a type of energy beam that can go through the body and onto film, making a picture of areas inside the body.

How Gastrointestinal Carcinoid Tumors Are Grouped

Gastrointestinal carcinoid tumors are grouped for treatment based on where they are in the body.

- **Localized:** Cancer is found in the appendix, colon, rectum, small intestine, and/or stomach only.
- **Regional:** Cancer has spread from the appendix, colon, rectum, stomach, and/or small intestine to nearby tissues or lymph nodes.
- **Metastatic:** Cancer has spread to other parts of the body.

Recurrent gastrointestinal carcinoid tumors: A recurrent gastrointestinal carcinoid tumor is a tumor that has recurred (come back) after it has been treated. The tumor may come back in the stomach or intestines or in other parts of the body.

Treatment Option Overview

Different types of treatment are available for patients with gastrointestinal carcinoid tumors. Some treatments are standard (the currently used treatment), and some are being tested in clinical trials. Before starting treatment, patients may want to think about taking part in a clinical trial. A treatment clinical trial is a research study meant to help improve current treatments or obtain information on new treatments for patients with cancer. When clinical trials show that a new treatment is better than the standard treatment, the new treatment may become the standard treatment.

Clinical trials are taking place in many parts of the country. Information about ongoing clinical trials is available from the National Cancer Institute (NCI)'s website at http://www.cancer.gov. Choosing the most appropriate cancer treatment is a decision that ideally involves the patient, family, and health care team.

Seven types of standard treatment are used:

Surgery: Treatment of gastrointestinal carcinoid tumors usually includes surgery. One of the following surgical procedures may be used:

- **Appendectomy:** Removal of the appendix.

- **Fulguration:** Use of an electric current to burn away the tumor using a special tool.

- **Cryosurgery:** A treatment that uses an instrument to freeze and destroy abnormal tissue, such as carcinoma in situ. This type of treatment is also called cryotherapy. The doctor may use ultrasound to guide the instrument.

- **Resection:** Surgery to remove part or all of the organ that contains cancer. Resection of the tumor and a small amount of normal tissue around it is called a local excision.

- **Bowel resection and anastomosis:** Removal of the bowel tumor and a small section of healthy bowel on each side. The healthy parts of the bowel are then sewn together (anastomosis). Lymph nodes are removed and checked by a pathologist to see if they contain cancer.

- **Radiofrequency ablation:** The use of a special probe with tiny electrodes that release high-energy radio waves (similar to microwaves) that kill cancer cells. The probe may be inserted through the skin or through an incision (cut) in the abdomen.

- **Hepatic resection:** Surgery to remove part or all of the liver.

- **Hepatic artery ligation or embolization:** A procedure to ligate (tie off) or embolize (block) the hepatic artery, the main blood vessel that brings blood into the liver. Blocking the flow of blood to the liver helps kill cancer cells growing there.

Radiation therapy: Radiation therapy is a cancer treatment that uses high-energy x-rays or other types of radiation to kill cancer cells. There are two types of radiation therapy. External radiation therapy uses a machine outside the body to send radiation toward the cancer. Internal radiation therapy uses a radioactive substance sealed in needles, seeds, wires, or catheters that are placed directly into or near the cancer. The way the radiation therapy is given depends on the type and stage of the cancer being treated.

Chemotherapy: Chemotherapy is a cancer treatment that uses drugs to stop the growth of cancer cells, either by killing the cells or by stopping the cells from dividing. When chemotherapy is taken by mouth or injected into a vein or muscle, the drugs enter the bloodstream and can reach cancer cells throughout the body (systemic chemotherapy). When chemotherapy is placed directly into the spinal column, an organ, or a body cavity such as the abdomen, the drugs mainly affect cancer cells in those areas (regional chemotherapy).

Chemoembolization of the hepatic artery is a type of regional chemotherapy that may be used to treat a gastrointestinal carcinoid tumor that has spread to the liver. The anticancer drug is injected into the hepatic artery through a catheter (thin tube). The drug is mixed with a substance that embolizes (blocks) the artery, cutting off blood flow to the tumor. Most of the anticancer drug is trapped near the tumor and only a small amount of the drug reaches other parts of the body. The blockage may be temporary or permanent, depending on the substance used to block the artery. The tumor is prevented from getting the oxygen and nutrients it needs to grow. The liver continues to receive blood from the hepatic portal vein, which carries blood from the stomach and intestine. The way the chemotherapy is given depends on the type and stage of the cancer being treated.

Percutaneous ethanol injection: Percutaneous ethanol injection is a cancer treatment in which a small needle is used to inject ethanol (alcohol) directly into a tumor to kill cancer cells. This procedure is also called intratumoral ethanol injection.

Biologic therapy: Biologic therapy is a treatment that uses the patient's immune system to fight cancer. Substances made by the body or made in a laboratory are used to boost, direct, or restore the body's natural defenses against cancer. This type of cancer treatment is also called biotherapy or immunotherapy.

Hormone therapy: Hormone therapy is a cancer treatment that removes hormones or blocks their action and stops cancer cells from growing. Hormones are substances produced by glands in the body and circulated in the bloodstream. The presence of some hormones can cause certain cancers to grow. If tests show that the cancer cells have places where hormones can attach (receptors), drugs, surgery, or radiation therapy are used to reduce the production of hormones or block them from working.

Other drug therapy: MIBG (metaiodobenzylguanidine) is sometimes used, with or without radioactive iodine (I-131), to lessen the symptoms of gastrointestinal carcinoid tumors.

Treatment Options for Gastrointestinal Carcinoid Tumors

Localized Gastrointestinal Carcinoid Tumors

Carcinoid tumors in the appendix: Treatment of localized gastrointestinal carcinoid tumors in the appendix may include the following:

- Appendectomy
- Appendectomy and local excision
- Appendectomy, bowel resection with anastomosis, and removal of lymph nodes

Rectal carcinoid tumors: Treatment of localized gastrointestinal carcinoid tumors in the rectum may include the following:

- Fulguration
- Local excision
- Resection
- Surgery that saves the sphincter muscles (the muscles that open and close the anus) may be possible

Small bowel carcinoid tumors: Treatment of localized gastrointestinal carcinoid tumors in the small intestine may include the following:

- Local excision
- Resection with removal of nearby lymph nodes

Gastric, colon, and pancreatic carcinoid tumors: Treatment of localized gastrointestinal carcinoid tumors in the stomach, colon, or pancreas is usually resection.

Regional Gastrointestinal Carcinoid Tumors

Treatment is usually surgery to remove all the cancer that can be seen at the site of the original tumor, as well as nearby tissues and lymph nodes. If the tumor cannot be completely removed by surgery, treatment is usually palliative therapy to relieve symptoms and improve the patient's quality of life. This may include the following:

- Resection, cryosurgery, or radiofrequency ablation to remove as much of the tumor as possible

- Chemoembolization to shrink tumors in the liver

Metastatic Gastrointestinal Carcinoid Tumors

Distant metastases: If the metastatic gastrointestinal carcinoid tumor is not causing symptoms, there may be a period of watchful waiting before treatment is given. Treatment of distant metastases of gastrointestinal carcinoid tumors is usually palliative therapy that may include the following:

- Surgery to bypass or remove part of a tumor blocking the small intestine
- Chemotherapy, which may include chemoembolization
- Radiation therapy, sometimes with radioisotopes such as radioactive iodine (I-131)
- MIBG (metaiodobenzylguanidine) therapy
- Biologic therapy and/or hormone therapy
- Clinical trials of new treatments

Carcinoid syndrome: Treatment of metastatic gastrointestinal carcinoid tumors that are causing carcinoid syndrome may include the following:

- Resection, cryosurgery, radiofrequency ablation, or percutaneous ethanol injection for tumors in the liver
- Hepatic artery ligation or embolization, with or without regional or systemic chemotherapy
- Hormone therapy
- Biologic therapy with or without chemotherapy
- Clinical trials of new combinations of chemotherapy
- A heart valve replacement

Recurrent gastrointestinal carcinoid tumors: Treatment of recurrent gastrointestinal carcinoid tumors may include the following:

- Surgery to remove part or all of the tumor
- A clinical trial

407

Chapter 40

Liver Cancer

Adult primary liver cancer is a disease in which malignant (cancer) cells form in the tissues of the liver. The liver is one of the largest organs in the body, filling the upper right side of the abdomen inside the rib cage. It has two parts, a right lobe and a smaller left lobe. The liver has many important functions, including the following:

- Filtering harmful substances from the blood so they can be passed from the body in stools and urine

- Making bile to help digest fats from food

- Storing glycogen (sugar), which the body uses for energy

The following are possible risk factors for adult primary liver cancer:

- Having hepatitis B and/or hepatitis C

- Having a close relative with both hepatitis and liver cancer

- Having cirrhosis

- Eating foods tainted with aflatoxin (poison from a fungus that can grow on foods, such as grains and nuts, that have not been stored properly)

PDQ® Cancer Information Summary. National Cancer Institute; Bethesda, MD. Adult Primary Liver Cancer (PDQ®): Treatment - Patient. Updated 01/2005. Available at: http://cancer.gov. Accessed April 30, 2006.

A doctor should be consulted if any of the following symptoms occur:

- A hard lump on the right side just below the rib cage
- Discomfort in the upper abdomen on the right side
- Pain around the right shoulder blade
- Unexplained weight loss
- Jaundice (yellowing of the skin and whites of the eyes)
- Unusual tiredness
- Nausea
- Loss of appetite

The following tests and procedures may be used to detect (find) and diagnose adult primary liver cancer:

Physical exam and history: An exam of the body to check general signs of health, including checking for signs of disease, such as lumps or anything else that seems unusual. A history of the patient's health habits and past illnesses and treatments will also be taken.

Serum tumor marker test: A procedure in which a sample of blood is examined to measure the amounts of certain substances released into the blood by organs, tissues, or tumor cells in the body. Certain substances are linked to specific types of cancer when found in increased levels in the blood. These are called tumor markers. An increased level of alpha-fetoprotein (AFP) in the blood may be a sign of liver cancer. Other cancers and certain noncancerous conditions, including cirrhosis and hepatitis, may also increase AFP levels.

Complete blood count (CBC): A procedure in which a sample of blood is drawn and checked for the following:

- The number of red blood cells, white blood cells, and platelets
- The amount of hemoglobin (the protein that carries oxygen) in the red blood cells
- The portion of the blood sample made up of red blood cells

Laparoscopy: A surgical procedure to look at the organs inside the abdomen to check for signs of disease. Small incisions (cuts) are made in the wall of the abdomen and a laparoscope (a thin, lighted tube) is inserted into one of the incisions. Other instruments may be inserted through the same or other incisions to perform procedures such as removing organs or taking tissue samples for biopsy.

Biopsy: The removal of cells or tissues so they can be viewed under a microscope by a pathologist to check for signs of cancer. The sample may be taken using a fine needle inserted into the liver during an x-ray or ultrasound. This is called needle biopsy or fine-needle aspiration. The biopsy may be done during a laparoscopy.

CT scan (CAT scan): A procedure that makes a series of detailed pictures of areas inside the body, taken from different angles. The pictures are made by a computer linked to an x-ray machine. A dye may be injected into a vein or swallowed to help the organs or tissues show up more clearly. This procedure is also called computed tomography, computerized tomography, or computerized axial tomography.

MRI (magnetic resonance imaging): A procedure that uses a magnet, radio waves, and a computer to make a series of detailed pictures of areas inside the body. This procedure is also called nuclear magnetic resonance imaging (NMRI).

Ultrasound: A procedure in which high-energy sound waves (ultrasound) are bounced off internal tissues or organs and make echoes. The echoes form a picture of body tissues called a sonogram.

Prognosis

The prognosis (chance of recovery) and treatment options depend on the following:

- The stage of the cancer (the size of the tumor, whether it affects part or all of the liver, or has spread to other places in the body)
- How well the liver is working
- The patient's general health, including whether there is cirrhosis of the liver
- The patient's alpha-fetoprotein (AFP) levels

Stages of Adult Primary Liver Cancer

After adult primary liver cancer has been diagnosed, tests are done to find out if cancer cells have spread within the liver or to other parts

411

of the body. The process used to find out if cancer has spread within the liver or to other parts of the body is called staging. The information gathered from the staging process determines the stage of the disease. It is important to know the stage in order to plan treatment. The following tests and procedures may be used in the staging process:

- **Chest x-ray:** An x-ray of the organs and bones inside the chest. An x-ray is a type of energy beam that can go through the body and onto film, making a picture of areas inside the body.

- **CT scan (CAT scan)**

- **MRI (magnetic resonance imaging)**

- **Bone scan:** A procedure to check if there are rapidly dividing cells, such as cancer cells, in the bone. A very small amount of radioactive material is injected into a vein and travels through the bloodstream. The radioactive material collects in the bones and is detected by a scanner.

- **Doppler ultrasound:** A type of ultrasound that uses differences in the ultrasound echoes to measure the speed and direction of blood flow.

The following stages are used for adult primary liver cancer:

Stage I: In stage I, there is one tumor and it has not spread to nearby blood vessels.

Stage II: In stage II, one of the following is found:

- One tumor that has spread to nearby blood vessels; or
- More than one tumor, none of which is larger than five centimeters.

Stage III: Stage III is divided into stage IIIA, IIIB, and IIIC.

- In stage IIIA, one of the following is found:
  - more than one tumor larger than five centimeters; or
  - one tumor that has spread to a major branch of blood vessels near the liver.

- In stage IIIB, there are one or more tumors of any size that have either:

- spread to nearby organs other than the gallbladder; or
- broken through the lining of the peritoneal cavity.
- In stage IIIC, the cancer has spread to nearby lymph nodes.

Stage IV: In stage IV, cancer has spread beyond the liver to other places in the body, such as the bones or lungs. The tumors may be of any size and may also have spread to nearby blood vessels and/or lymph nodes.

Liver Cancer Groups

For adult primary liver cancer, stages are also grouped according to how the cancer may be treated. There are 3 treatment groups:

- **Localized resectable:** The cancer is found in the liver only, has not spread, and can be completely removed by surgery.

- **Localized and locally advanced unresectable:** The cancer is found in the liver only and has not spread, but cannot be completely removed by surgery.

- **Advanced:** Cancer has spread throughout the liver or has spread to other parts of the body, such as the lungs and bone.

Recurrent adult primary liver cancer: Recurrent adult primary liver cancer is cancer that has recurred (come back) after it has been treated. The cancer may come back in the liver or in other parts of the body.

Treatment Option Overview

Different types of treatments are available for patients with adult primary liver cancer. Some treatments are standard (the currently used treatment), and some are being tested in clinical trials. Before starting treatment, patients may want to think about taking part in a clinical trial. A treatment clinical trial is a research study meant to help improve current treatments or obtain information on new treatments for patients with cancer. When clinical trials show that a new treatment is better than the standard treatment, the new treatment may become the standard treatment.

Clinical trials are taking place in many parts of the country. Information about ongoing clinical trials is available from the National Cancer Institute (NCI)'s website at http://www.cancer.gov. Choosing the most appropriate cancer treatment is a decision that ideally involves the patient, family, and health care team.

Four types of standard treatment are used:

Surgery: The following types of surgery may be used to treat liver cancer:

- **Cryosurgery:** A treatment that uses an instrument to freeze and destroy abnormal tissue, such as carcinoma in situ (cancer that involves only the cells in which it began and that has not spread to nearby tissues). This type of treatment is also called cryotherapy. The doctor may use ultrasound to guide the instrument.

- **Partial hepatectomy:** Removal of the part of the liver where cancer is found. The part removed may be a wedge of tissue, an entire lobe, or a larger portion of the liver, along with some of the healthy tissue around it. The remaining liver tissue takes over the functions of the liver.

- **Total hepatectomy and liver transplant:** Removal of the entire liver and replacement with a healthy donated liver. A liver transplant may be done when the disease is in the liver only and a donated liver can be found. If the patient has to wait for a donated liver, other treatment is given as needed.

- **Radiofrequency ablation:** The use of a special probe with tiny electrodes that kill cancer cells. Sometimes the probe is inserted directly through the skin and only local anesthesia is needed. In other cases, the probe is inserted through an incision in the abdomen. This is done in the hospital with general anesthesia.

Radiation therapy: Radiation therapy is a cancer treatment that uses high-energy x-rays or other types of radiation to kill cancer cells. Radiation therapy is given in different ways. The way the radiation therapy is given depends on the type and stage of the cancer being treated:

- External radiation therapy uses a machine outside the body to send radiation toward the cancer.

- Internal radiation therapy uses a radioactive substance sealed in needles, seeds, wires, or catheters that are placed directly into or near the cancer.

- Drugs called radiosensitizers may be given with the radiation therapy to make the cancer cells more sensitive to radiation therapy.

- Radiation may be delivered to the tumor using radiolabeled antibodies. Radioactive substances are attached to antibodies made in the laboratory. These antibodies, which target tumor cells, are injected into the body and the tumor cells are killed by the radioactive substance.

Chemotherapy: Chemotherapy is a cancer treatment that uses drugs to stop the growth of cancer cells, either by killing the cells or by stopping the cells from dividing. When chemotherapy is taken by mouth or injected into a vein or muscle, the drugs enter the bloodstream and can reach cancer cells throughout the body (systemic chemotherapy). When chemotherapy is placed directly into the spinal column, an organ, or a body cavity such as the abdomen, the drugs mainly affect cancer cells in those areas (regional chemotherapy). The way the chemotherapy is given depends on the type and stage of the cancer being treated.

Regional chemotherapy is usually used to treat liver cancer. A small pump containing anticancer drugs may be placed in the body. The pump puts the drugs directly into the blood vessels that go to the tumor.

Another type of regional chemotherapy is chemoembolization of the hepatic artery. The anticancer drug is injected into the hepatic artery through a catheter (thin tube). The drug is mixed with a substance that blocks the artery, cutting off blood flow to the tumor. Most of the anticancer drug is trapped near the tumor and only a small amount of the drug reaches other parts of the body. The blockage may be temporary or permanent, depending on the substance used to block the artery. The tumor is prevented from getting the oxygen and nutrients it needs to grow. The liver continues to receive blood from the hepatic portal vein, which carries blood from the stomach and intestine.

Percutaneous ethanol injection: Percutaneous ethanol injection is a cancer treatment in which a small needle is used to inject ethanol (alcohol) directly into a tumor to kill cancer cells. The procedure may be done once or twice a week. Usually local anesthesia is used, but if the patient has many tumors in the liver, general anesthesia may be needed.

New Treatments

Other types of treatment are being tested in clinical trials. These include the following:

Hyperthermia therapy: Hyperthermia therapy is a type of treatment in which body tissue is exposed to high temperatures to damage and kill cancer cells or to make cancer cells more sensitive to the effects of radiation and certain anticancer drugs. Because some cancer cells are more sensitive to heat than normal cells are, the cancer cells die and the tumor shrinks.

Biologic therapy: Biologic therapy is a treatment that uses the patient's immune system to fight cancer. Substances made by the body or made in a laboratory are used to boost, direct, or restore the body's natural defenses against cancer. This type of cancer treatment is also called biotherapy or immunotherapy.

Treatment Options for Adult Primary Liver Cancer

Localized resectable adult primary liver cancer: Treatment of localized resectable adult primary liver cancer may include the following:

- Surgery (partial hepatectomy)
- Surgery (total hepatectomy) and liver transplant
- A clinical trial of regional or systemic chemotherapy or biologic therapy following surgery

Localized and locally advanced unresectable adult primary liver cancer: Treatment of localized and locally advanced unresectable adult primary liver cancer may include the following:

- Surgery (cryosurgery or radiofrequency ablation)
- Chemotherapy (chemoembolization, regional chemotherapy, or systemic chemotherapy)
- Percutaneous ethanol injection
- Surgery (total hepatectomy) and liver transplant
- Radiation therapy with radiosensitizers
- A clinical trial of a combination of surgery, chemotherapy, and radiation therapy. Hyperthermia therapy may also be used.

Chemotherapy and radiation therapy may be used to shrink the tumor before surgery.

Advanced adult primary liver cancer: There is no standard treatment for advanced adult primary liver cancer. Patients may consider taking part in a clinical trial. Treatment may be a clinical trial of biologic therapy, chemotherapy, and/or radiation therapy with or without radiosensitizers. These treatments may be given as palliative therapy to help relieve symptoms and improve the quality of life.

Recurrent adult primary liver cancer: Treatment of recurrent adult primary liver cancer may include the following:

- Surgery (partial hepatectomy)
- Surgery (total hepatectomy) and liver transplant
- Chemotherapy (chemoembolization or systemic chemotherapy)
- Percutaneous ethanol injection
- A clinical trial of a new therapy

Chapter 41

Childhood Liver Cancer: Hepatoblastoma and Hepatocellular Carcinoma

Childhood liver cancer is a disease in which malignant (cancer) cells form in the tissues of the liver. The liver is one of the largest organs in the body, filling the upper right side of the abdomen, inside the rib cage. The liver has two parts, a right lobe and a smaller left lobe. The liver has many important functions, including the following:

- Filtering harmful substances from the blood so they can be passed from the body in stools and urine

- Making bile to help digest fats from food

- Storing glycogen (sugar), which the body uses for energy

There are two main types of childhood liver cancer:

- **Hepatoblastoma:** A type of liver cancer that usually does not spread outside the liver. This type usually affects children younger than three years old.

- **Hepatocellular carcinoma:** A type of liver cancer that often spreads to other places in the body. This type can affect children of any age.

PDQ® Cancer Information Summary. National Cancer Institute; Bethesda, MD. Childhood Liver Cancer (PDQ®): Treatment - Patient. Updated 12/2004. Available at: http://cancer.gov. Accessed April 30, 2006.

419

Risk factors for hepatoblastoma include the following:

- Being male
- Having familial adenomatous polyposis (FAP)
- Having Beckwith-Wiedemann syndrome
- Having had a very low weight at birth

Risk factors for hepatocellular carcinoma include the following:

- Being male
- Having hepatitis B or hepatitis C. The risk is greatest when the virus is passed from mother to child at birth
- Having liver damage caused by certain diseases, such as biliary cirrhosis or tyrosinemia

A doctor should be consulted if any of the following symptoms occur:

- A painless lump in the abdomen
- Swelling or pain in the abdomen
- Weight loss for no known reason
- Loss of appetite
- Early puberty in boys
- Nausea and vomiting

The following tests and procedures may be used:

Physical exam and history: An exam of the body to check general signs of health, including checking for signs of disease, such as lumps or anything else that seems unusual. A history of the patient's health habits and past illnesses and treatments will also be taken.

Serum tumor marker test: A procedure in which a blood sample is checked to measure the amounts of certain substances released into the blood by organs, tissues, or tumor cells in the body. Certain substances are linked to specific types of cancer when found in increased levels in the blood. These are called tumor markers. The blood of children who have liver cancer may have increased amounts of a protein called alpha-fetoprotein (AFP) or a hormone called beta-human chorionic gonadotropin (β-hCG). Other cancers and certain noncancerous conditions, including cirrhosis and hepatitis, may also increase AFP levels.

Complete blood count: A procedure in which a sample of blood is drawn and checked for the following:

- The number of red blood cells, white blood cells, and platelets

- The amount of hemoglobin (the protein that carries oxygen) in the red blood cells

- The portion of the blood sample made up of red blood cells

Liver function tests: A procedure in which a blood sample is checked to measure the amounts of certain substances released into the blood by the liver. A higher than normal amount of a substance can be a sign of liver cancer.

Abdominal x-ray: An x-ray of the organs in the abdomen. An x-ray is a type of energy beam that can go through the body onto film, making a picture of areas inside the body.

Ultrasound: A procedure in which high-energy sound waves (ultra-sound) are bounced off internal tissues or organs and make echoes. The echoes form a picture of body tissues called a sonogram.

CT scan (CAT scan): A procedure that makes a series of detailed pictures of areas inside the body, taken from different angles. The pictures are made by a computer linked to an x-ray machine. A dye may be injected into a vein or swallowed to help the organs or tissues show up more clearly. This procedure is also called computed tomography, computerized tomography, or computerized axial tomography. In childhood liver cancer, a CT scan of the chest and abdomen is usually done.

MRI (magnetic resonance imaging): A procedure that uses a magnet, radio waves, and a computer to make a series of detailed pictures of areas inside the body. This procedure is also called nuclear magnetic resonance imaging (NMRI).

Biopsy: The removal of cells or tissues so they can be viewed under a microscope to check for signs of cancer. The sample may be taken during surgery to remove or view the tumor. A pathologist views the sample under a microscope to determine the type of liver cancer.

Prognosis

The prognosis (chance of recovery) and treatment options depend on the following:

- The stage of the cancer (the size of the tumor, whether it affects part or all of the liver, and whether it has spread to other places in the body, such as the lungs)
- Whether the cancer can be removed completely by surgery
- The type of liver cancer (hepatoblastoma or hepatocellular)
- Whether the cancer has just been diagnosed or has recurred

Prognosis may also depend on these factors:

- Certain features of the cancer cell (how it looks under a microscope)
- Whether the AFP blood levels go down after chemotherapy begins
- Childhood liver cancer may be cured if the tumor is small and can be completely removed by surgery. Complete removal is possible more often for hepatoblastoma than for hepatocellular carcinoma.

Stages of Childhood Liver Cancer

After childhood liver cancer has been diagnosed, tests are done to find out if cancer cells have spread within the liver or to other parts of the body. he process used to find out if cancer has spread within the liver or to other parts of the body is called staging. The information gathered from the staging process determines the stage of the disease. It is important to know the stage in order to plan treatment.

There are 2 staging systems for childhood liver cancer:

- **Postsurgical (after surgery) staging:** The stage is based on the amount of tumor that remains after the patient has had surgery to look at or remove the tumor. Postsurgical staging is used for most childhood liver cancer.

- **Presurgical (before surgery) staging:** The stage is based on where the tumor has spread within the four parts (quadrants) of the liver, as shown by imaging procedures such as MRI or CT.

This staging system, called PRETEXT, may be used for childhood hepatoblastoma.

The following tests and procedures may be used in the staging process:

- **CT scan (CAT scan)**
- **MRI (magnetic resonance imaging)**
- **Ultrasound:** A procedure in which high-energy sound waves (ultrasound) are bounced off internal tissues or organs and make echoes. The echoes form a picture of body tissues called a sonogram.
- **Surgery:** An operation will be done to look at or remove the tumor. Tissues removed during surgery will be checked by a pathologist.

The following stages are used after surgery:

Stage I: In stage I, all of the cancer was removed by surgery.

Stage II: In stage II, all of the cancer that can be seen without a microscope was removed by surgery. A small amount of cancer remains in the liver, but it can be seen only with a microscope or the tumor cells may have spilled into the abdomen during surgery.

Stage III: In stage III:

- the tumor cannot be removed by surgery; or
- cancer that can be seen without a microscope remains after surgery; or
- the cancer has spread to nearby lymph nodes.

Stage IV: In stage IV, the cancer has spread to other parts of the body.

Other Stages

The following stages are used for childhood hepatoblastoma before surgery:

- **PRETEXT stage 1:** In stage 1, the cancer is found in one quadrant of the liver.

- **PRETEXT stage 2:** In stage 2, cancer is found in two quadrants of the liver that are next to each other.

- **PRETEXT stage 3:** In stage 3, cancer is found in three quadrants of the liver that are next to each other or two quadrants that are not next to each other.

- **PRETEXT stage 4:** In stage 4, cancer is found in all four quadrants.

Recurrent childhood liver cancer: Recurrent childhood liver cancer is cancer that has recurred (come back) after it has been treated. The cancer may come back in the liver or in other parts of the body.

Treatment Option Overview

Different types of treatments are available for children with liver cancer. Some treatments are standard (the currently used treatment), and some are being tested in clinical trials. A treatment clinical trial is a research study meant to help improve current treatments or obtain information on new treatments for patients with cancer. When clinical trials show that a new treatment is better than the standard treatment, the new treatment may become the standard treatment.

Because cancer in children is rare, a clinical trial should be considered for all children who have liver cancer. Clinical trials are taking place in many parts of the country. Information about ongoing clinical trials is available from the National Cancer Institute website (http://www.cancer.gov). Choosing the most appropriate cancer treatment is a decision that ideally involves the patient, family, and health care team.

Children with liver cancer should have their treatment planned by a team of doctors with expertise in treating this rare childhood cancer. Your child's treatment will be overseen by a pediatric oncologist, a doctor who specializes in treating children with cancer. The pediatric oncologist may refer you to other pediatric doctors who specialize in certain areas of medicine and who have experience and expertise in treating children who have liver cancer. It is especially important to have a pediatric surgeon with experience in liver surgery. Other specialists may include the following:

- Radiation oncologist
- Pediatric nurse specialist

- Rehabilitation specialist
- Psychologist
- Social worker

Three types of standard treatment are used:

Surgery: When possible, the cancer is removed by surgery.

- **Partial hepatectomy:** Removal of the part of the liver where cancer is found. The part removed may be a wedge of tissue, an entire lobe, or a larger part of the liver, along with a small amount of normal tissue around it.

- **Total hepatectomy and liver transplant:** Removal of the entire liver and replacement with a healthy liver from a donor. A liver transplant may be possible when cancer has not spread beyond the liver and a donated liver can be found. If the patient has to wait for a donated liver, other treatment is given as needed.

- **Resection of metastases:** Surgery to remove cancer that has spread outside of the liver, such as to nearby tissues, the lungs, or the brain.

Chemotherapy or radiation therapy is sometimes given before surgery, to shrink the tumor and make it easier to remove. This is called neoadjuvant therapy. Even if the doctor removes all the cancer that can be seen at the time of the surgery, some patients may be given chemotherapy after surgery to kill any cancer cells that are left. Treatment given after the surgery, to increase the chances of a cure, is called adjuvant therapy.

Chemotherapy: Chemotherapy is a cancer treatment that uses drugs to stop the growth of cancer cells, either by killing the cells or by stopping the cells from dividing. When chemotherapy is taken by mouth or injected into a vein or muscle, the drugs enter the bloodstream and can reach cancer cells throughout the body (systemic chemotherapy). When chemotherapy is placed directly into the spinal column, an organ, or a body cavity such as the abdomen, the drugs mainly affect cancer cells in those areas (regional chemotherapy).

Chemoembolization of the hepatic artery (the main artery that supplies blood to the liver) is a type of regional chemotherapy used to treat childhood liver cancer. The anticancer drug is injected into the hepatic artery through a catheter (thin tube). The drug is mixed with a substance that blocks the artery, cutting off blood flow to the tumor. Most of the anticancer drug is trapped near the tumor and only a small amount of the drug reaches other parts of the body. The blockage may be temporary or permanent, depending on the substance used to block the artery. The tumor is prevented from getting the oxygen and nutrients it needs to grow. The liver continues to receive blood from the hepatic portal vein, which carries blood from the stomach and intestine.

Treatment using more than one anticancer drug is called combination chemotherapy. The way the chemotherapy is given depends on the type and stage of the cancer being treated.

Radiation therapy: Radiation therapy is a cancer treatment that uses high-energy x-rays or other types of radiation to kill cancer cells. There are two types of radiation therapy. External radiation therapy uses a machine outside the body to send radiation toward the cancer. Internal radiation therapy uses a radioactive substance sealed in needles, seeds, wires, or catheters that are placed directly into or near the cancer. The way the radiation therapy is given depends on the type and stage of the cancer being treated.

Treatment Options by Stage

Stage I and II childhood liver cancer: Treatment for stages I and II and PRETEXT stages 1, 2, and 3 hepatoblastoma may include the following:

- Surgery to remove the tumor, followed by chemotherapy or watchful waiting (closely monitoring a patient's condition without giving any treatment until symptoms appear or change)
- Chemotherapy to shrink the tumor, followed by surgery to remove the tumor

Treatment for stage I and II hepatocellular carcinoma is usually surgery to remove the tumor, followed by combination chemotherapy.

Stage III childhood liver cancer: Treatment of stage III and PRETEXT stage 4 hepatoblastoma may include the following:

- Combination chemotherapy to shrink the tumor, followed by surgery to remove as much of the tumor as possible

- If the tumor cannot be removed by surgery after chemotherapy, further treatment may include the following:
  - High-dose chemotherapy
  - Radiation therapy
  - Chemoembolization of the hepatic artery
  - Liver transplant
  - A clinical trial of combination chemotherapy

Treatment of stage III hepatocellular carcinoma is usually combination chemotherapy to shrink the tumor, followed by surgery to remove as much of the tumor as possible.

Stage IV childhood liver cancer: Treatment of stage IV hepatoblastoma may include the following:

- Combination chemotherapy to shrink the tumor, followed by surgery to remove as much of the cancer as possible, including cancer that has spread to the lungs. If the cancer is completely removed, additional chemotherapy is given to kill any cancer cells that may remain.
- If the tumor cannot be removed by surgery after chemotherapy, further treatment may include the following:
  - High-dose chemotherapy
  - Radiation therapy followed by surgery to remove as much of the tumor as possible
  - Chemoembolization of the hepatic artery
  - Liver transplant
  - A clinical trial of chemotherapy

Treatment of stage IV hepatocellular carcinoma may be combination chemotherapy to reduce the size of the tumor, followed by surgery to remove as much of the tumor as possible.

Recurrent childhood liver cancer: Treatment of recurrent hepatoblastoma is usually surgery to remove isolated (single and separate) metastatic tumors.

Chapter 42

Small Intestine Cancer

There are five types of small intestine cancer. The types of cancer found in the small intestine are adenocarcinoma, sarcoma, carcinoid tumors, gastrointestinal stromal tumor, and lymphoma.

Adenocarcinoma starts in glandular cells in the lining of the small intestine and is the most common type of small intestine cancer. Most of these tumors occur in the part of the small intestine near the stomach. They may grow and block the intestine.

Leiomyosarcoma starts in the smooth muscle cells of the small intestine. Most of these tumors occur in the part of the small intestine near the large intestine.

Risk factors include the following:

- Eating a high-fat diet
- Having Crohn disease
- Having celiac disease
- Having familial adenomatous polyposis (FAP)

A doctor should be consulted if any of the following symptoms occur:

- Pain or cramps in the middle of the abdomen
- Weight loss with no known reason

Excerpted from PDQ® Cancer Information Summary. National Cancer Institute; Bethesda, MD. Small Intestine Cancer (PDQ®): Treatment - Patient. Updated 01/2005. Available at: http://cancer.gov. Accessed April 30, 2006.

- A lump in the abdomen
- Blood in the stool

Procedures that create pictures of the small intestine and the area around it help diagnose small intestine cancer and show how far the cancer has spread. The process used to find out if cancer cells have spread within and around the small intestine is called staging.

In order to plan treatment, it is important to know the type of small intestine cancer and whether the tumor can be removed by surgery. Tests and procedures to detect, diagnose, and stage small intestine cancer are usually done at the same time. In addition to a physical exam and history, the following tests and procedures may be used:

Blood chemistry studies: A procedure in which a blood sample is checked to measure the amounts of certain substances released into the blood by organs and tissues in the body. An unusual (higher or lower than normal) amount of a substance can be a sign of disease in the organ or tissue that produces it.

Liver function tests: A procedure in which a blood sample is checked to measure the amounts of certain substances released into the blood by the liver. A higher than normal amount of a substance can be a sign of liver disease that may be caused by small intestine cancer.

Abdominal x-ray: An x-ray of the organs in the abdomen. An x-ray is a type of energy beam that can go through the body onto film, making a picture of areas inside the body.

Barium enema: A series of x-rays of the lower gastrointestinal (GI) tract. A liquid that contains barium (a silver-white metallic compound) is put into the rectum. The barium coats the lower gastrointestinal tract and x-rays are taken. This procedure is also called a lower GI series.

Fecal occult blood test: A test to check stool (solid waste) for blood that can only be seen with a microscope. Small samples of stool are placed on special cards and returned to the doctor or laboratory for testing.

Upper endoscopy: A procedure to look at the inside of the esophagus, stomach, and duodenum (first part of the small intestine, near the stomach). An endoscope (a thin, lighted tube) is inserted through the mouth and into the esophagus, stomach, and duodenum. Tissue samples may be taken for biopsy.

Upper GI series with small bowel follow-through: A series of x-rays of the esophagus, stomach, and small bowel. The patient drinks a liquid that contains barium (a silver-white metallic compound). The liquid coats the esophagus, stomach, and small bowel. X-rays are taken at different times as the barium travels through the upper GI tract and small bowel.

Biopsy: The removal of cells or tissues so they can be viewed under a microscope to check for signs of cancer. This may be done during the endoscopy. The sample is checked by a pathologist to see if it contains cancer cells.

CT scan (CAT scan): A procedure that makes a series of detailed pictures of areas inside the body, taken from different angles. The pictures are made by a computer linked to an x-ray machine. A dye may be injected into a vein or swallowed to help the organs or tissues show up more clearly. This procedure is also called computed tomography, computerized tomography, or computerized axial tomography.

Lymph node biopsy: The removal of all or part of a lymph node. A pathologist views the tissue under a microscope to look for cancer cells.

Laparotomy: A surgical procedure in which an incision (cut) is made in the wall of the abdomen to check the inside of the abdomen for signs of disease. The size of the incision depends on the reason the laparotomy is being done. Sometimes organs are removed or tissue samples are taken for biopsy.

Treatment Option Overview

Three types of standard treatment are used:

Surgery: Surgery is the most common treatment of small intestine cancer. One of the following types of surgery may be done:

- **Resection:** Surgery to remove part or all of an organ that contains cancer. The resection may include the small intestine and nearby organs (if the cancer has spread). The doctor may remove the section of the small intestine that contains cancer and perform an anastomosis (joining the cut ends of the intestine together). The doctor will usually remove lymph nodes near the small intestine and examine them under a microscope to see whether they contain cancer.

- **Bypass:** Surgery to allow food in the small intestine to go around (bypass) a tumor that is blocking the intestine but cannot be removed.

Even if the doctor removes all the cancer that can be seen at the time of the surgery, some patients may be given radiation therapy after surgery to kill any cancer cells that are left. Treatment given after the surgery, to increase the chances of a cure, is called adjuvant therapy.

Radiation therapy: Radiation therapy is a cancer treatment that uses high-energy x-rays or other types of radiation to kill cancer cells. There are two types of radiation therapy. External radiation therapy uses a machine outside the body to send radiation toward the cancer. Internal radiation therapy uses a radioactive substance sealed in needles, seeds, wires, or catheters that are placed directly into or near the cancer. The way the radiation therapy is given depends on the type and stage of the cancer being treated.

Chemotherapy: Chemotherapy is a cancer treatment that uses drugs to stop the growth of cancer cells, either by killing the cells or by stopping the cells from dividing. When chemotherapy is taken by mouth or injected into a vein or muscle, the drugs enter the bloodstream and can reach cancer cells throughout the body (systemic chemotherapy). When chemotherapy is placed directly into the spinal column, an organ, or a body cavity such as the abdomen, the drugs mainly affect cancer cells in those areas (regional chemotherapy). The way the chemotherapy is given depends on the type and stage of the cancer being treated.

New Treatments

Other types of treatment are being tested in clinical trials. These include the following:

Biologic therapy: Biologic therapy is a treatment that uses the patient's immune system to fight cancer. Substances made by the body or made in a laboratory are used to boost, direct, or restore the body's natural defenses against cancer. This type of cancer treatment is also called biotherapy or immunotherapy.

Radiation therapy with radiosensitizers: Radiosensitizers are drugs that make tumor cells more sensitive to radiation therapy. Combining radiation therapy with radiosensitizers may kill more tumor cells.

Treatment Options for Small Intestine Cancer

Small intestine adenocarcinoma: When possible, treatment of small intestine adenocarcinoma will be surgery to remove the tumor and some of the normal tissue around it.

Treatment of small intestine adenocarcinoma that cannot be removed by surgery may include the following:

- Surgery to bypass the tumor
- Radiation therapy as palliative therapy to relieve symptoms and improve the patient's quality of life
- A clinical trial of radiation therapy with radiosensitizers, with or without chemotherapy
- A clinical trial of new anticancer drugs
- A clinical trial of biologic therapy

Small intestine leiomyosarcoma: When possible, treatment of small intestine leiomyosarcoma will be surgery to remove the tumor and some of the normal tissue around it.

Treatment of small intestine leiomyosarcoma that cannot be removed by surgery may include the following:

- Surgery (to bypass the tumor) and radiation therapy
- Surgery, radiation therapy, or chemotherapy as palliative therapy to relieve symptoms and improve the patient's quality of life
- A clinical trial of new anticancer drugs
- A clinical trial of biologic therapy

Recurrent small intestine cancer: Treatment of recurrent small intestine cancer that has spread to other parts of the body is usually a clinical trial of new anticancer drugs or biologic therapy.

Treatment of locally recurrent small intestine cancer may include the following:

- Surgery

- Radiation therapy or chemotherapy as palliative therapy to relieve symptoms and improve the patient's quality of life

- A clinical trial of radiation therapy with radiosensitizers, with or without chemotherapy

Chapter 43

Colorectal Cancer

Cancers of the colon and rectum, often referred to collectively as colorectal cancer, are life-threatening tumors that develop in the large intestine.

More than 80% of colorectal tumors evolve from adenomatous polyps. These are gland-like growths that develop on the mucous membrane that lines the large intestine. They are usually one of the following types:

- Tubular polyps, which protrude mushroom-like
- Villous adenomas, which are flat and spreading and are more apt to become malignant (cancerous)

It should be noted that these polyps are very common and almost always benign. Their numbers increase with age. Polyps are found in about 25% of people by age 50 and half of people by age 75. Fewer than one percent of polyps under one centimeter (slightly less than half an inch) become cancerous (malignant). About 10% of larger polyps become malignant within 10 years and about 25% of these larger polyps become cancerous after 20 years. Certain inherited polyps can become malignant more rapidly.

Causes

In most cases of colon or rectal cancers the cause or causes are unknown. Defects in genes that normally protect against cancer play

Excerpted from "Colon and Rectal Cancers," © 2006 A.D.A.M., Inc. Reprinted with permission.

the major role in causing polyp cells to continuously spread and become cancerous. Some of these cases are caused by inherited genetic defects, and such patients usually have family histories of colorectal cancer. Most of genetic mutations involved in colon cancers, however, appear to arise spontaneously (no strong family history) rather than being inherited. In such cases, environmental or other factors trigger genetic changes in the intestine that lead to cancer.

Inherited Genetic Factors

About 6% of cases of colon cancer are due to inherited facts.

APC gene and familial adenomatous polyposis (FAP): When the adenomatous polyposis coli (APC) gene is normal, it helps suppress tumor growth. In its defective form, it permits high levels of the protein beta-catenin to accumulate, which accelerates cell growth leading to polyps.

Hereditary nonpolyposis colorectal cancer (HNPCC): Hereditary nonpolyposis colorectal cancer (HNPCC), also known as Lynch syndrome, accounts for at least half of colorectal cancers that run in families. (However, only 3% or less of all colorectal cancers are due to this problem). About 50–80% of people who inherit the abnormal gene will develop colon cancer. HNPCC tends to develop in the right side of the colon, often in young individuals. (Left sided cancers can still occur as well.)

Biochemical Factors Involved in Colon and Rectal Cancers

Cyclooxygenases and prostaglandins: Cyclooxygenase 1 and 2 (COX-1 and COX-2) are enzymes involved in the production of prostaglandins, substances produced by the body that cause inflammation, widen and narrow blood vessels, control muscle contractions, and inhibit hormones that regulate fat metabolism. COX-2, but not COX-1, appears to play a role in the development and spread of colorectal tumors. COX-2 increases the levels of prostaglandin E2 (PGE2), which, in turn, stimulates factors that inhibit apoptosis, the natural process whereby all cells, including cancerous ones, self-destruct. It also activates interleukin-6 (IL-6), a factor in the immune system that is associated with cancer cell invasion.

C-reactive protein (CRP): CRP is another indicator of inflammation. In a case-control study published in the *Journal of the American*

Medical Association (*JAMA*) in 2004, elevated CRP levels predicted the development of colon—but not rectal—cancer.

Bile acid salts: Deoxycholic acid, which is found in the fat-digesting bile salts released by the gallbladder, appears to have carcinogenic properties. Its effects are now believed to play a role in some cases of colon cancer. Levels of the acid can rise as a result of high-fat diets or certain diseases.

Growth factors: Chronically higher circulating levels of growth factors, including insulin-like growth factor (IGF), have been associated with colorectal cancer.

Inflammatory Bowel Disease

Inflammatory bowel diseases (IBDs) include Crohn disease and ulcerative colitis. These chronic disorders cause persistent injuries in the intestinal tract that can, in some cases, produce cancerous changes.

Symptoms

It is possible to have colon or rectal cancer without symptoms. Many patients are free of symptoms until their tumors are quite advanced.

Weight Loss and Changes in Bowel Movements

Weight loss and changes in bowel movements are general symptoms for colon cancer but also occur in many other diseases.

Rectal Bleeding

Blood in the stools is a common sign of many intestinal cancers. It may appear red if it is fresh or black if it is old. It should be reported to a physician immediately, even though it is often caused by conditions other than cancer, including the following:

- Hemorrhoids
- Minor tears around the rectal or anal areas
- Diverticulosis
- Stools can turn red after eating certain red foods, such as beets or red licorice.

- Iron supplements and medications that have bismuth sub-salicylate, most commonly Pepto-Bismol, can cause stools to turn black.

Nevertheless, blood in the stools is an abnormal finding that should never be ignored. Always report it to your doctor for further advice.

Symptoms of Cancers in Specific Areas of the Colon

Symptoms of colorectal cancer vary widely depending on the location of the cancer within the large intestine.

Tumors in the cecum and ascending colon (right colon): The waste matter in the first portion of the colon is in liquid or semi-liquid form. Tumors that develop here do not change bowel habits or stool formation, but they may cause intermittent or chronic bleeding. Although the stools look normal, patients may develop symptoms of anemia from iron deficiency. Such symptoms include weakness, fatigue, heart palpitations, shortness of breath, and exercise intolerance.

Tumors in the transverse colon: As waste material passes across the upper quadrants of the abdomen (the transverse colon), the intestine absorbs water and the waste matter becomes more solid. In addition to bleeding, tumors here may cause cramps, gas, partial or complete obstruction, and even perforation of the bowel. Anemia as described above can also occur.

Tumors in the descending colon and rectum (left colon): When tumors partially block the lower intestine, thin, pencil-shaped stools may form. Bowel habits can change. Tumors in the rectum and lowest part of the intestine can cause pain and a feeling of fullness. Defecation may be painful or patients may feel the urge to defecate, but nothing happens. Bleeding from these locations may be brisk and bright red or maroon, but cancer is often detected before symptoms of chronic anemia develop.

Risk Factors

Colorectal cancer is the fourth most common cancer in the U.S., with Americans facing a lifetime risk of 6% for this cancer. An estimated 147,000 people in the U.S. are expected to be diagnosed with colon or rectal cancer in 2004.

- **Sex:** The risks overall are equal in men and women, but men have a higher risk for rectal cancers and women for colon cancers.

- **Age:** The most important risk factor for colon cancer is getting older. More than 90% of these cancers occur in people over 50. The rate of colorectal cancer in patients under 20 years is less than 1 in 100,000 per year.

- **Ethnicity:** Compared to Caucasians, African Americans are at higher risk of colon (but not rectal) cancer. The highest risks are in men of African descent, particularly in the sub-Saharan region. Ashkenazi Jews, of Eastern Europe descent, also have a higher incidence of colorectal cancer.

- **Family history:** About 25% of patients under 45 years old and 15% of everyone who develops colorectal cancer have a genetic risk. The average lifetime risk of developing colorectal cancer is approximately 2%. People who have a sibling or parent (first degree relative) who developed colorectal cancer have three times (6%) the lifetime risk of developing colorectal cancer. People who have a first degree relative who developed colorectal cancer before age 45 have an even higher, 10%, lifetime risk of developing colorectal cancer.

- **Lifestyle factors:** The risks for colon cancer are far higher in industrialized nations than less developed countries. A Western lifestyle, being sedentary, smoking, and excess weight have all been associated with increased risk for colorectal cancer. (It should be noted, however, that about 75% of cases occur without a known predisposing factor.)

- **Inflammatory bowel disease:** Crohn disease and ulcerative colitis are chronic afflictions of the large intestine known as inflammatory bowel diseases (IBDs). Both have been linked to increased risk for colorectal cancer.

Other Risk Factors

Polyps: Polyps are tissue growths, usually benign, that develop in the color or rectum, most often in patients over 50 years of age. When pathologists examine polyps removed from the colon, they classify them as either hyperplastic or adenomatous. Both types are benign, but some adenomas will become malignant. As a preventive measure, polyps should be removed (polypectomy).

Ureterosigmoidostomy: People who have had ureterosigmoidostomy, a surgical procedure to correct a birth defect in the bladder or to treat some bladder cancers, may develop tumors near the site of the defect, which is chronically exposed to urine and feces. Such patients have a 5% to 10% chance of developing colon cancer 15 to 30 years after the operation.

Diabetes: Many studies have identified a possible association between type 2 diabetes and colon cancer. Both diseases share common risk factors of obesity and physical inactivity, but diabetes may independently predispose for colon cancer. Data from a case control study of 50,000 U.S. veterans presented at the 2004 Digestive Disease Week conference found that patients with diabetes were 32 percent more likely to develop colon cancer than similar patients who did not have diabetes.

Dietary Factors

Previous research suggested that diets low in fruits and vegetables and high in meats pose a risk for colon cancer, and that those rich in fruits and vegetables are protective against many cancers.

Fruits, Vegetables, and Whole Grains

There has been a prevailing belief from a number of studies that high intake of fruits and vegetables can lower the risk for colorectal cancer. Studies have been mixed, however, on their benefits. A 2002 study, for example, reported that these foods do not prevent polyps from forming but may help prevent them from becoming cancerous.

It should be noted that it is nearly impossible to do controlled studies on dietary factors, since people's eating habits can rarely be made consistent. Dietary studies also use a variety of different approaches to obtain results that make comparisons very difficult. To help determine their specific effects researchers are studying the phytochemicals (plant chemicals) in fruits and vegetables and also fiber (which is also found in whole grains.)

Phytochemicals: Many studies have demonstrated the cancer-fighting effects of plant chemicals called phytochemicals. Fruits and vegetables that contain phytochemicals can often be identified by colors:

- Dark green (broccoli, spinach, kale, collard greens, mustard greens): These specific vegetables contain chemicals called isothiocyanates, which have been associated with a lower risk for cancer in general.

- Red (red pepper, tomatoes, watermelon, raspberries, pink grape-fruit): Lycopene is a chemical found in these foods that may have strong cancer-protective properties. Cooking tomatoes appears to increase their benefits.

- Yellow-orange (carrots, pumpkin, sweet potatoes, oranges, tan-gerines): The colors in these foods are due to carotenoids, which have been associated with health protection, although may not have much effect on colon cancer itself.

- Blue-black (many berries): Dark berries appear to have potent chemicals that may be protective against cancer. In one animal study, extracts from black raspberries reduced colon cancer tumors in rats.

Organosulfurs are important food chemicals that are part of the allium family and there have been studies reporting health benefits from foods containing them. These compounds are found in garlic, leeks, onions, chives, scallions, and shallots. A review of 300 studies concluded that people who eat raw or cooked garlic regularly experience about two-thirds the risk of colorectal cancer as people who eat little or none. Another analysis, however, found the available evidence about garlic to be inconclusive. Garlic supplements, in any case, do not appear to be protective.

Fiber: Studies have been mixed on whether fiber (found in fruits, vegetables, and whole grains) protects the colon from cancer. For example, three major studies in 2002 and 2003 reported no difference in the development of colorectal polyps or cancer recurrence with high intake of fiber. On the other hand, other studies have been positive. In fact, 2003 results of the European Prospective Investigation into Cancer and Nutrition (EPIC)—the largest study ever conducted on the role of diet in the development of cancer—suggested that fiber is protective regardless of its source. However, in the study, the greatest benefits were observed for the left side of the colon and the least for the rectum. In any case, fiber, which is only found in plant products, may be beneficial for the heart and have other health advantages.

Fats and Oils

The role of fats in inflammatory bowel disease is complex and not fully known. Any benefits or risks appear to depend on the type of compounds that make up fats (the fatty acids) or other nutrients or substances with fatty acids.

Saturated fats and trans-fatty oils: Some studies had found an association between colon cancer and consumption of saturated fats (found primarily in animal fats). The association is not altogether clear, however, and more recent evidence has not supported a strong link. Some experts suggest that the real hazard is iron from red meat, which is often high in saturated fats and may have confused study results.

Of further interest, however, is a 2001 study that reported a possible link between colon cancer and trans fatty acids, which are partially hydrogenated oils found in stick margarine, fried foods, and commercial baked goods. The association is supported by known chemical effects of these manufactured fats, and more research is warranted.

Monounsaturated fats: Monounsaturated fats are mostly present in olive, canola, and peanut oils and in most nuts. Olive oil, for example, may protect the colon. Some evidence suggests that it reduces levels of deoxycholic acid, an acid found in bile that has tumor-promoting properties.

Polyunsaturated fats: Polyunsaturated fats are found in both plant and fish oils, and are composed of essential fatty acids including omega-3 and omega-6 fatty acids. These fatty acids may play different roles in colon cancer.

- Omega-3 fatty acids are found in oily fish and canola oil, soybeans, flaxseed, and certain nuts and seeds. They have been associated with protection against inflammation in the intestinal tract. It should be noted, however, that not all studies show protection. For example, omega-3 fatty acids in fish are composed of docosahexaenoic (DHA) and eicosapentaenoic (EPA) acids. Some evidence suggests that EPA—although not DHA—may be protective.

- Omega-6 fatty acids, found in corn, safflower, soybean, and sunflower oil, constitute most of the oils consumed in the U.S. Some omega-6 fatty acids are important for health. However, a high intake has been associated with heart disease and certain cancers.

Currently it is reasonable to reduce saturated fats and transfatty acids and to favor monounsaturated oils and polyunsaturated oils, particularly containing omega-3 fatty acids.

Meat and High-Temperature Cooking

Some evidence suggests that red meat raises the risk for colon cancer. Red meat contains dietary iron, which has been associated with a higher risk for colon cancer. In fact, early results in 2000 from the largest study on diet and cancer to date have supported previous studies linking red meat with intestinal tumors.

High-temperature cooking (grilling, broiling, or pan-frying) has been specifically associated with increased risk for colon polyps and colon cancer. Over-cooking meat increases the amount of carcinogens called heterocyclic amines, which has been associated with cancerous changes.

Some research has been focusing on acrylamide, a chemical found in high amounts in certain foods cooked at high temperatures, especially fried potatoes, and also bread products. Animal studies have suggested that acrylamide is a carcinogen. A surprising 2003 study, however, found no evidence of risk for colorectal or other cancers with high intake of foods that contain large amounts of this chemical.

Dairy Products and Calcium

Milk, lactose, and probiotics: In a Finish 2001 population study, adults who drank the most milk had the lowest risk for colon cancer. A 2004 study published in the *Journal of the National Cancer Institute* supports this conclusion. In this review of 10 epidemiologic studies that included more than half a million people, people who consumed more milk and calcium had a lower risk of developing colorectal cancer. Milk not only contains calcium but also other compounds, such as lactose, that may help protect against colon cancer. Yogurt specifically has been associated with a lower risk for colon cancer if it contains live active bacterial cultures, such as *Lactobacillus acidophilus*, that are called probiotics. These "friendly bacteria" appear to protect the colon from cancerous changes. (Acidophilus and other probiotic capsules are also available in health food stores.) Results are mixed on other fermented milk products, such as buttermilk and cheese, which in one study were associated with a higher risk. The reasons for this were not clear.

Calcium: Calcium, which is found in dairy products, is also associated with colon cancer protection. Most studies show a possible protective effect from either high-calcium diets or calcium supplements. The protective effect has been observed as early as one year after calcium supplementation began. A large 2002 study concluded that daily intake of about 700 mg, from food or supplements, reduces the risk of colon cancer, but intake beyond this level does not add any further protection. Calcium supplements may even offset certain effects of dietary iron, found in red meat and other foods, which may increase the risk for colon cancer. More work in this area is needed, however.

Total Calories and Sugar

Obesity has been associated with colon cancer. In some studies of people under 67 years old, the amounts of fat and protein were less important than the total number of calories consumed: the higher the energy intake, the greater the risk for developing colon cancer. In older adults, high calorie intake did not make any significant difference. Other studies have indicated that excessive sugar intake may increase the risk for colon cancer.

Coffee and Tea

Studies conducted in a number of countries have found that drinking four or more cups of coffee a day is associated with a lower risk for colorectal cancer. Green tea may have beneficial properties, but more research is needed in both of these areas.

Vitamin and Mineral Supplements

Folate and B vitamins: There is evidence that the B vitamin folate (called folic acid) is protective. Both folate and vitamin B_{12} convert the amino acid homocysteine to methionine, a chemical that protects certain genes that help prevent cells from becoming malignant. Folate is found in beans, citrus fruits, and green vegetables, but benefits seem higher when taking supplements. The protective effect appears to be greatest for people who are genetically predisposed to colorectal cancer.

Antioxidant supplements: Antioxidants are chemicals the help eliminate harmful particles called oxygen-free radicals that have been associated with cancerous changes. Some studies have associated supplements of the antioxidants selenium and vitamins A, C, D, and E with lower colon cancer risk, but most studies have found no protective effect.

Diagnosis

Colon and rectal cancers are diagnosed using the screening tests discussed below. These tests can detect precancerous polyps and colorectal cancers at stages early enough for complete removal and cure.

Unfortunately, only 30% to 40% of adults over 50 years old (mostly in the upper socioeconomic group) have regular screening tests that could detect a cancer early enough for curative treatment. A survey reported that many people are not screened because they are too embarrassed and revealed that they would rather lose months off their life than face these tests. Those who had already had the tests were willing to have them again if they saved one additional day of their lives. There is some debate about what is the best screening modality. However almost all experts agree that not enough people are screened and that if these tests were adopted with the same regularity as other screening tests, such as Pap smears, they would save many lives. It is especially important that anyone at increased risk or with symptoms, such as rectal bleeding, undergo testing.

Digital Rectal Examination (DRE)

The digital rectal examination is used to detect tumors in the rectum, lower intestine, and prostate gland. The doctor inserts a lubricated-gloved finger into the patient's rectum and feels for lumps or other abnormalities. The exam is quick and painless but embarrassing for some. Fewer than 10% of colon cancers develop within the region that can be evaluated by a DRE, so it is not useful as a sole screening test.

Fecal Occult Blood Test (FOBT)

Blood in bowel movements is not always visible, in which case it is called occult blood. Fecal occult blood tests (FOBTs) are used to detect this hidden blood. The most common FOBT method is called the guaiac-based test. The patient is asked to supply up to six stool specimens in a specially prepared package. A small quantity of feces is smeared on specially treated paper, which reacts to hydrogen peroxide. If blood is present, the paper turns blue.

Visualizing the Colon: Colonoscopy, Sigmoidoscopy, and Barium Enema

If a digital rectal exam (DRE) or fecal occult blood test (FOBT) shows signs of trouble, several methods to visualize the colon are available. They include colonoscopy, sigmoidoscopy, and double-contrast barium enema. They have the following similarities and differences:

- Sigmoidoscopy can only view the rectum and the left side of the colon, while colonoscopy and barium enemas allow a view of the entire large intestine.

- Both flexible sigmoidoscopy and colonoscopy involve snaking a fiber optic tube through regions of the rectum and colon to view the walls of the intestine. The tube contains a tiny camera that transmits the image to a video screen. The use of an ultrasound (sound wave) scanner is proving to enhance viewing quality. Barium enemas simply use x-rays.

- During either sigmoidoscopy or colonoscopy, the physician is able to remove polyps or other abnormalities revealed by these procedures with surgical instruments inserted through the tube. It is not possible to remove polyps with a barium enema, which is not invasive.

Experimental Screening and Diagnostic Methods

Virtual colonoscopy: A promising experimental technique called virtual colonoscopy allows three-dimensional imaging of the colon without using invasive instruments. As with standard colonoscopy, the patient takes a laxative first to clear out the intestine. The procedure itself involves pumping air into the colon and scanning the intestine using computed tomography (CT). It is very safe and takes only about 10 minutes. The procedure is similar in accuracy to conventional colonoscopy for detection of larger polyps (6 mm or more in diameter) and is also potentially less expensive. Colonoscopy is required, however, if suspicious areas are found, which may occur frequently with the CT procedure, since it erroneously identifies a high number of nonexistent polyps.

A study published in April 2004 in the *Journal of the American Medical Association* (*JAMA*) compared results of standard colonoscopy versus virtual colonoscopy in over 600 patients at nine major medical centers. Virtual colonoscopy had much lower rates of successfully finding polyps than standard colonoscopy. Virtual colonoscopy detected polyps of at least 6 mm in 39% of patients and polyps of at least 10 mm in 55% of patients. By contrast, standard colonoscopy detected 99% of polyps of at least 6 mm, and 100% of polyps of at least 10 mm. In addition, accuracy rates varied widely among the different hospitals. The authors advised that until more improvement in training and technique is achieved, virtual colonoscopy "is not yet ready for widespread clinical application."

Magnetic resonance colonography (MRC): Magnetic resonance colonography (MRC) is another non-invasive technique for visualizing the colon. The patient receives an enema containing a contrast agent, and then magnetic resonance images are taken. MRC is fast, comfortable, and less invasive than colonoscopy. Currently, however, there is a poor detection rate for flat tumors and for polyp tumors less than 10 mm in diameter.

Encapsulated video camera: Researchers have developed a video camera that is small enough to be swallowed. It works its way through the digestive tract, beaming data to a receiver worn on the patient's waist, and is excreted in eight to 72 hours. The camera was not designed to replace standard visualization procedures and is currently being used to assess problems in the hard-to-reach small intestine. More testing is needed to determine whether it has value in colon cancer screening as well.

Staging

A diagnosis of cancer will lead to staging and other tests to help determine the outlook and the appropriate treatments.

Staging

Unlike many other cancers, the size of the tumor is not a major factor in determining the outcome of colorectal cancer. Of greater importance is how far the cancer has spread. To determine this, physicians will assign a stage to the tumor. There are several methods for staging. The older system, known as Dukes', categorizes four basic stages: A, B, C, and D. A more recent system refers to these stages as I, II, III, and IV but divides the categories slightly differently. The term "five-year survival" means that patients have lived at least five years since diagnosis. Most patients who live five years without a recurrence are considered to be cured of their disease.

Tumor Markers

Researchers are continually seeking to identify tumor markers, substances (usually found in blood samples) that will assist in the diagnosis of cancer and in monitoring effects of treatment.

Carcinoembryonic antigen (CEA): High blood levels of a protein called carcinoembryonic antigen (CEA) sometimes indicate the presence of colon cancer. Unfortunately, it is also elevated in other cancers and in some noncancerous conditions. CEA is not effective as a screening tool for healthy people, but might eventually be helpful for cancer patients.

- An advanced diagnostic technique called polymerase chain reaction (PCR) can detect genetic evidence of CEA. One study indicated that when these microscopic footprints of colon cancer are detected in the lymph nodes of Stage II patients (whose lymph nodes otherwise appear to be not involved with cancer), the outlook is similar to that of Stage III patients. Patients without this so-called micrometastasis have a very favorable prognosis. Further research is needed, however, before PCR can be used in widespread practice.

- In patients with a history of or active colon cancer, follow-up measuring of blood CEA levels may be helpful in detecting recurrence of the cancer and effectiveness of treatments.

Defective p53 gene: The presence of a defective p53 gene is a marker for very poor prognosis in patients with advanced colon cancer. In its normal state, the gene is important for regulation of cell growth. Testing for this abnormality, however, is not widely done because it is not clear how to use this information.

Other tumor markers: Other tumor markers under investigation include a protein called GLUT1, cancer antigen 19-9 (CA 19-9), matrix metalloproteinase-9 (MMP-9) RNA, HER-2/neu oncoprotein,

Table 43.1. Stages of Colorectal Cancer

Stage	Condition	Five-Year Survival
A or I	Tumor superficially involves the inner lining of the intestine.	More than 90%
B or II	Tumor has penetrated through the muscle wall of the intestine but has not reached the lymph nodes.	70% to 85%
C or III	Lymph nodes are involved.	65% or below
D or IV	Tumor has spread to other organs (metastasized), usually the liver first.	5% to 9%

transforming growth factor beta-1 (TGF-beta-1), and CD44. However, their role is unknown and they should not be used outside the setting of a clinical study.

Sentinel Node Biopsy

A technique known as a sentinel node biopsy is increasingly performed by experienced surgeons in selected patients. This procedure is used to determine if cancer has spread beyond the nodes and so possibly help reduce the need for complete axillary lymphadenectomies. It involves the following:

- The procedure uses an injection of a tiny amount of a tracer, either a radioactively-labeled substance (radioisotope) or a blue dye, into the tumor site.

- The tracer or dye then flows via the lymphatic system into the so-called sentinel node. This is the first lymph node to which any cancer would spread.

- The sentinel lymph node and possibly one or two others are then removed.

- If they do not show any signs of cancer, it is highly likely that the remainder of the lymph nodes will be cancer free, and further surgery becomes unnecessary.

It is still not known if the sentinel node biopsy has any survival advantages compared to the standard procedures with lymph nodes removal.

Of note, however, a 2002 study indicated that careful and complete removal of potentially cancerous lymph nodes is still very important for improving survival in Stage II and III patients.

Prognosis

Over 57,000 people are expected to die from colorectal cancer in 2003. Only lung cancer is responsible for more cancer deaths, despite the fact that colorectal cancer is almost always a preventable or curable disease when proper screening is used.

Survival Rates

Survival rates for colorectal cancer have been rising in recent years. The five-year survival rate for patients undergoing colon cancer surgery is as high as 90% for cancer that has not spread to the lymph nodes. When cancer has spread to lymph nodes, survival rates drop to 65% and below. Because many cancers are detected at later stages, the overall survival rate is currently about 60%. African-Americans and other minorities tend to have lower survival rates than Caucasians. Studies suggest, however, these higher mortality rates are largely due to less access to optimal health care, including appropriate surgical care and aggressive treatments.

Factors in Treatment Success

In most cases age is not a factor in treatment success; good survival rates are achieved in the elderly as well as in young people. Chances for survival are less in Stage II cancers if the intestine is obstructed or perforated. If cancer has spread to lymph nodes (Stage III), the outlook is better if three or fewer lymph nodes are involved. Treatment can prolong life even when cancer has spread.

Surgery

Surgical removal of the tumor ("resection") along with any affected surrounding tissue is the standard initial treatment for potentially curable colorectal cancers (cancers that have not spread beyond the colon or lymph nodes). Drug therapy, radiation, or both are often used for advanced cancers and are continuously being tested with surgery in different combinations and sequences.

Although choosing a qualified surgeon is critical, choosing a hospital experienced in procedures is also important. The more often colon cancer surgery is performed at a given hospital, the lower the mortality rate at that hospital is likely to be. In one 2000 study, the 30-day postoperative mortality rate for patients treated at hospitals in the top quartile of procedure volume was 3.5%. For hospitals in the bottom quartile, mortality was 5.5%. However, the differences were small, and significantly less than seen for more complex cancer surgeries.

Colectomy

Unless cancer is very advanced, most tumors are removed by an operation known as colectomy:

- Colectomy involves removing the cancerous part of the colon and nearby lymph nodes.

- The surgeon then reconnects the intestine by a procedure known as anastomosis.

- If the surgeon cannot reconnect the intestine, usually because of infection or obstruction, a colostomy is performed. The need for colostomies is higher after surgery for rectal cancer. In most cases of colon cancer, colostomies are not needed.

The surgical approach: The standard technique for a colectomy is open, invasive surgery. Laparoscopy, sometimes called "keyhole surgery" is a less invasive method. Laparoscopy is still considered an investigational technique for treating colon cancer, but it is gaining more acceptance and showing good results in clinical trials.

Open Surgery

- Open surgery uses a wide incision to open up the patient's abdomen. The surgeon then performs the procedures with standard surgical instruments. This is the usual method for performing colectomy.

Laparoscopy

- Laparoscopy uses a few small incisions through which the surgeon passes a fiber optic tube (laparoscope) containing a small camera or tiny instruments. It is generally used for early colon cancer (for tumors less than 2 centimeters or for well-defined tumors less than 3 centimeters).

- A 2004 study published in the *New England Journal of Medicine* found that patients who received laparoscopic colectomy had similar rates of surgical complications, cancer recurrence, and survival as those who received traditional open surgery. However, the patients who had laparoscopy recovered faster and did not need as many narcotic painkillers.

- Several 2005 studies indicated that laparoscopy works as well as conventional surgery for treatment of colon cancer. However, laparoscopy does not appear to be as effective for rectal cancer.

Other Investigative Measures: Some investigators are testing expandable metal tube-like devices called stents to keep the intestine open. It may used before a procedure to allow bowel cleansing or it may be used for long-term use to keep open colons that are inoperable.

451

Colostomy

A colostomy is performed in order to bypass or remove the lower colon and rectum. The procedure generally involves creating a passage, called a stoma, through the abdominal wall that is connected to the colon. The feces pass through this passage and are eliminated. Patients must learn how to care for the stoma and keep the area sanitary.

Usually the colostomy is temporary and can be reversed by a second operation after about three to six months. If the rectum and sphincter muscles in the rectum need to be removed, the colostomy is permanent. Permanent colostomies are more common when the cancerous regions are within two to three centimeters of the anus. Fortunately, surgical advances and knowledge of the extent of safe margins are reducing the need for permanent colostomies.

Managing permanent colostomies: In cases where the colostomy is permanent, the patient must wear a colostomy pouch, which sticks to the skin using a special glue. Pouches are available as one- or two-piece systems. The one-piece system is simpler, but the two piece system allows replacement of the pouch without removing the tape.

For best results, the pouch should be emptied when about one-third full. It should be replaced one or two times a week, depending on signs of leakage (itching or burning of the skin near the stoma). It is important to stress that the pouches are odor proof.

Surgical Treatments for Rectal Cancer

Surgical treatments for cancer in the rectum are complex since they involve muscles and tissue that are critical for urinary and sexual function.

Local excision or polypectomy for early stages: In order to preserve the function of the anal sphincter and prevent the need for colostomy, Stage I and Stage II tumors may be removed by local excision, sometimes followed by chemotherapy and radiation. In this procedure, the tumor is cut out without removal of a major section of rectum. In some cases cancer recurs, but a second operation may be possible. Another treatment for early-stage rectal cancer called electrocoagulation, which destroys tumors using a high frequency electric current, is being tested but should only be used in the setting of clinical trials.

Radical resection: In about a third of cases of rectal cancer, the cancer occurs in the lower part of the rectum, where between 70% and 80% of cancers have spread beyond the rectal wall. In such cases, a radical resection is required, in which surrounding structures, including the sphincter muscles that control bowel movements, must often be removed.

The use of chemotherapy and radiation prior to surgery may prevent the need for permanent colostomy in some patients. This is an active area of clinical research and current trials are under way to address this issue. An alternative technique called coloanal anastomosis reconstructs the area to avoid the need for colostomy, and may be appropriate in selected patients.

Total mesorectal excision: Total mesorectal excision (TME) involves dissection and removal of the entire cancerous area of the rectum along with surrounding fatty regions where the lymph nodes are located (the mesorectum). When successful, TME preserves the sphincter muscle, reducing the need for a permanent colostomy. Increasing use of this procedure is resulting in lower recurrence rates, lower levels of impotence and incontinence, and better overall survival rates compared to other resection techniques. Some experts now recommend that it be the first choice for certain patients with locally advanced rectal cancer.

Combining chemotherapy and radiation either before or after TME is yielding promising long-term results and a low risk for local recurrence. There are many questions, however, and it is not clear which approach is better for specific patients.

Managing Side Effects and Psychological Repercussions

Side effects of colon surgery include:

- **Sexual dysfunction:** This is of particular concern. In general, colostomy does not usually affect sexual function. However, wide rectal surgery can cause short- or long-term sexual dysfunction. Sildenafil (Viagra) may help men who experience this after surgery.

- **Irregular bowel movements.**

- **Gas and flatulence:** Pouching filters are available to reduce gas. Certain foods produce more gas than others—usually within six to eight hours for colostomy patients. They include beans, oat bran, most fruit, and certain vegetables (cabbage, cauliflower, Brussels sprouts, broccoli, and asparagus). To prevent swallowing air, patients should avoid sipping through straws, chewing gum, and chewing with their mouths open.

- **Diarrhea.**

- **Bladder complications.**

- **Sense of urinary urgency.**

- **Fecal incontinence:** Patients with rectal surgery have a higher risk for bowel dysfunction than those who had a colostomy.

- **Complications in or around the stoma:** These can occur early after surgery to many years after the procedure. They include skin infection or breakdown, hernias, narrowing of the stoma, bleeding, and collapse.

There are no dietary restrictions, although many patients avoid foods that can produce gas. Everyone should drink plenty of fluids and sufficient fiber.

The potential side effects of sexual and bowel dysfunction for colorectal surgical patients can be devastating, although many patients do very well and live normal productive lives. Positive emotions play a strong role in recovery. Patients who are depressed should discuss with a physician all aspects of treatment that affect the quality of life and possibly seek support groups.

Medications

Chemotherapy uses drugs that kill cancer cells throughout the body. There are two situations in which chemotherapy is used:

- **The adjuvant setting:** Adjuvant refers to the use of chemotherapy after surgery in patients with stage III tumors and selected patients with high-risk stage II tumors (that is disease that is potentially curable). The goal of this therapy is to eliminate any cancer cells that surgery may have missed, thereby preventing recurrence and increasing the chance of cure. Patients of all ages, including the elderly, can benefit.

- **In metastatic disease:** In patients with metastatic disease the goal of chemotherapy is to shrink tumors, improve symptoms and quality of life, and to lengthen life.

454

In the adjuvant setting, there are some differences in chemotherapy treatments between colon and rectal cancers:

- Chemotherapy for stage II patients is considered standard care for stage II rectal cancer but is under debate for colon cancer.

- Chemotherapy is standard for stage III colon cancer patients. Chemotherapy is also standard for stage III rectal cancer patients but is used in combination with radiation.

Chemotherapy for stage II patients with colon cancer: Adjuvant chemotherapy for Stage II colon cancer patients is controversial. Such patients tend to have a good outcome after surgery and the positive effects of chemotherapy have been difficult to demonstrate. To date, the survival advantage of adjuvant chemotherapy in this group has been reported to be only in the range of 2%. However, better trials are still needed to confirm or refute the benefits in specific patient groups.

Although not yet known with certainty, some data suggest that certain Stage II patients may be at higher risk of recurrence and would theoretically benefit from adjuvant therapy. These include patients with the following conditions:

- Cancers that have obstructed the bowel,

- Cancers that have perforated the wall of the colon, or

- Cancers that have adhered to structures outside the intestine.

Advanced diagnostic techniques are under investigation for helping to select appropriate Stage II candidates for adjuvant therapy. None of these methods, however, are ready to be used routinely to help make treatment decisions. The decision whether to pursue chemotherapy for stage II disease should be made after careful discussion between the patient and his or her oncologist, especially after features, such as bowel perforation or obstruction, are taken into account.

Chemotherapy for stage III patients with colon cancer: Since the early 1990s, adjuvant chemotherapy with 5-FU and leucovorin has been the standard of care for stage III colon cancer. Numerous trials have shown that adjuvant chemotherapy in this setting reduces the absolute risk of death from colon cancer by approximately one-third and improves survival by 10%. Current clinical trials are investigating whether the addition of new chemotherapy drugs, such as irinotecan, oxaliplatin, capecitabine, and antibody therapies, will improve cure rates over 5-FU and leucovorin alone. However, most of these new agents should currently not be used for adjuvant treatment of colon cancer unless as part of a clinical trial.

Chemotherapy for advanced colorectal cancer: Chemotherapy and radiation are generally used to reduce symptoms and prolong life in advanced colorectal cancer. Some experts suggest that chemotherapy should be considered for the following patients:

- Able to carry out all normal activity without restriction.

- Restricted in physically strenuous activity, but able to walk about and carry out light work.

- Able to walk about and capable of all self care, but unable to carry out any work. Out of bed or chair for more than 50% of waking hours.

Chemotherapy in most studies offers a modest improvement in survival and often relieves symptoms. One 2003 study suggested that for these patients chemotherapy given intermittently has fewer toxic or serious adverse effects and may be as beneficial as continuous administration.

The following patients are unlikely to benefit from chemotherapy:

- Those capable only of limited self care. Confined to bed or chair for more than 50% of waking hours.

- Those severely disabled. Cannot carry out any self care. Totally confined to bed or chair.

Specific Chemotherapy Agents

5-fluorouracil (5-FU) with leucovorin: Adjuvant therapy using 5-fluorouracil along with leucovorin (5-FU/LV) is currently the standard treatment for patients with high-risk colon cancer (Stage III or selected patients with Stage II tumors). Leucovorin, also called folinic acid, is a form of the B vitamin folic acid. Patients are given a series of cycles that usually continue for at least six months. 5-FU is given intravenously at present, but oral preparations are currently being tested in clinical trials.

There are many different ways of giving 5-FU, including intravenously over several hours once a week, intravenously daily for five consecutive days every month, or as continuous infusion with a portable pump.

The side effects can be quite different depending on the way 5-FU is given, and women may be more susceptible than men. In one analysis, 53% of women and 40% of men experienced severe side effects, while response rates and survival were similar for both sexes. Many patients, however, tolerate 5-FU with leucovorin well with manageable side effects.

Irinotecan: Irinotecan (Camptosar) inhibits an enzyme essential for cell division and works in combination with 5-FU and LV. This combination therapy (irinotecan plus 5-FU/LV) is also referred to as the "Salz regimen" or IFL. When it was approved in the mid 1990s, irinotecan was the first new drug developed for colon cancer in over 30 years. Two studies in 2000 reported that a combination of irinotecan along with 5-fluorouracil and leucovorin (5-FU/LV) significantly delays the time at which tumors progress and improves survival in metastatic cancer compared to 5-FU/LV alone. While the survival advantage is small, the combination has become the standard of care for metastatic cancer for many oncologists. Of concern, however, were 2001 studies reporting an increased risk of death from toxic effects with the use of the three-drug combination. Such deaths appeared to be related to blood clotting complications. Experts recommend careful monitoring and use of lower drug doses.

Capecitabine: Capecitabine (Xeloda) is the first pill approved for metastatic colorectal cancer. A major 2005 study, published in the *New England Journal of Medicine*, found that capecitabine worked as well as the standard 5-FU/leucovorin treatment and caused significantly fewer side effects. The study involved patients with stage III colon cancer who had undergone surgical removal of the tumor. Capecitabine is also showing promise in combination with radiation therapy for rectal cancers.

Oxaliplatin: Oxaliplatin (Eloxatin) is related to cisplatin, a widely used platinum-based chemotherapy drug. Oxaliplatin is used in combination with 5-FU and leucovorin. (This triple combination therapy is called the FOLFOX regimen.) Oxaliplatin was approved in 2002 for use in combination with 5-FU and leucovorin as a second-line treatment for cancer that has progressed after initial therapy. Since 2002, oxaliplatin has received additional approvals as a first-line treatment for advanced colorectal cancer, and as a post-surgical treatment for patients who have undergone tumor resection. Oxaliplatin can cause pain and tingling sensations in the hands and feet (neuropathy) that is worsened by exposure to cold.

Raltitrexed: Raltitrexed (Tomudex) may be effective and may have additive or synergistic effects with 5-FU.

Recently Approved Treatments[1]

Bevacizumab: Bevacizumab (Avastin) was approved in February 2004 as a first-line treatment for patients with metastatic colorectal cancer (advanced cancer that has spread in the body). It is used in combination with IFL (irinotecan, 5-FU, leucovorin). Bevacizumab is a genetically engineered monoclonal antibody that targets and inhibits vascular endothelial growth factor (VEGF), a protein that regulates angiogenesis (the development of new blood vessels that feed a tumor's blood supply). It is the first anti-angiogenic therapy approved for the treatment of colorectal cancer. In a study of 800 patients with metastatic colorectal cancer, bevacizumab administered intravenously along with IFL extended survival by approximately 5 months longer than IFL alone. Common side effects of bevacizumab are nosebleeds, fatigue, diarrhea, and high blood pressure. Less common side effects include stroke, heart attacks, angina, and formation of holes in the colon and stomach (gastrointestinal perforation).

Cetuximab: Cetuximab (Erbitux) was approved in February 2004 for the treatment of metastatic colorectal cancer. This monoclonal antibody drug targets epidermal growth factor receptor (EGFR), a protein required by cancer cells in order to proliferate. It can be used either in combination with irinotecan, or alone for patients who have not responded to irinotecan. Clinical research demonstrated that combination treatment delayed tumor growth by 4 months. For patients who received only cetuximab, tumor growth was delayed by 1.5 months.

Oxaliplatin: Oxaliplatin (Eloxatin) received a new indication approval in January 2004 as a first-line treatment for advanced colorectal cancer. The drug is used in combination with 5-FU and leucovorin (LV). In data submitted for the approval process, patients who received oxaliplatin in combination with 5-FU and LV survived an average of nearly 5 months longer than patients who received only 5-FU and LV.

Side Effects of Chemotherapy

Side effects occur with all chemotherapeutic drugs; they are more severe with higher doses and increase over the course of treatment. Because cancer cells grow and divide rapidly, anticancer drugs work by killing fast-growing cells. This means that healthy cells that multiply quickly can also be affected. The fast-growing normal cells most likely to be affected are blood cells forming in the bone marrow, and cells in the digestive tract, reproductive system, and hair follicles.

Targeted Therapies and Biologics

One of the most promising recent developments in cancer treatment research has been the emergence of so-called "targeted therapies." Traditional chemotherapeutic agents can be effective, but because they do not distinguish between healthy and cancerous cells their generalized toxicity can cause severe side effects. Targeted therapies work on a molecular level by blocking specific mechanisms associated with cancer cell growth and division. Because they selectively target cancerous cells, they may induce less severe side effects. In addition, these drugs hold the promise of creating options for more individualized cancer treatment based on a patient's genotype. In the future, diagnostic tests may help doctors identify which patients are more likely to respond successfully to specific drugs.

Biologic therapies use the body's immune system to attack the cancer (immunotherapy). These drugs are derived from biological sources and include vaccines, monoclonal antibodies (MAbs), and gene therapies. Many targeted therapies are classified as biologics.

Targeted therapies involve many different types of drugs and molecular pathways. These include:

Angiogenesis inhibitors: Anti-angiogenesis drugs inhibit the formation of new blood vessels that supply tumors with the blood, oxygen, and nutrients vital to tumor growth. Angiogenesis inhibitors, such as the monoclonal antibody bevacizumab (Avastin), target vascular endothelial growth factor (VEGF).

Tumor growth factor inhibitors: Tumor growth factors, such as epidermal growth factor, stimulate cell growth. Drugs that target the epidermal growth factor receptor (EGFR) include cetuximab (Erbitux).

Tyrosine kinase inhibitors: Tyrosine kinase is an enzyme associated with EGFR that is involved with the signaling mechanisms that prompt cell growth. Clinical trials are currently investigating the use of the lung cancer drug gefitinib (Iressa), in combination with oxaliplatin and standard chemotherapy agents, for the treatment of advanced colorectal cancer. Gefitinib blocks tyrosine kinase growth signaling capacities. Similarly, the EGFR/tyrosine kinase inhibitor erlotinib (Tarceva), which is in late-stage trials for the treatment of pancreatic and lung cancer, is also being investigated as an adjuvant treatment for metastatic colorectal cancer.

Vaccines: ALVAC is an experimental vaccine derived from the canarypox virus. It is designed to trigger the body's immune system to fight cancer cells. It is currently in early-stage clinical trials to determine its efficacy in combination with chemotherapy for treatment of metastatic colorectal cancer.

Radiation Treatment

Radiation therapy uses x-rays to kill cancer cells that might remain after an operation or to shrink large tumors before an operation so that they can be removed surgically. The object of radiation therapy is to damage the tumor as much as possible without harming surrounding tissues. Radiation may be administered in the following ways:

- Externally by an x-ray machine (external beam radiation)

- By passing radioactive pellets through thin plastic tubes inserted into the intestine

- By implanting tiny radiation seeds directly into the tumor (brachytherapy)

- Computer imaging techniques providing 3-dimensional pictures of the cancerous area are allowing precise targeting of radiation to the tumor

Postoperative Radiation with Chemotherapy for Rectal Cancer

Postoperative radiation treatment combined with chemotherapy is common practice for patients with rectal cancer in Stages II and III. Such patients are at risk of recurrence both at the site of their original tumor and elsewhere in the body. Although there can be significant long-term side effects, the combination of 5-FU and radiation is still considered standard after surgery.

Preoperative Radiation

The standard procedure in the U.S. is to apply radiation after surgery (postoperative). Preoperative chemotherapy and radiation, however, are sometimes used to preserve sphincter-muscle function and reduce the chance that a patient will require a colostomy. Furthermore, some studies suggest that the use of radiation before surgery reduces the likelihood of recurrences and may slightly prolong survival in some patients with rectal cancer. (It has no additional advantages, however, if the subsequent surgery does not completely remove the cancerous regions.) Studies comparing preoperative and postoperative chemotherapy and radiation are currently under way.

Intra-Operative Radiotherapy (IORT)

Radiation therapy is also being used during surgery (a procedure called intra-operative radiotherapy.) It allows the surgeon to move healthy tissue out of the path of the radiation beam.

Side Effects of Radiation Therapy

Short-term side effects of radiation include:

- Diarrhea;
- Skin irritation around the anus;
- Incontinence;
- Fatigue;
- Bowel movement problems.

Longer-term complications may include:

- Incontinence;
- Soiling;
- Hip and pelvic fractures;
- Diarrhea;
- Increased risk for bowel obstruction.

Treatment for Metastasized Colorectal Cancer

The liver is the most frequent site for metastasized colorectal cancers. Here, treatments may slow the spread of cancer and even prolong survival. Cure is very rare.

Surgery

When cancer has spread, surgery to remove or bypass obstructions in the intestine may be performed. In these circumstances, surgery is considered palliative in that it may improve symptoms but will not lead to cure. In rare cases, metastatic colon cancer may be cured with surgical removal of tumors in areas to which the cancer has spread, such as the liver, ovaries, and lung. The liver is the most common site of spread. Only selected patients may be eligible for such surgery, but in such patients five-year survival has been 25% and may be higher.

Chemotherapy

Chemotherapy may be used to improve symptoms and possibly a prolong survival in metastasized colorectal cancers. A number of investigative agents are being tested. Physicians are testing chemotherapy administered directly into the liver—a treatment called intrahepatic arterial chemotherapy. It is possible to shrink swollen, painful livers this way, but to date studies are not reporting any survival advantages with this approach compared to chemotherapy delivered intravenously.

Other Techniques

Other investigative techniques used to destroy liver tumors include:

- **Cryosurgery:** This approach freezes the tumor or surrounding tissue.

- **Embolization**: Embolization employs a catheter to deliver agents into the liver that block blood vessels and therefore starve the tumor. Chemotherapy is often delivered with these agents.

- **Radiation.**

For end-stage cancer, hospice care is a compassionate option.

References

Clinical Outcomes of Surgical Therapy Study Group. A comparison of laparoscopically assisted and open colectomy for colon cancer. *N Engl J Med*. 2004;350(20):2050–2059.

Guillou PJ, Quirke P, Thorpe H, et al. Short-term endpoints of conventional versus laparoscopic-assisted surgery in patients with colorectal cancer (MRC CLASICC trial): multicentre, randomized controlled trial. *Lancet.* 2005;365(9472):1718–1726.

Twelves C, Wong A, Nowacki MP, et al. Capecitabine as adjuvant treatment for stage III colon cancer. N *Engl J Med.* 2005;352(26):2696–2704.

Veldkamp R, Kuhry E, Hop WC, et al. Laparoscopic surgery versus open surgery for colon cancer: short-term outcomes of a randomized trial. *Lancet Oncol.* 2005;6(7):477–484.

Note

1. On September 27, 2006, the U.S. Food and Drug Administration approved Vectibix (panitumumab) for the treatment of patients with colorectal cancer that has metastasized following standard chemotherapy. Vectibix, a monoclonal antibody that binds to a protein called epidermal growth factor receptor (or EGFR) on some cancer cells, received an accelerated approval after showing effectiveness in slowing tumor growth, and in some cases, reducing the size of the tumor. The mean time to disease progression or death in patients receiving Vectibix was 96 days versus 60 days in patients receiving the best standard supportive care. In addition, 8 percent of the patients on Vectibix experienced a tumor shrinkage that in some cases exceeded 50 percent of the pre-treatment size of the tumor. Both study groups showed similar overall survival. The most serious adverse events in the studies of Vectibix included pulmonary fibrosis, severe skin rash complicated by infections, infusion reactions, abdominal pain, nausea, vomiting, and constipation. Vectibix is manufactured by Amgen, Inc. in Thousand Oaks, California. (Source: Information in this note was excerpted from "FDA Approves a New Drug for Colorectal Cancer, Vectibix," a U.S. Food and Drug Administration press release dated September 27, 2006.)

Chapter 44

Anal Cancer

Anal cancer is a disease in which malignant (cancer) cells form in the tissues of the anus. The anus is the end of the large intestine, below the rectum, through which stool (solid waste) leaves the body. The anus is formed partly from the outer, skin layers of the body and partly from the intestine. Two ring-like muscles, called sphincter muscles, open and close the anal opening to let stool pass out of the body. The anal canal, the part of the anus between the rectum and the anal opening, is about 1½ inches long.

The skin around the outside of the anus is called the perianal area. Tumors in this area are skin tumors, not anal cancer.

Risk factors include the following:

• Being over 50 years old

• Being infected with human papillomavirus (HPV)

• Having many sexual partners

• Having receptive anal intercourse (anal sex)

• Frequent anal redness, swelling, and soreness

• Having anal fistulas (abnormal openings)

• Smoking cigarettes

Excerpted from PDQ® Cancer Information Summary. National Cancer Institute; Bethesda, MD. Anal Cancer (PDQ®): Treatment - Patient. Updated 04/2005. Available at: http://cancer.gov. Accessed April 30, 2006.

A doctor should be consulted if any of the following symptoms occur:

- Bleeding from the anus or rectum
- Pain or pressure in the area around the anus
- Itching or discharge from the anus
- A lump near the anus
- A change in bowel habits

In addition to a physical exam and history, the following tests and procedures may be used to detect (find) and diagnose anal cancer:

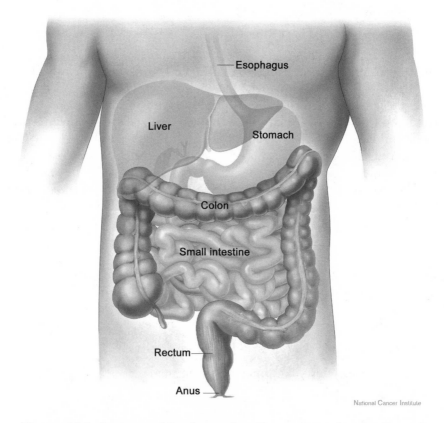

National Cancer Institute

Figure 44.1. Anatomy of the lower digestive system, showing the colon and other organs (Source: Image by Terese Winslow, National Cancer Institute, NCI Visuals Online, November 2005).

Digital rectal examination (DRE): An exam of the anus and rectum. The doctor or nurse inserts a lubricated, gloved finger into the lower part of the rectum to feel for lumps or anything else that seems unusual.

Anoscopy: An exam of the anus and lower rectum using a short, lighted tube called an anoscope.

Proctoscopy: An exam of the rectum using a short, lighted tube called a proctoscope.

Endo-anal or endorectal ultrasound: A procedure in which an ultrasound transducer (probe) is inserted into the anus or rectum and used to bounce high-energy sound waves (ultrasound) off internal tissues or organs and make echoes. The echoes form a picture of body tissues called a sonogram.

Biopsy: The removal of cells or tissues so they can be viewed under a microscope by a pathologist to check for signs of cancer. If an abnormal area is seen during the anoscopy, a biopsy may be done at that time.

Stages of Anal Cancer

The following stages are used for anal cancer:

Stage 0 (carcinoma in situ): In stage 0, cancer is found only in the innermost lining of the anus. Stage 0 cancer is also called carcinoma in situ.

Stage I: In stage I, the tumor is 2 centimeters or smaller.

Stage II: In stage II, the tumor is larger than 2 centimeters.

Stage IIIA: In stage IIIA, the tumor may be any size and has spread to either:

- lymph nodes near the rectum; or
- nearby organs, such as the vagina, urethra, and bladder.

Stage IIIB: In stage IIIB, the tumor may be any size and has spread:

- to nearby organs and to lymph nodes near the rectum; or

- to lymph nodes on one side of the pelvis and/or groin, and may have spread to nearby organs; or

- to lymph nodes near the rectum and in the groin, and/or to lymph nodes on both sides of the pelvis and/or groin, and may have spread to nearby organs.

Stage IV: In stage IV, the tumor may be any size and cancer may have spread to lymph nodes or nearby organs and has spread to distant parts of the body.

Recurrent anal cancer: Recurrent anal cancer is cancer that has recurred (come back) after it has been treated. The cancer may come back in the anus or in other parts of the body.

Treatment Option Overview

Three types of standard treatment are used:

Radiation therapy: Radiation therapy is a cancer treatment that uses high-energy x-rays or other types of radiation to kill cancer cells. There are two types of radiation therapy. External radiation therapy uses a machine outside the body to send radiation toward the cancer. Internal radiation therapy uses a radioactive substance sealed in needles, seeds, wires, or catheters that are placed directly into or near the cancer. The way the radiation therapy is given depends on the type and stage of the cancer being treated.

Chemotherapy: Chemotherapy is a cancer treatment that uses drugs to stop the growth of cancer cells, either by killing the cells or

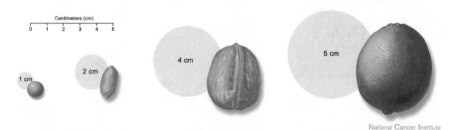

National Cancer Institute

Figure 44.2. Pea, peanut, walnut, and lime show tumor sizes (Source: Image by Terese Winslow, National Cancer Institute, NCI Visuals Online, November 2005).

by stopping the cells from dividing. When chemotherapy is taken by mouth or injected into a vein or muscle, the drugs enter the bloodstream and can reach cancer cells throughout the body (systemic chemotherapy). When chemotherapy is placed directly into the spinal column, an organ, or a body cavity such as the abdomen, the drugs mainly affect cancer cells in those areas (regional chemotherapy). The way the chemotherapy is given depends on the type and stage of the cancer being treated.

Surgery:

- **Local resection:** A surgical procedure in which the tumor is cut from the anus along with some of the healthy tissue around it. Local resection may be used if the cancer is small and has not spread. This procedure may save the sphincter muscles so the patient can still control bowel movements. Tumors that develop in the lower part of the anus can often be removed with local resection.

- **Abdominoperineal resection:** A surgical procedure in which the anus, the rectum, and part of the sigmoid colon are removed through an incision made in the abdomen. The doctor sews the end of the intestine to an opening, called a stoma, made in the surface of the abdomen so body waste can be collected in a disposable bag outside of the body. This is called a colostomy. Lymph nodes that contain cancer may also be removed during this operation.

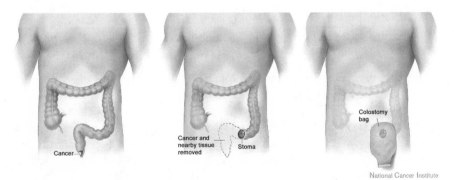

Figure 44.3. Anal cancer surgery with colostomy. The anus, rectum, and part of the colon are removed, a stoma is created, and a colostomy bag is attached to the stoma (Source: Image by Terese Winslow, National Cancer Institute, NCI Visuals Online, November 2005).

Cancer therapy can further damage the already weakened immune systems of patients who have the human immunodeficiency virus (HIV). For this reason, patients who have anal cancer and HIV are usually treated with lower doses of anticancer drugs and radiation than patients who do not have HIV.

New Treatments

Other types of treatment are being tested in clinical trials. These include the following:

Radiosensitizers: Radiosensitizers are drugs that make tumor cells more sensitive to radiation therapy. Combining radiation therapy with radiosensitizers may kill more tumor cells.

Treatment Options by Stage

Stage 0 anal cancer (carcinoma in situ): Treatment of stage 0 anal cancer is usually local resection.

Stage I anal cancer: Treatment of stage I anal cancer may include the following:

- Local resection
- External-beam radiation therapy with or without chemotherapy. If cancer remains after treatment, additional chemotherapy and radiation therapy may be given to avoid the need for a permanent colostomy.
- Internal radiation therapy
- Abdominoperineal resection, if cancer remains or comes back after treatment with radiation therapy and chemotherapy
- Internal radiation therapy for cancer that remains after treatment with external-beam radiation therapy

Patients who have had treatment that saves the sphincter muscles may receive follow-up exams every three months for the first two years, including rectal exams with endoscopy and biopsy, as needed.

Stage II anal cancer: Treatment of stage II anal cancer may include the following:

- Local resection

- External-beam radiation therapy with chemotherapy. If cancer remains after treatment, additional chemotherapy and radiation therapy may be given to avoid the need for a permanent colostomy.

- Internal radiation therapy

- Abdominoperineal resection, if cancer remains or comes back after treatment with radiation therapy and chemotherapy

- A clinical trial of new treatment options

Patients who have had treatment that saves the sphincter muscles may receive follow-up exams every three months for the first two years, including rectal exams with endoscopy and biopsy, as needed.

Stage IIIA anal cancer: Treatment of stage IIIA anal cancer may include the following:

- External-beam radiation therapy with chemotherapy. If cancer remains after treatment, additional chemotherapy and radiation therapy may be given to avoid the need for a permanent colostomy.

- Internal radiation therapy

- Abdominoperineal resection, if cancer remains or comes back after treatment with chemotherapy and radiation therapy

- A clinical trial of new treatment options

Stage IIIB anal cancer: Treatment of stage IIIB anal cancer may include the following:

- External-beam radiation therapy with chemotherapy

- Local resection or abdominoperineal resection, if cancer remains or comes back after treatment with chemotherapy and radiation therapy. Lymph nodes may also be removed.

- A clinical trial of new treatment options

Stage IV anal cancer: Treatment of stage IV anal cancer may include the following:

- Surgery as palliative therapy to relieve symptoms and improve the quality of life

- Radiation therapy as palliative therapy
- Chemotherapy with radiation therapy as palliative therapy
- A clinical trial of new treatment options

Recurrent anal cancer: Treatment of recurrent anal cancer may include the following:

- Radiation therapy and chemotherapy, for recurrence after surgery
- Surgery, for recurrence after radiation therapy and/or chemotherapy
- A clinical trial of radiation therapy with chemotherapy and/or radiosensitizers

Chapter 45

Renal Cell (Kidney) Cancer

Renal cell cancer is a disease in which malignant (cancer) cells form in tubules of the kidney. Renal cell cancer (also called kidney cancer or renal adenocarcinoma) is a disease in which malignant (cancer) cells are found in the lining of tubules (very small tubes) in the kidney. There are two kidneys, one on each side of the backbone, above the waist. The tiny tubules in the kidneys filter and clean the blood, taking out waste products and making urine. The urine passes from each kidney into the bladder through a long tube called a ureter. The bladder stores the urine until it is passed from the body.

Cancer that starts in the ureters or the renal pelvis (the part of the kidney that collects urine and drains it to the ureters) is different from renal cell cancer.)

Risk factors include the following:

- Smoking

- Misusing certain pain medicines, including over-the-counter pain medicines, for a long time

- Having certain genetic conditions, such as von Hippel-Lindau disease or hereditary papillary renal cell carcinoma

PDQ® Cancer Information Summary. National Cancer Institute; Bethesda, MD. Renal Cell Cancer (PDQ®): Treatment - Patient. Updated 06/2005. Available at: http://cancer.gov. Accessed August 17, 2006.

There may be no symptoms in the early stages. Symptoms may appear as the tumor grows. A doctor should be consulted if any of the following problems occur:

- Blood in the urine
- A lump in the abdomen
- A pain in the side that doesn't go away
- Loss of appetite
- Weight loss for no known reason
- Anemia

The following tests and procedures may be used:

Physical exam and history: An exam of the body to check general signs of health, including checking for signs of disease, such as lumps or anything else that seems unusual. A history of the patient's health habits and past illnesses and treatments will also be taken.

Blood chemistry studies: A procedure in which a blood sample is checked to measure the amounts of certain substances released into the blood by organs and tissues in the body. An unusual (higher or lower than normal) amount of a substance can be a sign of disease in the organ or tissue that produces it.

Urinalysis: A test to check the color of urine and its contents, such as sugar, protein, blood, and bacteria.

Liver function test: A procedure in which a sample of blood is checked to measure the amounts of enzymes released into it by the liver. An abnormal amount of an enzyme can be a sign that cancer has spread to the liver. Certain conditions that are not cancer may also increase liver enzyme levels.

Intravenous pyelogram (IVP): A series of x-rays of the kidneys, ureters, and bladder to find out if cancer is present in these organs. A contrast dye is injected into a vein. As the contrast dye moves through the kidneys, ureters, and bladder, x-rays are taken to see if there are any blockages.

Ultrasound exam: A procedure in which high-energy sound waves (ultrasound) are bounced off internal tissues or organs and make echoes. The echoes form a picture of body tissues called a sonogram.

CT scan (CAT scan): A procedure that makes a series of detailed pictures of areas inside the body, taken from different angles. The pictures are made by a computer linked to an x-ray machine. A dye may be injected into a vein or swallowed to help the organs or tissues show up more clearly. This procedure is also called computed tomography, computerized tomography, or computerized axial tomography.

MRI (magnetic resonance imaging): A procedure that uses a magnet, radio waves, and a computer to make a series of detailed pictures of areas inside the body. This procedure is also called nuclear magnetic resonance imaging (NMRI).

Biopsy: The removal of cells or tissues so they can be viewed under a microscope by a pathologist to check for signs of cancer. To do a biopsy for renal cell cancer, a thin needle is inserted into the tumor and a sample of tissue is withdrawn.

Stages of Renal Cell Cancer

After renal cell cancer has been diagnosed, tests are done to find out if cancer cells have spread within the kidney or to other parts of the body.

The process used to find out if cancer has spread within the kidney or to other parts of the body is called staging. The information gathered from the staging process determines the stage of the disease. It is important to know the stage in order to plan treatment. The following tests and procedures may be used in the staging process:

- **CT scan (CAT scan)**

- **MRI (magnetic resonance imaging)**

- **Chest x-ray:** An x-ray of the organs and bones inside the chest. An x-ray is a type of energy beam that can go through the body and onto film, making a picture of areas inside the body.

- **Bone scan:** A procedure to check if there are rapidly dividing cells, such as cancer cells, in the bone. A very small amount of radioactive material is injected into a vein and travels through the bloodstream. The radioactive material collects in the bones and is detected by a scanner.

The following stages are used for renal cell cancer:

Stage I: In stage I, the tumor is seven centimeters or smaller and is found only in the kidney.

Stage II: In stage II, the tumor is larger than seven centimeters and is found only in the kidney.

Stage III: In stage III, cancer is found:

* in the kidney and in one nearby lymph node; or
* in an adrenal gland or in the layer of fatty tissue around the kidney, and may be found in one nearby lymph node; or
* in the main blood vessels of the kidney and may be found in one nearby lymph node.

Stage IV: In stage IV, cancer has spread:

* beyond the layer of fatty tissue around the kidney and may be found in one nearby lymph node; or
* to two or more nearby lymph nodes; or
* to other organs, such as the bowel, pancreas, or lungs, and may be found in nearby lymph nodes.

Recurrent renal cell cancer: Recurrent renal cell cancer is cancer that has recurred (come back) after it has been treated. The cancer may come back many years after initial treatment, in the kidney or in other parts of the body.

Treatment Option Overview

Different types of treatments are available for patients with renal cell cancer. Some treatments are standard (the currently used treatment), and some are being tested in clinical trials. Before starting treatment, patients may want to think about taking part in a clinical trial. A treatment clinical trial is a research study meant to help improve current treatments or obtain information on new treatments for patients with cancer. When clinical trials show that a new treatment is better than the standard treatment, the new treatment may become the standard treatment.

Clinical trials are taking place in many parts of the country. Information about ongoing clinical trials is available from the National

Cancer Institute website (http://www.cancer.gov). Choosing the most appropriate cancer treatment is a decision that ideally involves the patient, family, and health care team.

Five types of standard treatment are used:

Surgery: Surgery to remove part or all of the kidney is often used to treat renal cell cancer. The following types of surgery may be used:

- **Partial nephrectomy:** A surgical procedure to remove the cancer within the kidney and some of the tissue around it. A partial nephrectomy may be done to prevent loss of kidney function when the other kidney is damaged or has already been removed.

- **Simple nephrectomy:** A surgical procedure to remove the kidney only.

- **Radical nephrectomy:** A surgical procedure to remove the kidney, the adrenal gland, surrounding tissue, and, usually, nearby lymph nodes.

A person can live with part of one working kidney, but if both kidneys are removed or not working, the person will need dialysis (a procedure to clean the blood using a machine outside of the body) or a kidney transplant (replacement with a healthy donated kidney). A kidney transplant may be done when the disease is in the kidney only and a donated kidney can be found. If the patient has to wait for a donated kidney, other treatment is given as needed.

When surgery to remove the cancer is not possible, a treatment called arterial embolization may be used to shrink the tumor. A small incision is made and a catheter (thin tube) is inserted into the main blood vessel that flows to the kidney. Small pieces of a special gelatin sponge are injected through the catheter into the blood vessel. The sponges block the blood flow to the kidney and prevent the cancer cells from getting oxygen and other substances they need to grow.

Even if the doctor removes all the cancer that can be seen at the time of the surgery, some patients may be given chemotherapy or radiation therapy after surgery to kill any cancer cells that are left. Treatment given after the surgery, to increase the chances of a cure, is called adjuvant therapy.

Radiation therapy: Radiation therapy is a cancer treatment that uses high-energy x-rays or other types of radiation to kill cancer cells. There are two types of radiation therapy. External radiation therapy uses a machine outside the body to send radiation toward the cancer.

Internal radiation therapy uses a radioactive substance sealed in needles, seeds, wires, or catheters that are placed directly into or near the cancer. The way the radiation therapy is given depends on the type and stage of the cancer being treated.

Chemotherapy: Chemotherapy is a cancer treatment that uses drugs to stop the growth of cancer cells, either by killing the cells or by stopping the cells from dividing. When chemotherapy is taken by mouth or injected into a vein or muscle, the drugs enter the bloodstream and can reach cancer cells throughout the body (systemic chemotherapy). When chemotherapy is placed directly into the spinal column, an organ, or a body cavity such as the abdomen, the drugs mainly affect cancer cells in those areas (regional chemotherapy). The way the chemotherapy is given depends on the type and stage of the cancer being treated.

Biologic therapy: Biologic therapy is a treatment that uses the patient's immune system to fight cancer. Substances made by the body or made in a laboratory are used to boost, direct, or restore the body's natural defenses against cancer. This type of cancer treatment is also called biotherapy or immunotherapy.

Targeted therapy: Targeted therapy uses drugs or other substances that can find and attack specific cancer cells without harming normal cells. Antiangiogenic agents are a type of targeted therapy that may be used to treat advanced renal cell cancer. They keep blood vessels from forming in a tumor, causing the tumor to starve and stop growing or to shrink.

New Treatments

New types of treatment are being tested in clinical trials. These include the following:

Stem cell transplant: Stem cells (immature blood cells) are removed from the blood or bone marrow of a donor and given to the patient through an infusion. These reinfused stem cells grow into (and restore) the body's blood cells.

Treatment Options by Stage

Stage I renal cell cancer: Standard treatment of stage I renal cell cancer may include the following:

478

- Surgery (radical nephrectomy, simple nephrectomy, or partial nephrectomy)

- Radiation therapy as palliative therapy to relieve symptoms in patients who cannot have surgery

- Arterial embolization as palliative therapy

- New treatments for stage I renal cell cancer are being studied in clinical trials

Stage II renal cell cancer: Standard treatment of stage II renal cell cancer may include the following:

- Surgery (radical nephrectomy or partial nephrectomy)

- Surgery (nephrectomy), before or after radiation therapy

- Radiation therapy as palliative therapy to relieve symptoms in patients who cannot have surgery

- Arterial embolization as palliative therapy

- New treatments for stage II renal cell cancer are being studied in clinical trials

Stage III renal cell cancer: Standard treatment of stage III renal cell cancer may include the following:

- Surgery (radical nephrectomy). Blood vessels of the kidney and some lymph nodes may also be removed

- Arterial embolization followed by surgery (radical nephrectomy)

- Radiation therapy as palliative therapy to relieve symptoms and improve the quality of life

- Arterial embolization as palliative therapy

- Surgery (nephrectomy) as palliative therapy

- Radiation therapy before or after surgery (radical nephrectomy)

- One of the treatments being studied in clinical trials for stage III renal cell cancer is biologic therapy following surgery.

Stage IV renal cell cancer: Standard treatment of stage IV renal cell cancer may include the following:

- Targeted therapy alone or after biologic therapy

479

- Biologic therapy alone or after surgery (nephrectomy) to reduce the size of the tumor

- Arterial embolization as palliative therapy to relieve symptoms and improve the quality of life

- Radiation therapy as palliative therapy to relieve symptoms and improve the quality of life

- Surgery (nephrectomy) as palliative therapy

- Surgery (radical nephrectomy, with or without removal of cancer from other areas where it has spread)

- New treatments for stage IV renal cell cancer are being studied in clinical trials.

Recurrent renal cell cancer: Standard treatment of recurrent renal cell cancer may include the following:

- Biologic therapy

- Radiation therapy as palliative therapy to relieve symptoms and improve the quality of life

- Chemotherapy

- Some of the treatments being studied in clinical trials for recurrent renal cell cancer include chemotherapy, biologic therapy, and stem cell transplant.

Chapter 46

Wilms Tumor and Other Childhood Kidney Tumors

Wilms tumor: Wilms tumor and other kidney tumors are diseases in which malignant (cancer) cells are found in the kidney. In Wilms tumor, one or more tumors may be found in one or both kidneys. There are two kidneys, one on each side of the backbone, above the waist. Tiny tubules in the kidneys filter and clean the blood, taking out waste products and making urine. The urine passes from each kidney through a long tube called a ureter into the bladder. The bladder holds the urine until it is passed from the body.

Wilms tumor may spread to the lungs, liver, or nearby lymph nodes.

Other kidney tumors: Clear cell sarcoma of the kidney, rhabdoid tumor of the kidney, neuroepithelial tumor of the kidney, and renal cell cancer are also childhood kidney tumors, but they are not related to Wilms tumor.

- Clear cell sarcoma of the kidney is a type of kidney tumor that may spread to the lung, bone, brain, and soft tissue.

- Rhabdoid tumor of the kidney is a type of cancer that occurs mostly in children under age two. It grows and spreads quickly, often to the lungs and brain.

PDQ® Cancer Information Summary. National Cancer Institute; Bethesda, MD. Wilms' Tumor and Other Childhood Kidney Tumors (PDQ®): Treatment - Patient. Updated 04/2006. Available at: http://cancer.gov. Accessed August 17, 2006.

- Neuroepithelial tumors of the kidney are rare and usually occur in young adults. They grow and spread quickly.

- Renal cell cancer occurs rarely in children. It may spread to the lungs, liver, or lymph nodes.

Anything that increases your risk of getting a disease is called a risk factor. Wilms tumor may be part of a genetic syndrome that affects growth or development. A genetic syndrome is a set of symptoms or conditions that occur together and is usually caused by abnormal genes. Certain birth defects can also increase a child's risk for developing Wilms tumor. The following genetic syndromes and birth defects have been linked to Wilms tumor:

- WAGR (Wilms tumor, aniridia, ambiguous genitalia, and mental retardation) syndrome
- Beckwith-Wiedemann syndrome
- Hemihypertrophy
- Denys-Drash syndrome
- Cryptorchidism
- Hypospadias

Children with these genetic syndromes and birth defects should be screened for Wilms tumor every three months until age eight. An ultrasound test may be used for screening.

A doctor should be consulted if any of the following symptoms occur in the child:

- A lump, swelling, or pain in the abdomen
- Blood in the urine
- Fever for no known reason

The following tests and procedures may be used:

Physical exam and history: An exam of the body to check general signs of health, including checking for signs of disease, such as lumps or anything else that seems unusual. A history of the patient's health habits and past illnesses and treatments will also be taken.

Complete blood count (CBC): A procedure in which a sample of blood is drawn and checked for the following:

- The number of red blood cells, white blood cells, and platelets
- The amount of hemoglobin (the protein that carries oxygen) in the red blood cells
- The portion of the blood sample made up of red blood cells

Blood chemistry studies: A procedure in which a blood sample is checked to measure the amounts of certain substances released into the blood by organs and tissues in the body. An unusual (higher or lower than normal) amount of a substance can be a sign of disease in the organ or tissue that makes it.

Liver function test: A procedure in which a blood sample is checked to measure the amounts of certain substances released into the blood by the liver. A higher than normal amount of a substance can be a sign that the liver is not working as it should.

Renal function test: A procedure in which blood or urine samples are checked to measure the amounts of certain substances released into the blood or urine by the kidneys. A higher or lower than normal amount of a substance can be a sign that the kidneys are not working as they should.

Urinalysis: A test to check the color of urine and its contents, such as sugar, protein, blood, and bacteria.

Ultrasound exam: A procedure in which high-energy sound waves (ultrasound) are bounced off internal tissues or organs and make echoes. The echoes form a picture of body tissues called a sonogram. An ultrasound of the abdomen is done to diagnose a kidney tumor.

CT scan (CAT scan): A procedure that makes a series of detailed pictures of areas inside the body, taken from different angles. The pictures are made by a computer linked to an x-ray machine. A dye may be injected into a vein or swallowed to help the organs or tissues show up more clearly. This procedure is also called computed tomography, computerized tomography, or computerized axial tomography.

Abdominal x-ray: An x-ray of the organs inside the abdomen. An x-ray is a type of energy beam that can go through the body and onto film, making a picture of areas inside the body.

Biopsy: The removal of cells or tissues so they can be viewed under a microscope by a pathologist to check for signs of cancer.

Prognosis

Wilms tumor and other childhood kidney tumors are usually diagnosed and removed in surgery. Once a kidney tumor is found, surgery is done to find out whether or not the tumor is cancer. If the tumor is only in the kidney, the surgeon will remove the whole kidney (nephrectomy). If there are tumors in both kidneys or if the tumor has spread outside the kidney, a piece of the tumor will be removed. In any case, a sample of tissue from the tumor is sent to a pathologist, who looks at it under a microscope to check for signs of cancer.

The prognosis (chance of recovery) and treatment options depend on the following:

- How different the tumor cells are from normal kidney cells
- The stage of the cancer
- The type and size of the tumor
- The age of the child
- Whether the tumor can be completely removed in surgery
- Whether the cancer has just been diagnosed or has recurred (come back)
- Whether there are any abnormal chromosomes or genes
- Whether the patient is treated by pediatric experts with experience in treating patients with Wilms tumor

Stages of Wilms Tumor and Other Childhood Kidney Tumors

The process used to find out if cancer has spread outside of the kidney to other parts of the body is called staging. The information gathered from the staging process determines the stage of the disease. It is important to know the stage in order to plan treatment.

For Wilms tumors, the stage is determined during the initial surgery and with the results from imaging tests. The following imaging tests may be done to see if cancer has spread to other places in the body:

- **CT scan (CAT scan)**

- **X-ray of the chest and bones:** An x-ray is a type of energy beam that can go through the body and onto film, making a picture of areas inside the body.

- **MRI (magnetic resonance imaging):** A procedure that uses a magnet, radio waves, and a computer to make a series of detailed pictures of areas inside the body, such as the brain. This procedure is also called nuclear magnetic resonance imaging (NMRI).

- **Bone scan:** A procedure to check if there are rapidly dividing cells, such as cancer cells, in the bone. A very small amount of radioactive material is injected into a vein and travels through the bloodstream. The radioactive material collects in the bones and is detected by a scanner.

- **Ultrasound exam:** An ultrasound of the major heart vessels is done to stage Wilms tumor.

In addition to the stages, Wilms tumors are described by their histology. The histology (how the cells look under a microscope) of the tumor affects the prognosis and may be favorable or unfavorable. Tumors with a favorable histology respond better to treatment than those with unfavorable histology.

- **Favorable histology:** The cancer cells look like normal kidney cells.

- **Unfavorable histology:** The cancer cells are anaplastic, which means they divide rapidly and look very different from normal kidney cells. Anaplastic tumors may be focal (in one area) or diffuse (spread widely throughout an area). Focal tumors have a better prognosis than diffuse tumors.

The following stages are used for both favorable and unfavorable histology Wilms tumors:

Stage I: In stage I, the tumor was completely removed by surgery and all of the following are true:

- Cancer was found only in the kidney and did not spread to blood vessels of the kidney.

- The outer layer of the kidney did not break open.

- The tumor did not break open.

• A biopsy of the tumor was not done.

• No cancer cells are found at the edges of the area where the tumor was removed.

Stage II: In stage II, the tumor was completely removed by surgery and no cancer cells are found at the edges of the area where the cancer was removed. Also, one of the following is true:

• Cancer spread out of the kidney to nearby soft tissue.

• Cancer spread to blood vessels of the kidney.

Stage III: In stage III, cancer remains in the abdomen after surgery and at least one of the following is true:

• Cancer spread to lymph nodes in the abdomen or pelvis (the part of the body between the hips).

• Cancer spread to or through the surface of the peritoneum (the layer of tissue that lines the abdominal cavity and covers most organs in the abdomen).

• A biopsy of the tumor was done during surgery to remove it.

• The tumor was removed in more than one piece.

Stage IV: In stage IV, cancer has spread through the blood to organs such as the lungs, liver, bone, or brain, or to lymph nodes outside of the abdomen and pelvis.

Stage V: In stage V, cancer cells are found in both kidneys when the disease is first diagnosed. Each kidney will be staged separately as I, II, III, or IV.

Recurrent Wilms tumor and other childhood kidney tumors: Recurrent cancer is cancer that has recurred (come back) after it has been treated.

Treatment Option Overview

Different types of treatment are available for children with Wilms and other childhood kidney tumors. Some treatments are standard (the currently used treatment), and some are being tested in clinical trials. A treatment clinical trial is a research study meant to help improve current treatments or obtain information on new treatments for patients with cancer. When clinical trials show that a new treatment is better than the standard treatment, the new treatment may become the standard treatment.

Because cancer in children is rare, taking part in a clinical trial should be considered. Clinical trials are taking place in many parts of the country. Information about ongoing clinical trials is available from the National Cancer Institute website (http://www.cancer.gov). Choosing the most appropriate cancer treatment is a decision that ideally involves the patient, family, and health care team.

Children with Wilms tumor or other childhood kidney tumors should have their treatment planned by a team of doctors with expertise in treating cancer in children. Your child's treatment will be overseen by a pediatric oncologist, a doctor who specializes in treating children with cancer. The pediatric oncologist may refer you to other doctors who have experience and expertise in treating children with Wilms tumor or other childhood kidney tumors and who specialize in certain areas of medicine. These may include the following specialists:

- Pediatric surgeon or urologist
- Radiation oncologist
- Rehabilitation specialist
- Pediatric nurse specialist
- Social worker

Four types of standard treatment are used:

Surgery: Wilms tumor and other childhood kidney tumors are usually treated with nephrectomy (surgery to remove the whole kidney). Nearby lymph nodes may also be removed.

If cancer is found in both kidneys, surgery may include a partial nephrectomy (removal of the cancer in the kidney and a small amount of normal tissue around it). Partial nephrectomy is done to keep the kidney working.

Even if the doctor removes all the cancer that can be seen at the time of the surgery, some patients may be given chemotherapy or radiation therapy after surgery to kill any cancer cells that are left. Treatment given after the surgery, to increase the chances of a cure, is called adjuvant therapy. Sometimes, a second-look surgery is done to see if cancer remains after chemotherapy or radiation therapy.

Radiation therapy: Radiation therapy is a cancer treatment that uses high-energy x-rays or other types of radiation to kill cancer cells. There are two types of radiation therapy. External radiation therapy uses a machine outside the body to send radiation toward the cancer. Internal radiation therapy uses a radioactive substance sealed in needles, seeds, wires, or catheters that are placed directly into or near the cancer. The way the radiation therapy is given depends on the type and stage of the cancer being treated.

Chemotherapy: Chemotherapy is a cancer treatment that uses drugs to stop the growth of cancer cells, either by killing the cells or by stopping the cells from dividing. When chemotherapy is taken by mouth or injected into a vein or muscle, the drugs enter the bloodstream and can reach cancer cells throughout the body (systemic chemotherapy). When chemotherapy is placed directly into the spinal column, an organ, or a body cavity such as the abdomen, the drugs mainly affect cancer cells in those areas (regional chemotherapy). The way the chemotherapy is given depends on the type and stage of the cancer being treated.

Combination chemotherapy is treatment using two or more anti-cancer drugs.

Biologic therapy: Biologic therapy is a treatment that uses the patient's immune system to fight cancer. Substances made by the body or made in a laboratory are used to boost, direct, or restore the body's natural defenses against cancer. This type of cancer treatment is also called biotherapy or immunotherapy.

New Treatments

New types of treatment are being tested in clinical trials. These include the following:

High-dose chemotherapy with stem cell transplant: High-dose chemotherapy with stem cell transplant is a method of giving high doses of chemotherapy and replacing blood-forming cells destroyed by the cancer treatment. Stem cells (immature blood cells) are removed from the blood or bone marrow of the patient or a donor and are frozen and stored. After the chemotherapy is completed, the stored stem cells are thawed and given back to the patient through an infusion. These re-infused stem cells grow into (and restore) the body's blood cells.

Late Effects

Some cancer treatments cause side effects that continue or appear months or years after cancer treatment has ended. These are called late effects. It is important that parents of children who are treated for cancer know about the possible late effects caused by certain treatments. After several years, some patients develop another form of cancer as a result of their treatment with chemotherapy and radiation. Clinical trials are ongoing to find out if lower doses of chemotherapy and radiation can be used.

Treatment Options for Wilms Tumor and Other Childhood Kidney Tumors

Stage I Wilms tumor: Treatment of stage I Wilms tumor with either favorable or unfavorable histology may include the following:

* Nephrectomy with lymph node removal, followed by combination chemotherapy

* A clinical trial of nephrectomy alone

Stage II Wilms tumor: Treatment of stage II Wilms tumor with favorable histology is usually nephrectomy with removal of lymph nodes, followed by combination chemotherapy.

Treatment of stage II Wilms tumor with unfavorable histology is usually nephrectomy with removal of lymph nodes, followed by radiation therapy to the abdomen and combination chemotherapy.

Stage III Wilms tumor: Treatment of stage III Wilms tumor with either favorable or unfavorable histology is usually nephrectomy with removal of lymph nodes, followed by radiation therapy to the abdomen and combination chemotherapy.

Stage IV Wilms tumor: Treatment of stage IV Wilms tumor with either favorable or unfavorable histology is usually nephrectomy with removal of lymph nodes, followed by radiation therapy to the abdomen and combination chemotherapy. Some patients may also receive radiation therapy to the lungs.

Stage V Wilms tumor: Treatment of stage V Wilms tumor may be different for each patient. Treatment is usually chemotherapy to shrink the tumor, followed by surgery to remove as much of the cancer as possible. This may be followed by more chemotherapy and/or radiation therapy if cancer remains after surgery.

Inoperable tumors: Sometimes the tumor is inoperable (cannot be removed by surgery) because it is too close to important organs or blood vessels or because it is too large to remove. In this case, chemotherapy may be given to reduce the size of the tumor so it may be removed in surgery. If the tumor does not shrink enough after chemotherapy, radiation therapy may be given to shrink it further so that surgery may be done. This may be followed by more chemotherapy and/or more radiation therapy.

Clear cell sarcoma of the kidney: There is no standard treatment for clear cell sarcoma of the kidney. Treatment is usually within a clinical trial and may include nephrectomy, followed by radiation therapy to the abdomen and combination chemotherapy. Some patients may also receive radiation therapy to the lungs.

Rhabdoid tumor of the kidney: There is no standard treatment for rhabdoid tumor of the kidney. Treatment may be within a clinical trial and may include combination chemotherapy.

Neuroepithelial tumor of the kidney: There is no standard treatment for neuroepithelial tumor of the kidney. Treatment is usually within a clinical trial. It may be treated in the same way that Ewing family of tumors or primitive neuroectodermal tumors are treated.

Renal cell cancer: Treatment of renal cell cancer is usually nephrectomy with removal of lymph nodes. If cancer has spread, treatment may include biologic therapy or surgery to remove the primary tumor.

Recurrent Wilms tumor and other childhood kidney tumors: Treatment of recurrent Wilms tumor may be within a clinical trial of combination chemotherapy, surgery, and radiation therapy, with or without stem cell transplant, using the child's own blood stem cells.

Treatment of recurrent clear cell sarcoma, rhabdoid tumor, and neuroepithelial tumor of the kidney is usually within a clinical trial.

Chapter 47

Transitional Cell Cancer of the Renal Pelvis and Ureter

Transitional cell cancer of the renal pelvis and ureter is a disease in which malignant (cancer) cells form in the renal pelvis and ureter. The renal pelvis is part of the kidney and the ureter connects the kidney to the bladder. There are two kidneys, one on each side of the backbone, above the waist. The kidneys of an adult are about five inches long and three inches wide and are shaped like a kidney bean. The kidneys clean the blood and produce urine to rid the body of waste. The urine collects in the middle of each kidney in a large cavity called the renal pelvis. Urine drains from each kidney through a long tube called the ureter, into the bladder, where it is stored until it is passed from the body through the urethra.

The renal pelvis and ureters are lined with transitional cells. These cells can change shape and stretch without breaking apart. Transitional cell cancer starts in these cells. Transitional cell cancer can form in the renal pelvis or the ureter or both. Renal cell cancer is a more common type of kidney cancer.

Risk factors include the following:

- Misusing certain pain medicines, including over-the-counter pain medicines, for a long time

- Being exposed to certain dyes and chemicals used in making leather goods, textiles, plastics, and rubber

PDQ® Cancer Information Summary. National Cancer Institute; Bethesda, MD. Transitional Cell Cancer of the Renal Pelvis and Ureter (PDQ®): Treatment - Patient. Updated 04/2005. Available at: http://cancer.gov. Accessed April 30, 2006.

- Smoking cigarettes

There may be no symptoms in the early stages. Symptoms may appear as the tumor grows. A doctor should be consulted if any of the following problems occur:

- Blood in the urine
- A pain in the back that doesn't go away
- Extreme tiredness
- Weight loss with no known reason
- Painful or frequent urination

The following tests and procedures may be used to detect (find) and diagnose transitional cell cancer of the renal pelvis and ureter:

Physical exam and history: An exam of the body to check general signs of health, including checking for signs of disease, such as lumps or anything else that seems unusual. A history of the patient's health habits and past illnesses and treatments will also be taken.

Urinalysis: A test to check the color of urine and its contents, such as sugar, protein, blood, and bacteria.

Ureteroscopy: A procedure to look inside the ureter and renal pelvis to check for abnormal areas. A ureteroscope (a thin, lighted tube) is inserted through the urethra into the bladder, ureter, and renal pelvis. Tissue samples may be taken for biopsy.

Urine cytology: Examination of urine under a microscope to check for abnormal cells. Cancer in the kidney, bladder, or ureter may shed cancer cells into the urine.

Intravenous pyelogram (IVP): A series of x-rays of the kidneys, ureters, and bladder to check for cancer. A contrast dye is injected into a vein. As the contrast dye moves through the kidneys, ureters, and bladder, x-rays are taken to see if there are any blockages.

CT scan (CAT scan): A procedure that makes a series of detailed pictures of areas inside the body, taken from different angles. The pictures are made by a computer linked to an x-ray machine. A dye may be injected into a vein or swallowed to help the organs or tissues show up more clearly. This procedure is also called computed tomography, computerized tomography, or computerized axial tomography.

Ultrasound: A procedure in which high-energy sound waves (ultrasound) are bounced off internal tissues or organs and make echoes. The echoes form a picture of body tissues called a sonogram. An ultrasound of the abdomen may be done to help diagnose cancer of the renal pelvis and ureter.

Stages of Transitional Cell Cancer of the Renal Pelvis and Ureter

After transitional cell cancer of the renal pelvis and ureter has been diagnosed, tests are done to find out if cancer cells have spread within the renal pelvis and ureter or to other parts of the body. The process used to find out if cancer has spread within the renal pelvis and ureter or to other parts of the body is called staging. The information gathered from the staging process determines the stage of the disease. It is important to know the stage in order to plan treatment. The following tests and procedures may be used in the staging process:

- **Intravenous pyelogram (IVP):** A series of x-rays of the kidneys, ureters, and bladder to find out if cancer has spread within these organs. A contrast dye is injected into a vein. As the contrast dye moves through the kidneys, ureters, and bladder, x-rays are taken to see if there are any blockages.

- **CT scan (CAT scan)**

- **Ultrasound**

- **Ureteroscopy:** A procedure to look inside the ureter and renal pelvis to check for abnormal areas. A ureteroscope (a thin, lighted tube) is inserted through the urethra into the bladder, ureter, and renal pelvis. Tissue samples may be taken for biopsy.

- **Surgery:** Tissues removed during surgery to treat the transitional cell cancer will be examined by a pathologist.

The following stages are used for transitional cell cancer of the renal pelvis and/or ureter:

Stage 0 (carcinoma in situ): In stage 0, the cancer is found only on tissue lining the inside of the renal pelvis or ureter. Stage 0 is divided into stage 0a and stage 0is, depending on the type of tumor:

- Stage 0a may look like tiny mushrooms growing from the lining. Stage 0a is also called noninvasive papillary carcinoma.

- Stage 0is is a flat tumor on the tissue lining the inside of the renal pelvis or ureter. Stage 0is is also called carcinoma in situ.

Stage I: In stage I, cancer has spread through the cells lining the renal pelvis and/or ureter, into the layer of connective tissue.

Stage II: In stage II, cancer has spread through the layer of connective tissue to the muscle layer of the renal pelvis and/or ureter.

Stage III: In stage III, cancer has spread:

- to the layer of fat outside the renal pelvis and/or ureter; or
- into the wall of the kidney.

Stage IV: In stage IV, cancer has spread to at least one of the following:

- A nearby organ
- The layer of fat surrounding the kidney
- One or more lymph nodes
- Other parts of the body

Transitional cell cancer of the renal pelvis and ureter is also described as localized, regional, or metastatic:

- **Localized:** The cancer is found only in the kidney.
- **Regional:** The cancer has spread to tissues around the kidney and to nearby lymph nodes and blood vessels in the pelvis.
- **Metastatic:** The cancer has spread to other parts of the body.

Recurrent transitional cell cancer of the renal pelvis and ureter: Recurrent transitional cell cancer of the renal pelvis and ureter is cancer that has recurred (come back) after it has been treated. The cancer may come back in the renal pelvis, ureter, or other parts of the body.

Treatment Option Overview

Different types of treatments are available for patients with transitional cell cancer of the renal pelvis and ureter. Some treatments are standard (the currently used treatment), and some are being tested in clinical trials. Before starting treatment, patients may want to think about taking part in a clinical trial. A treatment clinical trial is a research study meant to help improve current treatments or obtain information on new treatments for patients with cancer. When clinical trials show that a new treatment is better than the standard treatment, the new treatment may become the standard treatment.

Clinical trials are taking place in many parts of the country. Information about ongoing clinical trials is available from the National Cancer Institute website (http://www.cancer.gov). Choosing the most appropriate cancer treatment is a decision that ideally involves the patient, family, and health care team.

One type of standard treatment is used:

Surgery: One of the following surgical procedures may be used to treat transitional cell cancer of the renal pelvis and ureter:

- **Nephroureterectomy:** Surgery to remove the entire kidney, the ureter, and the bladder cuff (tissue that connects the ureter to the bladder).

- **Segmental resection of the ureter:** A surgical procedure to remove the part of the ureter that contains cancer and some of the healthy tissue around it. The ends of the ureter are then reattached. This treatment is used when the cancer is superficial and in the lower third of the ureter only, near the bladder.

Other types of treatment are being tested in clinical trials. These include the following:

Fulguration: Fulguration is a surgical procedure that destroys tissue using an electric current. A tool with a small wire loop on the end is used to remove the cancer or to burn away the tumor with electricity.

Segmental resection of the renal pelvis: This is a surgical procedure to remove localized cancer from the renal pelvis without removing the entire kidney. Segmental resection may be done to save kidney function when the other kidney is damaged or has already been removed.

Laser surgery: A laser beam (narrow beam of intense light) is used as a knife to remove the cancer. A laser beam can also be used to kill the cancer cells. This procedure may be called laser therapy or laser fulguration.

Regional chemotherapy and regional biologic therapy: Chemotherapy is a cancer treatment that uses drugs to stop the growth of cancer cells, either by killing the cells or by stopping the cells from dividing. Biologic therapy is a treatment that uses the patient's immune system to fight cancer; substances made by the body or made in a laboratory are used to boost, direct, or restore the body's natural defenses against cancer. Regional treatment means the anticancer drugs or biologic substances are placed directly into an organ or a body cavity such as the abdomen, so the drugs will affect cancer cells in that area. Clinical trials are studying the effectiveness of chemotherapy or biologic therapy using drugs placed directly into the renal pelvis or the ureter.

Treatment Options for Transitional Cell Cancer of the Renal Pelvis and Ureter

Localized transitional cell cancer of the renal pelvis and ureter: Treatment of localized transitional cell cancer of the renal pelvis and ureter may include the following:

- Surgery (nephroureterectomy or segmental resection of ureter)
- A clinical trial of fulguration
- A clinical trial of laser surgery
- A clinical trial of segmental resection of the renal pelvis
- A clinical trial of regional chemotherapy
- A clinical trial of regional biologic therapy

Regional transitional cell cancer of the renal pelvis and ureter: Treatment of regional transitional cell cancer of the renal pelvis and ureter is usually done in a clinical trial.

Metastatic transitional cell cancer of the renal pelvis and ureter: Treatment of metastatic transitional cell cancer of the renal pelvis and ureter is usually done in a clinical trial, which may include chemotherapy.

Recurrent transitional cell cancer of the renal pelvis and ureter: Treatment of recurrent transitional cell cancer of the renal pelvis and ureter is usually done in a clinical trial, which may include chemotherapy.

Chapter 48

Urethral Cancer

Urethral cancer is a disease in which malignant (cancer) cells form in the tissues of the urethra. The urethra is the tube that carries urine from the bladder to outside the body. In women, the urethra is about 1½ inches long and is just above the vagina. In men, the urethra is about 8 inches long, and goes through the prostate gland and the penis to the outside of the body. In men, the urethra also carries semen.

Urethral cancer is a rare cancer that occurs more often in women than in men. There are different types of urethral cancer that begin in cells that line the urethra. These cancers are named for the types of cells that become malignant (cancerous):

- Squamous cell carcinoma is the most common type of urethral cancer. It forms in cells in the part of the urethra near the bladder in women, and in the lining of the urethra in the penis in men.

- Transitional cell carcinoma forms in the area near the urethral opening in women, and in the part of the urethra that goes through the prostate gland in men.

- Adenocarcinoma forms in glands near the urethra in both men and women.

PDQ® Cancer Information Summary. National Cancer Institute; Bethesda, MD. Urethral Cancer PDQ®): Treatment - Patient. Updated 03/2006. Available at: http://cancer.gov. Accessed April 30, 2006.

- Urethral cancer can metastasize (spread) quickly to tissues around the urethra and is often found in nearby lymph nodes by the time it is diagnosed.

Risk factors include the following:

- Having a history of bladder cancer
- Having conditions that cause chronic inflammation in the urethra, including:
    - Sexually transmitted diseases (STDs)
    - Frequent urinary tract infections (UTIs)
- Being 60 or older
- Being a white female

Sometimes early cancer of the urethra does not cause any symptoms at all. A doctor should be consulted if any of the following symptoms occur:

- Bleeding from the urethra or blood in the urine
- Weak or interrupted ("stop-and-go") flow of urine
- Frequent urination
- A lump or thickness in the perineum or penis
- Discharge from the urethra
- Enlarged lymph nodes in the groin area

The following tests and procedures may be used:

Physical exam and history: An exam of the body to check general signs of health, including checking for signs of disease, such as lumps or anything else that seems unusual. A history of the patient's health habits and past illnesses and treatments will also be taken.

Laboratory tests: Medical procedures that test samples of tissue, blood, urine, or other substances in the body. These tests help to diagnose disease, plan and check treatment, or monitor the disease over time.

Urine cytology: Examination of urine under a microscope to check for abnormal cells.

Urinalysis: A test to check the color of urine and its contents, such as sugar, protein, blood, and white blood cells. If white blood cells (a sign of infection) are found, a urine culture is usually done to find out what type of infection it is.

Digital rectal exam: An exam of the rectum. The doctor or nurse inserts a lubricated, gloved finger into the lower part of the rectum to feel for lumps or anything else that seems unusual. This procedure may be done while the patient is under anesthesia.

Pelvic exam: An exam of the vagina, cervix, uterus, fallopian tubes, ovaries, and rectum. The doctor or nurse inserts one or two lubricated, gloved fingers of one hand into the vagina and places the other hand over the lower abdomen to feel the size, shape, and position of the uterus and ovaries. A speculum is also inserted into the vagina and the doctor or nurse looks at the vagina and cervix for signs of disease. This may be done while the patient is under anesthesia.

Cystoscopy: A procedure to look inside the urethra and bladder to check for abnormal areas. A cystoscope (a thin, lighted tube) is inserted through the urethra into the bladder. Tissue samples may be taken for biopsy.

Biopsy: The removal of cells or tissues from the urethra, bladder, and, sometimes, the prostate gland, so they can be viewed under a microscope by a pathologist to check for signs of cancer.

The prognosis (chance of recovery) depends on the following:

- The stage and size of the cancer (whether it is in only one area or has spread to other areas).
- Where in the urethra the cancer first formed.
- The patient's general health.
- Whether the cancer has just been diagnosed or has recurred (come back).

Treatment options depend on the following:

- The stage of the cancer and where it is in the urethra.
- The patient's sex and general health.
- Whether the cancer has just been diagnosed or has recurred.

Stages of Urethral Cancer

After urethral cancer has been diagnosed, tests are done to find out if cancer cells have spread within the urethra or to other parts of the body. The process used to find out if cancer has spread within the urethra or to other parts of the body is called staging. The information gathered from the staging process determines the stage of the disease. It is important to know the stage in order to plan treatment. The following procedures may be used in the staging process:

Chest x-ray: An x-ray of the organs and bones inside the chest. An x-ray is a type of energy beam that can go through the body and onto film, making a picture of areas inside the body.

CT scan (CAT scan) of the pelvis and abdomen: A procedure that makes a series of detailed pictures of the pelvis and abdomen, taken from different angles. The pictures are made by a computer linked to an x-ray machine. A dye may be injected into a vein or swallowed to help the organs or tissues show up more clearly. This procedure is also called computed tomography, computerized tomography, or computerized axial tomography.

MRI (magnetic resonance imaging): A procedure that uses a magnet, radio waves, and a computer to make a series of detailed pictures of the urethra, nearby lymph nodes, and other soft tissue and bones in the pelvis. A substance called gadolinium is injected into the patient through a vein. The gadolinium collects around the cancer cells so they show up brighter in the picture. This procedure is also called nuclear magnetic resonance imaging (NMRI).

Blood chemistry studies: A procedure in which a blood sample is checked to measure the amounts of certain substances released into the blood by organs and tissues in the body. An unusual (higher or lower than normal) amount of a substance can be a sign of disease in the organ or tissue that produces it.

Complete blood count (CBC): A procedure in which a sample of blood is drawn and checked for the following:

- The number of red blood cells, white blood cells, and platelets.
- The amount of hemoglobin (the protein that carries oxygen) in the red blood cells.

- The portion of the blood sample made up of red blood cells.

Urethral cancer is staged and treated based on the part of the urethra that is affected and how deeply the tumor has spread into tissue around the urethra. Urethral cancer can be described as anterior or posterior.

- **Anterior urethral cancer:** In anterior urethral cancer, the tumors are not deep and they affect the part of the urethra that is closest to the outside of the body.
- **Posterior urethral cancer:** In posterior urethral cancer, the tumors are deep and affect the part of the urethra closest to the bladder. In women, the entire urethra may be affected. In men, the prostate gland may be affected.

The following stages are also used to describe urethral cancer:

Stage 0 (carcinoma in situ): In stage 0, cancer is found only in the inside lining of the urethra. Stage 0 is also called carcinoma in situ.

Stage A: In stage A, cancer has spread into the layer of tissue beneath the lining of the urethra.

Stage B: In stage B, cancer is found in the muscle around the urethra. In men, the penile tissue surrounding the urethra may be affected.

Stage C: In stage C, cancer has spread beyond the tissue surrounding the urethra, and:

- in women, may be found in the vagina, vaginal lips, or nearby muscle;
- in men, may be found in the penis or in nearby muscle.

Stage D: Stage D is divided into stage D1 and stage D2, based on where the cancer has spread.

- In stage D1, cancer has spread to nearby lymph nodes in the pelvis and groin.
- In stage D2, cancer has spread to distant lymph nodes or to other organs in the body, such as the lungs, liver, and bone.

Recurrent urethral cancer: Recurrent urethral cancer is cancer that has recurred (come back) after it has been treated. The cancer may come back in the urethra or in other parts of the body.

Urethral cancer may be associated with invasive bladder cancer. A small number of patients who have bladder cancer are also diagnosed with cancer of the urethra, or will develop it in the future.

Treatment Option Overview

Different types of treatments are available for patients with urethral cancer. Some treatments are standard (the currently used treatment), and some are being tested in clinical trials. Before starting treatment, patients may want to think about taking part in a clinical trial. A treatment clinical trial is a research study meant to help improve current treatments or obtain information on new treatments for patients with cancer. When clinical trials show that a new treatment is better than the standard treatment, the new treatment may become the standard treatment.

Clinical trials are taking place in many parts of the country. Information about ongoing clinical trials is available from the National Cancer Institute website (http://www.cancer.gov). Choosing the most appropriate cancer treatment is a decision that ideally involves the patient, family, and health care team.

Three types of standard treatment are used:

Surgery: Surgery is the most common treatment for cancer of the urethra. One of the following types of surgery may be done:

- **Open excision:** Removal of the cancer by surgery.

- **Electro-resection with fulguration:** Surgery to remove the cancer by electric current. A lighted tool with a small wire loop on the end is used to remove the cancer or to burn the tumor away with high-energy electricity.

- **Laser surgery:** A surgical procedure that uses a laser beam (a narrow beam of intense light) as a knife to make bloodless cuts in tissue or to remove or destroy tissue.

- **Lymph node dissection:** Lymph nodes in the pelvis and groin may be removed.

- **Cystourethrectomy:** Surgery to remove the bladder and the urethra.

- **Cystoprostatectomy:** Surgery to remove the bladder and the prostate.

- **Anterior exenteration:** Surgery to remove the urethra, the bladder, and the vagina. Plastic surgery may be done to rebuild the vagina.

- **Partial penectomy:** Surgery to remove the part of the penis surrounding the urethra where cancer has spread. Plastic surgery may be done to rebuild the penis.

- **Radical penectomy:** Surgery to remove the entire penis. Plastic surgery may be done to rebuild the penis.

If the urethra is removed, the surgeon will make a new way for the urine to pass from the body. This is called urinary diversion. If the bladder is removed, the surgeon will make a new way for urine to be stored and passed from the body. The surgeon may use part of the small intestine to make a tube that passes urine through an opening (stoma). This is called an ostomy or urostomy. If a patient has an ostomy, a disposable bag to collect urine is worn under clothing. The surgeon may also use part of the small intestine to make a new storage pouch (continent reservoir) inside the body where the urine can collect. A tube (catheter) is then used to drain the urine through a stoma.

Even if the doctor removes all the cancer that can be seen at the time of the surgery, some patients may be given chemotherapy or radiation therapy after surgery to kill any cancer cells that are left. Treatment given after the surgery, to increase the chances of a cure, is called adjuvant therapy.

Radiation therapy: Radiation therapy is a cancer treatment that uses high-energy x-rays or other types of radiation to kill cancer cells. There are two types of radiation therapy. External radiation therapy uses a machine outside the body to send radiation toward the cancer. Internal radiation therapy uses a radioactive substance sealed in needles, seeds, wires, or catheters that are placed directly into or near the cancer. The way the radiation therapy is given depends on the type and stage of the cancer being treated.

Watchful waiting: Watchful waiting is closely monitoring a patient's condition without giving any treatment until symptoms appear or change.

New Treatments

New types of treatment are being tested in clinical trials. These include the following:

Chemotherapy: Chemotherapy is a cancer treatment that uses drugs to stop the growth of cancer cells, either by killing the cells or by stopping the cells from dividing. When chemotherapy is taken by mouth or injected into a vein or muscle, the drugs enter the bloodstream and can reach cancer cells throughout the body (systemic chemotherapy). When chemotherapy is placed directly into the spinal column, an organ, or a body cavity such as the abdomen, the drugs mainly affect cancer cells in those areas (regional chemotherapy). The way the chemotherapy is given depends on the type and stage of the cancer being treated.

Treatment Options for Urethral Cancer

Anterior urethral cancer: Treatment of anterior urethral cancer is different for men and women.

For women, treatment may include the following:

- Radiation therapy followed by surgery (anterior exenteration and urinary diversion)
- Surgery (open excision, electro-resection with fulguration, lymph node dissection, or anterior exenteration and urinary diversion)
- Laser surgery
- External and/or internal radiation therapy

For men, treatment may include the following:

- Surgery (open excision, electro-resection with fulguration, lymph node dissection, or partial or radical penectomy)
- Laser surgery
- Radiation therapy

Posterior urethral cancer: Treatment of posterior urethral cancer is different for men and women.

For women, treatment may include the following:

- Radiation therapy followed by surgery (anterior exenteration with lymph node dissection and urinary diversion)

- Radiation therapy with or without surgery (other than anterior exenteration and urinary diversion)
- Surgery (other than anterior exenteration and urinary diversion) alone

For men, treatment may be radiation therapy followed by surgery (cystoprostatectomy, penectomy, lymph node dissection, and urinary diversion).

Urethral cancer associated with invasive bladder cancer: Treatment of urethral cancer that develops with invasive bladder cancer may include the following:

- Surgery (cystourethrectomy or cystoprostatectomy)
- Watchful waiting

Recurrent urethral cancer: Treatment of recurrent urethral cancer that comes back near the urethra depends on the type of treatment the patient received before, as follows:

- Surgery: For patients who were first treated with radiation therapy
- Radiation therapy with surgery: For patients who were first treated with surgery alone

Treatment of recurrent urethral cancer that comes back in distant parts of the body is usually a clinical trial of chemotherapy.

Chapter 49

Bladder Cancer

Bladder cancer is a disease in which malignant (cancer) cells form in the tissues of the bladder. The bladder is a hollow organ in the lower part of the abdomen. It is shaped like a small balloon and has a muscular wall that allows it to get larger or smaller. The bladder stores urine until it is passed out of the body. Urine is the liquid waste that is made by the kidneys when they clean the blood. The urine passes from the two kidneys into the bladder through two tubes called ureters. When the bladder is emptied during urination, the urine goes from the bladder to the outside of the body through another tube called the urethra.

There are three types of bladder cancer that begin in cells in the lining of the bladder. These cancers are named for the type of cells that become malignant (cancerous):

- **Transitional cell carcinoma:** Cancer that begins in cells in the innermost tissue layer of the bladder. These cells are able to stretch when the bladder is full and shrink when it is emptied. Most bladder cancers begin in the transitional cells.

- **Squamous cell carcinoma:** Cancer that begins in squamous cells, which are thin, flat cells that may form in the bladder after long-term infection or irritation.

PDQ® Cancer Information Summary. National Cancer Institute; Bethesda, MD. Bladder Cancer (PDQ®): Treatment - Patient. Updated 04/2006. Available at: http://cancer.gov. Accessed June 23, 2006.

- **Adenocarcinoma:** Cancer that begins in glandular (secretory) cells. Glandular cells in the lining of the bladder make substances such as mucus.

Cancer that is confined to the lining of the bladder is called superficial bladder cancer. Cancer that begins in the transitional cells may spread through the lining of the bladder and invade the muscle wall of the bladder or spread to nearby organs and lymph nodes; this is called invasive bladder cancer.

Anything that increases your chance of getting a disease is called a risk factor. Risk factors for bladder cancer include the following:

- Smoking
- Being exposed to certain substances at work, such as rubber, certain dyes and textiles, paint, and hairdressing supplies
- A diet high in fried meats and fat
- Being older, male, or white
- Having an infection caused by a certain parasite

A doctor should be consulted if any of the following symptoms occur:

- Blood in the urine (slightly rusty to bright red in color)
- Frequent urination, or feeling the need to urinate without being able to do so
- Pain during urination
- Lower back pain

The following tests and procedures may be used to help detect (find) and diagnose bladder cancer:

CT scan (CAT scan): A procedure that makes a series of detailed pictures of areas inside the body, taken from different angles. The pictures are made by a computer linked to an x-ray machine. A dye may be injected into a vein or swallowed to help the organs or tissues show up more clearly. This procedure is also called computed tomography, computerized tomography, or computerized axial tomography.

Urinalysis: A test to check the color of urine and its contents, such as sugar, protein, blood, and bacteria.

Internal exam: An exam of the vagina and/or rectum. The doctor inserts gloved fingers into the vagina and/or rectum to feel for lumps.

Intravenous pyelogram (IVP): A series of x-rays of the kidneys, ureters, and bladder to find out if cancer is present in these organs. A contrast dye is injected into a vein. As the contrast dye moves through the kidneys, ureters, and bladder, x-rays are taken to see if there are any blockages.

Cystoscopy: A procedure to look inside the bladder and urethra to check for abnormal areas. A cystoscope (a thin, lighted tube) is inserted through the urethra into the bladder. Tissue samples may be taken for biopsy.

Biopsy: The removal of cells or tissues so they can be viewed under a microscope by a pathologist to check for signs of cancer. A biopsy for bladder cancer is usually done during cystoscopy. It may be possible to remove the entire tumor during biopsy.

Urine cytology: Examination of urine under a microscope to check for abnormal cells.

Prognosis

The prognosis (chance of recovery) depends on the following:

- The stage of the cancer (whether it is superficial or invasive bladder cancer, and whether it has spread to other places in the body). Bladder cancer in the early stages can often be cured.
- The type of bladder cancer cells and how they look under a microscope.
- The patient's age and general health.

Stages of Bladder Cancer

After bladder cancer has been diagnosed, tests are done to find out if cancer cells have spread within the bladder or to other parts of the body. The process used to find out if cancer has spread within the bladder lining and muscle or to other parts of the body is called staging. The information gathered from the staging process determines the stage of the disease. It is important to know the stage in order to plan treatment. The following tests and procedures may be used in the staging process:

- **Cystoscopy**

- **CT scan (CAT scan)**

- **MRI (magnetic resonance imaging):** A procedure that uses a magnet, radio waves, and a computer to make a series of detailed pictures of areas inside the body. This procedure is also called nuclear magnetic resonance imaging (NMRI).

- **Physical exam and history:** An exam of the body to check general signs of health, including checking for signs of disease, such as lumps or anything else that seems unusual. A history of the patient's health habits and past illnesses and treatments will also be taken.

- **Chest x-ray:** An x-ray of the organs and bones inside the chest. An x-ray is a type of energy beam that can go through the body and onto film, making a picture of areas inside the body.

- **Bone scan:** A procedure to check if there are rapidly dividing cells, such as cancer cells, in the bone. A very small amount of radioactive material is injected into a vein and travels through the bloodstream. The radioactive material collects in the bones and is detected by a scanner.

The following stages are used for bladder cancer:

Stage 0: In stage 0, the cancer is found only on tissue lining the inside of the bladder. Stage 0 is divided into stage 0a and stage 0is, depending on the type of the tumor:

- Stage 0a is also called papillary carcinoma, which may look like tiny mushrooms growing from the lining of the bladder.

- Stage 0is is also called carcinoma in situ, which is a flat tumor on the tissue lining the inside of the bladder.

Stage I: In stage I, the cancer has spread to the layer below the inner lining of the bladder.

Stage II: In stage II, cancer has spread to either the inner half or outer half of the muscle wall of the bladder.

Stage III: In stage III, cancer has spread from the bladder to the fatty layer of tissue surrounding it, and may have spread to the reproductive organs (prostate, uterus, and vagina).

Stage IV: In stage IV, cancer has spread from the bladder to the wall of the abdomen or pelvis. Cancer may have spread to one or more lymph nodes or to other parts of the body.

Recurrent bladder cancer: Recurrent bladder cancer is cancer that has recurred (come back) after it has been treated. The cancer may come back in the bladder or in other parts of the body.

Treatment Option Overview

Different types of treatment are available for patients with bladder cancer. Some treatments are standard (the currently used treatment), and some are being tested in clinical trials. Before starting treatment, patients may want to think about taking part in a clinical trial. A treatment clinical trial is a research study meant to help improve current treatments or obtain information on new treatments for patients with cancer. When clinical trials show that a new treatment is better than the standard treatment, the new treatment may become the standard treatment.

Clinical trials are taking place in many parts of the country. Information about ongoing clinical trials is available from the National Cancer Institute website (http://www.cancer.gov). Choosing the most appropriate cancer treatment is a decision that ideally involves the patient, family, and health care team.

Four types of standard treatment are used:

Surgery: One of the following types of surgery may be done:

- **Transurethral resection (TUR) with fulguration:** Surgery in which a cystoscope (a thin lighted tube) is inserted into the bladder through the urethra. A tool with a small wire loop on the end is then used to remove the cancer or to burn the tumor away with high-energy electricity. This is known as fulguration.

- **Radical cystectomy:** Surgery to remove the bladder and any lymph nodes and nearby organs that contain cancer. This surgery may be done when the bladder cancer invades the muscle wall, or when superficial cancer involves a large part of the bladder. In men, the nearby organs that are removed are the prostate and the seminal vesicles. In women, the uterus, the ovaries, and part of the vagina are removed. Sometimes, when the cancer has spread outside the bladder and cannot be completely removed, surgery to remove only the bladder may be done to reduce urinary symptoms caused by the cancer. When the bladder must be removed, the surgeon creates another way for urine to leave the body.

- **Segmental cystectomy:** Surgery to remove part of the bladder. This surgery may be done for patients who have a low-grade tumor that has invaded the wall of the bladder but is limited to one area of the bladder. Because only a part of the bladder is removed, patients are able to urinate normally after recovering from this surgery.

- **Urinary diversion:** Surgery to make a new way for the body to store and pass urine.

Even if the doctor removes all the cancer that can be seen at the time of the surgery, some patients may be given chemotherapy after surgery to kill any cancer cells that are left. Treatment given after surgery, to increase the chances of a cure, is called adjuvant therapy.

Radiation therapy: Radiation therapy is a cancer treatment that uses high-energy x-rays or other types of radiation to kill cancer cells. There are two types of radiation therapy. External radiation therapy uses a machine outside the body to send radiation toward the cancer. Internal radiation therapy uses a radioactive substance sealed in needles, seeds, wires, or catheters that are placed directly into or near the cancer. The way the radiation therapy is given depends on the type and stage of the cancer being treated.

Chemotherapy: Chemotherapy is a cancer treatment that uses drugs to stop the growth of cancer cells, either by killing the cells or by stopping the cells from dividing. When chemotherapy is taken by mouth or injected into a vein or muscle, the drugs enter the bloodstream and can reach cancer cells throughout the body (systemic chemotherapy). When chemotherapy is placed directly into the spinal column, an organ, or a body cavity such as the abdomen, the drugs mainly affect cancer cells in those areas (regional chemotherapy). Bladder cancer may be treated with intravesical (into the bladder through a tube inserted into the urethra) chemotherapy. The way the chemotherapy is given depends on the type and stage of the cancer being treated.

Biologic therapy: Biologic therapy is a treatment that uses the patient's immune system to fight cancer. Substances made by the body or made in a laboratory are used to boost, direct, or restore the body's natural defenses against cancer. This type of cancer treatment is also called biotherapy or immunotherapy.

New Treatments

New types of treatment are being tested in clinical trials. These include the following:

Chemoprevention: Chemoprevention is the use of drugs, vitamins, or other substances to reduce the risk of developing cancer or to reduce the risk that cancer will recur (come back).

Photodynamic therapy: Photodynamic therapy (PDT) is a cancer treatment that uses a drug and a certain type of laser light to kill cancer cells. A drug that is not active until it is exposed to light is injected into a vein. The drug collects more in cancer cells than in normal cells. Fiberoptic tubes are then used to deliver the laser light to the cancer cells, where the drug becomes active and kills the cells. Photodynamic therapy causes little damage to healthy tissue.

Treatment Options by Stage

Stage 0 bladder cancer (carcinoma in situ): Treatment of stage 0 bladder cancer may include the following:

- Transurethral resection with fulguration
- Transurethral resection with fulguration followed by intravesical biologic therapy or chemotherapy
- Segmental cystectomy
- Radical cystectomy
- A clinical trial of photodynamic therapy
- A clinical trial of biologic therapy
- A clinical trial of chemoprevention therapy given after treatment to stop cancer from recurring (coming back)

Stage I bladder cancer: Treatment of stage I bladder cancer may include the following:

- Transurethral resection with fulguration
- Transurethral resection with fulguration followed by intravesical biologic therapy or chemotherapy

- Segmental or radical cystectomy
- Radiation implants with or without external radiation therapy
- A clinical trial of chemoprevention therapy given after treatment to stop cancer from recurring (coming back)
- A clinical trial of intravesical therapy

Stage II bladder cancer: Treatment of stage II bladder cancer may include the following:

- Radical cystectomy with or without surgery to remove pelvic lymph nodes
- Combination chemotherapy followed by radical cystectomy
- External radiation therapy combined with chemotherapy
- Radiation implants before or after external radiation therapy
- Transurethral resection with fulguration
- Segmental cystectomy

Stage III bladder cancer: Treatment of stage III bladder cancer may include the following:

- Radical cystectomy with or without surgery to remove pelvic lymph nodes
- Combination chemotherapy followed by radical cystectomy
- External radiation therapy combined with chemotherapy
- External radiation therapy with radiation implants
- Segmental cystectomy

Stage IV bladder cancer: Treatment of stage IV bladder cancer may include the following:

- Radical cystectomy with surgery to remove pelvic lymph nodes
- External radiation therapy (may be as palliative therapy to relieve symptoms and improve quality of life)
- Urinary diversion as palliative therapy to relieve symptoms and improve quality of life
- Cystectomy as palliative therapy to relieve symptoms and improve quality of life

- Chemotherapy alone or after local treatment (surgery or radiation therapy)
- A clinical trial of chemotherapy

Treatment options for recurrent bladder cancer: Treatment of recurrent bladder cancer depends on previous treatment and where the cancer has recurred. Treatment for recurrent bladder cancer may include the following:

- Surgery
- Chemotherapy
- Radiation therapy
- A clinical trial of chemotherapy

Chapter 50

Breast Cancer

The Breasts

The breasts sit on the chest muscles that cover the ribs. Each breast is made of 15 to 20 lobes. Lobes contain many smaller lobules. Lobules contain groups of tiny glands that can produce milk. Milk flows from the lobules through thin tubes called ducts to the nipple. The nipple is in the center of a dark area of skin called the areola. Fat fills the spaces between the lobules and ducts.

The breasts also contain lymph vessels. These vessels lead to small, round organs called lymph nodes. Groups of lymph nodes are near the breast in the axilla (underarm), above the collarbone, in the chest behind the breastbone, and in many other parts of the body. The lymph nodes trap bacteria, cancer cells, or other harmful substances.

When breast cancer cells spread, the cancer cells are often found in lymph nodes near the breast. Also, breast cancer can spread to almost any other part of the body. The most common are the bones, liver, lungs, and brain. The new tumor has the same kind of abnormal cells and the same name as the primary tumor. For example, if breast cancer spreads to the bones, the cancer cells in the bones are actually breast cancer cells. The disease is metastatic breast cancer, not bone cancer. For that reason, it is treated as breast cancer, not bone cancer. Doctors call the new tumor "distant" or metastatic disease.

Excerpted from "What You Need to Know about™ Breast Cancer," National Cancer Institute, July 30, 2005.

Risk Factors

No one knows the exact causes of breast cancer. Doctors often cannot explain why one woman develops breast cancer and another does not. They do know that bumping, bruising, or touching the breast does not cause cancer. And breast cancer is not contagious. You cannot "catch" it from another person.

Studies have found the following risk factors for breast cancer:

- **Age:** The chance of getting breast cancer goes up as a woman gets older. Most cases of breast cancer occur in women over 60. This disease is not common before menopause.

- **Personal history of breast cancer:** A woman who had breast cancer in one breast has an increased risk of getting cancer in her other breast.

- **Family history:** A woman's risk of breast cancer is higher if her mother, sister, or daughter had breast cancer. The risk is higher if her family member got breast cancer before age 40. Having other relatives with breast cancer (in either her mother's or father's family) may also increase a woman's risk.

- **Certain breast changes:** Some women have cells in the breast that look abnormal under a microscope. Having certain types of abnormal cells (atypical hyperplasia and lobular carcinoma in situ [LCIS]) increases the risk of breast cancer.

- **Gene changes:** Changes in certain genes increase the risk of breast cancer. These genes include BRCA1, BRCA2, and others. Tests can sometimes show the presence of specific gene changes in families with many women who have had breast cancer. Health care providers may suggest ways to try to reduce the risk of breast cancer, or to improve the detection of this disease in women who have these changes in their genes.

- **Reproductive and menstrual history:**
  - The older a woman is when she has her first child, the greater her chance of breast cancer.
  - Women who had their first menstrual period before age 12 are at an increased risk of breast cancer.
  - Women who went through menopause after age 55 are at an increased risk of breast cancer.

- Women who never had children are at an increased risk of breast cancer.

- Women who take menopausal hormone therapy with estrogen plus progestin after menopause also appear to have an increased risk of breast cancer.

- Large, well-designed studies have shown no link between abortion or miscarriage and breast cancer.

- **Race:** Breast cancer is diagnosed more often in white women than Latina, Asian, or African American women.

- **Radiation therapy to the chest:** Women who had radiation therapy to the chest (including breasts) before age 30 are at an increased risk of breast cancer. This includes women treated with radiation for Hodgkin lymphoma. Studies show that the younger a woman was when she received radiation treatment, the higher her risk of breast cancer later in life.

- **Breast density:** Breast tissue may be dense or fatty. Older women whose mammograms (breast x-rays) show more dense tissue are at increased risk of breast cancer.

- **Taking DES (diethylstilbestrol):** DES was given to some pregnant women in the United States between about 1940 and 1971. (It is no longer given to pregnant women.) Women who took DES during pregnancy may have a slightly increased risk of breast cancer. The possible effects on their daughters are under study.

- **Being overweight or obese after menopause:** The chance of getting breast cancer after menopause is higher in women who are overweight or obese.

- **Lack of physical activity:** Women who are physically inactive throughout life may have an increased risk of breast cancer. Being active may help reduce risk by preventing weight gain and obesity.

- **Drinking alcohol:** Studies suggest that the more alcohol a woman drinks, the greater her risk of breast cancer.

Other possible risk factors are under study. Researchers are studying the effect of diet, physical activity, and genetics on breast cancer risk. They are also studying whether certain substances in the environment can increase the risk of breast cancer.

Many risk factors can be avoided. Others, such as family history, cannot be avoided. Women can help protect themselves by staying away from known risk factors whenever possible.

But it is also important to keep in mind that most women who have known risk factors do not get breast cancer. Also, most women with breast cancer do not have a family history of the disease. In fact, except for growing older, most women with breast cancer have no clear risk factors.

If you think you may be at risk, you should discuss this concern with your doctor. Your doctor may be able to suggest ways to reduce your risk and can plan a schedule for checkups.

Screening

Screening for breast cancer before there are symptoms can be important. Screening can help doctors find and treat cancer early. Treatment is more likely to work well when cancer is found early.

Your doctor may suggest the following screening tests for breast cancer:

- Screening mammogram
- Clinical breast exam
- Breast self-exam

You should ask your doctor about when to start and how often to check for breast cancer.

Screening Mammogram

To find breast cancer early, it is recommended that:

- Women in their 40s and older should have mammograms every one to two years. A mammogram is a picture of the breast made with x-rays.

- Women who are younger than 40 and have risk factors for breast cancer should ask their health care provider whether to have mammograms and how often to have them.

Mammograms can often show a breast lump before it can be felt. They also can show a cluster of tiny specks of calcium. These specks are called microcalcifications. Lumps or specks can be from cancer, precancerous cells, or other conditions. Further tests are needed to find out if abnormal cells are present.

If an abnormal area shows up on your mammogram, you may need to have more x-rays. You also may need a biopsy. A biopsy is the only way to tell for sure if cancer is present.

Clinical Breast Exam

During a clinical breast exam, your health care provider checks your breasts. You may be asked to raise your arms over your head, let them hang by your sides, or press your hands against your hips.

Your health care provider looks for differences in size or shape between your breasts. The skin of your breasts is checked for a rash, dimpling, or other abnormal signs. Your nipples may be squeezed to check for fluid.

Using the pads of the fingers to feel for lumps, your health care provider checks your entire breast, underarm, and collarbone area. A lump is generally the size of a pea before anyone can feel it. The exam is done on one side, then the other. Your health care provider checks the lymph nodes near the breast to see if they are enlarged.

A thorough clinical breast exam may take about 10 minutes.

Breast Self-Exam

You may perform monthly breast self-exams to check for any changes in your breasts. It is important to remember that changes can occur because of aging, your menstrual cycle, pregnancy, menopause, or taking birth control pills or other hormones. It is normal for breasts to feel a little lumpy and uneven. Also, it is common for your breasts to be swollen and tender right before or during your menstrual period.

You should contact your health care provider if you notice any unusual changes in your breasts.

Breast self-exams cannot replace regular screening mammograms and clinical breast exams. Studies have not shown that breast self-exams alone reduce the number of deaths from breast cancer.

Symptoms

Common symptoms of breast cancer include:

- A change in how the breast or nipple feels
  - A lump or thickening in or near the breast or in the underarm area
  - Nipple tenderness

521

- A change in how the breast or nipple looks

  - A change in the size or shape of the breast

  - A nipple turned inward into the breast

  - The skin of the breast, areola, or nipple may be scaly, red, or swollen. It may have ridges or pitting so that it looks like the skin of an orange

- Nipple discharge (fluid)

Early breast cancer usually does not cause pain. Still, a woman should see her health care provider about breast pain or any other symptom that does not go away. Most often, these symptoms are not due to cancer. Other health problems may also cause them. Any woman with these symptoms should tell her doctor so that problems can be diagnosed and treated as early as possible.

Diagnosis

If you have a symptom or screening test result that suggests cancer, your doctor must find out whether it is due to cancer or to some other cause. Your doctor may ask about your personal and family medical history. You may have a physical exam. Your doctor also may order a mammogram or other imaging procedure. These tests make pictures of tissues inside the breast. After the tests, your doctor may decide no other exams are needed. Your doctor may suggest that you have a follow-up exam later on. Or you may need to have a biopsy to look for cancer cells.

Ultrasound

An ultrasound device sends out sound waves that people cannot hear. The waves bounce off tissues. A computer uses the echoes to create a picture. Your doctor can view these pictures on a monitor. The pictures may show whether a lump is solid or filled with fluid. A cyst is a fluid-filled sac. Cysts are not cancer. But a solid mass may be cancer. After the test, your doctor can store the pictures on video or print them out. This exam may be used along with a mammogram.

Magnetic Resonance Imaging

Magnetic resonance imaging (MRI) uses a powerful magnet linked to a computer. MRI makes detailed pictures of breast tissue. Your doctor can view these pictures on a monitor or print them on film. MRI may be used along with a mammogram.

Biopsy

Your doctor may refer you to a surgeon or breast disease specialist for a biopsy. Fluid or tissue is removed from your breast to help find out if there is cancer.

Some suspicious areas can be seen on a mammogram but cannot be felt during a clinical breast exam. Doctors can use imaging procedures to help see the area and remove tissue. Such procedures include ultrasound-guided, needle-localized, or stereotactic biopsy.

Doctors can remove tissue from the breast in different ways:

- **Fine-needle aspiration:** Your doctor uses a thin needle to remove fluid from a breast lump. If the fluid appears to contain cells, a pathologist at a lab checks them for cancer with a microscope. If the fluid is clear, it may not need to be checked by a lab.

- **Core biopsy:** Your doctor uses a thick needle to remove breast tissue. A pathologist checks for cancer cells. This procedure is also called a needle biopsy.

- **Surgical biopsy:** Your surgeon removes a sample of tissue. A pathologist checks the tissue for cancer cells.

  - An incisional biopsy takes a sample of a lump or abnormal area.

  - An excisional biopsy takes the entire lump or area.

If cancer cells are found, the pathologist can tell what kind of cancer it is. The most common type of breast cancer is ductal carcinoma. Abnormal cells are found in the lining of the ducts. Lobular carcinoma is another type. Abnormal cells are found in the lobules.

Staging

To plan your treatment, your doctor needs to know the extent (stage) of the disease. The stage is based on the size of the tumor and whether the cancer has spread. Staging may involve x-rays and lab tests. These tests can show whether the cancer has spread and, if so, to what parts of your body. When breast cancer spreads, cancer cells are often found in lymph nodes under the arm (axillary lymph nodes).

The stage often is not known until after surgery to remove the tumor in your breast and the lymph nodes under your arm.

These are the stages of breast cancer:

Stage 0: Stage 0 is carcinoma in situ.

- **Lobular carcinoma in situ (LCIS):** Abnormal cells are in the lining of a lobule. LCIS seldom becomes invasive cancer. However, having LCIS in one breast increases the risk of cancer for both breasts.

- **Ductal carcinoma in situ (DCIS):** Abnormal cells are in the lining of a duct. DCIS is also called intraductal carcinoma. The abnormal cells have not spread outside the duct. They have not invaded the nearby breast tissue. DCIS sometimes becomes invasive cancer if not treated.

Stage I: Stage I is an early stage of invasive breast cancer. The tumor is no more than 2 centimeters (three-quarters of an inch) across. Cancer cells have not spread beyond the breast.

Stage II: Stage II is one of the following:

- The tumor in the breast is no more than 2 centimeters (three-quarters of an inch) across. The cancer has spread to the lymph nodes under the arm.

- The tumor is between 2 and 5 centimeters (three-quarters of an inch to 2 inches). The cancer may have spread to the lymph nodes under the arm.

- The tumor is larger than 5 centimeters (2 inches). The cancer has not spread to the lymph nodes under the arm.

Stage III: Stage III may be a large tumor, but the cancer has not spread beyond the breast and nearby lymph nodes. It is locally advanced cancer.

- Stage IIIA is one of the following:

  - The tumor in the breast is smaller than 5 centimeters (2 inches). The cancer has spread to underarm lymph nodes that are attached to each other or to other structures.

  - The tumor is more than 5 centimeters across. The cancer has spread to the underarm lymph nodes.

- Stage IIIB is one of the following:
  - The tumor has grown into the chest wall or the skin of the breast.
  - The cancer has spread to lymph nodes behind the breastbone.
  - Inflammatory breast cancer is a rare type of Stage IIIB breast cancer. The breast looks red and swollen because cancer cells block the lymph vessels in the skin of the breast.
- Stage IIIC is a tumor of any size. It has spread in one of the following ways:
  - The cancer has spread to the lymph nodes behind the breastbone and under the arm.
  - The cancer has spread to the lymph nodes under or above the collarbone.

Stage IV: Stage IV is distant metastatic cancer. The cancer has spread to other parts of the body.

Recurrent: Recurrent cancer is cancer that has come back (recurred) after a period of time when it could not be detected. It may recur locally in the breast or chest wall. Or it may recur in any other part of the body, such as the bone, liver, or lungs.

Treatment Methods

Women with breast cancer have many treatment options. These include surgery, radiation therapy, chemotherapy, hormone therapy, and biological therapy. These options are described below. Many women receive more than one type of treatment.

Surgery

Surgery is the most common treatment for breast cancer. There are several types of surgery. Your doctor can explain each type, discuss and compare the benefits and risks, and describe how each will change the way you look:

- **Breast-sparing surgery:** An operation to remove the cancer but not the breast is breast-sparing surgery. It is also called breast-conserving surgery, lumpectomy, segmental mastectomy, and partial mastectomy. Sometimes an excisional biopsy serves as a lumpectomy because the surgeon removes the whole lump. The surgeon often removes the underarm lymph nodes as well. A separate incision is made. This procedure is called an axillary lymph node dissection. It shows whether cancer cells have entered the lymphatic system. After breast-sparing surgery, most women receive radiation therapy to the breast. This treatment destroys cancer cells that may remain in the breast.

- **Mastectomy:** An operation to remove the breast (or as much of the breast tissue as possible) is a mastectomy. In most cases, the surgeon also removes lymph nodes under the arm. Some women have radiation therapy after surgery.

Studies have found equal survival rates for breast-sparing surgery (with radiation therapy) and mastectomy for Stage I and Stage II breast cancer.

You may choose to have breast reconstruction. This is plastic surgery to rebuild the shape of the breast. It may be done at the same time as a mastectomy or later. If you are considering reconstruction, you may wish to talk with a plastic surgeon before having a mastectomy.

The time it takes to heal after surgery is different for each woman. Surgery causes pain and tenderness. Medicine can help control the pain. Before surgery, you should discuss the plan for pain relief with your doctor or nurse. After surgery, your doctor can adjust the plan if you need more relief. Any kind of surgery also carries a risk of infection, bleeding, or other problems. You should tell your health care provider right away if you develop any problems.

You may feel off balance if you've had one or both breasts removed. You may feel more off balance if you have large breasts. This imbalance can cause discomfort in your neck and back. Also, the skin where your breast was removed may feel tight. Your arm and shoulder muscles may feel stiff and weak. These problems usually go away. The doctor, nurse, or physical therapist can suggest exercises to help you regain movement and strength in your arm and shoulder. Exercise can also reduce stiffness and pain. You may be able to begin gentle exercises within days of surgery.

Because nerves may be injured or cut during surgery, you may have numbness and tingling in your chest, underarm, shoulder, and upper arm. These feelings usually go away within a few weeks or months. But for some women, numbness does not go away.

Removing the lymph nodes under the arm slows the flow of lymph fluid. The fluid may build up in your arm and hand and cause swelling. This swelling is lymphedema. Lymphedema can develop right after surgery or months to years later.

If lymphedema occurs, the doctor may suggest raising your arm above your heart whenever you can. The doctor may show you hand and arm exercises. Some women with lymphedema wear an elastic sleeve to improve lymph circulation. Medication, manual lymph drainage (massage), or use of a machine that gently compresses the arm may also help. You may be referred to a physical therapist or another specialist.

Radiation Therapy

Radiation therapy (also called radiotherapy) uses high-energy rays to kill cancer cells. Most women receive radiation therapy after breast-sparing surgery. Some women receive radiation therapy after a mastectomy. Treatment depends on the size of the tumor and other factors. The radiation destroys breast cancer cells that may remain in the area.

Some women have radiation therapy before surgery to destroy cancer cells and shrink the tumor. Doctors use this approach when the tumor is large or may be hard to remove. Some women also have chemotherapy or hormone therapy before surgery.

Doctors use two types of radiation therapy to treat breast cancer. Some women receive both types:

- **External radiation:** The radiation comes from a large machine outside the body. Most women go to a hospital or clinic for treatment. Treatments are usually five days a week for several weeks.

- **Internal radiation (implant radiation):** Thin plastic tubes (implants) that hold a radioactive substance are put directly in the breast. The implants stay in place for several days. A woman stays in the hospital while she has implants. Doctors remove the implants before she goes home.

Side effects depend mainly on the dose and type of radiation and the part of your body that is treated. It is common for the skin in the treated area to become red, dry, tender, and itchy. Your breast may feel heavy and tight. These problems will go away over time. Toward the end of treatment, your skin may become moist and "weepy." Exposing this area to air as much as possible can help the skin heal.

Bras and some other types of clothing may rub your skin and cause soreness. You may want to wear loose-fitting cotton clothes during this time. Gentle skin care also is important. You should check with your doctor before using any deodorants, lotions, or creams on the treated area. These effects of radiation therapy on the skin will go away. The area gradually heals once treatment is over. However, there may be a lasting change in the color of your skin.

You are likely to become very tired during radiation therapy, especially in the later weeks of treatment. Resting is important, but doctors usually advise patients to try to stay as active as they can.

Although the side effects of radiation therapy can be distressing, your doctor can usually relieve them.

Chemotherapy

Chemotherapy uses anticancer drugs to kill cancer cells. Chemotherapy for breast cancer is usually a combination of drugs. The drugs may be given as a pill or by injection into a vein (IV). Either way, the drugs enter the bloodstream and travel throughout the body.

Women with breast cancer can have chemotherapy in an outpatient part of the hospital, at the doctor's office, or at home. Some women need to stay in the hospital during treatment.

Side effects depend mainly on the specific drugs and the dose. The drugs affect cancer cells and other cells that divide rapidly:

- **Blood cells:** These cells fight infection, help your blood to clot, and carry oxygen to all parts of the body. When drugs affect your blood cells, you are more likely to get infections, bruise or bleed easily, and feel very weak and tired. Years after chemotherapy, some women have developed leukemia (cancer of the blood cells).

- **Cells in hair roots:** Chemotherapy can cause hair loss. Your hair will grow back, but it may be somewhat different in color and texture.

- **Cells that line the digestive tract:** Chemotherapy can cause poor appetite, nausea and vomiting, diarrhea, or mouth and lip sores.

Your doctor can suggest ways to control many of these side effects.

Some drugs used for breast cancer can cause tingling or numbness in the hands or feet. This problem usually goes away after treatment is over. Other problems may not go away. In some women, the drugs used for breast cancer may weaken the heart.

Some anticancer drugs can damage the ovaries. The ovaries may stop making hormones. You may have symptoms of menopause. The symptoms include hot flashes and vaginal dryness. Your menstrual periods may no longer be regular or may stop. Some women become infertile (unable to become pregnant). For women over the age of 35, infertility is likely to be permanent.

On the other hand, you may remain fertile during chemotherapy and be able to become pregnant. The effects of chemotherapy on an unborn child are not known. You should talk to your doctor about birth control before treatment begins.

Hormone Therapy

Some breast tumors need hormones to grow. Hormone therapy keeps cancer cells from getting or using the natural hormones they need. These hormones are estrogen and progesterone. Lab tests can show if a breast tumor has hormone receptors. If you have this kind of tumor, you may have hormone therapy.

This treatment uses drugs or surgery:

- **Drugs:** Your doctor may suggest a drug that can block the natural hormone. One drug is tamoxifen, which blocks estrogen. Another type of drug prevents the body from making the female hormone estradiol. Estradiol is a form of estrogen. This type of drug is an aromatase inhibitor. If you have not gone through menopause, your doctor may give you a drug that stops the ovaries from making estrogen.

- **Surgery:** If you have not gone through menopause, you may have surgery to remove your ovaries. The ovaries are the main source of the body's estrogen. A woman who has gone through menopause does not need surgery. (The ovaries produce less estrogen after menopause.)

The side effects of hormone therapy depend largely on the specific drug or type of treatment. Tamoxifen is the most common hormone treatment. In general, the side effects of tamoxifen are similar to some of the symptoms of menopause. The most common are hot flashes and vaginal discharge. Other side effects are irregular menstrual periods, headaches, fatigue, nausea, vomiting, vaginal dryness or itching, irritation of the skin around the vagina, and skin rash. Not all women who take tamoxifen have side effects.

When the ovaries are removed, menopause occurs at once. The side effects are often more severe than those caused by natural menopause. Your health care provider can suggest ways to cope with these side effects.

Biological Therapy

Biological therapy helps the immune system fight cancer. The immune system is the body's natural defense against disease.

Some women with breast cancer that has spread receive a biological therapy called Herceptin® (trastuzumab). It is a monoclonal antibody. It is made in the laboratory and binds to cancer cells.

Treatment Choices by Stage

Below are brief descriptions of common treatments for each stage. Other treatments may be appropriate for some women.

Stage 0: Stage 0 breast cancer refers to lobular carcinoma in situ (LCIS) or ductal carcinoma in situ (DCIS):

- **LCIS:** Most women with LCIS do not have treatment. Instead, the doctor may suggest regular checkups to watch for signs of breast cancer. Some women take tamoxifen to reduce the risk of developing breast cancer. Others may take part in studies of promising new preventive treatments. Having LCIS in one breast increases the risk of cancer for both breasts. A very small number of women with LCIS try to prevent cancer with surgery to remove both breasts. This is a bilateral prophylactic mastectomy. The surgeon usually does not remove the underarm lymph nodes.

- **DCIS:** Most women with DCIS have breast-sparing surgery followed by radiation therapy. Some women choose to have a total mastectomy. Underarm lymph nodes are not usually removed. Women with DCIS may receive tamoxifen to reduce the risk of developing invasive breast cancer.

Stages I, II, IIIA, and operable IIIC: Women with stage I, II, IIIA, and operable (can treat with surgery) IIIC breast cancer may have a combination of treatments. Some may have breast-sparing surgery followed by radiation therapy to the breast. This choice is common for women with stage I or II breast cancer. Others decide to have a mastectomy.

With either approach, women (especially those with stage II or IIIA breast cancer) often have lymph nodes under the arm removed. The doctor may suggest radiation therapy after mastectomy if cancer cells are found in one to three lymph nodes under the arm, or if the tumor in the breast is large. If cancer cells are found in more than three lymph nodes under the arm, the doctor usually will suggest radiation therapy after mastectomy.

Some women have chemotherapy before surgery. This is neoadjuvant therapy (treatment before the main treatment). Chemotherapy before surgery may shrink a large tumor so that breast-sparing surgery is possible. Women with large stage II or IIIA breast tumors often choose this treatment.

After surgery, many women receive adjuvant therapy. Adjuvant therapy is treatment given after the main treatment to increase the chances of a cure. Radiation treatment can kill cancer cells in and near the breast. Women also may have systemic treatment such as chemotherapy, hormone therapy, or both. This treatment can destroy cancer cells that remain anywhere in the body. It can prevent the cancer from coming back in the breast or elsewhere.

Stages IIIB and Inoperable IIIC: Women with Stage IIIB (including inflammatory breast cancer) or inoperable Stage IIIC breast cancer usually have chemotherapy. (Inoperable cancer means it cannot be treated with surgery.)

If the chemotherapy shrinks the tumor, the doctor then may suggest further treatment:

- **Mastectomy:** The surgeon removes the breast. In most cases, the lymph nodes under the arm are removed. After surgery, a woman may receive radiation therapy to the chest and underarm area.

- **Breast-sparing surgery:** The surgeon removes the cancer but not the breast. In most cases, the lymph nodes under the arm are removed. After surgery, a woman may receive radiation therapy to the breast and underarm area.

- **Radiation therapy instead of surgery:** Some women have radiation therapy but no surgery. The doctor also may recommend more chemotherapy, hormone therapy, or both. This therapy may help prevent the disease from coming back in the breast or elsewhere.

Stage IV: In most cases, women with Stage IV breast cancer have hormone therapy, chemotherapy, or both. Some also may have biological therapy. Radiation may be used to control tumors in certain parts of the body. These treatments are not likely to cure the disease, but they may help a woman live longer.

Many women have supportive care along with anticancer treatments. Anticancer treatments are given to slow the progress of the disease. Supportive care helps manage pain, other symptoms, or side effects (such as nausea). It does not aim to extend a woman's life. Supportive care can help a woman feel better physically and emotionally. Some women with advanced cancer decide to have only supportive care.

Recurrent breast cancer: Recurrent cancer is cancer that has come back after it could not be detected. Treatment for the recurrent disease depends mainly on the location and extent of the cancer. Another main factor is the type of treatment the woman had before.

If breast cancer comes back only in the breast after breast-sparing surgery, the woman may have a mastectomy. Chances are good that the disease will not come back again.

If breast cancer recurs in other parts of the body, treatment may involve chemotherapy, hormone therapy, or biological therapy. Radiation therapy may help control cancer that recurs in the chest muscles or in certain other areas of the body.

Treatment can seldom cure cancer that recurs outside the breast. Supportive care is often an important part of the treatment plan. Many patients have supportive care to ease their symptoms and anticancer treatments to slow the progress of the disease. Some receive only supportive care to improve their quality of life.

Breast Reconstruction

Some women who plan to have a mastectomy decide to have breast reconstruction. Other women prefer to wear a breast form (prosthesis). Others decide to do nothing. All of these options have pros and cons. What is right for one woman may not be right for another. What is important is that nearly every woman treated for breast cancer has choices.

Breast reconstruction may be done at the same time as the mastectomy, or later on. If you are thinking about breast reconstruction, you should talk to a plastic surgeon before the mastectomy, even if you plan to have your reconstruction later on.

There are many ways to reconstruct the breast. Some women choose to have implants. Implants may be made of saline or silicone. The safety of silicone breast implants has been under review by the U.S. Food and Drug Administration (FDA) for several years. If you are thinking about having silicone implants, you may want to talk with your doctor about the FDA findings.

You also may have breast reconstruction with tissue that the plastic surgeon moves from another part of your body. Skin, muscle, and fat can come from your lower abdomen, back, or buttocks. The surgeon uses this tissue to create a breast shape.

Which type of reconstruction is best depends on your age, body type, and the type of surgery you had. The plastic surgeon can explain the risks and benefits of each type of reconstruction.

Chapter 51

Male Breast Cancer

Breast cancer may occur in men. Men at any age may develop breast cancer, but it is usually detected (found) in men between 60 and 70 years of age. Male breast cancer makes up less than 1% of all cases of breast cancer.

The following types of breast cancer are found in men:

- **Infiltrating ductal carcinoma:** Cancer that has spread beyond the cells lining ducts in the breast. Most men with breast cancer have this type of cancer.

- **Ductal carcinoma in situ:** Abnormal cells that are found in the lining of a duct; also called intraductal carcinoma.

- **Inflammatory breast cancer:** A type of cancer in which the breast looks red and swollen and feels warm.

- **Paget disease of the nipple:** A tumor that has grown from ducts beneath the nipple onto the surface of the nipple.

Lobular carcinoma in situ (abnormal cells found in one of the lobes or sections of the breast), which sometimes occurs in women, has not been seen in men.

PDQ® Cancer Information Summary. National Cancer Institute; Bethesda, MD. Male Breast Cancer (PDQ®): Treatment - Patient. Updated 06/2006. Available at: http://cancer.gov. Accessed August 18, 2006.

Risk Factors and Diagnosis

Anything that increases your risk of getting a disease is called a risk factor. Risk factors for breast cancer in men may include the following:

- Being exposed to radiation

- Having a disease related to high levels of estrogen in the body, such as cirrhosis (liver disease) or Klinefelter syndrome (a genetic disorder)

- Having several female relatives who have had breast cancer, especially relatives who have an alteration of the BRCA2 gene

Male breast cancer is sometimes caused by inherited gene mutations (changes). The genes in cells carry the hereditary information that is received from a person's parents. Hereditary breast cancer makes up approximately 5% to 10% of all breast cancer. Some altered genes related to breast cancer are more common in certain ethnic groups. Men who have an altered gene related to breast cancer have an increased risk of developing this disease.

Tests have been developed that can detect altered genes. These genetic tests are sometimes done for members of families with a high risk of cancer.

Lumps and other symptoms may be caused by male breast cancer. Other conditions may cause the same symptoms. A doctor should be seen if changes in the breasts are noticed.

The following tests and procedures may be used to detect (find) and diagnose breast cancer in men:

Biopsy: The removal of cells or tissues so they can be viewed under a microscope by a pathologist to check for signs of cancer. The following are different types of biopsies:

- **Needle biopsy:** The removal of part of a lump, suspicious tissue, or fluid, using a thin needle. This procedure is also called a fine-needle aspiration biopsy.

- **Core biopsy:** The removal of part of a lump or suspicious tissue using a wide needle.

- **Excisional biopsy:** The removal of an entire lump or suspicious tissue.

Estrogen and progesterone receptor test: A test to measure the amount of estrogen and progesterone (hormones) receptors in cancer tissue. If cancer is found in the breast, tissue from the tumor is checked in the laboratory to find out whether estrogen and progesterone could affect the way cancer grows. The test results show whether hormone therapy may stop the cancer from growing.

HER2 test: A test to measure the amount of HER2 in cancer tissue. HER2 is a growth factor protein that sends growth signals to cells. When cancer forms, the cells may make too much of the protein, causing more cancer cells to grow. If cancer is found in the breast, tissue from the tumor is checked in the laboratory to find out if there is too much HER2 in the cells. The test results show whether monoclonal antibody therapy may stop the cancer from growing.

Prognosis

Survival for men with breast cancer is similar to that for women with breast cancer when their stage at diagnosis is the same. Breast cancer in men, however, is often diagnosed at a later stage. Cancer found at a later stage may be less likely to be cured.

The prognosis (chance of recovery) and treatment options depend on the following:

- The stage of the cancer (whether it is in the breast only or has spread to other places in the body)

- The type of breast cancer

- Estrogen-receptor and progesterone-receptor levels in the tumor tissue

- Whether the cancer is also found in the other breast

- The patient's age and general health

Stages of Male Breast Cancer

After breast cancer has been diagnosed, tests are done to find out if cancer cells have spread within the breast or to other parts of the body. This process is called staging. The information gathered from the staging process determines the stage of the disease. It is important to know the stage in order to plan treatment. Breast cancer in men is staged the same as it is in women (see Chapter 50—Breast Cancer for more information). The spread of cancer from the breast to lymph nodes and other parts of the body appears to be similar in men and women.

Recurrent male breast cancer: Recurrent breast cancer is cancer that has recurred (come back) after it has been treated. The cancer may come back in the breast, in the chest wall, or in other parts of the body.

Treatment Option Overview

Different types of treatment are available for men with breast cancer. Some treatments are standard (the currently used treatment), and some are being tested in clinical trials. Before starting treatment, patients may want to think about taking part in a clinical trial. A treatment clinical trial is a research study meant to help improve current treatments or obtain information on new treatments for patients with cancer. When clinical trials show that a new treatment is better than the standard treatment, the new treatment may become the standard treatment.

Clinical trials are taking place in many parts of the country. Information about ongoing clinical trials is available from the National Cancer Institute website (http://www.cancer.gov). Choosing the most appropriate cancer treatment is a decision that ideally involves the patient, family, and health care team.

Four types of standard treatment are used to treat men with breast cancer:

Surgery: Surgery for men with breast cancer is usually a modified radical mastectomy (removal of the breast, many of the lymph nodes under the arm, the lining over the chest muscles, and sometimes part of the chest wall muscles).

Chemotherapy: Chemotherapy is a cancer treatment that uses drugs to stop the growth of cancer cells, either by killing the cells or by stopping the cells from dividing. When chemotherapy is taken by mouth or injected into a vein or muscle, the drugs enter the bloodstream and can reach cancer cells throughout the body (systemic chemotherapy). When chemotherapy is placed directly into the spinal column, an organ, or a body cavity such as the abdomen, the drugs mainly affect cancer cells in those areas (regional chemotherapy). The way the chemotherapy is given depends on the type and stage of the cancer being treated.

Hormone therapy: Hormone therapy is a cancer treatment that removes hormones or blocks their action and stops cancer cells from growing. Hormones are substances made by glands in the body and circulated in the bloodstream. Some hormones can cause certain cancers to grow. If tests show that the cancer cells have places where hormones can attach (receptors), drugs, surgery, or radiation therapy are used to reduce the production of hormones or block them from working.

Radiation therapy: Radiation therapy is a cancer treatment that uses high-energy x-rays or other types of radiation to kill cancer cells. There are two types of radiation therapy. External radiation therapy uses a machine outside the body to send radiation toward the cancer. Internal radiation therapy uses a radioactive substance sealed in needles, seeds, wires, or catheters that are placed directly into or near the cancer. The way the radiation therapy is given depends on the type and stage of the cancer being treated.

New Treatments

New types of treatment are being tested in clinical trials. These include the following:

Monoclonal antibodies as adjuvant therapy: Monoclonal antibody therapy is a cancer treatment that uses antibodies made in the laboratory, from a single type of immune system cell. These antibodies can identify substances on cancer cells or normal substances that may help cancer cells grow. The antibodies attach to the substances and kill the cancer cells, block their growth, or keep them from spreading. Monoclonal antibodies are given by infusion. They may be used alone or to carry drugs, toxins, or radioactive material directly to cancer cells. Monoclonal antibodies are also used in combination with chemotherapy as adjuvant therapy (treatment given after surgery to increase the chances of a cure).

Trastuzumab (Herceptin) is a monoclonal antibody that blocks the effects of the growth factor protein HER2.

Treatment Options for Male Breast Cancer

Breast cancer in men is treated the same as breast cancer in women.

Initial surgery: Treatment for men diagnosed with breast cancer is usually modified radical mastectomy.

Adjuvant therapy: Therapy given after an operation when cancer cells can no longer be seen is called adjuvant therapy. Even if the doctor removes all the cancer that can be seen at the time of the operation, the patient may be given radiation therapy, chemotherapy, hormone therapy, and/or monoclonal antibody therapy after surgery to try to kill any cancer cells that may be left.

- **Node-negative:** For men whose cancer is node-negative (cancer has not spread to the lymph nodes), adjuvant therapy should be considered on the same basis as for a woman with breast cancer because there is no evidence that response to therapy is different for men and women.

- **Node-positive:** For men whose cancer is node-positive (cancer has spread to the lymph nodes), adjuvant therapy may include the following:

  - Chemotherapy plus tamoxifen (to block the effect of estrogen)
  - Other hormone therapy
  - A clinical trial of trastuzumab (Herceptin)

These treatments appear to increase survival in men as they do in women. The patient's response to hormone therapy depends on whether there are hormone receptors (proteins) in the tumor. Most breast cancers in men have these receptors. Hormone therapy is usually recommended for male breast cancer patients, but it can have many side effects, including hot flashes and impotence (the inability to have an erection adequate for sexual intercourse).

Distant metastases: Treatment for men with distant metastases (cancer that has spread to other parts of the body) may be hormone therapy, chemotherapy, or both. Hormone therapy may include the following:

- Orchiectomy (the removal of the testicles to decrease hormone production)

- Luteinizing hormone-releasing hormone agonist with or without total androgen blockade (to decrease the production of sex hormones)

- Tamoxifen for cancer that is estrogen-receptor positive

- Progesterone (a female hormone)

- Aromatase inhibitors (to lessen the amount of estrogen produced)

- Hormone therapies may be used in sequence (one after the other). Standard chemotherapy regimens may be used if hormone therapy does not work. Men usually respond to therapy in the same way as women who have breast cancer.

Treatment options for locally recurrent male breast cancer: For men with locally recurrent disease (cancer that has come back in a limited area after treatment), treatment is usually either:

- surgery combined with chemotherapy; or
- radiation therapy combined with chemotherapy.

Chapter 52

Cancers of the Female Reproductive Organs

Each year, approximately 77,000 women are diagnosed with one of the gynecologic cancers:

- ovarian
- uterine
- cervical
- vulvar
- vaginal
- tubal

Cancer is a word used to define a collection of diseases that share one unique characteristic—the uncontrolled growth of cells. Our bodies are made up of cells, with each one containing 23 pairs of chromosomes. Distributed amongst the 46 chromosomes are approximately 300,000–500,000 genes. The genes contribute to how we grow, what we look like, and how we behave. In normal cells, the chromosomes reproduce every time the cell divides. Occasionally, something goes wrong and a number of genes are altered. When this happens, the cells escape from the normal growth control mechanisms, and they multiply until they form a mass of cells, usually referred to as a tumor.

Some tumors are benign and are composed of cells which resemble the normal cells of that organ. Although they may form a large mass, they do not spread. However, when cells undergo malignant change, they look "wild" under a microscope. These cells can invade nearby normal tissue and spread to other parts of the body: the condition is

From "Maintain Your Gynecologic Health with Education and Early Detection," reprinted with permission from the Gynecologic Cancer Foundation, http://www.gcf.org. © 2006. All rights reserved.

known as cancer. Metastasis is the word used to define the spreading of cancer from where it started to a new location.

Cancers that develop in the various organs manifest themselves in different ways, which is why each cancer has a unique way of being diagnosed. For example, breast cancer is detected by changes seen on mammograms, and cervical cancers usually produce abnormalities detected by Pap tests. Once a cancer is diagnosed, it is given a stage indicating how advanced the tumor is. How a cancer is treated depends on the type and stage of the cancer.

Gynecologic cancers attack a woman's reproductive organ(s) including the cervix, uterus, ovaries, fallopian tubes, vagina, and vulva. They are named according to the organ of origin and can also be classified by the kind of tissue in which they arise. Each year approximately 77,000 women in the United States are diagnosed with cancers affecting the reproductive organs. Although they are often discussed as a group, gynecologic cancers have a spectrum of different causes, prevention and detection methods, treatment, and likelihood of a cure.

Why do women get these cancers?

Biomedical research has discovered that some genes, called oncogenes, promote the growth of cancer. You can acquire these genetic mutations during life (for example, through smoking, aging, or environmental influences) or you can inherit these mutations from your parents or grandparents. Many cancers of the cervix, vagina, and vulva are caused by a virus that blocks normal gene function. So far, only a few of the specific genes leading to reproductive cancers have been identified. Knowing your family history can increase your chance of early diagnosis and can help you take action toward prevention. The knowledge that some cancers are linked together and run in your family can help you know what other diseases you should be screened for, such as breast or colon cancers. Your physician can determine an appropriate screening and prevention program based on your family's history of cancer and other factors.

Who should take care of me?

Detection and treatment of gynecologic cancers require physicians who are trained specifically in this area. Gynecologic oncologists are cancer specialists whose training is first that of an obstetrician-gynecologist. These physicians then train for an additional three to four years in the treatment of gynecologic cancers (surgery, radiation therapy, chemotherapy, and experimental treatments).

This training is available in a number of medical centers around the country. Physicians who complete this training are able to offer patients the therapy or combination of therapies most likely to be successful, without fragmenting care among many physicians. Gynecologic oncologists practice in a variety of settings including teaching hospitals, cancer centers, regional and local hospitals, and private offices.

What are the warning signs?

Gynecologic oncologists advise women to seek medical attention if these symptoms persist for two weeks:

- A change in bowel or bladder habits
- A genital sore that does not heal
- Unusual vaginal discharge
- A thickening or lump that either causes pain or can be seen or felt
- Persistent indigestion
- Pain in the pelvic area
- Persistent or progressive fullness, bloating, or pressure in the abdomen or pelvis

In addition, women should seek medical attention immediately if they have vaginal bleeding after menopause, a new onset of heavy menstrual periods, or bleeding between periods.

Ovarian Cancer

What is ovarian cancer?

The most deadly of the gynecologic malignancies, ovarian cancers, usually arise on the surface of the ovary. When this happens, the ovaries frequently become enlarged. The cancer cells often fall off of the ovary's surface and implant throughout the abdominal cavity. Each one of these seedlings can then grow into a separate ovarian cancer tumor nodule.

What are the common symptoms?

The most common symptoms are a pressure or fullness in the pelvis, abdominal bloating, or changes in bowel and bladder patterns which are constant and progressive. For women over 40, persistent digestive problems such as stomach discomfort, distention, and gas might indicate the need to be checked for ovarian cancer, usually involving a pelvic ultrasound and a blood test called a CA 125.

How is screening done for ovarian cancer

There are no established tests to screen for ovarian cancer for average-risk women. Studies are underway to evaluate blood tests and ultrasound, but so far neither have proven that a screening method can save lives. For the highest risk women, ultrasound and a CA 125 test every 6–12 months is often advised.

How is it treated?

The cornerstone of therapy is surgery. Therefore, it is vitally important that a patient be operated on by the right doctor. A gynecologic oncologist has special surgical training which enables him/her to perform the appropriate and optimal surgical procedure. Furthermore, he/she understands the biology of ovarian cancer and can appropriately address each of the metastatic sites and remove all of the visible tumor whenever possible. For women who don't have access to these specialists, it is important to determine that their surgeon understands that the key to success is removal of as much tumor as possible. After surgery, most patients receive chemotherapy for approximately six months.

What are the risk factors?

The risk of ovarian cancer increases with age, especially around the time of menopause. There are cases of ovarian cancer in women as young as teens, but it is most often a disease of women older than 50. A family history of ovarian cancer is one of the most important risk factors. It is important for women to find out if members of their family have been affected by cancers of the ovaries, uterus, colon, or breast because there may be a hereditary tendency linking these cancers.

The genes for ovarian cancer are not "sex linked," which means that familial cancer risk can be transmitted by either the mother or the father. For example, if your father's sister had ovarian cancer, you are at a higher risk. Still, it is important to remember that most women with ovarian cancer do not have a family history of this disease. Infertility and not bearing children are additional risk factors, whereas pregnancy can decrease the risk of developing ovarian cancer. Birth control pills provide an incremental reduction in risk each year they are taken. Tubal ligation has also been found to significantly reduce the ovarian cancer risk.

Uterine Cancer

What is uterine cancer?

Most uterine cancers begin in the lining of the uterus (endometrium). The endometrium is the tissue shed each month with the menstrual cycle. After menopause, the endometrium flattens out. With uterine cancer, it is typically the cells in the lining that grow out of control and invade the muscle of the uterus (the myometrium). From there, the cancer can spread to lymph nodes or surrounding organs. Another type of uterine cancer is uterine sarcoma. These tumors develop in the walls of the uterus and are less common than endometrial cancers.

What are common symptoms?

Bleeding after menopause and irregular, or excessive vaginal bleeding before menopause, may be a warning sign of uterine cancer. Uterine cancer is frequently diagnosed at an early stage because the bleeding is a trigger that prompts women to see a physician. Enlarging fibroids after menopause may be a warning sign for uterine sarcoma.

How is it treated?

A diagnosis of uterine cancer is typically made by an endometrial biopsy, and is frequently treated by hysterectomy and surgical staging. This involves removing selected lymph nodes and performing biopsies to find the extent of the cancer. Many patients are cured by surgery alone. For some uterine cancers, including sarcomas, radiation treatments or chemotherapy may be added to the surgical treatments.

What are the risk factors?

For endometrial cancers, the risk factors include obesity, hypertension, diabetes, tamoxifen use, and late menopause. Women who have not been pregnant have a slightly higher risk. Use of estrogen medications without the balancing effect of the other female hormone, progesterone, causes increased risk. Pelvic radiation and tamoxifen use are associated with increased risk for uterine sarcomas.

Cervical Cancer

What is cervical cancer?

Cervical cancer is the most preventable gynecologic cancer. The Pap test has significantly reduced the incidence and death rates of cervical cancer for women who get regular tests. A new cervical cancer vaccine holds promise for further reducing the risks of this cancer. The Pap test can detect dysplasias (abnormal cells) or precancerous changes in the cervix that precede the development of cancer, thereby allowing physicians to intervene. When cervical cancer arises, the tumor replaces the normal cervix and can spread to the lymph nodes, bladder, rectum, or other distant sites.

Since 2005 women age 30 and older have had an additional option for screening for cervical cancer. The new test checks directly for the HPV virus that can cause cervical cancer. The main advantage of combining the HPV test with a Pap test is that women with both a negative HPV test and a normal Pap test are at very low risk for cervical cancer and can be screened less often (no more than every three years).

A vaccine to prevent cervical cancer became available in the United States in 2006. The vaccine is most effective when given before a women starts to have sex. The vaccine is not a substitute for cervical cancer screening, which should still be scheduled according to the American Cancer Society guidelines.

What are the common symptoms?

Cervical cancer typically has no symptoms in the early stages. That is why Pap tests are important. Bleeding after intercourse, excessive discharge, and abnormal bleeding between periods are the most frequent symptoms. Cervical cancer is easily diagnosed by a magnified view of the cervix, called colposcopy, and cervical biopsies that are done in the doctor's office. Sometimes a minor surgical procedure called a LEEP (loop electrocautery excision procedure) or cone biopsy makes the diagnosis.

How is it treated?

Most cervical cancers are diagnosed when they are still within the cervix. Most tumors within the cervix can be successfully treated with a radical hysterectomy or radiation therapy. Both forms of treatment have similar cure rates but different side effects. In a radical hysterectomy, the cervix, uterus, and surrounding tissues and lymph nodes are removed, but not necessarily the ovaries. This is important for young women since the loss of fertility does not have to be compounded by early menopause. Some patients may opt for radiation therapy and avoid surgery, but they may have later side effects such as bowel and bladder problems, and vaginal dryness. When cervical cancer has spread outside the cervix, radiation therapy is most effective. Some of the earliest tumors may be treated with a cone biopsy or a radical trachelectomy (the removal of the cervix without removal of the upper uterus). These surgeries have the advantage of preserving fertility. If fertility is not important, the early tumors may be treated with a simple hysterectomy.

What are the risk factors?

Socioeconomic class is a significant risk factor, since a lack of access to medical care often eliminates the opportunity for early diagnosis by Pap test screening. A sexually transmitted virus called HPV (human papilloma virus) is the cause of most cervical cancer. HPV infection is common in all sexually active women, but causes cancer only in a few. Smoking, a high number of sexual partners, and early age of first intercourse are other risk factors. HIV infection is also associated with cervical cancer.

Vulvar Cancer

Vulvar cancer is typically a disease of older women and is often heralded by itching in the vulvar area. Women in their 70s, 80s, and 90s should not attribute perineal itching only to yeast and other infections and should have a physician examine them if these symptoms persist. Most vulvar lesions in older women should be biopsied. It is encouraging to note that this is usually a very curable type of cancer, typically with surgical removal of the vulvar lesions and the groin lymph nodes. Risk factors include diabetes, advanced age, and chronic vulvar irritation.

Vaginal Cancer

Vaginal cancers are very rare. They are usually diagnosed in elderly women and treated with radiation. One exception occurs in women who were exposed to a drug called DES. DES is a hormone medication that was used years ago to try to prevent miscarriage. Decades later scientists realized that daughters born of mothers who took DES had an abnormal risk of developing a rare form of vaginal cancer called clear cell cancer. DES has not been used in pregnancy since the 1960's. Discharge or bleeding are symptoms of vaginal cancer.

Cancer of the Fallopian Tubes

The fallopian tubes will rarely develop cancer. Symptoms, treatments, and risk factors for fallopian tube cancer are similar to ovarian cancer.

Typical Questions to Ask your Doctor

You will probably have many questions for your doctor if you have been diagnosed with a gynecologic cancer. The following are typical questions you'll want answered:

- Has the cancer spread? What does that mean?
- What happens in surgery?
- What happens with chemotherapy? How is it given and how often?
- Will I lose my hair?
- What happens with radiation therapy?
- Can I still work?
- How will this affect my family?
- Is it hereditary? Should I see a genetic specialist?
- Will I be infertile?
- How will this affect my sex life?
- What alternative treatments should I consider?
- How important is nutrition?
- Are you the appropriate doctor to be taking care of me?
- Have you had special training in the management of gynecologic cancers?
- Where should I go for additional information?

What Now?

You have just received a great deal of information, much of it sounding scary. Relax—the good news is the more you know the better you'll be at protecting yourself. We recommend that you log onto the Women's Cancer Network at www.wcn.org to learn more. Try taking the personal cancer risk assessment to learn if you are high risk for any gynecologic cancer. Keep asking questions and keep learning. It is for your health.

Chapter 53

Gestational Trophoblastic Tumors

Gestational trophoblastic tumor, a rare cancer in women, is a disease in which cancer (malignant) cells grow in the tissues that are formed following conception (the joining of sperm and egg). Gestational trophoblastic tumors start inside the uterus, the hollow, muscular, pear-shaped organ where a baby grows. This type of cancer occurs in women during the years when they are able to have children. There are two types of gestational trophoblastic tumors: hydatidiform mole and choriocarcinoma.

If a patient has a hydatidiform mole (also called a molar pregnancy), the sperm and egg cells have joined without the development of a baby in the uterus. Instead, the tissue that is formed resembles grape-like cysts. Hydatidiform mole does not spread outside of the uterus to other parts of the body.

If a patient has a choriocarcinoma, the tumor may have started from a hydatidiform mole or from tissue that remains in the uterus following an abortion or delivery of a baby. Choriocarcinoma can spread from the uterus to other parts of the body. A very rare type of gestational trophoblastic tumor starts in the uterus where the placenta was attached. This type of cancer is called placental-site trophoblastic disease.

PDQ® Cancer Information Summary. National Cancer Institute; Bethesda, MD. Gestational Trophoblastic Tumors (PDQ®): Treatment - Patient. Updated 06/2005. Available at: http://cancer.gov. Accessed June 23, 2006.

Gestational trophoblastic tumor is not always easy to find. In its early stages, it may look like a normal pregnancy. A doctor should be seen if the there is vaginal bleeding (not menstrual bleeding) and if a woman is pregnant and the baby hasn't moved at the expected time.

If there are symptoms, a doctor may use several tests to see if the patient has a gestational trophoblastic tumor. An internal (pelvic) examination is usually the first of these tests. The doctor will feel for any lumps or strange feeling in the shape or size of the uterus. The doctor may then do an ultrasound, a test that uses sound waves to find tumors. A blood test will also be done to look for high levels of a hormone called beta-hCG (beta human chorionic gonadotropin) which is present during normal pregnancy. If a woman is not pregnant and hCG is in the blood, it can be a sign of gestational trophoblastic tumor.

The chance of recovery (prognosis) and choice of treatment depend on the type of gestational trophoblastic tumor, whether it has spread to other places, and the patient's general state of health.

Stages of Gestational Trophoblastic Tumors

Once gestational trophoblastic tumor has been found, more tests will be done to find out if the cancer has spread from inside the uterus to other parts of the body (staging). A doctor needs to know the stage of the disease to plan treatment. The following stages are used for gestational trophoblastic tumor:

Hydatidiform mole: Cancer is found only in the space inside the uterus. If the cancer is found in the muscle of the uterus, it is called an invasive mole (choriocarcinoma destruens).

Placental-site gestational trophoblastic tumors: Cancer is found in the place where the placenta was attached and in the muscle of the uterus.

Nonmetastatic: Cancer cells have grown inside the uterus from tissue remaining following treatment of a hydatidiform mole or following an abortion or delivery of a baby. Cancer has not spread outside the uterus.

Metastatic, good prognosis: Cancer cells have grown inside the uterus from tissue remaining following treatment of a hydatidiform mole or following an abortion or delivery of a baby. The cancer has spread from the uterus to other parts of the body. Metastatic gestational trophoblastic tumors are considered good prognosis or poor prognosis.

Metastatic gestational trophoblastic tumor is considered good prognosis if all of the following are true:

1. The last pregnancy was less than 4 months ago

2. The level of beta-hCG in the blood is low

3. Cancer has not spread to the liver or brain

4. The patient has not received chemotherapy earlier

Metastatic, poor prognosis: Cancer cells have grown inside the uterus from tissue remaining following treatment of a hydatidiform mole or following an abortion or delivery of a baby. The cancer has spread from the uterus to other parts of the body. Metastatic gestational trophoblastic tumors are considered good prognosis or poor prognosis.

Metastatic gestational trophoblastic tumor is considered poor prognosis if any the following are true:

1. The last pregnancy was more than 4 months ago

2. The level of beta-hCG in the blood is high

3. Cancer has spread to the liver or brain

4. The patient received chemotherapy earlier and the cancer did not go away

5. The tumor began after the completion of a normal pregnancy

Recurrent: Recurrent disease means that the cancer has come back (recurred) after it has been treated. It may come back in the uterus or in another part of the body.

Treatment Option Overview

There are treatments for all patients with gestational trophoblastic tumor. Two kinds of treatment are used: surgery (taking out the cancer) and chemotherapy (using drugs to kill cancer cells). Radiation therapy (using high-energy x-rays to kill cancer cells) may be used in certain cases to treat cancer that has spread to other parts of the body.

The doctor may take out the cancer using one of the following operations:

1. Dilation and curettage (D & C) with suction evacuation is stretching the opening of the uterus (the cervix) and removing the material inside the uterus with a small vacuum-like device. The walls of the uterus are then scraped gently to remove any material that may remain in the uterus. This is used only for molar pregnancies.

2. Hysterectomy is an operation to take out the uterus. The ovaries usually are not removed in the treatment of this disease.

Chemotherapy uses drugs to kill cancer cells. It may be taken by pill or put into the body by a needle in a vein or muscle. It is called a systemic treatment because the drugs enter the bloodstream, travel through the body, and can kill cancer cells outside the uterus. Chemotherapy may be given before or after surgery or alone.

Radiation therapy uses high-energy x-rays to kill cancer cells and shrink tumors. Radiation may come from a machine outside the body (external-beam radiation therapy) or from putting materials that produce radiation (radioisotopes) through thin plastic tubes into the area where the cancer cells are found (internal radiation).

Treatment by Stage

Treatment of gestational trophoblastic tumor depends on the stage of the disease, and the patient's age and overall condition.

Standard treatment may be considered because of its effectiveness in patients in past studies, or participation in a clinical trial may be considered. Not all patients are cured with standard therapy and some standard treatments may have more side effects than are desired. For these reasons, clinical trials are designed to find better ways to treat cancer patients and are based on the most up-to-date information. Clinical trials are ongoing in most parts of the country for most stages of gestational trophoblastic tumor. To learn more about clinical trials, call the Cancer Information Service at 800-4-CANCER (800-422-6237); TTY at 800-332-8615.

Hydatidiform mole: Treatment may be one of the following:

1. Removal of the mole using dilation and curettage (D & C) and suction evacuation

2. Surgery to remove the uterus (hysterectomy)

Following surgery, the doctor will follow the patient closely with regular blood tests to make sure the level of beta-hCG in the blood falls to normal levels. If the blood level of beta-hCG increases or does not go down to normal, more tests will be done to see whether the tumor has spread. Treatment will then depend on whether the patient has nonmetastatic disease or metastatic disease.

Placental-site gestational trophoblastic tumors: Treatment will probably be surgery to remove the uterus (hysterectomy).

Nonmetastatic gestational trophoblastic tumors: Treatment may be one of the following:

1. Chemotherapy

2. Surgery to remove the uterus (hysterectomy) if the patient no longer wishes to have children

Good prognosis metastatic gestational trophoblastic tumors: Treatment may be one of the following:

1. Chemotherapy

2. Surgery to remove the uterus (hysterectomy) followed by chemotherapy

3. Chemotherapy followed by hysterectomy if cancer remains following chemotherapy

Poor prognosis metastatic gestational trophoblastic tumors: Treatment will probably be chemotherapy. Radiation therapy may also be given to places where the cancer has spread, such as the brain.

Recurrent gestational trophoblastic tumors: Treatment will probably be chemotherapy.

Chapter 54

Germ Cell Tumors

What are germ cell tumors?

Germ cells are reproductive cells that develop in the testicles in males and the ovaries in females. Sometimes these cells migrate to other areas of the body, such as the chest, abdomen, or brain, and may cause a rare type of cancer called a germ cell tumor. Germ cell tumors form in developing cells and usually contain normal tissues that are located in abnormal areas.

Germ cell tumors can be classified as benign teratomas or malignant (cancerous) germ cell tumors. Teratomas can be either mature (tissue that is less likely to become cancer) or immature (tissue that can spread and become cancer). Germ cell tumors of early childhood have biological characteristics that are different than those that occur in adolescents and young adults. The major types of germ cell tumors are:

- Testicular germ cell tumors of early childhood—form within the testes of boys younger than 4 years of age. Treatment includes a radical inguinal orchiectomy (removal of the testicle).

- Testicular germ cell tumors of adolescence and young adulthood—form within the testes of older boys. Are classified as either

"Germ Cell Tumors for the Pediatric Patient," reprinted with permission from the University of Texas M.D. Anderson Cancer Center. © 2004 M.D. Anderson Cancer Center.

seminoma or nonseminoma. Seminomas are more sensitive to radiation therapy.

• Extragonadal germ cell tumors of early childhood—germ cell tumors that are not located in the reproductive organs (testicles or ovaries) or in the brain. These tumors are usually located in the sacrum and the coccyx (tailbone). They occur more frequently in girls than in boys, and can be present at birth.

• Extragonadal germ cell tumors of adolescence and young adulthood—usually located within the chest.

• Ovarian germ cell tumors, a rare type of cancer that affects teenage girls and young women—cancer cells are found in egg making cells in an ovary. Treatment includes a unilateral salpingo-oophorectomy (removal of ovary and fallopian tube).

What are the symptoms of germ cell tumors?

The first symptoms will correspond to the site of the tumor. A solid mass or lump may be noticed. If the mass interferes with a function of the body it may cause other symptoms.

How are germ cell tumors diagnosed and treated?

If a germ cell tumor is suspected, the doctor may order laboratory tests, x-rays, and other tests to find out if the cancer cells have spread to other parts of the body. This is called staging. It is important to know the stage of the disease to plan treatment. Many malignant germ cell tumors produce substances (alpha-fetoprotein or human chorionic gonadotropin) that allow the tumor to be monitored with blood tests. Treatment for germ cell tumors depends upon the location, stage, and type of tumor. Complete or near complete surgical removal of the tumor is often possible. If the tumor cannot be completely removed, chemotherapy or radiation will also be given.

Chapter 55

Testicular and Penile Cancers

Testicular Cancer

Testicular cancer is a disease in which malignant (cancer) cells form in the tissues of one or both testicles. The testicles are two egg-shaped glands located inside the scrotum (a sac of loose skin that lies directly below the penis). The testicles are held within the scrotum by the spermatic cord, which also contains the vas deferens and vessels and nerves of the testicles.

The testicles are the male sex glands and produce testosterone and sperm. Germ cells within the testicles produce immature sperm that travel through a network of tubules (tiny tubes) and larger tubes into the epididymis (a long coiled tube next to the testicles) where the sperm mature and are stored.

Almost all testicular cancers start in the germ cells. The two main types of testicular germ cell tumors are seminomas and nonseminomas. These two types grow and spread differently and are treated differently. Nonseminomas tend to grow and spread more quickly than seminomas. Seminomas are more sensitive to radiation. A testicular tumor that contains both seminoma and nonseminoma cells is treated as a nonseminoma.

This chapter includes PDQ® Cancer Information Summary. National Cancer Institute; Bethesda, MD. Testicular Cancer (PDQ®): Treatment - Patient. Updated 01/2006. Available at: http://cancer.gov. Accessed April 30, 2006. And, PDQ® Cancer Information Summary. National Cancer Institute; Bethesda, MD. Penile Cancer (PDQ®): Treatment - Patient. Updated 07/2006. Available at: http://cancer.gov. Accessed December 2, 2006.

Risks and Diagnosis

Testicular cancer is the most common cancer in men 20 to 35 years old. Health history can affect the risk of developing testicular cancer. Anything that increases the chance of getting a disease is called a risk factor. Risk factors for testicular cancer include the following:

- Having had an undescended testicle
- Having had abnormal development of the testicles
- Having a personal or family history of testicular cancer
- Having Klinefelter syndrome
- Being white

Possible signs of testicular cancer include swelling or discomfort in the scrotum. These and other symptoms may be caused by testicular cancer. Other conditions may cause the same symptoms. A doctor should be consulted if any of the following problems occur:

- A painless lump or swelling in either testicle
- A change in how the testicle feels
- A dull ache in the lower abdomen or the groin
- A sudden build-up of fluid in the scrotum
- Pain or discomfort in a testicle or in the scrotum

Tests that examine the testicles and blood are used to detect (find) and diagnose testicular cancer. The following tests and procedures may be used:

Physical exam and history: An exam of the body to check general signs of health, including checking for signs of disease, such as lumps or anything else that seems unusual. The testicles will be examined to check for lumps, swelling, or pain. A history of the patient's health habits and past illnesses and treatments will also be taken.

Ultrasound exam: A procedure in which high-energy sound waves (ultrasound) are bounced off internal tissues or organs and make echoes. The echoes form a picture of body tissues called a sonogram.

Serum tumor marker test: A procedure in which a sample of blood is examined to measure the amounts of certain substances released into the blood by organs, tissues, or tumor cells in the body. Certain substances are linked to specific types of cancer when found in increased levels in the blood. These are called tumor markers. The following tumor markers are used to detect testicular cancer: alpha-fetoprotein (AFP); beta-human chorionic gonadotropin (beta-hCG); and lactate dehydrogenase (LDH). Tumor marker levels are measured before radical inguinal orchiectomy and biopsy, to help diagnose testicular cancer.

Radical inguinal orchiectomy and biopsy: A procedure to remove the entire testicle through an incision in the groin. A tissue sample from the testicle is then viewed under a microscope to check for cancer cells. (The surgeon does not cut through the scrotum into the testicle to remove a sample of tissue for biopsy, because if cancer is present, this procedure could cause it to spread into the scrotum and lymph nodes.) If cancer is found, the cell type (seminoma or nonseminoma) is determined in order to help plan treatment.

Prognosis

Certain factors affect prognosis (chance of recovery) and treatment options. The prognosis (chance of recovery) and treatment options depend on the following:

- Stage of the cancer (whether it is in or near the testicle or has spread to other places in the body, and blood levels of AFP, beta-hCG, and LDH)
- Type of cancer
- Size of the tumor
- Number and size of retroperitoneal lymph nodes

Testicular cancer is often curable, but certain treatments for testicular cancer can cause infertility that may be permanent. Patients who may wish to have children should consider sperm banking before having treatment. Sperm banking is the process of freezing sperm and storing it for later use.

Stages of Testicular Cancer

After testicular cancer has been diagnosed, tests are done to find out if cancer cells have spread within the testicles or to other parts of the body. The process used to find out if cancer has spread within the testicles or to other parts of the body is called staging. The information gathered from the staging process determines the stage of the disease. It is important to know the stage in order to plan treatment. The following tests and procedures may be used in the staging process:

- **Chest x-ray:** An x-ray of the organs and bones inside the chest. An x-ray is a type of energy beam that can go through the body and onto film, making a picture of areas inside the body.

- **CT scan (CAT scan):** A procedure that makes a series of detailed pictures of areas inside the body, taken from different angles. The pictures are made by a computer linked to an x-ray machine. A dye may be injected into a vein or swallowed to help the organs or tissues show up more clearly. This procedure is also called computed tomography, computerized tomography, or computerized axial tomography.

- **Lymphangiography:** A procedure used to x-ray the lymph system. A dye is injected into the lymph vessels in the feet. The dye travels upward through the lymph nodes and lymph vessels, and x-rays are taken to see if there are any blockages. This test helps find out whether cancer has spread to the lymph nodes.

- **Abdominal lymph node dissection:** A procedure to examine lymph nodes in the abdomen. Lymph nodes are removed and a pathologist checks them for cancer cells. For patients with non-seminoma, removing the lymph nodes may help stop the spread of disease. Cancer cells in the lymph nodes of seminoma patients can be treated with radiation therapy.

- **Radical inguinal orchiectomy and biopsy**

- **Serum tumor marker test**

The following stages are used for testicular cancer:

Stage 0: In stage 0, abnormal cells are found only in the tiny tubules where the sperm cells begin to develop. The cells do not invade normal tissues. This is sometimes called a "precancerous condition." Stage 0 cancer is also called carcinoma in situ. All tumor marker levels are normal.

Stage I: Stage I is divided into stage IA, stage IB, and stage IS and is determined after a radical inguinal orchiectomy is done.

- **In stage IA:** The cancer is in the testicle and epididymis and may have spread to the inner layer of the membrane surrounding the testicle. All tumor marker levels are normal.

- **In stage IB:** The cancer is in the testicle and the epididymis and has spread to the blood or lymph vessels in the testicle; or has spread to the outer layer of the membrane surrounding the testicle; or is in the spermatic cord or the scrotum and may be in the blood or lymph vessels of the testicle. All tumor marker levels are normal.

- **In stage IS:** The cancer is found anywhere within the testicle, spermatic cord, or the scrotum and either: all tumor marker levels are slightly above normal; or one or more tumor marker levels are moderately above normal or high.

Stage II: Stage II is divided into stage IIA, stage IIB, and stage IIC and is determined after a radical inguinal orchiectomy is done.

- **In stage IIA:** The cancer is anywhere within the testicle, spermatic cord, or scrotum; and has spread to up to 5 lymph nodes in the abdomen, none larger than 2 centimeters. All tumor marker levels are normal or slightly above normal.

- **In stage IIB:** The cancer is anywhere within the testicle, spermatic cord, or scrotum; and either: has spread to up to 5 lymph nodes in the abdomen; at least one of the lymph nodes is larger than 2 centimeters, but none are larger than 5 centimeters; or has spread to more than 5 lymph nodes; the lymph nodes are not larger than 5 centimeters. All tumor markers levels are normal or slightly above normal.

- **In stage IIC:** The cancer: is anywhere within the testicle, spermatic cord, or scrotum; and has spread to a lymph node in the abdomen that is larger than 5 centimeters. All tumor marker levels are normal or slightly above normal.

Stage III: Stage III is divided into stage IIIA, stage IIIB, and stage IIIC and is determined after a radical inguinal orchiectomy is done.

- **In stage IIIA:** The cancer is anywhere within the testicle, spermatic cord, or scrotum; and may have spread to one or more lymph nodes in the abdomen; and has spread to distant lymph nodes or to the lungs. The level of one or more tumor markers may range from normal to slightly above normal.

- **In stage IIIB:** The cancer is anywhere within the testicle, spermatic cord, or scrotum; and may have spread to one or more nearby or distant lymph nodes or to the lungs. The level of one or more tumor markers may range from normal to high.

- **In stage IIIC:** The cancer is anywhere within the testicle, spermatic cord, or scrotum; and may have spread to one or more nearby or distant lymph nodes or to the lungs or anywhere else in the body. The level of one or more tumor markers may range from normal to very high.

Recurrent testicular cancer: Recurrent testicular cancer is cancer that has recurred (come back) after it has been treated. The cancer may come back many years after the initial cancer, in the other testicle or in other parts of the body.

Treatment Option Overview

Different types of treatments are available for patients with testicular cancer. Some treatments are standard (the currently used treatment), and some are being tested in clinical trials. Before starting treatment, patients may want to think about taking part in a clinical trial. A treatment clinical trial is a research study meant to help improve current treatments or obtain information on new treatments for patients with cancer. When clinical trials show that a new treatment is better than the standard treatment, the new treatment may become the standard treatment.

Clinical trials are taking place in many parts of the country. Information about ongoing clinical trials is available from the National Cancer Institute website (http://www.cancer.gov). Choosing the most appropriate cancer treatment is a decision that ideally involves the patient, family, and health care team.

Testicular tumors are divided into three groups, based on how well the tumors are expected to respond to treatment.

Good prognosis: For nonseminoma, all of the following must be true:

- The tumor is found only in the testicle or in the retroperitoneum (area outside or behind the abdominal wall); and

- The tumor has not spread to organs other than the lungs; and

- The levels of all the tumor markers are slightly above normal.

For seminoma, all of the following must be true:

- The tumor has not spread to organs other than the lungs; and
- The level of alpha-fetoprotein (AFP) is normal. Beta-human chorionic gonadotropin (beta-hCG) and lactate dehydrogenase (LDH) may be at any level.

Intermediate prognosis: For nonseminoma, all of the following must be true:

- The tumor is found in one testicle only or in the retroperitoneum (area outside or behind the abdominal wall); and
- The tumor has not spread to organs other than the lungs; and
- The level of any one of the tumor markers is more than slightly above normal.

For seminoma, all of the following must be true:

- The tumor has spread to organs other than the lungs; and
- The level of AFP is normal. beta-hCG and LDH may be at any level.

Poor prognosis: For nonseminoma, at least one of the following must be true:

- The tumor is in the center of the chest between the lungs; or
- The tumor has spread to organs other than the lungs; or
- The level of any one of the tumor markers is high.

There is no poor prognosis grouping for seminoma testicular tumors.

Standard Treatment

Three types of standard treatment are used:

Surgery: Surgery to remove the testicle (radical inguinal orchiectomy) and some of the lymph nodes may be done at diagnosis and staging. Tumors that have spread to other places in the body may be partly or entirely removed by surgery. Even if the doctor removes all the cancer that can be seen at the time of the surgery, some patients may be given chemotherapy or radiation therapy after surgery to kill any cancer cells that are left. Treatment given after the surgery, to increase the chances of a cure, is called adjuvant therapy.

Radiation therapy: Radiation therapy is a cancer treatment that uses high-energy x-rays or other types of radiation to kill cancer cells. There are two types of radiation therapy. External radiation therapy uses a machine outside the body to send radiation toward the cancer. Internal radiation therapy uses a radioactive substance sealed in needles, seeds, wires, or catheters that are placed directly into or near the cancer. The way the radiation therapy is given depends on the type and stage of the cancer being treated.

Chemotherapy: Chemotherapy is a cancer treatment that uses drugs to stop the growth of cancer cells, either by killing the cells or by stopping the cells from dividing. When chemotherapy is taken by mouth or injected into a vein or muscle, the drugs enter the bloodstream and can reach cancer cells throughout the body (systemic chemotherapy). When chemotherapy is placed directly into the spinal column, an organ, or a body cavity such as the abdomen, the drugs mainly affect cancer cells in those areas (regional chemotherapy). The way the chemotherapy is given depends on the type and stage of the cancer being treated.

Other Treatment Issues

New types of treatment are being tested in clinical trials. These include the following:

- **High-dose chemotherapy with stem cell transplant:** High-dose chemotherapy with stem cell transplant is a method of giving high doses of chemotherapy and replacing blood-forming cells destroyed by the cancer treatment. Stem cells (immature blood cells) are removed from the blood or bone marrow of the patient or a donor and are frozen and stored. After the chemotherapy is completed, the stored stem cells are thawed and given back to the patient through an infusion. These reinfused stem cells grow into (and restore) the body's blood cells.

Lifelong follow-up exams are very important for men who have had testicular cancer. Men who have had testicular cancer have an increased risk of developing cancer in the other testicle. A patient is advised to regularly check the other testicle and report any unusual symptoms to a doctor right away. Lifelong clinical exams are very important. The patient will probably have checkups once per month during the first year after surgery, every other month during the next year, and less often after that.

Treatment Options by Stage

Stage I: Treatment of stage I testicular cancer depends on whether the cancer is a seminoma or a nonseminoma. Treatment of seminoma is usually surgery to remove the testicle, with or without radiation therapy to lymph nodes in the abdomen after the surgery, with life-long follow-up.

Treatment of nonseminoma may include the following:

- Surgery to remove the testicle and lymph nodes in the abdomen, with lifelong follow-up

- Surgery to remove the testicle, followed by chemotherapy and lifelong follow-up

- Surgery to remove the testicle, with lifelong follow-up

Stage II: Treatment of stage II testicular cancer depends on whether the cancer is a seminoma or a nonseminoma. Treatment of seminoma may include the following:

- When the tumor is 5 centimeters or smaller, treatment is usually surgery to remove the testicle followed by radiation therapy to lymph nodes in the abdomen and pelvis, with lifelong follow-up.

- When the tumor is larger than 5 centimeters, treatment is usually surgery to remove the testicle followed by combination chemotherapy or radiation therapy to lymph nodes in the abdomen and pelvis, with lifelong follow-up.

Treatment of nonseminoma may include the following:

- Surgery to remove the testicle and lymph nodes, with lifelong follow-up

- Surgery to remove the testicle and lymph nodes, followed by combination chemotherapy and lifelong follow-up

- Surgery to remove the testicle followed by combination chemotherapy and a second surgery if cancer remains, with lifelong follow-up

- Combination chemotherapy before surgery to remove the testicle, for cancer that has spread and is thought to be life-threatening
- A clinical trial of combination chemotherapy instead of removing the lymph nodes

Stage III: Treatment of stage III testicular cancer depends on whether the cancer is a seminoma or a nonseminoma. Treatment of seminoma may include the following:

- Surgery to remove the testicle followed by combination chemotherapy. Any tumor remaining after treatment will need lifelong follow-up.
- A clinical trial of a new therapy
- A clinical trial of high-dose chemotherapy with bone marrow transplant

Treatment of nonseminoma may include the following:

- Surgery to remove the testicle, followed by combination chemotherapy
- Combination chemotherapy followed by surgery to remove any remaining tumor. Additional chemotherapy may be given if the tumor tissue removed contains cancer cells that are growing.
- Combination chemotherapy combined with radiation therapy to the brain for cancer that has spread to the brain.
- Combination chemotherapy before surgery to remove the testicle, for cancer that has spread and is thought to be life-threatening
- A clinical trial of a new therapy
- A clinical trial of high-dose chemotherapy with bone marrow transplant

Recurrent testicular cancer: Treatment of recurrent testicular cancer may include the following:

- Combination chemotherapy
- High-dose chemotherapy with bone marrow transplant
- Surgery to remove cancer that has either come back more than

two years after complete remission; or come back in only one place and does not respond to chemotherapy

- A clinical trial of a new therapy.

Penile Cancer

Penile cancer is a disease in which malignant (cancer) cells form in the tissues of the penis. The penis is a rod-shaped male reproductive organ that passes sperm and urine from the body. It contains two types of erectile tissue (spongy tissue with blood vessels that fill with blood to make an erection):

- **Corpora cavernosa:** The two columns of erectile tissue that form most of the penis

- **Corpus spongiosum:** The single column of erectile tissue that forms a small portion of the penis. The corpus spongiosum surrounds the urethra (the tube through which urine and sperm pass from the body).

The erectile tissue is wrapped in connective tissue and covered with skin. The glans (head of the penis) is covered with loose skin called the foreskin.

Risk Factors and Possible Signs of Penile Cancer

Anything that increases your chance of getting a disease is called a risk factor. Human papillomavirus infection may increase the risk of developing penile cancer. Circumcision may help prevent infection with the human papillomavirus (HPV). A circumcision is an operation in which the doctor removes part or all of the foreskin from the penis. Many boys are circumcised shortly after birth. Men who were not circumcised at birth may have a higher risk of developing penile cancer.

Other risk factors for penile cancer include the following:

- Being age 60 or older
- Having phimosis (a condition in which the foreskin of the penis cannot be pulled back over the glans)
- Having poor personal hygiene
- Having many sexual partners
- Using tobacco products

Possible signs of penile cancer include sores, discharge, and bleeding. These and other symptoms may be caused by penile cancer. Other conditions may cause the same symptoms. A doctor should be consulted if any of the following problems occur:

- Redness, irritation, or a sore on the penis
- A lump on the penis

Stages of Penile Cancer

Stage 0: In stage 0, abnormal cells are found only on the surface of the skin of the penis. Stage 0 is also called carcinoma in situ.

Stage I: In stage I, cancer has formed and spread to connective tissue just under the skin of the penis.

Stage II: In stage II, cancer has spread to:

- connective tissue just under the skin of the penis and to one lymph node in the groin; or
- erectile tissue (spongy tissue that fills with blood to make an erection) and may have spread to one lymph node in the groin.

Stage III: In stage III, cancer has spread to:

- connective tissue or erectile tissue of the penis and to more than one lymph node on one or both sides of the groin; or
- the urethra or prostate, and may have spread to one or more lymph nodes on one or both sides of the groin.

Stage IV: In stage IV, cancer has spread:

- to tissues near the penis and may have spread to lymph nodes in the groin or pelvis; or
- anywhere in or near the penis and in one or more lymph nodes deep in the pelvis or groin; or
- to distant parts of the body.

Recurrent: Recurrent penile cancer is cancer that has recurred (come back) after it has been treated. The cancer may come back in the penis or in other parts of the body.

Treatment Option Overview

Three types of standard treatment are used: surgery, radiation therapy, and chemotherapy. Topical chemotherapy may be used to treat stage 0 penile cancer.

Surgery: Surgery is the most common treatment for all stages of penile cancer. A doctor may remove the cancer using one of the following operations:

- **Mohs microsurgery:** A procedure in which the tumor is cut from the skin in thin layers. During the surgery, the edges of the tumor and each layer of tumor removed are viewed through a microscope to check for cancer cells. Layers continue to be removed until no more cancer cells are seen. This type of surgery removes as little normal tissue as possible and is often used to remove cancer on the skin. It is also called Mohs surgery.

- **Laser surgery:** A surgical procedure that uses a laser beam (a narrow beam of intense light) as a knife to make bloodless cuts in tissue or to remove a surface lesion such as a tumor.

- **Cryosurgery:** A treatment that uses an instrument to freeze and destroy abnormal tissue. This type of treatment is also called cryotherapy.

- **Circumcision:** Surgery to remove part or all of the foreskin of the penis.

- **Wide local excision:** Surgery to remove only the cancer and some normal tissue around it.

- **Amputation of the penis:** Surgery to remove part or all of the penis. If part of the penis is removed, it is a partial penectomy. If all of the penis is removed, it is a total penectomy.

Lymph nodes in the groin may be taken out during surgery.

Even if the doctor removes all the cancer that can be seen at the time of the surgery, some patients may be given chemotherapy or radiation therapy after surgery to kill any cancer cells that are left. Treatment given after the surgery, to increase the chances of a cure, is called adjuvant therapy.

New Treatments

New types of treatment are being tested in clinical trials. These include the following:

Biologic therapy: Biologic therapy is a treatment that uses the patient's immune system to fight cancer. Substances made by the body or made in a laboratory are used to boost, direct, or restore the body's natural defenses against cancer. This type of cancer treatment is also called biotherapy or immunotherapy. Topical biologic therapy may be used to treat stage 0 penile cancer.

Radiosensitizers: Radiosensitizers are drugs that make tumor cells more sensitive to radiation therapy. Combining radiation therapy with radiosensitizers helps kill more tumor cells.

Treatment Options by Stage

Stage 0: Treatment of stage 0 may be one of the following:

- Mohs microsurgery
- Topical chemotherapy
- Topical biologic therapy
- Laser surgery
- Cryosurgery

Stage I: If the cancer is only in the foreskin, wide local excision and circumcision may be the only treatment needed. Treatment of stage I penile cancer may include the following:

- Surgery (partial or total penectomy with or without removal of lymph nodes in the groin
- External or internal radiation therapy
- Mohs microsurgery
- A clinical trial of laser therapy

Stage II: Treatment of stage II penile cancer may include the following:

- Surgery (partial or total penectomy, with or without removal of lymph nodes in the groin)
- External or internal radiation therapy followed by surgery
- A clinical trial of laser surgery

Stage III: Treatment of stage III penile cancer may include the following:

- Surgery (penectomy and removal of lymph nodes in the groin) with or without radiation therapy
- Radiation therapy
- A clinical trial of radiosensitizers
- A clinical trial of chemotherapy before or after surgery

Stage IV: Treatment of stage IV penile cancer is usually palliative (to relieve symptoms and improve the quality of life). Treatment may include the following:

- Surgery (wide local excision and removal of lymph nodes in the groin)
- Radiation therapy
- A clinical trial of chemotherapy before or after surgery

Recurrent: Treatment of recurrent penile cancer may include the following:

- Surgery (penectomy)
- Radiation therapy
- A clinical trial of biologic therapy
- A clinical trial of chemotherapy

Chapter 56

Prostate Cancer

The Prostate

The prostate is part of a man's reproductive system. It is located in front of the rectum and under the bladder. It surrounds the urethra, the tube through which urine flows. A healthy prostate is about the size of a walnut.

The prostate makes part of seminal fluid. During ejaculation, seminal fluid helps carry sperm out of the man's body as part of semen.

Male hormones (androgens) make the prostate grow. The testicles are the main source of male hormones, including testosterone. The adrenal gland also makes testosterone, but in small amounts. If the prostate grows too large, it squeezes the urethra. This may slow or stop the flow of urine from the bladder to the penis.

Benign prostatic hyperplasia (BPH) is the abnormal growth of benign prostate cells. The prostate grows larger and squeezes the urethra. This prevents the normal flow of urine. BPH is a very common problem. In the United States, most men over the age of 50 have symptoms of BPH. For some men, symptoms may be severe enough to need treatment. BPH is not cancer.

Risk Factors

No one knows the exact causes of prostate cancer. Doctors often cannot explain why one man develops prostate cancer and another does

From "What You Need to Know about™ Prostate Cancer," National Cancer Institute, August 1, 2005.

not. However, we do know that prostate cancer is not contagious. You cannot "catch" it from another person.

Research has shown that men with certain risk factors are more likely than others to develop prostate cancer. A risk factor is something that may increase the chance of developing a disease. Studies have found the following risk factors for prostate cancer:

- **Age:** Age is the main risk factor for prostate cancer. This disease is rare in men younger than 45. The chance of getting it goes up sharply as a man gets older. In the United States, most men with prostate cancer are older than 65.

- **Family history:** A man's risk is higher if his father or brother had prostate cancer.

- **Race:** Prostate cancer is more common in African American men than in white men, including Hispanic white men. It is less common in Asian and American Indian men.

- **Certain prostate changes:** Men with cells called high-grade prostatic intraepithelial neoplasia (PIN) may be at increased risk for prostate cancer. These prostate cells look abnormal under a microscope.

- **Diet:** Some studies suggest that men who eat a diet high in animal fat or meat may be at increased risk for prostate cancer. Men who eat a diet rich in fruits and vegetables may have a lower risk.

Many of these risk factors can be avoided. Others, such as family history, cannot be avoided. You can help protect yourself by staying away from known risk factors whenever possible.

Scientists have also studied whether BPH, obesity, smoking, a virus passed through sex, or lack of exercise might increase the risk for prostate cancer. At this time, these are not clear risk factors. Also, most studies have not found an increased risk of prostate cancer for men who have had a vasectomy. A vasectomy is surgery to cut or tie off the tubes that carry sperm out of the testicles.

Most men who have known risk factors do not get prostate cancer. On the other hand, men who do get the disease often have no known risk factors, except for growing older. If you think you may be at risk, you should talk with your doctor. Your doctor may be able to suggest ways to reduce your risk and can plan a schedule for checkups.

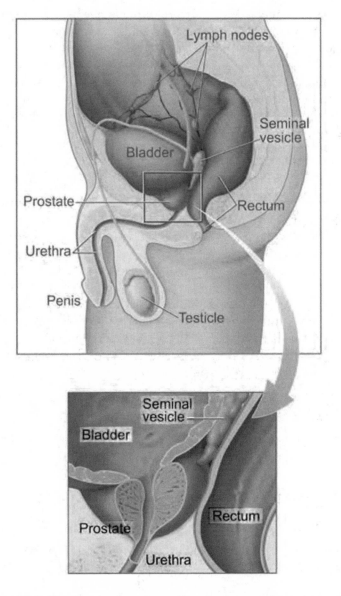

Figure 56.1. *The top image shows the prostate and nearby organs. The detailed image below shows the inside of the prostate, urethra, rectum, and bladder.*

Screening

Your doctor can check you for prostate cancer before you have any symptoms. Screening can help doctors find and treat cancer early. But studies so far have not shown that screening tests reduce the number of deaths from prostate cancer. You may want to talk with your doctor about the possible benefits and harms of being screened. The decision to be screened, like many other medical decisions, is a personal one. You should decide after learning the pros and cons of screening. Your doctor can explain more about these tests:

- **Digital rectal exam:** The doctor inserts a lubricated, gloved finger into the rectum and feels the prostate through the rectal wall. The prostate is checked for hard or lumpy areas.

- **Blood test for prostate-specific antigen (PSA):** A lab checks the level of PSA in a man's blood sample. A high PSA level is commonly caused by BPH or prostatitis (inflammation of the prostate). Prostate cancer may also cause a high PSA level.

The digital rectal exam and PSA test can detect a problem in the prostate. They cannot show whether the problem is cancer or a less serious condition. Your doctor will use the results of these tests to help decide whether to check further for signs of cancer. Information about other tests is in the "Diagnosis" section.

Symptoms

A man with prostate cancer may not have any symptoms. For men who have symptoms of prostate cancer, common symptoms include the following:

- Urinary problems
- Not being able to urinate
- Having a hard time starting or stopping the urine flow
- Needing to urinate often, especially at night
- Weak flow of urine
- Urine flow that starts and stops
- Pain or burning during urination
- Difficulty having an erection

- Blood in the urine or semen

- Frequent pain in the lower back, hips, or upper thighs

Most often, these symptoms are not due to cancer. BPH, an infection, or another health problem may cause them. Any man with these symptoms should tell his doctor so that problems can be diagnosed and treated as early as possible. He may see his regular doctor or a urologist. A urologist is a doctor whose specialty is diseases of the urinary system.

Diagnosis

If you have a symptom or test result that suggests cancer, your doctor must find out whether it is due to cancer or to some other cause. Your doctor will ask about your personal and family medical history. You will have a physical exam. You may have lab tests. Your visit may include a digital rectal exam, a urine test to check for blood or infection, and a blood test to measure PSA level. You also may have other exams:

- **Transrectal ultrasound:** The doctor inserts a probe into the man's rectum to check for abnormal areas. The probe sends out sound waves that people cannot hear (ultrasound). The waves bounce off the prostate. A computer uses the echoes to create a picture called a sonogram.

- **Cystoscopy:** The doctor uses a thin, lighted tube to look into the urethra and bladder.

- **Transrectal biopsy:** A biopsy is the removal of tissue to look for cancer cells. It is the only sure way to diagnose prostate cancer. The doctor inserts a needle through the rectum into the prostate. The doctor takes small tissue samples from many areas of the prostate. Ultrasound may be used to guide the needle. A pathologist checks for cancer cells in the tissue.

If Cancer Is Not Found

If the physical exam and test results do not suggest cancer, your doctor may suggest medicine to reduce symptoms caused by an enlarged prostate. Surgery also can relieve these symptoms. The surgery most often used in such cases is transurethral resection of the prostate (TURP or TUR). In TURP, an instrument is inserted through the urethra to remove prostate tissue that is pressing against the upper part of the urethra and restricting the flow of urine. You should talk to your doctor about the best treatment option.

If Cancer Is Found

If cancer is present, the pathologist studies tissue samples from the prostate under a microscope to report the grade of the tumor. The grade tells how much the tumor tissue differs from normal prostate tissue. It suggests how fast the tumor is likely to grow. Tumors with higher grades tend to grow faster than those with lower grades. They are also more likely to spread.

One system of grading prostate cancer uses G1 through G4. Another way of grading is with the Gleason score. The pathologist gives each area of cancer a grade of 1 through 5. The pathologist adds the two most common grades together to make a Gleason score. Or the pathologist may add the most common grade and the highest (most abnormal) grade to get the score. Gleason scores can range from 2 to 10.

Staging

To plan your treatment, your doctor needs to know the extent (stage) of the disease. The stage is based on the size of the tumor, whether the cancer has spread outside the prostate and, if so, where it has spread. You may have blood tests to see if the cancer has spread. Some men also may need imaging tests:

- **Bone scan:** The doctor injects a small amount of a radioactive substance into a blood vessel. It travels through the bloodstream and collects in the bones. A machine called a scanner detects and measures the radiation. The scanner makes pictures of the bones on a computer screen or on film. The pictures may show cancer that has spread to the bones.

- **CT scan:** An x-ray machine linked to a computer takes a series of detailed pictures of areas inside your body. Doctors often use CT scans to see the pelvis or abdomen.

- **Magnetic resonance imaging (MRI):** A strong magnet linked to a computer is used to make detailed pictures of areas inside your body.

These are the stages of prostate cancer:

578

- **Stage I:** The cancer cannot be felt during a digital rectal exam. It is found by chance when surgery is done for another reason, usually for BPH. The cancer is only in the prostate.

- **Stage II:** The cancer is more advanced, but it has not spread outside the prostate.

- **Stage III:** The cancer has spread outside the prostate. It may be in the seminal vesicles. It has not spread to the lymph nodes.

- **Stage IV:** The cancer may be in nearby muscles and organs (beyond the seminal vesicles). It may have spread to the lymph nodes. It may have spread to other parts of the body.

Recurrent cancer is cancer that has come back (recurred) after a time when it could not be detected. It may recur in or near the prostate. Or it may recur in any other part of the body, such as the bones.

Treatment

Men with prostate cancer have many treatment options. The treatment that is best for one man may not be best for another. Treatment may involve surgery, radiation therapy, or hormone therapy. You may have a combination of treatments. If your doctor recommends watchful waiting, your health will be monitored closely. You will have treatment only if symptoms occur or get worse.

Surgery

Surgery is a common treatment for early stage prostate cancer. Your doctor may remove the whole prostate or only part of it. In some cases, your doctor can use a method known as nerve-sparing surgery. This type of surgery may save the nerves that control erection. But if you have a large tumor or a tumor that is very close to the nerves, you may not be able to have this surgery. Each type of surgery has benefits and risks. Your doctor can further describe these types:

- **Radical retropubic prostatectomy:** The doctor removes the entire prostate and nearby lymph nodes through an incision (cut) in the abdomen.

- **Radical perineal prostatectomy:** The doctor removes the entire prostate through a cut between the scrotum and the anus. Nearby lymph nodes may be removed through a separate cut in the abdomen.

- **Laparoscopic prostatectomy:** The doctor removes the entire prostate and nearby lymph nodes through small incisions, rather than a single long cut in the abdomen. A thin, lighted tube (a laparoscope) is used to help remove the prostate.

- **Transurethral resection of the prostate (TURP):** The doctor removes part of the prostate with a long, thin device that is inserted through the urethra. The cancer is cut from the prostate. TURP may not remove all of the cancer. But it can remove tissue that blocks the flow of urine.

- **Cryosurgery:** This type of surgery for prostate cancer is under study at some medical centers.

- **Pelvic lymphadenectomy:** This is routinely done during prostatectomy. The doctor removes lymph nodes in the pelvis to see if cancer has spread to them. If there are cancer cells in the lymph nodes, the disease may have spread to other parts of the body. In this case, the doctor may suggest other types of treatment.

The time it takes to heal after surgery is different for each man and depends on the type of surgery he has had. You may be uncomfortable for the first few days. However, medicine can help control the pain. Before surgery, you should discuss the plan for pain relief with your doctor or nurse. After surgery, your doctor can adjust the plan if you need more pain relief.

After surgery, the urethra needs time to heal. You will have a catheter. A catheter is a tube put through the urethra into the bladder to drain urine. You will have the catheter for 5 days to 3 weeks. Your nurse or doctor will show you how to care for it.

Surgery may cause short-term problems, such as incontinence. After surgery, some men may lose control of the flow of urine (urinary incontinence). Most men regain bladder control after a few weeks.

Some men may become impotent. Nerve-sparing surgery is an attempt to avoid the problem of impotence. If a man can have nerve-sparing surgery and the operation is a success, impotence may not last. In some cases, men become permanently impotent. You can talk with your doctor about medicine and other ways to help manage the sexual effects of cancer treatment.

If your prostate is removed, you will no longer produce semen. You will have dry orgasms. If you wish to father children, you may consider sperm banking or a sperm retrieval procedure.

Radiation Therapy

Radiation therapy (also called radiotherapy) uses high-energy rays to kill cancer cells. It affects cells only in the treated area. For early stage prostate cancer, radiation treatment may be used instead of surgery. It also may be used after surgery to destroy any cancer cells that remain in the area. In later stages of prostate cancer, radiation treatment may be used to help relieve pain.

Doctors use two types of radiation therapy to treat prostate cancer. Some men receive both types:

- **External radiation:** The radiation comes from a large machine outside the body. Men go to a hospital or clinic for treatment. Treatments are usually 5 days a week for several weeks. Many men receive 3-dimensional conformal radiation therapy. This type of treatment more closely targets the cancer. It spares healthy tissue.

- **Internal radiation (implant radiation or brachytherapy):** The radiation comes from radioactive material usually contained in small seeds. The seeds are put into the tissue. They give off radiation for months. The seeds are harmless and do not need to be removed.

Side effects depend mainly on the dose and type of radiation. You are likely to be very tired during radiation therapy, especially in the later weeks of treatment. Resting is important, but doctors usually advise patients to try to stay as active as they can.

If you have external radiation, you may have diarrhea or frequent and uncomfortable urination. Some men have lasting bowel or urinary problems. Your skin in the treated area may become red, dry, and tender. You may lose hair in the treated area. The hair may not grow back.

Internal radiation treatment may cause incontinence. This side effect usually goes away. Lasting side effects from internal radiation are not common. Both internal and external radiation can cause impotence. Internal radiation is less likely to have this effect.

Hormone Therapy

Hormone therapy keeps prostate cancer cells from getting the male hormones (androgens) they need to grow. The testicles are the body's main source of the male hormone testosterone. The adrenal gland

581

makes a small amount of testosterone. Hormone treatment uses drugs or surgery:

- **Drugs:** Your doctor may suggest a drug that can block natural hormones.

  - **Luteinizing hormone-releasing hormone (LH-RH) agonists:** These drugs can prevent the testicles from making testosterone. Examples are leuprolide and goserelin.

  - **Antiandrogens:** These drugs can block the action of male hormones. Examples are flutamide, bicalutamide, and nilutamide.

  - **Other drugs:** Some drugs can prevent the adrenal gland from making testosterone. Examples are ketoconazole and aminoglutethimide.

- **Surgery:** Surgery to remove the testicles is called orchiectomy.

After orchiectomy or treatment with an LH-RH agonist, your body no longer gets testosterone from the testicles. However, the adrenal gland still produces a small amount of male hormones. You may receive an antiandrogen to block the action of the male hormones that remain. This combination of treatments is known as total androgen blockade. Studies have not shown whether total androgen blockade is more effective than surgery or an LH-RH agonist alone.

Doctors can usually control prostate cancer that has spread to other parts of the body with hormone therapy. The cancer often does not grow for several years. But in time, most prostate cancers can grow with very little or no male hormones. Hormone therapy is no longer helpful. At that time, your doctor may suggest other forms of treatment that are under study.

Hormone therapy is likely to affect your quality of life. It often causes side effects such as impotence, hot flashes, loss of sexual desire, and weaker bones. An LH-RH agonist may make your symptoms worse for a short time when you first take it. This temporary problem is called "flare." The treatment gradually causes your testosterone level to fall. Without testosterone, tumor growth slows. Your condition may improve. (To prevent flare, your doctor may give you an antiandrogen for a while along with the LH-RH agonist.)

Antiandrogens (such as nilutamide) can cause nausea, diarrhea, or breast growth or tenderness. Rarely, they may cause liver problems (pain in the abdomen, yellow eyes, or dark urine). Some men who use nilutamide may have difficulty breathing. Some may have trouble adjusting to sudden changes in light.

If used for a long time, ketoconazole may cause liver problems, and aminoglutethimide can cause skin rashes. If you receive total androgen blockade, you may have more side effects than if you have just one type of hormone treatment.

Any treatment that lowers hormone levels can weaken your bones. Your doctor can suggest medicines or dietary supplements that can reduce your risk of bone fractures.

Watchful Waiting

You may choose watchful waiting if the risks and possible side effects of treatment outweigh the possible benefits. Your doctor may offer this choice if you are older or have other serious health problems. Your doctor may also suggest watchful waiting if you are diagnosed with early stage prostate cancer that seems to be slowly growing. Your doctor will offer you treatment if symptoms occur or get worse.

Watchful waiting avoids or delays the side effects of surgery and radiation, but this choice has risks. It may reduce the chance to control cancer before it spreads. Also, it may be harder to cope with surgery and radiation therapy as you age.

You may decide against watchful waiting if you do not want to live with an untreated cancer. If you choose watchful waiting but grow concerned later, you should discuss your feelings with your doctor. A different approach is nearly always available.

You may want to ask your doctor these questions before choosing watchful waiting:

- If I choose watchful waiting, can I change my mind later on?

- Will the cancer be harder to treat later?

- How often will I have checkups?

- Between checkups, what problems should I report?

Complementary and Alternative Medicine

Some men with prostate cancer use complementary and alternative medicine (CAM):

- An approach is generally called complementary medicine when it is used along with standard treatment.

- An approach is called alternative medicine when it is used instead of standard treatment.

Acupuncture, massage therapy, herbal products, vitamins or special diets, visualization, meditation, and spiritual healing are types of CAM. Many men say that CAM helps them feel better. However, some types of CAM may change the way standard treatment works. These changes could be harmful. And some types of CAM could be harmful even if used alone. Some types of CAM are expensive. Health insurance may not cover the cost.

Follow-Up Care

Follow-up care after treatment for prostate cancer is important. Even when the cancer seems to have been completely removed or destroyed, the disease sometimes returns because undetected cancer cells remained somewhere in the body after treatment. Your doctor will monitor your recovery and check for recurrence of the cancer. Checkups help ensure that any changes in your health are noted and treated if needed. Checkups may include lab tests, x-rays, biopsies, or other tests. Between scheduled visits, you should contact your doctor if you have any health problems.

Chapter 57

Leukemia

Chapter Contents

Section 57.1

Leukemia Facts and Statistics

Leukemia (facts and statistics from *Leukemia, Lymphoma, Myeloma, Facts 2005-2006*, June 2005) is a malignant disease (cancer) of the bone marrow and blood. It is characterized by the uncontrolled accumulation of blood cells. Leukemia is divided into four categories: myelogenous or lymphocytic, each of which can be acute or chronic. The terms myelogenous or lymphocytic denote the cell type involved. Thus, the four major types of leukemia are:

- Acute lymphocytic leukemia (ALL)
- Chronic lymphocytic leukemia (CLL)
- Acute myelogenous leukemia (AML)
- Chronic myelogenous leukemia (CML)

Acute leukemia is a rapidly progressing disease that results in the accumulation of immature, functionless cells in the marrow and blood. The marrow often can no longer produce enough normal red blood cells, white blood cells, and platelets. Anemia, a deficiency of red cells, develops in virtually all leukemia patients. The lack of normal white cells impairs the body's ability to fight infections. A shortage of platelets results in bruising and easy bleeding.

Chronic leukemia progresses more slowly and allows greater numbers of more mature, functional cells to be made.

New Cases

An estimated 34,810 new cases of leukemia will be diagnosed in the United States in 2005. Acute leukemias account for nearly 11 percent more of the cases than chronic leukemias. Most cases occur in older adults; more than half of all cases occur after age 67. Leukemia is expected to strike 9 times as many adults as children in 2004.

(About 31,289 adults compared with 3,521 children, ages 0–19). About 30 percent of cancers in children ages 0–14 years are leukemia. The most common form of leukemia among children under 19 years of age is acute lymphocytic leukemia (ALL).

The most common types of leukemia in adults are acute myelogenous leukemia (AML), with an estimated 11,960 new cases this year, and chronic lymphocytic leukemia (CLL), with some 9,730 new cases this year. Chronic myelogenous leukemia (CML) is estimated to affect about 4,600 persons this year. Acute lymphocytic leukemia (ALL) will account for about 3,970 cases this year. Other unclassified forms of leukemia account for the 4,550 remaining cases.

Incidence by Gender

Incidence rates for all types of leukemia are higher among males than among females. In 2005, males are expected to account for more than 56 percent of the cases of leukemia. (Note: Incidence rates are the number of new cases in a given year not counting the pre-existing cases. The incidence rates are usually presented as a specific number per 100,000 population.)

Incidence by Race and Ethnicity

Incidence rates for all types of cancer are 7 percent higher among Americans of African descent than among those of European descent. The incidence rate for all cancers among African Americans, from 1973–2002, was 505.2 per 100,000 population, averaging about 175,093 cases each year.

Leukemia is one of the top 15 most frequently occurring cancers in minority groups. Leukemia incidence is highest among whites and lowest among American Indians/Alaskan natives.

Leukemia rates are substantially higher for white children than for black children.

Hispanic children of all races under the age of 20 have the highest rates of leukemia.

Incidence by Age Group

Incidence rates by age differ for each of the leukemias. The leukemias represented 25 percent of all cancers occurring among children younger than 20 years from 1997–2002. In the 13 SEER areas of the United States, there were 1,490 children under the age of 20 diagnosed with leukemia from 1998–2002, including 1,113 with ALL. From this data, it is estimated that 3,521 children will be diagnosed with leukemia in 2005 throughout the United States. Nearly 2,455 new cases of childhood ALL are expected to occur in 2005.

The most common form of leukemia among children under 19 years of age is ALL. The incidence of ALL among 1- to 4-year-old children is more than 10 times greater than the rate for young adults ages 20–24.

There is optimism within centers that specialize in the treatment of children because survival statistics have dramatically improved over the past 30 years. Most children with ALL are cured.

CLL and AML incidence increase dramatically among people who are over the age of 50, and CML incidence increases dramatically among people who are over the age of 60. These cancers are most prevalent in the seventh, eighth, and ninth decades of life.

Signs and Symptoms

Signs of acute leukemia may include easy bruising or bleeding (as a result of platelet deficiency), paleness or easy fatigue (as a result of anemia), and recurrent minor infections or poor healing of minor cuts (because of inadequate white cell count).

These symptoms and signs are not specific to leukemia and may be caused by other disorders. They do, however, warrant medical evaluation. A proportion of people with chronic leukemia may not have major symptoms and are diagnosed during a periodic medical examination. The diagnosis of leukemia requires examination of the cells in blood or marrow.

Possible Causes

Anyone can get leukemia. Leukemia affects all ages and sexes. The cause of leukemia is not known. Chronic exposure to benzene in the workplace and exposure to extraordinary doses of irradiation can be causes of the disease, although neither explains most cases.

Treatment

The aim of treatment is to bring about a complete remission. Complete remission means that there is no evidence of the disease, and the patient returns to good health with normal blood and marrow cells. Relapse indicates a return of the cancer cells and return of other signs and symptoms of the disease. For acute leukemia, a complete remission (no evidence of disease in the blood or marrow) that lasts five years after treatment often indicates cure. Treatment centers report increasing numbers of patients with leukemia who are in complete remission at least five years after diagnosis of their disease.

Survival

The relative five-year survival rate has more than tripled in the past 45 years for patients with leukemia. In 1960–1963, when compared to a person without leukemia, a patient had a 14 percent chance of living five years. By 1970–1973, the five year relative survival rate had jumped to 22 percent, and in 1995–2001 the overall relative survival rate was 48 percent. The relative survival rates differ by the age of the patient at diagnosis, gender, race, and type of leukemia.

During 1995–2001 relative survival rates overall were as follows:

- Acute lymphocytic leukemia (ALL): 64.6 percent overall; 88.4 percent for children under 5

- Chronic lymphocytic leukemia (CLL): 74.2 percent

- Acute myelogenous leukemia (AML): 19.8 percent overall; 52 percent for children under 15

- Chronic myelogenous leukemia (CML): 39.3 percent

At the present time (2006) there are approximately 198,257 people living with leukemia in the United States.

Deaths

It is anticipated that approximately 22,570 deaths in the United States will be attributed to leukemia in 2005 (12,540 males and 10,030 females).

There will be an estimated 4,600 deaths from chronic lymphocytic leukemia and 1,490 deaths from acute lymphocytic leukemia. There will be an estimated 9,000 deaths from acute myelogenous leukemia and 850 deaths from chronic myelogenous leukemia. Unclassified forms of leukemia will account for 6,630 additional deaths.

The estimated numbers of deaths attributed to leukemia in the United States are about 25 percent higher for males than females.

The leukemia death rate for children 0–14 years of age in the United States has declined 60 percent over the past three decades. Despite this decline, leukemia causes more deaths than any other cancer among children under age 20. Approximately 413 children from 0–14 years of age are expected to die from leukemia in 2005.

Section 57.2

Diagnosing Acute Leukemia

Approach to Diagnosis

- Medical history and physical examination
- Complete blood counts
- Bone marrow examination
- Cytogenetics
- Immunophenotyping

To diagnose leukemia, the blood and marrow cells must be examined. In addition to low red cell and platelet counts, examination of the stained (dyed) blood cells with a light microscope will usually show the presence of leukemic blast cells. This is confirmed by examination of the marrow which almost always shows leukemia cells. The blood or marrow cells are also used for studies of the number and shape of chromosomes (cytogenetic examination), immunophenotyping, and other special studies, if required.

Blood and bone marrow samples are used to diagnose and classify the disease. The following tests are used in the further classification of the disease. Examination of leukemic cells by cytogenetic techniques permits identification of chromosomes or gene abnormalities in the cells. The immunophenotype and chromosome abnormalities in the leukemic cells are very important guides in determining the approach to treatment and the intensity of the drug combinations to be used.

Immunophenotyping

This is a laboratory test that enable the physician to determine the type of disease that is present in the patient. It uses the antigens (proteins) on the cell surface and the antibodies produced by the body that match the antigen.

A method that uses the reaction of antibodies with cell antigens to determine a specific type of cell in a sample of blood cells, marrow cells, or lymph node cells. The antibodies react with specific antigens on the cell. A tag is attached to an antibody so that it can be detected. The tag can be identified by the laboratory equipment used for the test. As cells carrying their array of antigens are tagged with specific antibodies they can be identified; for example, myelogenous leukemic cells can be distinguished from lymphocytic leukemic cells. Normal lymphocytes may be distinguished from leukemic lymphocytes. This method also helps to subclassify cell types, which may, in turn, help to decide on the best treatment to apply in that type of leukemia or lymphoma. The antigen on a cell is referred to as cluster of differentiation or "CD" with an associated number. For example, CD7 and 19 may be present on leukemic lymphoblasts and CD13 and 33 on leukemic myeloblasts.

Cytogenetic Examination

Cytogenetic examination of tissue is the process of analyzing the number and shape of the chromosomes of cells. The individual, who prepares, examines and interprets the number and shape of chromosomes in cells is called a cytogeneticist. In addition to identifying chromosome alterations, the specific genes affected can be identified in some cases. These findings are very helpful in diagnosing specific types of leukemia and lymphoma, in determining treatment approaches, and in following the response to treatment.

Section 57.3

Acute Lymphocytic Leukemia

About 3,970 new cases of acute lymphocytic leukemia (ALL) are diagnosed each year in the United States. It is the most common type of leukemia under the age of 19. Children are most likely to develop the disease, but it can occur at any age. Acute lymphocytic leukemia may be called by several names, including acute lymphoid leukemia and acute lymphoblastic leukemia.

ALL results from an acquired (not inherited) genetic injury to the DNA of a single cell in the bone marrow. The disease is often referred to as acute lymphoblastic leukemia because the leukemic cell that replaces the normal marrow is the (leukemic) lymphoblast. The effects are the uncontrolled and exaggerated growth and accumulation of cells called "lymphoblasts" or "leukemic blasts," which fail to function as normal blood cells, and the blockade of the production of normal marrow cells, leading to a deficiency of red cells (anemia), platelets (thrombocytopenia), and normal white cells (especially neutrophils, or neutropenia) in the blood.

Causes and Risk Factors

In most cases, the cause of acute lymphocytic leukemia is not evident. Few factors have been associated with an increased risk of developing the disease. Exposure to high doses of irradiation, as carefully studied in the Japanese survivors of atomic bomb detonations, is one such factor. Unlike other forms of leukemia, acute lymphocytic leukemia occurs at different rates in different locations. There are higher leukemia rates in more developed countries and in higher socioeconomic groups.

The current causes of acute lymphoblastic leukemia in children or adults are not known. Scientists continue to explore possible relationships with lifestyle or environmental factors but no firm conclusions have yet been reached. Given the amount of study, this suggests that multifaceted complex factors may be involved. It is extremely disconcerting to patients and their families to wonder what they may have done differently to avoid the disease. Unfortunately, at the present time there is no known way to prevent the disease. Acute lymphocytic leukemia occurs most often in the first decade of life but increases in frequency again in older individuals.

Subtypes of Acute Lymphocytic Leukemia

Acute lymphocytic leukemia can develop from primitive lymphocytes that are in various stages of development. The principal subtypes are uncovered by special tests on the leukemic lymphoblasts called "immunophenotyping." Phenotype is the physical characteristics of the cells and these are measured using immune tools. The subclassification of cell types is important since it helps to determine the best treatment to apply in each type of leukemia. The principle subtypes are T lymphocyte and B lymphocyte types, so named because the cell has features that are similar to normal T or B lymphocytes. In addition, the B cell type can be divided into a precursor B cell type, as well. Once these features are determined the term used may be acute T lymphoblastic leukemia or acute precursor (or pre) B cell lymphoblastic leukemia. Other markers on the lymphoblasts that can be detected with immunophenotyping and may be useful to the physician include the common acute lymphoblastic leukemia antigen, cALLa, now called CD 10.

Immunophenotypes

B lymphocytic lineage subtypes: These cases are identified by finding cell surface markers on the leukemic blast cells that are identical to those that develop on normal B lymphocytes. About 85 percent of cases are of the precursor B or B cell subtype.

T lymphocytic lineage subtypes: These cases are identified by finding cell surface markers on the leukemic blast cells that are identical to those that develop in normal T lymphocytes. About 15 percent of cases are of the T cell subtype.

Chromosome Abnormalities

Injury to chromosomes can be assessed by cytogenetic methods, and the specific alteration in chromosomes also aids in subclassifying acute lymphocytic leukemia. For example, a change in chromosome number

22, referred to as the Philadelphia or Ph chromosome, which occurs in a small percentage of children and a larger percentage of adults with acute lymphocytic leukemia, places the patient in a higher risk category. Thus, the approach to therapy would be intensified in those subsets of patients.

Symptoms and Signs

Most patients feel a loss of well-being. They tire more easily and may feel short of breath when physically active. They may have a pale complexion from anemia. Signs of bleeding because of a very low platelet count may be noticed. These include black-and-blue marks occurring for no reason or because of a minor injury, the appearance of pinhead-sized, red spots under the skin, called petechiae, or prolonged bleeding from minor cuts. Discomfort in the bones and joints may occur. Fever in the absence of an obvious cause is common. Leukemic lymphoblasts may accumulate in the lymphatic system, and the lymph nodes can become enlarged. The leukemia cells can also collect on the lining of the brain and spinal cord and lead to headache or vomiting.

Section 57.4

Acute Myelogenous Leukemia

About 11,920 new cases of acute myelogenous leukemia are diagnosed each year in the United States. Acute myelogenous leukemia (AML) may be called by several names, including: acute myelocytic leukemia, acute myeloblastic leukemia, acute granulocytic leukemia, or acute nonlymphocytic leukemia.

AML results from acquired (not inherited) genetic damage to the DNA of developing cells in the bone marrow. The effects are the uncontrolled, exaggerated growth and accumulation of cells called "leukemic blasts" which fail to function as normal blood cells, and the blockade of the production of normal marrow cells, leading to a deficiency of red cells (anemia), platelets (thrombocytopenia), and normal white cells (especially neutrophils, or neutropenia) in the blood.

Causes and Risk Factors

In most cases the cause of AML is not evident. Several factors have been associated with an increased risk of disease. These include the following:

- Exposure to high doses of irradiation, as carefully studied in the Japanese survivors of atomic bomb detonations

- Exposure to the chemical benzene, usually in the work place

- Exposure to chemotherapy used to treat cancers such as breast cancer, cancer of the ovary or the lymphomas. Alkylating agents and topoisomerase inhibitors are most frequently associated with higher risk

- Therapeutic radiation, depending on the dose and setting

AML is not contagious and is not inherited. Uncommon genetic disorders such as Fanconi anemia, Schwachman-Diamond syndrome, Down syndrome and others are associated with an increased risk of AML. Older people are more likely to develop the disease.

Very rarely, AML may occur in unexpectedly high frequencies in certain families. It is thought that these families transmit a susceptibility gene to offspring through the germ-line. AML incidence increases dramatically among people who are over the age of 40. It is most prevalent in the sixth, seventh, eighth, and ninth decades of life.

Subtypes of Acute Myelogenous Leukemia

Leukemia is a malignant disease (cancer) of the bone marrow and blood. AML can occur in a variety of ways; different types of cells may be seen by the physician in blood or marrow.

Since most patients have one of seven different patterns of blood cell involvement, these patterns have formed a subclassification which is shown in Table 57.1.

If there are cells that are developing features of monocytes (monocytic type) or red cells (erythroleukemic), these designations are used and so forth.

Even though the leukemia cells look somewhat like blood cells, the process of their formation is incomplete. Normal, healthy blood cells are insufficient in quantity.

The subclassification of the disease is important. Different types of therapy may be used and the likely course of the disease and prognosis may be different. Additional features may be important in guiding the choice of therapy, including: abnormalities of chromosomes, the cell immunophenotype, the age and the general health of the patient, and others.

Table 57.1. Acute Myelogenous Leukemia Subtypes

Designation	Cell Subtype
M0	Myeloblastic, on special analysis
M1	Myeloblastic, without maturation
M2	Myeloblastic, with maturation
M3	Promyelocytic
M4	Myelomonocytic
M5	Monocytic
M6	Erythroleukemia
M7	Megakaryocytic

Symptoms and Signs

Most patients feel a loss of well-being. They tire more easily and may feel short of breath when physically active. They may have a pale complexion from anemia. Several signs of bleeding caused by a very low platelet count may be noticed. They include black-and-blue marks or bruises occurring for no reason or because of a minor injury, the appearance of pin-head sized spots under the skin, called petechiae, or prolonged bleeding from minor cuts. Mild fever, swollen gums, frequent minor infections like pustules or perianal sores, slow healing of cuts, or discomfort in bones or joints may occur.

Section 57.5

Chronic Lymphocytic Leukemia

Each year, nearly 9,730 people in the United States learn that they have chronic lymphocytic leukemia. The disease may be referred to as chronic lymphoid leukemia or as CLL.

CLL results from an acquired injury to the DNA of a single cell, a lymphocyte, in the bone marrow. This injury is not present at birth. Scientists do not yet understand what produces this change in the DNA of CLL patients.

The change in the cell's DNA gives the CLL cell a growth and survival advantage. The result is the uncontrolled growth of CLL cells in the marrow, leading to an increased concentration in the blood. The CLL cells that accumulate in the marrow do not impede normal blood cell production to the extent that is the case with acute lymphocytic leukemia. This important distinction from acute leukemia accounts for the less severe early course of the disease.

Causes and Risk Factors

Chronic lymphocytic leukemia is not associated with high-dose radiation or benzene exposures, as is the case with the other three major types of leukemia. CLL is very uncommon in individuals under 45 years of age. At the time of diagnosis, about 95 percent of patients are over age 50, and the incidence of the disease increases dramatically thereafter. The risk of chronic lymphocytic leukemia becomes measurable after age 35 and increases dramatically over succeeding decades.

Symptoms and Signs

Early in the disease, chronic lymphocytic leukemia may have little effect on a person's well-being. The symptoms of CLL usually develop gradually:

• Patients tire more easily.

597

- They may feel short of breath when physically active.

- They may lose weight.

- They may experience frequent infections of the skin, lungs, kidneys, or other sites.

Many CLL patients say they learned they had CLL after a routine check-up. When an enlarged lymph node or an enlarged spleen is found during a physical examination, or when a routine blood test shows a higher than normal number of lymphocytes, a physician will order lab tests to get more information.

Approach to Diagnosis

Diagnosis begins with a medical history and physical examination by the physician. To complete the diagnosis, the blood and, in most cases, the marrow cells must be examined. Physicians use a number of lab tests to look at cells in blood and marrow.

A test called flow cytometry is used to find out if a patient has CLL. This test is also called immunophenotyping. Flow cytometry shows if CLL is causing the high number of lymphocytes in the blood. Flow cytometry can also show if the CLL began with a B lymphocyte or a T lymphocyte. B lymphocyte (or B-cell CLL) is most common.

Other lab tests are done if flow cytometry shows the patient has CLL. A cytogenetic analysis looks to see if there are changes in the chromosomes of the CLL cells. (Every cell in the body has chromosomes that carry genes. Genes contain the instructions that tell each cell what to do.)

FISH (fluorescence in situ hybridization) is another test that is used to check for chromosome changes. After CLL treatment begins it can be used to see if treatment is working. This is done by measuring the number of cells with abnormal chromosomes that remain after treatment.

A bone marrow biopsy is used to look at the amount and pattern of CLL cells in the marrow. In patients with more advanced CLL a bone marrow biopsy is usually done as a baseline. The results from the baseline are compared to a repeat bone marrow biopsy after treatment. This is one way to tell how the patient is doing after treatment. This test is not always done for low-risk CLL patients.

Doctors also may check the blood for immunoglobulins (gamma globulins.) Immunoglobulins are proteins that help the body fight infection. CLL patients may not have enough of these proteins. With more advanced CLL, low levels of immunoglobulins may be a cause of repeated infections.

Section 57.6

Chronic Myelogenous Leukemia

About 4,600 new cases of chronic myelogenous leukemia (CML) are diagnosed each year in the United States. Chronic myelogenous leukemia may be called by several names, including chronic granulocytic, chronic myelocytic or chronic myeloid leukemia.

CML results from an acquired (not inherited) injury to the DNA of a stem cell in the marrow. This injury is not present at birth. Scientists do not yet understand what produces this change in the DNA in patients with CML.

This change in the stem cell's DNA confers a growth and survival advantage on the malignant stem cell. The result of this injury is the uncontrolled growth of white cells leading, if unchecked, to a massive increase in their concentration in the blood. Unlike acute myelogenous leukemia (AML), chronic myelogenous leukemia permits the development of mature white blood cells that generally can function normally. This important distinction from acute leukemia accounts for the less severe early course of the disease.

Most cases of chronic myelogenous leukemia occur in adults. Only 2.6 percent of leukemias in children ages 0–19 are CML. The frequency of the disease increases with age from about one in 1 million children in the first 10 years of life to nearly two in 100,000 people at age 50, to one in 10,000 people at age 80 and above. The disease in children is similar in behavior to that of adults; however, the outcome of stem cell transplantation is better in younger individuals.

Causes and Risk Factors

Chronic myelogenous leukemia is distinguished from other leukemias by the presence of a genetic abnormality in blood cells, called the Philadelphia chromosome. The changes that result in this chromosome "causing" chronic myelogenous leukemia have been studied intensively. In 1960, two physicians studying chromosomes in cancer cells noticed that a chromosome in CML patients was shorter in length than that of the same chromosome in normal cells. They named this shortened chromosome the Philadelphia chromosome, because the observation was made at the University of Pennsylvania School of Medicine in that city.

The total of 46 chromosomes in normal human cells is composed of 22 pairs of chromosomes numbered 1 to 22 and two sex chromosomes (either an X and Y in males or two Xs in females).

The Philadelphia chromosome (No. 22), which is an abnormally short chromosome, is usually referred to as the Ph-chromosome.

Further studies established that two chromosomes, usually chromosome No. 9 and 22, were abnormal. Pieces of the chromosomes, which are broken off in the blood cells of patients with chronic myelogenous leukemia, switch with each other. The detached portion of chromosome 9 sticks to the broken end of chromosome 22, and the detached portion of chromosome 22 sticks to the broken end of chromosome 9. This abnormal exchange of parts of chromosomes is called a translocation. This translocation of chromosome pieces occurs only in the stem cell and in the various blood cells derived from that stem cell. The chromosomes of the cells in other tissues are normal.

The breakage on chromosome 9 disrupts a gene referred to as "ABL" (for Abelson). The breakage on chromosome 22 involves a gene referred to as "BCR" (for breakpoint cluster region). The human ABL gene is mutated by the breakage of chromosome 9. The mutated gene is translocated to chromosome 22 and fuses with the remaining part of the BCR gene. This fusion between BCR and ABL leads to an abnormal fused gene, called BCR-ABL.

Despite these changes, the BCR-ABL gene can function. The function of a gene is to direct the production of a protein in the cell. In chronic myelogenous leukemia, the protein produced by the BCR-ABL gene is abnormal. The protein produced is an enzyme called tyrosine kinase. The ABL when fused to BCR results in an elongated protein when compared to the protein made by the normal ABL gene. This elongated protein (enzyme) functions abnormally and leads to dysfunctional regulation of cell growth and survival. Evidence points to the abnormal protein as the cause of the leukemic conversion of the hematopoietic stem cell. The mutated gene results in an abnormal or mutated protein, which is responsible for the development of the disease.

The cause of the chromosomal breakage in virtually all CML patients is not known. In a small proportion of patients, the cause of the breakage is exposure to very high doses of radiation. This effect has been most carefully studied in the Japanese survivors of the atomic bomb, whose leukemia risk was significantly increased. A slight increase in risk also occurs in some individuals treated with high dose radiotherapy for other cancers, such as lymphoma. Exposures to diagnostic dental or medical x-rays have not been associated with a heightened risk of chronic myelogenous leukemia.

Symptoms and Signs

The onset of chronic myelogenous leukemia is associated with symptoms that usually develop gradually. Most patients feel a loss of well-being. They tire more easily and may feel short of breath when physically active. They may have a pale complexion from anemia. Discomfort on the left side of the abdomen from an enlarged spleen is a frequent complaint. Patients may experience excessive sweating, weight loss, and inability to tolerate warm temperatures. Increasingly, the disease is discovered during the course of a "routine" medical examination. Since the disease worsens over weeks or months, most patients would have symptoms develop soon after such a medical examination in any case.

Approach to Diagnosis

To diagnose the disease, the blood and, in most cases, the marrow cells must be examined. The white cell count invariably increases, often to very high levels. Examination of the stained (dyed) blood cells with a light microscope shows a characteristic pattern of white cells: a small proportion of very immature cells (leukemic blast cells) and a larger proportion of maturing and fully-matured white cells (myelocytes and neutrophils).

In addition, a sample of marrow is examined to confirm the blood findings and to determine if there is an abnormality of chromosomes. This test, which measures the number and normalcy of chromosomes, is referred to as a cytogenetic analysis. The presence of the Philadelphia chromosome in the marrow cells, a shortened chromosome number 22, high white blood cell counts, and other characteristic blood and marrow findings, confirm that the disorder is chronic myelogenous leukemia.

Cytogenetic Analysis

Cytogenetic examination of tissue is the process of analyzing the number and shape of the chromosomes of cells. The individual, who prepares, examines, and interprets the number and shape of chromosomes in cells is called a cytogeneticist. In addition to identifying chromosome alterations, the specific genes affected can be identified in some cases. These findings are essential in verifying that the disease is BCR-ABL positive CML.

The chromosome abnormalities that characterize chronic myelogenous leukemia can be detected by other techniques as well. Fluorescence in situ hybridization (FISH) is another method to identify cells in which the nucleus that contains chromosomes with the 9:22 translocation characteristic of CML. FISH is also useful to follow the effects of treatment since it can reveal whether there has been a significant decrease of CML cells in the blood.

Polymerase Chain Reaction (PCR)

A very sensitive test of blood cells, the polymerase chain reaction or PCR, can increase very small amounts of either RNA or DNA and make them easier to detect. The alteration in DNA caused by the chromosome breakage in CML can be detected by this very sensitive method. PCR is more sensitive than FISH and can detect one BCR-ABL-positive cell in a background of about 500,000 normal cells.

Section 57.7

Hairy Cell Leukemia

Hairy cell leukemia is a type of chronic lymphocytic leukemia (CLL). CLL is one of the four major categories of leukemia. Based on the category and subset, the physician can determine what treatment will work best for the patient. Hairy cell leukemia is a slow-growing malignant disorder that affects white blood cells called lymphocytes. The disease is called hairy cell leukemia because the leukemic lymphocytes have short, thin projections from their surface that look like hairs when examined under a microscope. The hairy cells accumulate in the bone marrow and spleen and to a lesser extent in lymph nodes. The accumulation of these functionless leukemic lymphocytes in the marrow prevents the production of normal blood cells by the marrow. These normal cells are of great importance to the well-being of the patient. Researchers do not understand the ways in which leukemic cells get their competitive advantage, overgrow the marrow, and prevent normal cells from being made.

Causes and Risk Factors

The cause of hairy cell leukemia and the means to prevent it are unknown. There seems to be no direct link between the disease and exposure to environmental toxins. The disease has very occasionally occurred in members of the same family. However, no hereditary pattern has been established.

Symptoms and Signs

Hairy cell leukemia may be difficult to diagnose early because its symptoms are vague and resemble those of other illnesses. The disease may be discovered during a medical evaluation because of an enlarged spleen or an unexpected decrease in normal blood cell counts. Patients may experience a feeling of discomfort or fullness in the upper left side of their abdomen as a result of the enlarged spleen. Unexplained weight loss and loss of a sense of well-being may bring patients to their physician.

Hairy cells accumulate in the bone marrow preventing the marrow from producing sufficient normal blood cells. The disruption of normal blood cell production leads to anemia (deficiency of red cells), thrombocytopenia (deficiency of platelets) and increased risk of infection (deficiency of white cells called neutrophils and monocytes which fight infection). Often all three blood cell types are deficient (referred to as pancytopenia). Although the hairy cells are abnormal types of lymphocytes, enlargement of lymph nodes is uncommon. Hairy cells accumulate in the marrow and spleen (probably where these cells grow best) but less so in the lymph nodes.

A marked decrease in phagocytes (neutrophils and monocytes) results in an increased chance of developing an infection. Some patients are first aware of the disease because of fever, chills, and other signs of infection. Black and blue marks, as a result of the low concentration of blood platelets, may occur on the skin without injury or after a minor injury.

Approach to Diagnosis

An accurate diagnosis is made by an evaluation of the cells in the blood and marrow. A physician may suspect hairy cell leukemia after performing a preliminary examination of the blood. The normal blood cell counts are low and there may be hairy cells detected in the blood. Occasionally, the hairy cells are numerous in the blood, resulting in an increase in the white cell counts. A bone marrow sample is often needed to confirm the disease. Obtaining a marrow sample from the hipbone can be done in a physician's office.

Special testing, called immunophenotyping, is also performed on the blood and marrow cells. Certain proteins are located on the surface of cells. Each type of cell has its own characteristic pattern of these proteins. Like other cells, hairy cells have a pattern that helps in their identification. Examination of these surface proteins (antigens) with antibodies that combine with their specific antigens and light up using special detection equipment, helps the doctor confirm the type of leukemia that is present. This method also helps to subclassify cell types, which may, in turn, help to decide on the best treatment to apply in that type of leukemia or lymphoma. The antigen on a cell is referred to as cluster of differentiation or "CD" with an associated number. For example, CD11c, 22, and 256 may be present on leukemic hairy cells.

Other tests include a computed tomography (CT) scan which uses multiple images in the computer to create a two dimensional image of the body at several levels. This is a technique for imaging body tissues and organs. The resulting images are displayed as a cross-section of the body at any level from the head to the feet. A CT scan of the chest or abdomen permits detection of an enlarged lymph node, liver or spleen. A CT scan can be used to measure the size of these and other structures during and after treatment. Use of the CT scan for staging enables the physician to determine the extent of enlarged nodes and other organ involvement in the thorax or abdomen. CT scans are more sensitive than x-rays in finding tumors. These studies can be repeated after treatment to determine if the abdominal lymph node or spleen enlargement has decreased or returned to normal size.

Chapter 58

Myelodysplastic Syndromes

Myelodysplastic syndromes (MDS) are a group of diseases that affect the bone marrow and blood. Some types of MDS are mild and easily managed, while other types are severe and life-threatening. Mild MDS can grow more severe over time. It can also develop into a fast-growing, severe leukemia called acute myelogenous leukemia.

About 10,000 to 15,000 people are diagnosed with myelodysplastic syndromes in the United States each year. Although MDS can affect people of any age, more than 80% of cases are in people over age 60. MDS is more common in men than in women.

Causes of MDS

In MDS, the bone marrow does not make enough normal blood cells for the body. One, two, or all three types of blood cells—red blood cells, white blood cells, and platelets—may be affected. The marrow may also make unformed cells called blasts. Blasts normally develop into red blood cells, white blood cells, or platelets. In MDS, the blasts are abnormal and do not develop or function normally.

Most often the cause of the changes to the bone marrow is unknown. This is called de novo MDS. In a small number of people, MDS might be linked to heavy exposure to some chemicals, such as certain

"Myelodysplastic Syndromes (MDS),"© 2006 National Marrow Donor Program; reprinted with permission. For additional information from the National Marrow Donor Program, visit http://www.marrow.org.

solvents or pesticides, or to radiation. MDS can also be caused by treatment with chemotherapy or radiation therapy for other diseases. This is called treatment-related MDS or secondary MDS. Treatment-related MDS is often more severe and difficult to treat than de novo MDS.

MDS Symptoms

The symptoms of MDS depend on how severe the disease is. Many people with MDS have no symptoms when they are diagnosed. Their disease is found through a routine blood test. If a person does have symptoms, they are caused by low numbers of blood cells:

- Red blood cells carry oxygen throughout the body. Low numbers can lead to anemia—feeling tired or weak, being short of breath, and looking pale. Anemia is the most common symptom of MDS.

- White blood cells fight infection. Low numbers can lead to fever and frequent infections.

- Platelets control bleeding. Low numbers can lead to easy bleeding or bruising.

In severe MDS, infection or uncontrolled bleeding can be life-threatening.

Diagnosis

MDS is one of several diseases with these symptoms. Doctors look at samples of blood and bone marrow to diagnose MDS. They also look for changes in the chromosomes of bone marrow cells (cytogenetics).

MDS can be hard to diagnose. Careful study of blood and marrow samples is needed to tell MDS apart from other diseases with similar signs and symptoms, such as aplastic anemia. Blood and marrow samples are often tested several times over two or more months to find out whether the disease is stable or getting worse.

MDS is a group of diseases that have many differences. It is important to diagnose the type of MDS to make the best treatment choices. With some types of MDS, a person may live with few symptoms for years, while other types can be life-threatening within months. In addition, some types of MDS are more likely than others to develop into acute myelogenous leukemia (AML). AML that develops from MDS can be hard to treat.

Types of MDS

The likely course of MDS can be very different for different people. Experience has shown that certain disease factors affect a person's prognosis—his or her chances of long-term survival and risk of developing AML. Researchers use these factors to classify MDS into types.

The system that has been used for decades to classify MDS is called the FAB system because it was developed by a team of French, American, and British researchers. In the FAB system, there are five types of MDS.

The FAB system uses several disease factors to classify MDS. One important factor is the percent of blasts in the bone marrow. A higher percent of blasts is linked to a higher likelihood of developing AML and a poorer prognosis.

The two more common types of MDS are refractory anemia (RA) and refractory anemia with ringed sideroblasts (RARS). These are also the less severe forms of MDS. They have a lower risk of turning into AML. Some patients with these forms of MDS may live with few symptoms and need little treatment for many years.

The other types of MDS tend to be more severe and more difficult to treat successfully. The refractory anemia with excess blasts (RAEB) and refractory anemia with excess blasts in transformation (RAEB-t) forms of MDS also have a high risk of turning into AML.

Table 58.1. MDS Types in the FAB System

Type of MDS	Percent of blasts in marrow (less than 5% is normal)
Refractory anemia (RA)	Less than 5% (normal amount)
Refractory anemia with ringed sideroblasts (RARS)	Less than 5% (normal amount), plus more than 15% of abnormal red blood cells called ringed sideroblasts
Refractory anemia with excess blasts (RAEB)	5% to 20%
Refractory anemia with excess blasts in transformation (RAEB-t)	21% to 30%
Chronic myelomonocytic leukemia (CMML)	5% to 20%, plus a large number of a type of white blood cell called monocytes

Although the type of MDS can help predict the course of a person's disease, people with the same type of MDS may respond to the disease and to treatment differently.

To try to better predict people's outcomes, researchers developed another system for defining types of MDS. The newer World Health Organization (WHO) system divides MDS into eight types. Today a doctor may use either the FAB or WHO system to determine the type of MDS a person has. Either system can be helpful in planning a patient's treatment.

MDS Risk Scores

Researchers have developed one other system for classifying MDS. This system is called the international prognostic scoring system (IPSS). The IPSS risk score describes the risk that a person's disease will develop into AML or become life-threatening.

A doctor may use the IPSS risk score along with the MDS type to plan treatment. The IPSS risk score is based on three factors that have been shown to affect a patient's prognosis:

- The percent of cells in the bone marrow that are blasts

- Whether one, two, or all three types of blood cells are low (also called cytopenias). The three types are red blood cells, white blood cells, and platelets.

- Changes in the chromosomes of bone marrow blood cells. This may be called cytogenetics (the study of chromosome abnormalities). It may also be called the karyotype (a picture of the chromosomes that shows whether they are abnormal).

A person may have an IPSS risk score of low, intermediate-1, intermediate-2, or high risk. Doctors can use the risk score to plan treatment. Someone with low-risk disease may be likely to survive for years with few symptoms. That person may need less intense treatment. Someone with intermediate-1, intermediate-2, or high-risk disease may be likely to survive only if he or she receives aggressive treatment, such as a transplant.

However, people with the same risk score and type of MDS can still respond differently to treatment. A person's age, overall health and other factors all influence his or her response to the disease and treatment. A doctor will also look at all these factors when planning treatment. If you have MDS, it is important to talk with your doctor about what type of MDS you have and your risk score. Ask how this information affects your treatment options.

Treatment Options

The best treatment for a person with MDS depends on his or her type of MDS, risk level, age, overall health, and his or her own preferences. The treatment options include the following:

- Supportive care
- Bone marrow or cord blood transplant (BMT)
- Chemotherapy
- Newer drug therapies

Whichever treatment you and your doctor decide on, you may choose to be part of a clinical trial. Even standard treatments continue to be studied in clinical trials. These studies help doctors improve treatments so that more patients can have better results.

Supportive Care

Supportive care will be part of the treatment plan for all people with MDS. The goal of supportive care is to manage disease symptoms and related problems.

For some people, supportive care may be the only treatment needed. Some people with few symptoms may need only regular doctor visits. The doctor will watch for any signs the disease is getting more severe.

Some people with more severe MDS may also choose supportive care as their only treatment. People who are older or who have other health problems may be unable to tolerate stronger treatment. Other people weigh the possible risks and benefits of different treatment options and choose supportive care. Supportive care does not offer the possibility of a long-term remission from MDS, but it may offer a way to manage a person's symptoms.

Blood Transfusions

Many people with MDS need blood transfusions to manage symptoms caused by low numbers of red blood cells or platelets.

- Red blood cell transfusions reduce problems with being very tired and short of breath.

- Platelet transfusions reduce risks of bleeding problems caused by very low numbers of platelets.

If you have MDS, your doctor will determine when you need transfusions and manage the possible risks. To manage transfusion risks, your doctor may:

- Give you additional treatment to remove iron from the body (iron chelation therapy). After many red blood cell transfusions, iron builds up in the body, causing organ damage.

- Give as few platelet transfusions as possible to limit the risk of the immune system developing antibodies (immune cells) that attack transfused platelets. If this happens, platelet transfusions must be closely matched to the patient.

- Treat blood cells with radiation and filter out white blood cells before transfusion. This reduces the risks of an immune system reaction against transfused platelets.

Growth Factors

Growth factors are drugs that help the body make more blood cells. A person with MDS may be given growth factors to try to reduce the need for red blood cell transfusions. However, in many cases of MDS, the marrow does not respond to growth factors.

Growth factors may also be given after a transplant. In this case, growth factors often are effective. They can help speed up new blood cell production, reducing a person's need for transfusions and risk of infection.

Bone Marrow or Cord Blood Transplant for MDS

The only known treatment that can bring a long-term remission from MDS is a bone marrow or cord blood transplant (also called a BMT). A transplant replaces the abnormal cells in the bone marrow with healthy blood-forming cells from a family member or unrelated donor or cord blood unit.

The standard transplant for MDS is allogeneic, which uses blood-forming cells from a family member, an unrelated donor, or a cord blood unit. The donor for a transplant must closely match the patient's tissue type. The best donor is usually a matched sibling. For patients who do not have a suitable donor in their family, doctors may search the National Marrow Donor Program (NMDP) Registry for a matching adult volunteer donor or cord blood unit.

A transplant can offer some people the chance for a long-term remission of disease and a longer life, but it is not an option for all patients. A transplant may be a good option for people who have a suitable donor or cord blood unit and are healthy enough to tolerate a transplant. In general, younger patients tend to do better after a transplant than older patients. However, advances in transplant have enabled more older patients to undergo a transplant successfully.

Reduced-intensity transplant for MDS: Before a transplant, a patient receives a preparative regimen of high-dose chemotherapy with or without radiation therapy. Many patients with MDS are older and have other health problems that may make them unable to tolerate this high-dose regimen. However, some may be able to tolerate a reduced-intensity regimen, which uses lower doses of chemotherapy and low-dose or no radiation therapy.

Reduced-intensity transplant is a newer approach to transplant for MDS, and early results have been encouraging. The use of reduced-intensity transplant to treat MDS is growing. This approach may offer the chance for long-term survival to some patients, especially those who are older or have other health problems.

Autologous transplant for MDS: The standard transplant for MDS is allogeneic, which uses blood-forming cells from a family member, an unrelated donor or a cord blood unit. Another type of transplant is an autologous transplant, which uses the patient's own blood-forming cells. An autologous transplant is a standard treatment for some diseases and is being studied in clinical trials as a treatment for MDS. An autologous transplant may be an option for patients who do not have a suitable donor for an allogeneic transplant.

In an autologous transplant, blood-forming cells are collected from the patient. After treatment with high-dose chemotherapy and possibly radiation therapy, the patient receives his or her own cells back.

Autologous transplants have risks of serious side effects, but these risks are lower than for allogeneic transplants. However, a patient has higher risks of a relapse of MDS after an autologous transplant. This may be because disease cells may be returned to the patient along with his or her blood-forming cells.

Transplant success rates: Transplants have risks of serious complications, but a transplant offers some patients the best chance for a long-term remission. If transplant is an option for you, talk with your about the possible risks and benefits of a transplant.

Induction Chemotherapy

Chemotherapy uses drugs to destroy abnormal cells or stop them from growing. A treatment option for some people with severe MDS may be induction chemotherapy. Induction chemotherapy is very intense. The goal is to bring the disease into remission (no more signs of disease).

Induction chemotherapy may be an option for patients with high IPSS risk scores who are in good overall health but do not have a suitable donor for a transplant. Induction chemotherapy is also sometimes used to bring MDS into remission before a patient receives a transplant.

About half of patients treated with induction chemotherapy may reach a remission, but relapse is common and the rate of long-term survival is low, particularly in older patients. Because of the high relapse rate, patients may be given further treatment, such as a transplant or more chemotherapy.

In addition, many people with MDS, especially those who are older or who have other health problems, may be unable to tolerate intensive induction chemotherapy. Different chemotherapy regimens for MDS, some low-intensity and some high-intensity, are being studied in clinical trials to try to find a more effective approach.

Newer Drug Therapies

Much research is being done to find better treatment options for patients with MDS. Many newer drug therapies have been shown to bring a response in some patients with MDS. These therapies have either been approved by the U.S. Food and Drug Administration (FDA) or continue to be studied in clinical trials.

For some drug therapies, the goal is a long-term remission of the disease and long-term survival. For many other drug therapies, the goal is to improve a person's blood counts and symptoms. Managing the symptoms and related problems of MDS may offer a higher quality of life and a somewhat longer life than supportive care alone.

If you have MDS, talk with your doctor about the many newer drug therapies available. Your doctor can help you determine which, if any, are good options for you. Your doctor can also help you find clinical trials offering these treatments, if they are appropriate for you.

Making Treatment Choices

If you are diagnosed with MDS, it is important to talk with a doctor who has experience treating MDS. Ask about the type of MDS you have, your risk factors and treatment options, and discuss your own treatment goals. There are a variety of treatment options available, including newer treatments being studied in clinical trials. The best treatment for you will depend on your type of MDS, risk score, age, overall health and your own preferences.

Planning for Possible Transplant

If a transplant may be a treatment option for you, your doctor will refer you to a transplant doctor for a consultation. A transplant doctor can determine whether a transplant is a good treatment option for you.

The NMDP and American Society of Blood and Marrow Transplantation (ASBMT) recommend a patient be referred to a transplant doctor for consultation based on IPSS risk scores. Referral is recommended for patients with an intermediate-1, intermediate-2, or high risk score who have one or more of the following factors:

- More than 5% blasts in the bone marrow

- Intermediate or high-risk cytogenetic factors

- Low blood counts for more than one type of blood cell (red blood cells, white blood cells and platelets)

A transplant doctor can also help determine the best time for a transplant. An early consultation with a transplant doctor enables your doctors to plan ahead even if a transplant is not your first treatment choice. The transplant doctor can begin the search for a suitable donor among family members and the National Marrow Donor Program Registry of unrelated donor and cord blood units. Taking the first steps of the donor search early may enable a quicker transplant if you need one.

Information to Share with Your Doctor

The Physician Resources section of the National Marrow Donor Program (http://www.marrow.org) includes information for doctors about timing and outcomes of transplants for MDS, as well as references to related medical journal articles. You may want to share some of this information with your doctor.

More Information on MDS

You can get further information about MDS from disease-specific organizations, such as:

Aplastic Anemia & MDS International Foundation—Request an information packet:
https://www.toad.net/~aafa/aplastic/disease_information/educational
_material/index.php

Leukemia and Lymphoma Society—MDS:
http://www.leukemia-lymphoma.org/all_page?item_id=55442

National Cancer Institute—MDS (PDQ®): Treatment:
http://www.cancer.gov/cancertopics/pdq/treatment/myelodysplastic

American Cancer Society—How are MDS and MDS/MPD treated?:
http://www.cancer.org/docroot/CRI/content/CRI_2_2_4x_How_Are_
MDS_and_MDSMPD_Treated_65.asp

Chapter 59

Multiple Myeloma

Introduction to Myeloma

Multiple myeloma, a cancer of the plasma cell, is an incurable but treatable disease. While a myeloma diagnosis can be overwhelming, it is important to remember that there are several promising new therapies that are helping patients live longer, healthier lives. The estimated frequency of multiple myeloma is 5–6 new cases per 100,000 persons per year. Accordingly, in the U.S. 15,980 new cases were expected to be diagnosed in 2005. At present there are more than 50,000 people in the United States living with multiple myeloma.

Definition

Multiple myeloma (also known as myeloma or plasma cell myeloma) is a progressive hematologic (blood) disease. It is a cancer of the plasma cell, an important part of the immune system that produces immunoglobulins (antibodies) to help fight infection and disease. Multiple myeloma is characterized by excessive numbers of abnormal plasma cells in the bone marrow and overproduction of intact monoclonal immunoglobulin (IgG, IgA, IgD, or IgE) or Bence-Jones

This chapter includes text from "Intro to Myeloma," reviewed by Sagar Lonial, M.D., Emory University School of Medicine, September 9, 2005; and "Knowing Your Treatment Options," reviewed by Mohamad Hussein, M.D., Cleveland Clinic, November 11, 2004. © Multiple Myeloma Research Foundation; reprinted with permission. For additional information online visit www.multiplemyeloma.org.

protein (free monoclonal κ and λ light chains). Hypercalcemia, anemia, renal damage, increased susceptibility to bacterial infection, and impaired production of normal immunoglobulin are common clinical manifestations of multiple myeloma. It is often also characterized by diffuse osteoporosis, usually in the pelvis, spine, ribs, and skull.

Cells destined to become immune cells, like all blood cells, arise in the bone marrow from stem cells. Some stem cells develop into the small white blood cells called lymphocytes. The two major classes of lymphocytes are B cells (B lymphocytes) and T cells (T lymphocytes). Plasma cells develop from B cells.

Normal Plasma Cell Function in the Immune System

Plasma cells develop from B cells when foreign substances (antigens), such as bacteria, enter the body. In response to invasion by foreign substances, groups of plasma cells produce proteins called immunoglobulins

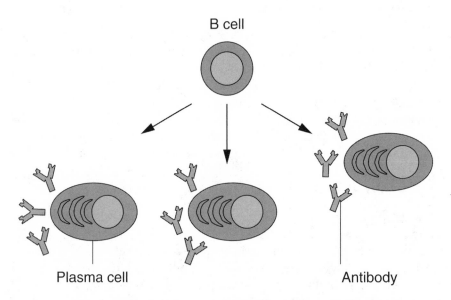

B cell

Plasma cell   Antibody

Figure 59.1. Like most blood cells, plasma cells develop from stem cells in the bone marrow. Stem cells can develop into B cells (B lymphocytes), which travel to the lymph nodes, mature, and then travel throughout the body. When foreign substances (antigens) enter the body, B cells develop into plasma cells that produce immunoglobulins (antibodies) to help fight infection and disease. (The image shown here is from the National Institute of Allergy and Infectious Diseases, NIH Publication No. 03-5423.)

(Ig), also known as antibodies that help fight disease and infection. Each plasma cell develops in response to a particular foreign substance within the body, and it produces immunoglobulins specific to that substance. Thus, there are many different immunoglobulins produced in the body.

Immunoglobulins are made up of protein chains, two long chains called heavy chains and two shorter chains known as light chains.

There are five major classes of immunoglobulins. Each class has a unique type of heavy chain that is defined by use of a Greek letter: gamma (IgG), alpha (IgA), mu (IgM), epsilon (IgE), or delta (IgD). Each type has a slightly different function in the body. Normally, a plasma cell makes one of these five major classes of immunoglobulin. The immunoglobulin class normally present in the largest amounts in blood is IgG, followed by IgA and IgM. IgD and IgE are present in very small amounts in the blood. Immunoglobulin light chains are defined by use of the Greek letters kappa (κ) or lambda (λ).

Development of Malignant Plasma Cells (Myeloma Cells)

It is normal for plasma cells to develop from B cells in lymph nodes as an immune response to disease or infection. Transformation of a normal B cell into a malignant plasma cell involves a multi-step process that includes multiple genetic abnormalities. Finally, the resulting plasma cells become malignant, meaning they continue to divide unchecked, generating more malignant plasma cells. These myeloma

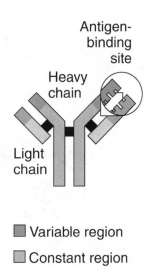

Figure 59.2. Immunoglobulins (antibodies) are made up of two heavy chains and two light chains. The variable region, which differs from one antibody to the next, allows an antibody to recognize its matching antigen. (The image shown here is from the National Institute of Allergy and Infectious Diseases, NIH Publication No. 03-5423.)

cells travel through the bloodstream and collect in the bone marrow, where they cause permanent damage to healthy tissue. We have recently learned that the interaction between the plasma cells and the bone marrow microenvironment is as important as the genetic changes in the development of these malignant cells.

Normally, plasma cells make up a very small portion (less than 5%) of cells in the bone marrow. Myeloma plasma cells, however, have specific adhesion molecules on their surface allowing them to target bone marrow where they attach to structural cells called stromal cells. Once myeloma cells attach to bone marrow stromal cells, several interactions cause myeloma cells to grow:

- Chemical messengers called cytokines are produced by both myeloma cells and stromal cells. These cytokines, such as interleukin 6 (IL-6), receptor for activation of NF-κB (RANK) ligand, and tumor necrosis factor (TNF), stimulate the growth of myeloma cells

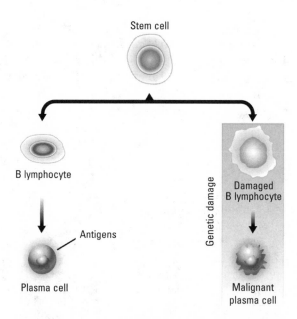

Figure 59.3. In multiple myeloma, the B cell is damaged and gives rise to too many plasma cells (myeloma cells). These malignant cells do not function properly and their increased numbers produce excess immunoglobulins of a single type that the body does not need along with reduced amounts of normal immunoglobulins.

and inhibit (prevent) natural cell death (called apoptosis), leading to proliferation of myeloma cells and ultimately resulting in bone destruction.

- Myeloma cells also produce growth factors that promote angiogenesis, the creation of new blood vessels. These new blood vessels provide the oxygen and nutrients that promote tumor growth. A growth factor called vascular endothelial growth factor (VEGF) plays a key role in angiogenesis. Angiogenesis encourages reproduction of myeloma cells, which increase in number and begin to infiltrate the bone marrow, eventually comprising more than 10% of the cells present.

- Mature myeloma cells may fail to activate the immune system and may produce substances that decrease the body's normal immune response to a foreign body. Thus, the cells can grow unchecked.

As tumors grow, they invade the hard outer part of the bone, the solid tissue. In most cases, the myeloma cells spread into the cavities of all the large bones of the body, forming multiple small lesions. This is why the disease is known as "multiple" myeloma. In some cases, collections of plasma cells arise either within bone or in soft tissues as masses or tumors. These collections are called plasmacytomas, and may represent a more aggressive form of myeloma.

Myeloma cells are identical and produce the same immunoglobulin protein, called monoclonal (M) protein or paraprotein, in large quantities. Although the specific M protein varies from patient to patient, it is always exactly the same in any one patient. When blood or urine is processed in a laboratory test called electrophoresis, these M proteins show up as a "spike" in the results.

Unlike normal immunoglobulin, M protein does not benefit the body. Instead, it crowds out normal, functional immunoglobulins. In addition, levels of functional immunoglobulin are depressed in individuals with myeloma. Although the process is not completely understood, it appears that the functional immunoglobulin made by existing normal plasma cells breaks down more quickly in patients with myeloma than in healthy individuals.

Myeloma Types

Myeloma is often referred to by the particular type of immunoglobulin or light chain (kappa or lambda type) produced by the cancerous plasma cell. The frequency of the various immunoglobulin types of myeloma parallels the normal serum concentrations of the immunoglobulins. The most common myeloma types are IgG and IgA. IgG myeloma accounts for about 60% to 70% of all cases of myeloma and IgA accounts for about 20% of cases. Few cases of IgD and IgE myeloma have been reported.

Although a high level of M protein in the blood is a hallmark of myeloma disease, about 15% to 20% of patients with myeloma produce incomplete immunoglobulins, containing only the light chain portion of the immunoglobulin (also known as Bence Jones proteins, after the chemist who discovered them). These patients are said to have light chain myeloma, or Bence Jones myeloma. In these patients, M protein is found primarily in the urine, rather than in the blood. These Bence Jones proteins may deposit in the kidney and clog the tiny tubules that make up the kidney's filtering system, which can eventually cause kidney damage and result in kidney failure. Bence Jones proteins will not be detected by routine urinalysis. A more complex test called immunoelectrophoresis can measure the exact amount of Bence Jones proteins in the urine.

A rare form of myeloma called nonsecretory myeloma affects about 1% of myeloma patients. In this form of the disease, plasma cells do not produce M protein or light chains.

Causes and Incidence

Multiple myeloma is the second most prevalent blood cancer after non-Hodgkin lymphoma. It represents approximately 1% of all cancers and 2% of all cancer deaths.

Statistics indicate both increasing incidence and earlier age of onset. The average age at diagnosis is about 68 years, and only 1% of cases are diagnosed in individuals under the age of 40. Approximately 50,000 Americans have myeloma, and the American Cancer Society estimates that approximately 15,980 new cases of myeloma were diagnosed during 2005.

Multiple myeloma occurs more frequently in men than women (of the estimated 15,980 new cases referenced above, 8,600 are expected to occur in men versus 7,380 in women). African Americans and Native Pacific Islanders have the highest reported incidence of this disease and Asians the lowest. A recent study found the incidence of myeloma to be 9.5 cases per 100,000 African Americans and 4.1 cases per 100,000 Caucasian Americans. Among African Americans, myeloma is one of the leading causes of cancer death.

Although a tremendous amount of work has gone into the search for the cause of multiple myeloma, to date no cause for this disease has been identified. However, the search for a cause has suggested possible associations between myeloma and a decline in the immune system, genetic factors, certain occupations, certain viruses, exposure to certain chemicals including Agent Orange, and exposure to radiation.

Age is the most significant risk factor for multiple myeloma, as 99% of cases are diagnosed in people over the age of 40, and more than 50% occur in people over the age of 71. Because the peak age for multiple myeloma is among the elderly it is thought that susceptibility may increase with the aging process and the consequent reduction in immune surveillance of evolving cancer, or that myeloma may result from a lifelong accumulation of toxic insults or antigenic challenges.

The higher incidence of myeloma in African Americans and the much less frequent occurrence in Asians suggest genetic factors. While it is uncommon for myeloma to develop in more than one family member, there is a slight increased risk among children and siblings of those with myeloma.

People in agricultural occupations, petroleum workers, workers in leather industries, and cosmetologists all seem to have a higher-than-average chance of developing multiple myeloma. Exposure to herbicides, insecticides, petroleum products, heavy metals, plastics, and various dusts including asbestos also appear to be risk factors for the disease. In addition, individuals exposed to large amounts of radiation, such as survivors of the atomic bomb explosions in Japan, have an increased risk for myeloma, although this accounts for a very small number of cases.

Chromosomal changes including chromosomal translocations (generally involving the Ig heavy chain gene), and chromosomal gains and losses are very frequent in myeloma. These abnormalities have an important influence on disease outcome.

It is important to remember that in most cases, individuals who develop multiple myeloma have no clear risk factors. Myeloma may be the result of several factors acting together.

Knowing Your Treatment Options

There is tremendous progress in the field of myeloma research and scientific advances now offer and unprecedented opportunity to treat myeloma patients.

Information regarding treatments for the disease is constantly changing. The Multiple Myeloma Research Foundation (MMRF), advises patients and caregivers to work with their physicians regarding specific questions relating to treatment and urges health care professionals to share this information with their patients.

Treatment Decisions in Myeloma

Deciding on a particular treatment for myeloma is a complex process. Treatment is tailored to each patient according to several factors, including:

- results of the physical exam;
- results of laboratory tests;
- the specific stage or classification of their disease;
- their age and general health;
- their symptoms;
- whether complications of the disease are present;
- whether they have previously received treatment for their disease;
- their lifestyle and their view and philosophy on quality of life.

Goals of Treatment

Treatment regimens may be designed to meet one or more different therapeutic goals, which can include:

1. Eradicating all evidence of disease, which may require accepting higher levels of toxicity;

2. Controlling disease activity to prevent damage to other organs of the body, using a regimen with an acceptable toxicity level;

3. Preserving normal performance and quality of life for as long as possible with minimal intervention;

4. Providing lasting relief of pain and other disease symptoms;

5. When applicable, managing myeloma that is in remission over the long-term.

With the many promising therapies in clinical trials, MMRF hopes to include the goal of a cure for myeloma in the near future.

Potential Outcomes of Treatment

There are several potential outcomes of treatment in myeloma, which are summarized in the following table. Although cures have not been documented in patients with myeloma, molecular complete responses have been achieved with some of the new therapies in clinical trials. Relapses still occur after molecular complete response, usually after a longer period of event-free survival. Evolving therapies may offer patients a greater chance of achieving a molecular complete response. However, there is currently no evidence that the quality of a response affects how long a patient lives.

Medical researchers have made much progress in the understanding of myeloma and in these promising therapies. However, they have yet to achieve the maximal benefit possible with regard to patient survival and improvement in quality of life. For these reasons, patients with myeloma should strongly consider participating in a clinical trial if it is an appropriate option for them.

Management Options for Myeloma

Myeloma therapy is tailored to each patient. It is important to note that there is no one "standard therapy" for active myeloma. The treatment regimens that are often referred to as standard therapies are those that have been traditionally used for the treatment of the disease and have an established track record of usefulness as documented through publication in reputable scientific journals.

Treatment of myeloma can be a complex process because many variables must be taken into account, such as the patient's overall state of health, other medical issues/diseases, and how well the disease is currently controlled, as well as the type, number, and response to previous therapy. Moreover, there is no single test result that can lead to a diagnosis of myeloma and determine its prognosis; many factors must be considered.

Many centers have developed their own guidelines for treating myeloma and these may vary from center to center. The National Comprehensive Cancer Network (NCCN) has also developed a set of general practice guidelines to aid physicians in treating myeloma. These guidelines indicate particular therapies that have been deemed appropriate based on a review of the literature and on the expertise and clinical experience of a panel of experts. (*NCCN Practice Guidelines in Oncology—Version 1.2004. Multiple Myeloma*; available at http://www.nccn.org).

623

To further advance therapy for multiple myeloma, it is highly suggested that all eligible patients be included on clinical trials. Clinical trials, especially Phase II and Phase III trials, are designed to be at least as effective as what is considered standard therapy.

Management options depend on a patient's disease classification and disease status.

Disease classification: Patients with myeloma can be classified as having either inactive disease or active disease.

Inactive disease is asymptomatic disease that does not require immediate treatment. Patients with inactive disease do not have evidence of any myeloma-related organ or tissue impairment (also known as end-organ damage). Inactive disease includes the following classifications subtypes of myeloma:

• Monoclonal gammopathy of undetermined significance (MGUS)

• Smoldering myeloma (SMM)

• Indolent myeloma (IMM)

• Stage I disease

Active disease is symptomatic disease that requires treatment. Patients with Stage II and Stage III disease fall into this category.

Disease status: The treatment options available to a patient also take into account their disease status, that is, whether they have already received therapy and if so, what was the outcome.

Patients with newly diagnosed disease are individuals who have myeloma that has not yet been treated.

Patients who have received therapy may fall into several categories:

• Responsive disease refers to myeloma that is responding to therapy. There has been a decrease in M protein of at least 50%. Some myeloma groups consider a decrease in M protein between 25% and 50% to be a minimal response whereas others consider this to be stable disease.

• Stable disease refers to myeloma that has not responded to treatment (that is the decrease in M protein has not reached 50%), but has not progressed (gotten worse). Some myeloma groups consider a decrease in M protein between 25% and 50% to be a minimal response.

- A plateau is reached when the outcome of therapy, be it a response or stable disease, has leveled off and disease parameters remain at a stable level.

- Progressive disease refers to active myeloma that is worsening (increasing M protein and worsening organ or tissue impairment [end organ damage]). In most cases, relapsed and/or refractory disease can be considered to be progressive disease.

- Relapsed disease refers to myeloma disease that initially responded to therapy but has then begun to progress again. Patients

Table 59.1. Potential Outcomes of Treatment in Myeloma

Treatment Outcome*	Definition
Cure	Complete and lasting recovery from disease (this has not yet been achieved in myeloma)
Molecular complete response	No evidence of disease using the most sensitive techniques available. These techniques continue to evolve and become more sensitive, so this definition is constantly changing and becoming more stringent.
Complete response (CR)	No detectable M protein in the serum and urine (using negative immunofixation electrophoresis test) **and** Normal percentage of plasma cells in the bone marrow **or** Absence of myeloma cells by staining techniques
Near complete	As listed for CR, but with a positive immunofixation test response
Very good partial response	Greater than 90% decrease in M protein
Partial response (PR)	Greater than 50% decrease in M protein
Minimal response (or minor response)	Less than 50% decrease in M protein. Note that some myeloma groups consider minimal response to be part of the definition of stable disease.
Stable disease (SD)	Stable disease parameters (including number and extent of lesions) with some decrease in M protein
Progressive disease	Greater than 25% increase in M protein, new bony lesions, or a new plasmacytoma

* Note that in all outcomes, response may also be referred to as remission. These terms are interchangeable.

may be further classified as having relapsed after initial therapy or after subsequent therapy.

- Refractory disease refers to myeloma that has not responded to initial therapy, as well as relapsed myeloma that does not respond to subsequent treatment. In this last instance, the myeloma may also be referred to as relapsed and refractory disease. Refractory disease can be of two types:

  - Non-responding progressing refractory disease, which refers to refractory disease that is progressing. This is a difficult type of myeloma to treat and some form of innovative therapy is usually suggested as a treatment option.

  - Non-responding non-progressing refractory disease, which refers to refractory disease that is not worsening. Patient with this type of disease often do as well as patients with responsive disease.

Treatment Approaches

Treatment approaches to myeloma depend on whether a patient has inactive or active disease. This section provides an overview of the various treatment approaches and therapeutic options for myeloma.

Inactive disease: Patients with inactive (asymptomatic) disease are typically observed and not treated unless their disease begins to progress. No therapy is recommended outside of a clinical trial unless there is evidence of active disease with end organ damage. However, in some cases, bisphosphonates and other forms of supportive care may be appropriate for patients with smoldering or indolent myeloma or Stage 1 disease. Participation in a clinical trial is also an option. For example, agents such as thalidomide are being tested in patients with inactive disease. You can access the MMRF Clinical Trials Monitor (CTM) to see what clinical trial options might be appropriate for you (online, go to http://www.multiplemyeloma.org/clinical _trials/4.04.html).

Active disease: Patients with newly diagnosed, active (symptomatic) myeloma typically receive some form of initial therapy, as well as bisphosphonates and supportive care as required to treat bone disease and other complications of the disease. Subsequent treatment options are often decided based on previous treatments received and the outcome.

The choice of initial therapy is dependent on whether a patient is a candidate for high-dose chemotherapy and autologous stem cell transplant, a therapeutic strategy that offers improved response rates and survival in myeloma. Patients under the age of 65 in good physical condition with adequate kidney, lung, and heart function are potential transplant candidates. However, older patients may be eligible if they are in very good health.

Non-transplant candidates: If a patient is not a candidate for an autologous transplant, the most common initial treatment is a combination of melphalan, a type of chemotherapy, and prednisone, a type of corticosteroid. Cyclophosphamide and prednisone (CP) or other combinations of agents may also be used. High-dose dexamethasone (another corticosteroid) is often used in older patients who may be unable to tolerate other therapies, as is combination Thalomid® (thalidomide, Celgene) and dexamethasone.

Non-transplant candidates typically continue initial therapy for about a year or until their response reaches a plateau. At that time they may receive some form of maintenance therapy, such as corticosteroids, and continue to receive bisphosphonates and supportive care as required. Patients who initially respond to therapy, however, eventually relapse (that is, disease begins to progress again). Patients who relapse shortly following completion of initial therapy may no longer respond to the initial medications used. These patients, as well as those who do not respond to initial therapy, are said to have refractory disease.

Transplant candidates: Certain chemotherapy agents, such as melphalan (which is also known as an alkylating agent) may impair the ability to collect stem cells for use in an autologous transplant and should be used with care. For this reason, patients who are candidates for autologous transplant often receive other agents as initial therapy or receive melphalan for only a brief period before their stem cells are collected. Options include combination thalidomide and dexamethasone, which is now the most frequently used initial therapy in transplant candidates, as well as dexamethasone or the chemotherapy regimen known as VAD (vincristine, doxorubicin, dexamethasone). A modification of the VAD regimen known as DVd (Doxil® [liposomal doxorubicin, Ortho Biotech], vincristine, short-schedule Decadron [dexamethasone]), which can be administered on an outpatient basis, may also be used. After three or four cycles of therapy, which minimizes the tumor burden, transplant candidates have their stem cells collected for use in their transplant.

627

After stem cell collection, transplant candidates may proceed directly to an autologous transplant ("early transplant"). Alternatively, they can continue to receive their initial therapy until plateau and then receive their transplant at the time of relapse ("late transplant"). Some prefer early transplantation because it minimizes a patient's time on chemotherapy and overall quality of life may be improved.

Treatments for relapsed or refractory disease: Treatments for relapsed and/or refractory disease are often referred to as salvage therapy. If a relapse occurs after six months of discontinuing therapy, the initial therapy may be reconsidered. Other options for treating relapsed or refractory disease include participation in a clinical trial, various salvage chemotherapy agents or combinations, thalidomide-based regimens, bortezomib (Velcade®), or stem cell transplant if possible.

Chapter 60

Hodgkin Lymphoma

Chapter Contents

Section 60.1

What Is Hodgkin Lymphoma?

Excerpted from "What You Need to Know about™ Hodgkin's Disease,"
National Cancer Institute, September 2002.

Hodgkin Disease (Lymphoma)

Hodgkin disease is one of a group of cancers called lymphomas.
Lymphoma is a general term for cancers that develop in the lymphatic
system. Hodgkin disease, an uncommon lymphoma, accounts for less
than 1 percent of all cases of cancer in this country. Other cancers of
the lymphatic system are called non-Hodgkin lymphomas.

The lymphatic system is part of the body's immune system. It helps
the body fight disease and infection. The lymphatic system includes
a network of thin lymphatic vessels that branch, like blood vessels,
into tissues throughout the body. Lymphatic vessels carry lymph, a
colorless, watery fluid that contains infection-fighting cells called lymphocytes. Along this network of vessels are small organs called lymph
nodes. Clusters of lymph nodes are found in the underarms, groin,
neck, chest, and abdomen. Other parts of the lymphatic system are
the spleen, thymus, tonsils, and bone marrow. Lymphatic tissue is also
found in other parts of the body, including the stomach, intestines, and
skin.

Cancer is a group of many related diseases that begin in cells, the
body's basic unit of life. To understand Hodgkin disease, it is helpful
to know about normal cells and what happens when they become cancerous. The body is made up of many types of cells. Normally, cells
grow and divide to produce more cells only when the body needs them.
This orderly process helps keep the body healthy. Sometimes cells keep
dividing when new cells are not needed, creating a mass of extra tissue. This mass is called a growth or tumor. Tumors can be either benign (not cancerous) or malignant (cancerous).

In Hodgkin disease, cells in the lymphatic system become abnormal. They divide too rapidly and grow without any order or control.
Because lymphatic tissue is present in many parts of the body, Hodgkin
disease can start almost anywhere. Hodgkin disease may occur in a

630

single lymph node, a group of lymph nodes, or, sometimes, in other parts of the lymphatic system such as the bone marrow and spleen. This type of cancer tends to spread in a fairly orderly way from one group of lymph nodes to the next group. For example, Hodgkin disease that arises in the lymph nodes in the neck spreads first to the nodes above the collarbones, and then to the lymph nodes under the arms and within the chest. Eventually, it can spread to almost any other part of the body.

Risk Factors Associated with Hodgkin Disease

Scientists at hospitals and medical centers all across the country are studying Hodgkin disease. They are trying to learn more about what causes the disease and more effective methods of treatment.

At this time, the cause or causes of Hodgkin disease are not known, and doctors can seldom explain why one person gets this disease and another does not. It is clear, however, that Hodgkin disease is not caused by an injury, and it is not contagious; no one can "catch" this disease from another person.

By studying patterns of cancer in the population, researchers have found certain risk factors that are more common in people who get Hodgkin disease than in those who do not. However, most people with these risk factors do not get Hodgkin disease, and many who do get this disease have none of the known risk factors. The following are some of the risk factors associated with this disease:

- **Age/Sex:** Hodgkin disease occurs most often in people between 15 and 34 and in people over the age of 55. It is more common in men than in women.

- **Family History:** Brothers and sisters of those with Hodgkin disease have a higher-than-average chance of developing this disease.

- **Viruses:** Epstein-Barr virus is an infectious agent that may be associated with an increased chance of getting Hodgkin disease.

People who are concerned about the chance of developing Hodgkin disease should talk with their doctor about the disease, the symptoms to watch for, and an appropriate schedule for checkups. The doctor's advice will be based on the person's age, medical history, and other factors.

Section 60.2

Diagnosing Hodgkin Lymphoma

A number of different examinations and tests are usually required to diagnose Hodgkin's lymphoma, as well as to assess how far the disease has spread and how well your body systems are working. Depending on your situation, the physician may use some or all of these tests to determine the best way to treat your disease.

The information from a patient's history, physical examinations, x-rays, scans, laboratory tests, and biopsy is analyzed to allow the doctor to determine the extent of disease and recommend the treatment (or treatments) that have the best chance of either producing a remission or cure.

Signs and Symptoms of Hodgkin's Lymphoma

A sign or symptom is anything out of the ordinary that the patient experiences that could be caused by a disease. Symptoms are not specific to lymphomas and are, in fact, similar to those of many other illnesses. People often first go to the doctor because they think they have a cold, the flu, or some other respiratory infection that does not go away.

The most common sign of Hodgkin's lymphoma is usually a swelling of lymph nodes, that may or may not be painful, and most often occurs in the neck. Some people may also experience swelling of lymph nodes in other parts of the body. Other symptoms of Hodgkin's lymphoma may include unexplained fever, weight loss, or sweating (usually at night), or a lack of energy. Coughing, shortness of breath, or chest discomfort may be signs of Hodgkin's lymphoma in the chest. There is usually no pain involved, especially when Hodgkin's lymphoma is in the early stages of development. About 5% of patients may experience pain at the tumor site after drinking alcoholic beverages. While this symptom is rare, it is characteristic for Hodgkin's lymphoma. The cause of this symptom is unknown.

Most people who have non-specific complaints such as these will not have Hodgkin's lymphoma. However, it is important that anyone who has persistent symptoms be seen by a doctor to make sure that Hodgkin's lymphoma is not present. Serious illnesses do not simply come and go, they persist.

What the doctor looks for during a physical examination: If you have symptoms suggesting Hodgkin's lymphoma, a complete physical examination will be performed. During this examination, the doctor will look for swollen lymph nodes under the chin, in the neck and tonsil area, under the arms, and in the groin. The doctor will also examine other parts of the body to see whether there is swelling or fluid in your chest or abdomen that could be caused by swollen lymph nodes. You will be asked about pain and examined for any weakness or paralysis that could be caused by an enlarged lymph node against nerves or the spinal cord. Your abdomen will be examined to see whether any internal organs are enlarged, especially the spleen and liver. If the doctor suspects Hodgkin's lymphoma after reviewing your symptoms and performing a physical examination, he or she may order other tests to help confirm the diagnosis. These tests should include a biopsy, and may also include blood tests, x-rays and other imaging tests, scans, or a bone marrow evaluation.

Biopsies and How They Are Performed

A biopsy is a procedure in which a piece of tissue from an area of suspected cancer is removed from the body for examination under a microscope. Hodgkin's lymphoma is diagnosed by looking for the characteristics of this disease in the lymph nodes or other tissues. The information provided by this tissue sample is crucial to diagnosing and treating Hodgkin's lymphoma.

There are several types of biopsies. One is called a core, or needle biopsy, in which a needle is inserted into a lymph node suspected of being cancerous and a small tissue sample is removed. This type of biopsy can be done under local anesthesia and stitches are usually not required.

Core biopsies are usually inadequate to diagnose properly and classify Hodgkin's lymphoma. It is usually much more accurate and informative to have an open biopsy (also called a surgical biopsy), in which an entire abnormal lymph node is removed. This procedure can usually be done under local anesthesia, but a general (whole body) anesthetic may sometimes be needed and a few stitches are often required.

When the only signs of lymphoma are in the abdomen or the pelvis, a core needle biopsy, laparoscopy(inserting a tube) or even abdominal surgery may be necessary to obtain a sample of the tumor for examination.

After a tissue sample has been removed, it is examined by a pathologist (a doctor who studies tissues and cells to identify diseases). Pathologists look at the tissue under a microscope and then provide the oncologist with a detailed report. Information obtained from a biopsy indicates the type of Hodgkin's lymphoma. If the pathologist's interpretation of the biopsy is uncertain, it should be reviewed by another pathologist who is an expert in lymphoma (hematopathologist). Specialized molecular tests can also help distinguish Hodgkin's lymphoma from non-Hodgkin's lymphoma or even from reactive (noncancerous) lymph nodes.

Tests and How They Help Evaluate the Cancer

Physicians often will order imaging tests that provide pictures of the inside of the body. Most of these tests are painless, and no anesthetic is required. Several types of imaging procedures may be needed, and the necessary tests will be chosen to help best evaluate your cancer, including:

- **X-rays:** X-rays use radiation to take pictures of areas inside the body. The amount of radiation used in most diagnostic tests are so small that it poses little risk to the patient.

- **CT or CAT (computerized axial tomography) scan:** A CAT scan takes x-rays from different angles around the body. The pictures that are obtained are then combined using a computer to give a detailed image. People with Hodgkin's lymphoma often have CAT scans of the neck, chest, abdomen, and pelvis. These tests are useful in determining the extent of nodal involvement and whether internal organs are affected by Hodgkin's lymphoma.

- **MRI (magnetic resonance imaging):** An MRI is similar to a CAT scan but uses magnets and radio frequency waves instead of x-rays. An MRI can provide important information about tissues and organs, particularly the nervous system, that is not available from other imaging techniques. An MRI may be ordered when the physician wants to get clear images of the brain and spinal cord to see whether the cancer has spread to these areas.

- **Gallium (radioisotope) scan:** Radioactive gallium is a chemical that collects in some tumors. Gallium scans are sometimes used when a patient is diagnosed with Hodgkin's lymphoma. This scan is performed by injecting a small amount of radioactive gallium into the body. The small amount of chemical used is not harmful. The body is then scanned from several angles to see whether the gallium has collected in a tumor. If the tumor attracts this chemical, the scan can be repeated after treatment is completed to help determine if the tumor has completely disappeared or become inactive.

- **PET (positron emission tomography) scan:** PET scans are now often replacing gallium scans in many cancer centers, because the technique is more convenient and more sensitive, particularly in the abdomen. This test evaluates Hodgkin's lymphoma activity in different parts of the body. To perform the test, a radioactive tracer substance is first injected. A positron camera is then used to detect the radioactivity and produce cross-sectional images of the body. Like gallium scans, PET scans are very useful in determining response to treatment. While CAT scans shows the size of a lymph node, gallium and PET scans show if the lymph node is active (still has disease).

Blood tests: Blood tests are performed to determine whether different types of blood cells are normal in number and appearance when viewed under the microscope. These include tests of red blood cells, white blood cells, platelets, and sedimentation rate. Abnormalities in these blood cells may sometimes be the first sign of lymphoma. Certain blood tests can be used to determine how aggressive a tumor may behave or whether a tumor is affecting the liver, kidneys, or other parts of the body.

Bone marrow examination: Bone marrow, is the spongy material found inside our bones. Bone marrow contains immature cells called stem cells, which develop into three main types of cells found in the body: red blood cells that deliver oxygen and take away the waste product carbon dioxide; white blood cells that protect the body from infection; and platelets that help blood clot. Hodgkin's lymphoma can spread to the bone marrow; therefore, doctors may want to examine the marrow to see whether cancer is present. Bone marrow is obtained by numbing the skin, tissue, and surface of the bone with a local anesthetic, and then inserting a thin needle into the pelvis or other large bone and withdrawing a small sample. The procedure can be briefly painful at the moment when the marrow is withdrawn. Patients should talk with their doctor and nurse if they would like a calming medication before the procedure.

Molecular diagnostic tests: Over the past decade, scientists have gained a deeper understanding of how disease works at the level of molecules such as genes and proteins. This understanding has led to powerful new diagnostic tools and treatments. These tools include PCR (polymerase chain reaction), which can detect small amounts of genetic material DNA and a variety of immunological techniques that detect the expression of specific proteins (antigens or markers) on the surface of tumor cells. Using these tests, doctors can sometimes detect cancer earlier, and they can more accurately classify tumor types. This information may help the physician choose the most appropriate treatment for the disease. Immunological and genetic tests can find evidence of cancer unseen by a pathologist's microscope. An advantage of molecular diagnostic tests is that they are usually highly accurate and require only very small amounts of tissue obtained from biopsies, fine-needle aspirates, or sometimes blood.

Researchers are currently developing ways to measure the activity of genes within the cells of a lymphoma sample. This technique, microarray analysis, may lead to even more accurate diagnoses based on a tumor's individual genetic characteristics and behavior. Currently, this method is being used in an experimental setting for assessing non-Hodgkin's lymphoma tumors, but in the future the technique may be useful for the routine diagnosis and treatment of Hodgkin's lymphoma as well.

Other tests: Doctors may also order other tests to evaluate the health of organs that could be affected by treatments. Examples include echocardiograms or radionuclide tests to evaluate the heart, and pulmonary function tests to evaluate the lungs.

Different Types of Hodgkin's Lymphoma

Hodgkin's lymphoma has been divided into subtypes according to how it looks under the microscope. The type of tumor provides important information that may affect treatment choices. In each type of Hodgkin's lymphoma, the tumor cells and the Reed-Sternberg cells (abnormal lymphocytes) are mixed with many normal cells. The abnormal cells are usually in the minority. In all types of Hodgkin's lymphoma, the cancerous cells are thought to be abnormal B-lymphocytes.

The most common subtype of Hodgkin's lymphoma is nodular sclerosis, followed by mixed cellularity. Two rare subtypes are lymphocyte predominant, which is indolent, and lymphocyte depletion, which is aggressive. A recently described fifth subtype is lymphocyte-rich classical Hodgkin's lymphoma. Hodgkin's lymphoma is now divided into "classical" lymphoma and lymphocyte predominant Hodgkin's lymphoma as follows:

Classical Hodgkin's Lymphoma

- **Nodular sclerosis:** In this type of Hodgkin's lymphoma, the involved lymph nodes contain areas composed of Reed-Sternberg cells mixed with normal white blood cells. The lymph nodes often contain prominent scar tissue, hence the name nodular sclerosis (scarring). This subtype is the most common, making up 60% to 75% of all cases of Hodgkin's lymphoma. It is more common in women than men, and it usually affects adolescents and young adults. The majority of patients are cured with current treatments.

- **Mixed cellularity:** In this type of Hodgkin's lymphoma, the involved lymph nodes contain many Reed-Sternberg cells in addition to several other cell types. Scarring is not apparent. Mixed cellularity accounts for about 5% to 15% of all cases of Hodgkin's lymphoma. It primarily affects older adults. More extensive disease is usually present by the time this subtype is diagnosed.

- **Lymphocyte-rich:** This disease is characterized by the presence of very few abnormal cells and classical Reed-Sternberg cells, but numerous normal lymphocytes. This recently identified form of Hodgkin's lymphoma is rare, accounting for only 5% of all Hodgkin's lymphoma cases. It is usually diagnosed at an early stage, in adults.

- **Lymphocyte depletion:** This Hodgkin's lymphoma subtype has few normal lymphocytes, but abundant Reed-Sternberg cells. It is found in less than 5% of Hodgkin's lymphoma cases and is usually not diagnosed until the disease is widespread.

Lymphocyte Predominant Hodgkin's Lymphoma

In this type of Hodgkin's lymphoma, most of the lymphocytes found in the lymph nodes are normal (not cancerous), hence the name lymphocyte predominant. This subtype makes up about 5% to 10% of cases. Typical Reed-Sternberg cells are not found in this subtype, but abnormal cells, sometimes referred to as popcorn cells, can be seen. Lymphocyte predominant affects more men than women and is usually diagnosed in people under 35 years of age. This subtype is usually diagnosed at an early stage and is not very aggressive. In many ways this form of Hodgkin's lymphoma resembles low-grade non-Hodgkin's lymphoma.

Tumor Bulk

Tumor bulk refers to how much tumor is present. In general, the smaller the tumor, the better the chances that it will be completely eliminated by treatment. Patients with small tumors (called non-bulky disease) generally have a better prognosis than those with large tumors (bulky disease).

Cancer Staging and What It Means

Stage is the term used to describe the extent of tumor spread in the body. Hodgkin's lymphoma is divided into four stages, depending on how far the disease has spread. Stages I and II are localized, while stages III and IV are considered advanced, widespread, or disseminated. Stage is an important piece of information that helps to predict outcome or prognosis and determine approaches to treatment.

Stages of Hodgkin's Lymphoma

- **Stage I (early disease):** The cancer is found only in a single lymph node or region.

- **Stage II (locally advanced disease):** The cancer is found in two or more lymph node regions on one side of the diaphragm (the breathing muscle that separates the abdomen from the chest).

- **Stage III (advanced disease):** The disease involves lymph nodes both above and below the diaphragm.

- **Stage IV (widespread disease):** The lymphoma is outside the lymph nodes and spleen AND has spread to one or more organs such as bone, bone marrow, skin or liver.

Meaning of the Letters "A," "B," or, "E" after the Stage

Each stage of Hodgkin's lymphoma is further divided into "A" and "B" categories, depending on the symptoms patients have when they are diagnosed. Some patients have symptoms that affect their entire body (called systemic symptoms systemic symptoms). Examples of these include fever, night sweats, and weight loss. Patients who have these symptoms will have the letter "B" after the stage of their disease. The "A" category is used to designate a person with no systemic symptoms.

The category "E" is used when the Hodgkin's lymphoma spreads locally from a lymph into the closely surrounding tissue.

Section 60.3

Hodgkin Lymphoma in Children

Excerpted from: PDQ® Cancer Information Summary. National Cancer Institute; Bethesda, MD. Childhood Hodgkin's Lymphoma (PDQ®): Treatment - Patient. Updated 12/2004. Available at: http://cancer.gov. Accessed April 30, 2006.

Treatment Option Overview

There are different types of treatment for children with Hodgkin lymphoma. Some treatments are standard and some are being tested in clinical trials. A treatment clinical trial is a research study meant to help improve current treatments or obtain information on new treatments for patients with cancer. When clinical trials show that a new treatment is better than the standard treatment, the new treatment may become the standard treatment.

Because cancer in children is rare, taking part in a clinical trial should be considered. Clinical trials are taking place in many parts of the country. Information about ongoing clinical trials is available from the National Cancer Institute website (http://www.cancer.gov). Choosing the most appropriate cancer treatment is a decision that ideally involves the patient, family, and health care team.

Children with Hodgkin lymphoma should have their treatment planned by a team of doctors with expertise in treating childhood cancer.

Your child's treatment will be overseen by a pediatric oncologist, a doctor who specializes in treating children with cancer. The pediatric oncologist may refer you to other pediatric doctors who have experience and expertise in treating children with Hodgkin lymphoma and who specialize in certain areas of medicine. These may include the following specialists:

- Medical oncologist/hematologist
- Pediatric surgeon
- Radiation oncologist
- Endocrinologist
- Pediatric nurse specialist
- Rehabilitation specialist
- Psychologist
- Social worker

Two types of standard treatment are used:

- **Chemotherapy:** Chemotherapy is a cancer treatment that uses drugs to stop the growth of cancer cells, either by killing the cells or by stopping the cells from dividing. When chemotherapy is taken by mouth or injected into a vein or muscle, the drugs enter the bloodstream and can reach cancer cells throughout the body (systemic chemotherapy). When chemotherapy is placed directly into the spinal column, an organ, or a body cavity such as the abdomen, the drugs mainly affect cancer cells in those areas. Combination chemotherapy is treatment using more than one anticancer drug. The way the chemotherapy is given depends on the type and stage of the cancer being treated.

- **Radiation therapy:** Radiation therapy is a cancer treatment that uses high-energy x-rays or other types of radiation to kill cancer cells. There are two types of radiation therapy. External radiation therapy uses a machine outside the body to send radiation toward the cancer. Internal radiation therapy uses a radioactive substance sealed in needles, seeds, wires, or catheters that are placed directly into or near the cancer. The way the radiation therapy is given depends on the type and stage of the cancer being treated.

Other types of treatment are being tested in clinical trials. These include the following:

- **High-dose chemotherapy with stem cell transplant:** High-dose chemotherapy with stem cell transplant is a method of replacing blood-forming cells destroyed by high doses of anticancer drugs or radiation therapy. Stem cells (immature blood cells) are removed from the bone marrow or blood of the patient or a donor and are frozen and stored. After therapy is completed, the stored stem cells are thawed and given back to the patient through an infusion. These reinfused stem cells grow into (and restore) the body's blood cells.

- **Surgery:** Surgery may be done to remove as much of the tumor as possible.

Treatment Options for Children and Adolescents with Hodgkin Lymphoma

Treatment of low-risk childhood Hodgkin lymphoma may include the following:

- Combination chemotherapy with low-dose radiation therapy to involved areas
- A clinical trial of combination chemotherapy with or without low-dose radiation therapy to involved areas

Treatment of intermediate-risk childhood Hodgkin lymphoma may include the following:

- Combination chemotherapy with low-dose radiation therapy to involved areas
- A clinical trial of combination chemotherapy with or without low-dose radiation therapy to involved areas
- A clinical trial of new combinations of chemotherapy before low-dose radiation therapy to involved areas

Treatment of high-risk childhood Hodgkin lymphoma may include intensive or high-dose combination chemotherapy with low-dose radiation therapy to involved areas.

Treatment of nodular lymphocyte predominant childhood Hodgkin lymphoma may include the following:

- Combination chemotherapy with low-dose radiation therapy to involved areas

- A clinical trial of surgery only, when the lymphoma is stage I and no cancer remains after the surgery

- A clinical trial of combination chemotherapy with or without low-dose radiation therapy to involved areas for patients with stage I or stage II

Treatment of primary progressive or recurrent childhood Hodgkin lymphoma may include the following:

- Chemotherapy with low-dose radiation therapy to involved areas for stage I or stage II non-bulky disease. Adolescent patients who have reached full growth may be treated with standard-dose radiation therapy.

- High-dose chemotherapy with stem cell transplant with or without radiation therapy

Late Effects from Childhood and Adolescent Hodgkin Lymphoma Treatment

Children and adolescents may have treatment-related side effects that appear months or years after treatment for Hodgkin lymphoma. Because of these late effects on health and development, regular follow-up exams are important. Late effects may include problems with the following:

- Development of sex organs in males
- Fertility (ability to have children)
- Thyroid, heart, or lungs
- An increased risk of developing a second primary cancer
- Bone growth and development

The risk of these long-term side effects will be considered when treatment decisions are made.

Section 60.4

Hodgkin Lymphoma in Adults

Excerpted from: PDQ® Cancer Information Summary. National Cancer Institute; Bethesda, MD. Adult Hodgkin's Lymphoma PDQ®): Treatment - Patient. Updated 02/2006. Available at: http://cancer.gov. Accessed April 30, 2006.

Treatment Option Overview

There are different types of treatment for patients with adult Hodgkin lymphoma. Some treatments are standard (the currently used treatment), and some are being tested in clinical trials. Before starting treatment, patients may want to think about taking part in a clinical trial. A treatment clinical trial is a research study meant to help improve current treatments or obtain information on new treatments for patients with cancer. When clinical trials show that a new treatment is better than the standard treatment, the new treatment may become the standard treatment.

Clinical trials are taking place in many parts of the country. Information about ongoing clinical trials is available from the National Cancer Institute website (http://www.cancer.gov). Choosing the most appropriate cancer treatment is a decision that ideally involves the patient, family, and health care team.

Patients with Hodgkin lymphoma should have their treatment planned by a team of doctors with expertise in treating lymphomas. Treatment will be overseen by a medical oncologist, a doctor who specializes in treating cancer. The medical oncologist may refer you to other doctors who have experience and expertise in treating adult Hodgkin lymphoma and who specialize in certain areas of medicine. These may include the following specialists:

- Neurosurgeon
- Neurologist
- Rehabilitation specialist
- Radiation oncologist
- Endocrinologist

- Hematologist
- Other oncology specialists

Three types of standard treatment are used:

- Chemotherapy
- Radiation therapy
- Surgery: Laparotomy is a procedure in which an incision (cut) is made in the wall of the abdomen to check the inside of the abdomen for signs of disease. The size of the incision depends on the reason the laparotomy is being done. Sometimes organs are removed or tissue samples are taken for biopsy. If cancer is found, the tissue or organ is removed during the laparotomy.

New types of treatment are being tested in clinical trials. These include high-dose chemotherapy and radiation therapy with stem cell transplant.

Treatment Options for Adult Hodgkin Lymphoma

Treatment of early favorable Hodgkin lymphoma may include the following:

- Combination chemotherapy with or without radiation therapy to parts of the body with cancer
- Radiation therapy alone to areas of the body with cancer or to the mantle field (neck, chest, armpits)
- Clinical trials of new combinations of chemotherapy and/or radiation therapy

Treatment of early unfavorable Hodgkin lymphoma may include the following:

- Combination chemotherapy with or without radiation therapy to parts of the body with cancer
- Clinical trials of new combinations of chemotherapy and/or radiation therapy

Treatment of advanced favorable Hodgkin lymphoma may include the following:

- Combination chemotherapy with or without radiation therapy to parts of the body with cancer

- Clinical trials of new combinations of chemotherapy

Treatment of advanced unfavorable Hodgkin lymphoma may include the following:

- Combination chemotherapy

- Clinical trials of new combinations of chemotherapy

- A clinical trial of high-dose chemotherapy and stem cell transplant using the patient's own stem cells

Treatment of recurrent Hodgkin lymphoma may include the following:

- Combination chemotherapy

- Combination chemotherapy followed by high-dose chemotherapy and stem cell transplant with or without radiation therapy

- Radiation therapy with or without chemotherapy

- Chemotherapy as palliative therapy to relieve symptoms and improve quality of life

- A clinical trial of high-dose chemotherapy and stem cell transplant

Section 60.5

Hodgkin Lymphoma during Pregnancy

PDQ® Cancer Information Summary. National Cancer Institute; Bethesda, MD. Hodgkin's Lymphoma during Pregnancy (PDQ®): Treatment - Patient. Updated 09/2005. Available at: http://cancer.gov. Accessed April 30, 2006.

There are different types of treatment for pregnant patients with Hodgkin lymphoma. Treatment is carefully chosen to protect the fetus. Treatment decisions are based on the mother's wishes, the stage of the Hodgkin lymphoma, and the age of the fetus. The treatment plan may change as the symptoms, cancer, and pregnancy change. Choosing the most appropriate cancer treatment is a decision that ideally involves the patient, family, and health care team.

Four types of standard treatment are used:

- **Radiation therapy:** Radiation therapy is a cancer treatment that uses high-energy x-rays or other types of radiation to kill cancer cells. To avoid any risk to the fetus, radiation therapy should be postponed until after delivery, if possible. If immediate treatment is needed, pregnant women with Hodgkin lymphoma may decide to continue the pregnancy and receive radiation therapy. However, lead used to shield the fetus may not protect it from scattered radiation that could possibly cause cancer in the future.

- **Chemotherapy:** Chemotherapy is a cancer treatment that uses drugs to stop the growth of cancer cells, either by killing the cells or by stopping the cells from dividing. The fetus cannot be protected from being exposed to chemotherapy when the mother is treated. Some chemotherapy regimens may cause birth defects when given in the first trimester. Vinblastine is an anticancer drug that has not been linked with birth defects in the second half of pregnancy.

- **Watchful waiting:** Watchful waiting is closely monitoring a patient's condition without giving any treatment unless symptoms appear or change. Delivery may be induced when the fetus is 32 to 36 weeks old, so that the mother can begin treatment.

- **Steroid therapy:** Steroids are hormones naturally produced in the body by the adrenal glands and by reproductive organs. Some types of steroids are made in a laboratory. Certain steroid drugs have been found to help chemotherapy work better and help stop the growth of cancer cells. Steroids can also help the lungs of the fetus develop faster than normal. This is important when delivery is induced early.

Treatment of Hodgkin Lymphoma during Pregnancy

When Hodgkin lymphoma is diagnosed in the first trimester of pregnancy, it does not necessarily mean that the patient will be advised to end the pregnancy. Each patient's treatment will depend on the stage of the lymphoma, how fast it is growing, and the patient's wishes. For women who choose to continue the pregnancy, treatment of Hodgkin lymphoma during the first trimester of pregnancy may include the following:

- Watchful waiting when the cancer is above the diaphragm and is slow-growing. Delivery may be induced when the fetus is 32 to 36 weeks old so the mother can begin treatment.

- Radiation therapy above the diaphragm, with the fetus shielded

- Systemic chemotherapy using one or more drugs

When Hodgkin lymphoma is diagnosed in the second half of pregnancy, most patients can delay treatment until after the baby is born. Treatment of Hodgkin lymphoma during the second half of pregnancy may include the following:

- Watchful waiting, with plans to induce delivery when the fetus is 32 to 36 weeks old

- Systemic chemotherapy using one or more drugs

- Steroid therapy

- Radiation therapy to relieve breathing problems caused by a large tumor in the chest

Chapter 61

Non-Hodgkin Lymphoma

What Is Non-Hodgkin Lymphoma?

Non-Hodgkin lymphoma (also called NHL) is cancer that begins in the lymphatic system. To understand this disease, it is helpful to know about the lymphatic system.

The Lymphatic System

The lymphatic system is part of the body's immune system. The immune system fights infections and other diseases.

In the lymphatic system, a network of lymph vessels carries clear fluid called lymph. Lymph vessels lead to small, round organs called lymph nodes. Lymph nodes are filled with lymphocytes (a type of white blood cell). The lymph nodes trap and remove bacteria or other harmful substances that may be in the lymph. Groups of lymph nodes are found in the neck, underarms, chest, abdomen, and groin.

Other parts of the lymphatic system include the tonsils, spleen, and thymus. Lymphatic tissue is also found in other parts of the body including the stomach, skin, and small intestine.

Non-Hodgkin Lymphoma

There are many types of non-Hodgkin lymphoma. All types of lymphoma begin in cells of the lymphatic system. Normally, cells grow

From "What You Need to Know about™ Non-Hodgkin Lymphoma," National Cancer Institute, June 17, 2005.

and divide to form new cells as the body needs them. When cells grow old, they die, and new cells take their place. Sometimes this process goes wrong. New cells form when the body does not need them, and old cells do not die when they should. These extra cells can form a mass of tissue called a growth or tumor.

Non-Hodgkin lymphoma begins when a lymphocyte (a B cell or T cell) becomes abnormal. Usually, non-Hodgkin lymphoma starts in a B cell in a lymph node. The abnormal cell divides to make copies of itself. The new cells divide again and again, making more and more abnormal cells. The abnormal cells are cancer cells. They do not die when they should. They do not protect the body from infections or other diseases. Also, the cancer cells can spread to nearly any other part of the body.

Risk Factors

Doctors can seldom explain why one person develops non-Hodgkin lymphoma and another does not. But research shows that certain risk factors increase the chance that a person will develop this disease. In general, the risk factors for non-Hodgkin lymphoma include the following:

- **Weak immune system:** Having a weak immune system (from an inherited condition, HIV infection, or certain drugs) increases the risk of developing non-Hodgkin lymphoma.

- **Certain infections:** Having certain types of infections increases the risk of developing lymphoma. However, lymphoma is not contagious. You cannot "catch" lymphoma from another person. The following are the main types of infection that can increase the risk of lymphoma:

  - **Human immunodeficiency virus (HIV):** HIV is the virus that causes AIDS. People who have HIV infection are at much greater risk of some types of non-Hodgkin lymphoma.

  - **Epstein-Barr virus (EBV):** Infection with EBV has been linked to an increased risk of lymphoma. In Africa, EBV infection is linked to Burkitt lymphoma.

  - ***Helicobacter pylori:*** *H. pylori* are bacteria that can cause stomach ulcers. They also increase a person's risk of lymphoma in the stomach lining.

  - **Human T-cell leukemia/lymphoma virus (HTLV-1):** Infection with HTLV-1 increases a person's risk of lymphoma and leukemia.

- **Hepatitis C virus:** Some studies have found an increased risk of lymphoma in people with hepatitis C virus. More research is needed to understand the role of hepatitis C virus.

- **Age:** Although non-Hodgkin lymphoma can occur in young people, the chance of developing this disease goes up with age. Most people with non-Hodgkin lymphoma are older than 60.

Researchers are studying obesity and other possible risk factors for non-Hodgkin lymphoma. People who work with herbicides or certain other chemicals may be at increased risk of this disease. Researchers are also looking at a possible link between using hair dyes before 1980 and non-Hodgkin lymphoma.

Most people who have known risk factors do not get non-Hodgkin lymphoma. On the other hand, people who do get the disease often have no known risk factors. If you think you may be at risk, you should discuss this concern with your doctor.

Symptoms

Non-Hodgkin lymphoma can cause many symptoms:

- Swollen, painless lymph nodes in the neck, armpits, or groin
- Unexplained weight loss
- Fever
- Soaking night sweats
- Coughing, trouble breathing, or chest pain
- Weakness and tiredness that don't go away
- Pain, swelling, or a feeling of fullness in the abdomen

Most often, these symptoms are not due to cancer. Infections or other health problems may also cause these symptoms. Anyone with symptoms that do not go away within two weeks should see a doctor so that problems can be diagnosed and treated.

Diagnosis

If you have swollen lymph nodes or other symptoms that suggest non-Hodgkin lymphoma, your doctor will help you find out whether they are from cancer or some other cause. Your doctor may ask about your personal and family medical history.

You may have some of the following exams and tests:

- **Physical exam:** Your doctor checks for swollen lymph nodes in your neck, underarms, and groin. Your doctor also checks your spleen and liver to see if they are swollen.

- **Blood tests:** The lab does a complete blood count to check the number of blood cells. The lab also checks for other substances, such as lactate dehydrogenase (LDH). Lymphoma may cause a high level of LDH.

- **Chest x-rays:** You may have x-rays to check for swollen lymph nodes or other signs of disease in your chest.

- **Biopsy:** Your doctor removes tissue to look for lymphoma cells. A biopsy is the only sure way to diagnose lymphoma. Your doctor may remove an entire lymph node (excisional biopsy) or only part of a lymph node (incisional biopsy). A pathologist checks the tissue for lymphoma cells with a microscope.

Types of Lymphoma

When lymphoma is found, the pathologist will report the type. The most common types are diffuse large B-cell lymphoma and follicular lymphoma.

Lymphomas may be grouped by how quickly they are likely to grow:

- Indolent (also called low-grade) lymphomas grow slowly. They tend to cause few symptoms.

- Aggressive (also called intermediate-grade and high-grade) lymphomas grow and spread more quickly. They tend to cause severe symptoms. Over time, many indolent lymphomas become aggressive lymphomas.

Staging

Your doctor needs to know the extent (stage) of non-Hodgkin lymphoma to plan the best treatment. Staging may involve some of these tests:

- **Bone marrow biopsy:** The doctor uses a thick needle to remove a small sample of bone and bone marrow from your hipbone or another large bone. Local anesthesia can help control pain. A pathologist then looks for lymphoma cells in the sample.

- **CT (computed tomography) scan:** An x-ray machine linked to a computer takes a series of detailed pictures of your chest, abdomen, or pelvis. You may receive an injection of contrast material. Also, you may be asked to drink another type of contrast material. The contrast material makes it easier for the doctor to see swollen lymph nodes and other abnormal areas on the x-ray.

- **MRI (magnetic resonance imaging):** A powerful magnet linked to a computer is used to make detailed pictures of your spinal cord, bone marrow, or brain. Your doctor can view these pictures on a monitor and can print them on film.

- **Ultrasound:** An ultrasound device sends out sound waves that people cannot hear. The small hand-held device is held against your body. The waves bounce off nearby tissues, and a computer uses the echoes to create a picture. Tumors may produce echoes that are different from the echoes made by healthy tissues. The picture can show possible tumors.

- **Spinal tap:** The doctor uses a long, thin needle to remove fluid from the spinal column. Local anesthesia can help control pain. You must lie flat for a few hours afterward so that you will not get a headache. The lab checks the fluid for lymphoma cells or other problems.

- **PET (positron emission tomography) scan:** You receive an injection of a small amount of radioactive sugar. A machine makes computerized pictures of the sugar being used by cells in the body. Cancer cells sometimes show up in the pictures as areas of high activity.

The stage is based on where lymphoma cells are found (in the lymph nodes or in other organs or tissues). The stage also depends on how many areas are affected. The stages of non-Hodgkin lymphoma are as follows:

Stage I: The lymphoma cells are in a single lymph node group (such as in the neck or underarm). Or, if the abnormal cells are not in the lymph nodes, they are in only one part of a tissue or organ (such as the lung, but not the liver or bone marrow).

Stage II: The lymphoma cells are in at least two lymph node groups on the same side of (either above or below) the diaphragm. Or, the lymphoma cells are in an organ and the lymph nodes near that organ (on the same side of the diaphragm). There may be lymphoma cells in other lymph node groups on the same side of the diaphragm.

Stage III: The lymphoma is in groups of lymph nodes above and below the diaphragm. It also may be found in an organ or tissue near these lymph node groups.

Stage IV: The lymphoma is throughout at least one organ or tissue (in addition to the lymph nodes). Or, it is in the liver, blood, or bone marrow.

Treatment

Your doctor may refer you to a specialist, or you may ask for a referral. Specialists who treat non-Hodgkin lymphoma include hematologists, medical oncologists, and radiation oncologists. Your doctor may suggest that you choose an oncologist who specializes in the treatment of lymphoma. Often, such doctors are associated with major academic centers.

Getting a Second Opinion

Before starting treatment, you might want a second opinion about your diagnosis and your treatment plan.

It is a good idea to get a second opinion about the type of lymphoma that you have. The treatment plan varies by the type of lymphoma. A pathologist at a major referral center can review your biopsy.

You also may want a second opinion about your treatment plan. Many insurance companies cover a second opinion if you or your doctor requests it. It may take some time and effort to gather your medical records and arrange to see another doctor. Most of the time, it is not a problem to take several weeks to get a second opinion. The delay in starting treatment usually will not make treatment less effective. To be sure, you should discuss this delay with your doctor. Some people with non-Hodgkin lymphoma need treatment right away.

There are a number of ways to find a doctor for a second opinion:

- Your doctor may refer you to one or more lymphoma specialists. At cancer centers, many specialists often work together as a team.

- The National Cancer Institute (NCI)'s Cancer Information Service, at 800-4-CANCER, can tell you about nearby treatment centers. Information Specialists also can help you online through LiveHelp at http://www.cancer.gov.

- A local or state medical society, a nearby hospital, or a medical school can usually provide the names of specialists in your area.

- The American Board of Medical Specialties (ABMS) has a list of doctors who have had training and passed exams in their specialty. You can find this list in the *Official ABMS Directory of Board Certified Medical Specialists.* This Directory is in most public libraries. Or you can look up doctors at http://www.abms.org (click on "Who's Certified").

- The NCI provides a helpful fact sheet called "How To Find a Doctor or Treatment Facility If You Have Cancer." (To get a copy of this fact sheet visit www.cancer.gov or call 800-4-CANCER).

- Nonprofit groups with an interest in lymphoma may be of help. Many such groups are listed in the NCI fact sheet "National Organizations That Offer Services to People with Cancer and Their Families."

Preparing for Treatment

The choice of treatment depends on many factors, including the following:

- Which type of non-Hodgkin lymphoma you have (for example, follicular lymphoma)

- The stage of your cancer (where the lymphoma is found)

- How quickly the cancer is growing (whether it is indolent or aggressive lymphoma)

- Your age

- Whether you have other health problems

Your doctor can describe your treatment choices and their expected results. You and your doctor can work together to develop a treatment plan that meets your needs.

You may want to ask the doctor these questions before treatment begins:

- What is the stage of my cancer? Where are the tumors?

- What are my treatment choices? Which do you recommend for me?

- What are the expected benefits of each kind of treatment? How will we know the treatment is working? What tests will be used to check its effectiveness? How often will I get these tests?

- What are the risks and possible side effects of each treatment? What can we do to control my side effects?

- How long will treatment last?

- Will I have to stay in the hospital?

- How will treatment affect my normal activities?

- What can I do to take care of myself during treatment?

- What is the treatment likely to cost? Will my insurance cover this treatment?

- How often will I need checkups?

- Would a clinical trial (research study) be appropriate for me?

Treatment Methods

If you have indolent non-Hodgkin lymphoma without symptoms, you may not need treatment for the cancer right away. The doctor watches your health closely so that treatment can start when you begin to have symptoms. Not getting cancer treatment right away is called watchful waiting.

If you have indolent lymphoma with symptoms, you will probably receive chemotherapy and biological therapy. Radiation therapy may be used for patients with Stage I or Stage II lymphoma.

If you have aggressive lymphoma, the treatment is usually chemotherapy and biological therapy. Radiation therapy also may be used.

If non-Hodgkin lymphoma comes back after treatment, doctors call this a relapse or recurrence. People whose lymphoma comes back after treatment may receive stem cell transplantation.

Because cancer treatments often harm healthy cells and tissues, side effects are common. Side effects depend mainly on the type and extent of the treatment. Side effects may not be the same for each person, and they may change from one treatment session to the next. The younger a person is, the easier it may be to cope with treatment and its side effects.

Before treatment starts, the health care team will explain possible side effects and suggest ways to help you manage them.

At any stage of the disease, you can have treatments to control pain and other symptoms, to relieve the side effects of therapy, and to ease emotional and practical problems. This kind of treatment is called supportive care.

You may want to talk to your doctor about taking part in a clinical trial, a research study of new treatment methods.

Watchful waiting: People who choose watchful waiting put off having cancer treatment until they have symptoms. Doctors sometimes suggest watchful waiting for a patient with indolent lymphoma. A person with indolent lymphoma may not have problems that require cancer treatment for a long time. Sometimes the tumor may even shrink for a while without therapy. By putting off treatment, a patient can avoid the side effects of chemotherapy or radiation therapy.

If you and your doctor agree that watchful waiting is a good idea, the doctor will check you regularly (every 3 months). You will receive treatment if symptoms occur or get worse.

Some people do not choose watchful waiting because they don't want to worry about having cancer that is not treated. Those who choose watchful waiting but later become worried should discuss their feelings with the doctor.

You may want to ask the doctor these questions before choosing watchful waiting:

- If I choose watchful waiting, can I change my mind later on?

- Will the disease be harder to treat later?

- How often will I have checkups?

- Between checkups, what problems should I report?

Chemotherapy: Chemotherapy uses drugs to kill cancer cells. It is called systemic therapy because the drugs travel through the bloodstream. The drugs can reach cancer cells in almost all parts of the body.

You may receive chemotherapy by mouth, through a vein, or in the space around the spinal cord. Treatment is usually in an outpatient part of the hospital, at the doctor's office, or at home. Some patients need to stay in the hospital during treatment.

If a patient has lymphoma in the stomach caused by *H. pylori* infection, the doctor may treat this lymphoma with antibiotics. After the drug cures the infection, the cancer also may go away.

The side effects of chemotherapy depend mainly on the specific drugs and the dose. The drugs affect cancer cells and other cells that divide rapidly:

- **Blood cells:** When drugs affect your healthy blood cells, you are more likely to get infections, bruise or bleed easily, and feel very weak and tired.

- **Cells in hair roots:** Chemotherapy can cause you to lose your hair. Your hair will grow back, but sometimes the new hair is somewhat different in color and texture.

- **Cells that line the mouth, stomach, and other parts of the digestive tract:** Chemotherapy can cause poor appetite, nausea and vomiting, diarrhea, trouble swallowing, or mouth and lip sores.

The drugs used for non-Hodgkin lymphoma also may cause skin rashes or blisters, and headaches or other aches. Your skin may become darker. Your nails may develop ridges or dark bands.

Your doctor can suggest ways to control many of these side effects.

You may want to ask the doctor these questions before starting chemotherapy:

- Which drug or drugs will I have?

- How do the drugs work?

- What are the expected benefits of the treatment?

- What are the risks and possible side effects of treatment? What can we do about them?

- Are there any long-term effects from the drugs?

- When will treatment start? When will it end?

- How will treatment affect my normal activities?

Biological therapy: People with certain types of non-Hodgkin lymphoma may have biological therapy. This type of treatment helps the immune system fight cancer.

Monoclonal antibodies are the type of biological therapy used for lymphoma. They are proteins made in the lab that can bind to cancer cells. They help the immune system kill lymphoma cells. Patients receive this treatment through a vein at the doctor's office, clinic, or hospital.

Flu-like symptoms such as fever, chills, headache, weakness, and nausea may occur. Most side effects are easy to treat. Rarely, a patient may have more serious side effects, such as breathing problems, low blood pressure, or severe skin rashes. Your doctor or nurse can tell you about the side effects that you can expect and how to manage them.

You may want to ask the doctor these questions before having biological therapy:

- What will the treatment do?

- Will I have to stay in the hospital?

- How will we know if the treatment is working?

- How long will I be on biological therapy?

- Will I have side effects during treatment? How long will they last? What can we do about them?

Radiation therapy: Radiation therapy (also called radiotherapy) uses high-energy rays to kill non-Hodgkin lymphoma cells. It can shrink tumors and help control pain.

Two types of radiation therapy are used for people with lymphoma:

- **External radiation:** A large machine aims the rays at the part of the body where lymphoma cells have collected. This is local therapy because it affects cells in the treated area only. Most people go to a hospital or clinic for treatment 5 days a week for several weeks.

- **Systemic radiation:** Some people with lymphoma receive an injection of radioactive material that travels throughout the body. The radioactive material is bound to antibodies that seek out lymphoma cells. The radiation destroys the lymphoma cells.

The side effects of radiation therapy depend mainly on the type of radiation therapy, the dose of radiation, and the part of the body that is treated. For example, external radiation to your abdomen can cause nausea, vomiting, and diarrhea. Radiation to the lung can cause coughing or shortness of breath. In addition, your skin in the treated area may become red, dry, and tender. You also may lose your hair in the treated area.

You are likely to become very tired during external radiation therapy, especially in the later weeks of treatment. Resting is important, but doctors usually advise patients to try to stay as active as they can.

People who get systemic radiation also may feel very tired. They may be more likely to get infections.

If you have radiation therapy and chemotherapy at the same time, your side effects may be worse. The side effects can be distressing. You can talk with your doctor about ways to relieve them.

You may want to ask the doctor these questions before starting radiation therapy:

- Why do I need this treatment?

- What are the expected benefits of radiation therapy?

- What are the risks and side effects of this treatment? What can we do about them?

- Are there any long-term effects?
- When will the treatments begin? When will they end?
- How will I feel during therapy?
- How will treatment affect my normal activities?

Stem cell transplantation: A person with lymphoma who has relapsed may receive stem cell transplantation. A transplant of blood-forming stem cells allows a person to receive high doses of chemotherapy, radiation therapy, or both. The high doses destroy both lymphoma cells and healthy blood cells in the bone marrow. Later, the patient receives healthy blood-forming stem cells through a flexible tube placed in a large vein in the neck or chest area. New blood cells develop from the transplanted stem cells.

Stem cell transplants take place in the hospital. The stem cells may come from the patient or from a donor:

- **Autologous stem cell transplantation:** This type of transplant uses the patient's own stem cells. The stem cells are removed from the patient, and the cells may be treated to kill lymphoma cells that may be present. The stem cells are frozen and stored. After the patient receives high-dose treatment, the stored stem cells are thawed and returned to the patient.

- **Allogeneic stem cell transplantation:** Sometimes healthy stem cells from a donor are available. The patient's brother, sister, or parent may be the donor. Or the stem cells may come from an unrelated donor. Doctors use blood tests to be sure the donor's cells match the patient's cells.

- **Syngeneic stem cell transplantation:** This type of transplant uses stem cells from the patient's healthy identical twin.

You may want to ask the doctor these questions before having a stem cell transplant:

- What are the possible benefits and risks of different types of transplants?
- What kind of stem cell transplant will I have? If I need a donor, how will we find one?
- How long will I need to be in the hospital? Will I need special care?
- How will we know if the treatment is working?

- What can we do about side effects?
- How will treatment affect my normal activities?
- What is my chance of a full recovery?

Supportive Care

Non-Hodgkin lymphoma and its treatment can lead to other health problems. You may receive supportive care to prevent or control these problems and to improve your comfort and quality of life during treatment.

You may receive antibiotics and other drugs to help protect you from infections. Your health care team may advise you to stay away from crowds and from people with colds and other contagious diseases. If an infection develops, it can be serious, and you will need treatment right away.

Non-Hodgkin lymphoma and its treatment also can lead to anemia, which may make you feel very tired. Drugs or blood transfusions can help with this problem.

Complementary and Alternative Medicine

Some people with cancer use complementary and alternative medicine (CAM):

- An approach is generally called complementary medicine when it is used along with standard treatment.
- An approach is called alternative medicine when it is used instead of standard treatment.

Acupuncture, massage therapy, herbal products, vitamins or special diets, visualization, meditation, and spiritual healing are types of CAM. Some people report that such approaches help them feel better.

However, some types of CAM can create health problems. An alternative medicine may not work as well as standard treatment. Patients with aggressive lymphoma who use alternative medicine instead of standard treatment may reduce the chance to control or cure their disease.

It is important to keep in mind that some complementary medicines may interfere with standard treatment. Combining CAM with standard treatment may even be harmful. Before trying any type of CAM, you should discuss its possible benefits and risks with your doctor.

Some types of CAM are expensive. Health insurance may not cover the cost.

You may want to ask the doctor these questions before you choose CAM:

- What benefits can I expect from this therapy?

- What are its risks?

- Do the expected benefits outweigh the risks?

- What side effects should I watch for?

- Will the therapy change the way my cancer treatment works? Could this be harmful?

- Is this therapy under study in a clinical trial? If so, who sponsors the trial?

- Will my health insurance pay for this therapy?

Nutrition

It is important for you to eat well. Eating well means getting enough calories to maintain a good weight and enough protein to keep up your strength. Good nutrition may help people with cancer feel better and have more energy.

But eating well can be hard. You may not feel like eating if you are tired or in pain. Also, the side effects of treatment (such as nausea, vomiting, or mouth sores) can be a problem. Some people find that foods do not taste as good during cancer treatment.

Follow-Up Care

Follow-up care for non-Hodgkin lymphoma is important. Your doctor will watch your recovery closely and check for recurrence of the lymphoma. Checkups help make sure that any changes in your health are noted and treated as needed. Checkups may include a physical exam, lab tests, chest x-rays, and other procedures. Between scheduled visits, you should contact the doctor right away if you have any health problems.

Sources of Support

Living with non-Hodgkin lymphoma is not easy. You may worry about caring for your family, keeping your job, or continuing daily activities. Concerns about treatments and managing side effects, hospital stays, and medical bills are also common. Doctors, nurses, and other members of the health care team can answer questions about treatment, working, or other activities. Meeting with a social worker, counselor, or member of the clergy can be helpful if you want to talk about your feelings or concerns. Often, a social worker can suggest resources for financial aid, transportation, home care, or emotional support.

Support groups also can help. In these groups, patients or their family members meet with other patients or their families to share what they have learned about coping with the disease and the effects of treatment. Groups may offer support in person, over the telephone, or on the internet. You may want to talk with a member of your health care team about finding a support group.

Information Specialists at 800-4-CANCER and at LiveHelp (http://www.cancer.gov) can provide information to help you locate programs, services, and publications.

The Promise of Cancer Research

Scientists are searching for causes of non-Hodgkin lymphoma. Also, doctors all over the country are studying new ways to treat lymphoma. Clinical trials (research studies in which people volunteer to take part) find out whether promising approaches to treatment are safe and effective. Research already has led to advances.

Researchers are studying many types of treatments for lymphoma:

- **Chemotherapy:** Doctors are testing new drugs that kill cancer cells. They are working with many drugs and drug combinations. They also are looking at ways of combining drugs with other treatments, such as biological therapy.

- **Radiation therapy:** Doctors are testing radiation treatment alone and with chemotherapy.

- **Biological therapy:** New types of biological therapy are under study. For example, researchers are making cancer vaccines that may help the immune system kill lymphoma cells. Also, doctors are studying a type of biological therapy that delivers radiation directly to cancer cells.

- **Stem cell transplantation:** Doctors are studying stem cell transplantation in people with newly diagnosed lymphoma and those who have already been treated.

People who join clinical trials may be among the first to benefit if a new approach is effective. And even if participants do not benefit directly, they still help doctors learn more about the disease and how to control it. Although clinical trials may pose some risks, researchers do all they can to protect their patients.

If you are interested in being part of a clinical trial, you should talk with your doctor.

NCI's website includes a section on clinical trials at http://www.cancer.gov/clinicaltrials. It has general information about clinical trials as well as detailed information about specific ongoing studies of new treatments for non-Hodgkin lymphoma. Information Specialists at 800-4-CANCER or at LiveHelp can answer questions and provide information about clinical trials.

Chapter 62

AIDS-Related Lymphoma

AIDS-related lymphoma is a disease in which malignant (cancer) cells form in the lymph system of patients who have acquired immunodeficiency syndrome (AIDS).

AIDS is caused by the human immunodeficiency virus (HIV), which attacks and weakens the body's immune system. The immune system is then unable to fight infection and diseases that invade the body. People with HIV disease have an increased risk of developing infections, lymphoma, and other types of cancer. A person with HIV disease who develops certain types of infections or cancer is then diagnosed with AIDS. Sometimes, people are diagnosed with AIDS and AIDS-related lymphoma at the same time.

Lymphomas are cancers that affect the white blood cells of the lymph system, part of the body's immune system. The lymph system is made up of the following:

- **Lymph:** Colorless, watery fluid that travels through the lymph system and carries white blood cells called lymphocytes. Lymphocytes protect the body against infections and the growth of tumors.

- **Lymph vessels:** A network of thin tubes that collect lymph from different parts of the body and return it to the bloodstream.

PDQ® Cancer Information Summary. National Cancer Institute; Bethesda, MD. AIDS-Related Lymphoma (PDQ®): Treatment - Patient. Updated 02/2006. Available at: http://cancer.gov. Accessed April 30, 2006.

- **Lymph nodes:** Small, bean-shaped structures that filter substances in lymph and help fight infection and disease. Lymph nodes are located along the network of lymph vessels found throughout the body. Clusters of lymph nodes are found in the underarm, pelvis, neck, abdomen, and groin.

- **Spleen:** An organ that produces lymphocytes, filters the blood, stores blood cells, and destroys old blood cells. It is located on the left side of the abdomen near the stomach.

- **Thymus:** An organ in which lymphocytes grow and multiply. The thymus is in the chest behind the breastbone.

- **Tonsils:** Two small masses of lymph tissue at the back of the throat. The tonsils produce lymphocytes.

- **Bone marrow:** The soft, spongy tissue in the center of large bones. Bone marrow produces white blood cells, red blood cells, and platelets.

There are many different types of lymphoma. Lymphomas are divided into two general types: Hodgkin lymphoma and non-Hodgkin lymphoma. Both Hodgkin lymphoma and non-Hodgkin lymphoma may occur in AIDS patients, but non-Hodgkin lymphoma is more common. When a person with AIDS has non-Hodgkin lymphoma, it is called an AIDS-related lymphoma.

Non-Hodgkin lymphomas are grouped by the way their cells look under a microscope. They may be indolent (slow-growing) or aggressive (fast-growing). AIDS-related lymphoma is usually aggressive. There are three main types of AIDS-related lymphoma:

- Diffuse large B-cell lymphoma

- B-cell immunoblastic lymphoma

- Small non-cleaved cell lymphoma

A doctor should be consulted if any of the following symptoms occur:

- Weight loss or fever for no known reason

- Night sweats

- Painless, swollen lymph nodes in the neck, chest, underarm, or groin

- A feeling of fullness below the ribs

The following tests and procedures may be used to help detect (find) and diagnose AIDS-related lymphoma:

Physical exam and history: An exam of the body to check general signs of health, including checking for signs of disease, such as lumps or anything else that seems unusual. A history of the patient's health habits and past illnesses and treatments will also be taken.

Complete blood count (CBC): A procedure in which a sample of blood is drawn and checked for the following:

- The number of red blood cells, white blood cells, and platelets
- The amount of hemoglobin (the protein that carries oxygen) in the red blood cells
- The portion of the sample made up of red blood cells

Lymph node biopsy: The removal of all or part of a lymph node. A pathologist views the tissue under a microscope to look for cancer cells. One of the following types of biopsies may be done:

- **Excisional biopsy:** The removal of an entire lymph node
- **Incisional biopsy or core biopsy:** The removal of part of a lymph node
- **Needle biopsy or fine-needle aspiration:** The removal of a sample of tissue from a lymph node with a needle

Bone marrow biopsy: The removal of a small piece of bone and bone marrow by inserting a needle into the hipbone or breastbone. A pathologist views both the bone and bone marrow samples under a microscope to look for signs of cancer.

HIV test: A test to measure the level of HIV antibodies in a sample of blood. Antibodies are made by the body when it is invaded by a foreign substance. A high level of HIV antibodies may mean the body has been infected with HIV.

Epstein-Barr virus (EBV) test: A test to measure the level of EBV antibodies in a sample of blood, tissue, or cerebrospinal fluid (CSF). Antibodies are made by the body when it is invaded by a foreign substance. A high level of EBV antibodies may mean the body has been infected with EBV.

Chest x-ray: An x-ray of the organs and bones inside the chest. An x-ray is a type of energy beam that can go through the body and onto film, making a picture of areas inside the body.

Prognosis

The prognosis (chance of recovery) and treatment options depend on the following:

- The stage of the cancer
- The number of CD4 lymphocytes (a type of white blood cell) in the blood
- Whether the patient has ever had AIDS-related infections
- The patient's ability to carry out regular daily activities

Stages of AIDS-Related Lymphoma

After AIDS-related lymphoma has been diagnosed, tests are done to find out if cancer cells have spread within the lymph system or to other parts of the body. The process used to find out if cancer cells have spread within the lymph system or to other parts of the body is called staging. The information gathered from the staging process determines the stage of the disease. It is important to know the stage in order to plan treatment, but AIDS-related lymphoma is usually advanced when it is diagnosed. The following tests and procedures may be used in the staging process:

- **CT scan (CAT scan):** A procedure that makes a series of detailed pictures of areas inside the body, taken from different angles. The pictures are made by a computer linked to an x-ray machine. A dye may be injected into a vein or swallowed to help the organs or tissues show up more clearly. This procedure is also called computed tomography, computerized tomography, or computerized axial tomography.

- **PET scan (positron emission tomography scan):** A procedure to find malignant tumor cells in the body. A small amount of radionuclide glucose (sugar) is injected into a vein. The PET scanner rotates around the body and makes a picture of where glucose is being used in the body. Malignant tumor cells show up brighter in the picture because they are more active and take up more glucose than normal cells.

- **MRI (magnetic resonance imaging):** A procedure that uses a magnet, radio waves, and a computer to make a series of detailed pictures of areas inside the body. A substance called gadolinium is injected into the patient through a vein. The gadolinium collects around the cancer cells so they show up brighter in the picture. This procedure is also called nuclear magnetic resonance imaging (NMRI).

- **Bone marrow biopsy:** The removal of a small piece of bone and bone marrow by inserting a needle into the hipbone or breastbone. A pathologist views both the bone and the bone marrow samples under a microscope to look for signs of cancer.

- **Lumbar puncture:** A procedure used to collect cerebrospinal fluid from the spinal column. This is done by placing a needle into the spinal column. This procedure is also called an LP or spinal tap.

- **Blood chemistry studies:** A procedure in which a blood sample is checked to measure the amounts of certain substances released into the blood by organs and tissues in the body. An unusual (higher or lower than normal) amount of a substance can be a sign of disease in the organ or tissue that produces it. The blood sample will be checked for the level of LDH (lactate dehydrogenase).

AIDS-related lymphoma may be described as follows:

- **E:** "E" stands for extranodal and means the cancer is found in an area or organ other than the lymph nodes or has spread to tissues beyond, but near, the major lymphatic areas.

- **S:** "S" stands for spleen and means the cancer is found in the spleen.

The following stages are used for AIDS-related lymphoma:

Stage I: Stage I AIDS-related lymphoma is divided into stage I and stage IE.

- **Stage I:** Cancer is found in one lymph node group.

- **Stage IE:** Cancer is found in an area or organ other than the lymph nodes.

Stage II: Stage II AIDS-related lymphoma is divided into stage II and stage IIE.

- **Stage II:** Cancer is found in two or more lymph node groups on the same side of the diaphragm (the thin muscle below the lungs that helps breathing and separates the chest from the abdomen).

- **Stage IIE:** Cancer is found in an area or organ other than the lymph nodes and in lymph nodes near that area or organ, and may have spread to other lymph node groups on the same side of the diaphragm.

Stage III: Stage III AIDS-related lymphoma is divided into stage III, stage IIIE, stage IIIS, and stage IIIS+E.

- **Stage III:** Cancer is found in lymph node groups on both sides of the diaphragm (the thin muscle below the lungs that helps breathing and separates the chest from the abdomen).

- **Stage IIIE:** Cancer is found in lymph node groups on both sides of the diaphragm and in an area or organ other than the lymph nodes.

- **Stage IIIS:** Cancer is found in lymph node groups on both sides of the diaphragm and in the spleen.

- **Stage IIIS+E:** Cancer is found in lymph node groups on both sides of the diaphragm, in an area or organ other than the lymph nodes, and in the spleen.

Stage IV: In stage IV AIDS-related lymphoma, the cancer either:

- is found throughout one or more organs other than the lymph nodes and may be in lymph nodes near those organs; or

- is found in one organ other than the lymph nodes and has spread to lymph nodes far away from that organ.

Patients who are infected with the Epstein-Barr virus or whose AIDS-related lymphoma affects the bone marrow have an increased risk of the cancer spreading to the central nervous system (CNS).

For treatment, AIDS-related lymphomas are grouped based on where they started in the body, as follows:

- **Peripheral/systemic lymphoma:** Lymphoma that starts in lymph nodes or other organs of the lymph system is called peripheral/systemic lymphoma. The lymphoma may spread throughout the body, including to the brain or bone marrow.

- **Primary CNS lymphoma:** Primary CNS lymphoma starts in the central nervous system (brain and spinal cord). Lymphoma that starts somewhere else in the body and spreads to the central nervous system is not primary CNS lymphoma.

Treatment Option Overview

Different types of treatment are available for patients with AIDS-related lymphoma. Some treatments are standard (the currently used treatment), and some are being tested in clinical trials. Before starting treatment, patients may want to think about taking part in a clinical trial. A treatment clinical trial is a research study meant to help improve current treatments or obtain information on new treatments for patients with cancer. When clinical trials show that a new treatment is better than the standard treatment, the new treatment may become the standard treatment.

Clinical trials are taking place in many parts of the country. Information about ongoing clinical trials is available from the National Cancer Institute website (http://www.cancer.gov). Choosing the most appropriate cancer treatment is a decision that ideally involves the patient, family, and health care team.

Treatment of AIDS-related lymphoma combines treatment of the lymphoma with treatment for AIDS. Patients with AIDS have weakened immune systems and treatment can cause further damage. For this reason, patients who have AIDS-related lymphoma are usually treated with lower doses of drugs than lymphoma patients who do not have AIDS.

Highly-active antiretroviral therapy (HAART) is used to slow progression of HIV (which is a retrovirus). Treatment with HAART may allow some patients to safely receive anticancer drugs in standard or higher doses. Medicine to prevent and treat infections, which can be serious, is also used.

AIDS-related lymphoma usually grows faster than lymphoma that is not AIDS-related and it is more likely to spread to other parts of the body. In general, AIDS-related lymphoma is harder to treat.

Three types of standard treatment are used:

Chemotherapy: Chemotherapy is a cancer treatment that uses drugs to stop the growth of cancer cells, either by killing the cells or by stopping the cells from dividing. When chemotherapy is taken by mouth or injected into a vein or muscle, the drugs enter the bloodstream and can reach cancer cells throughout the body (systemic chemotherapy).

When chemotherapy is placed directly into the spinal column (intrathecal chemotherapy), an organ, or a body cavity such as the abdomen, the drugs mainly affect cancer cells in those areas (regional chemotherapy). Combination chemotherapy is treatment using more than one anticancer drug. The way the chemotherapy is given depends on the type and stage of the cancer being treated.

Intrathecal chemotherapy may be used in patients who are more likely to have lymphoma in the central nervous system (CNS).

Colony-stimulating factors are sometimes given together with chemotherapy. This helps lessen the side effects chemotherapy may have on the bone marrow.

Radiation therapy: Radiation therapy is a cancer treatment that uses high-energy x-rays or other types of radiation to kill cancer cells. There are two types of radiation therapy. External radiation therapy uses a machine outside the body to send radiation toward the cancer. Internal radiation therapy uses a radioactive substance sealed in needles, seeds, wires, or catheters that are placed directly into or near the cancer. The way the radiation therapy is given depends on the type and stage of the cancer being treated.

High-dose chemotherapy with stem cell transplant: High-dose chemotherapy with stem cell transplant is a method of giving high doses of chemotherapy and replacing blood-forming cells destroyed by the cancer treatment. Stem cells (immature blood cells) are removed from the blood or bone marrow of the patient or a donor and are frozen and stored. After the chemotherapy is completed, the stored stem cells are thawed and given back to the patient through an infusion. These reinfused stem cells grow into (and restore) the body's blood cells.

New Treatments

New types of treatment are being tested in clinical trials. These include the following:

Monoclonal antibody therapy: Monoclonal antibody therapy is a cancer treatment that uses antibodies made in the laboratory from a single type of immune system cell. These antibodies can identify substances on cancer cells or normal substances that may help cancer cells grow. The antibodies attach to the substances and kill the cancer cells, block their growth, or keep them from spreading. Monoclonal antibodies are given by infusion. These may be used alone or to carry drugs, toxins, or radioactive material directly to cancer cells.

Treatment Options for AIDS-Related Lymphoma

AIDS-related peripheral/systemic lymphoma: There is no standard treatment plan for AIDS-related peripheral/systemic lymphoma. Treatment is adjusted for each patient and is usually one or more of the following:

- Combination chemotherapy
- High-dose chemotherapy and stem cell transplant
- A clinical trial of monoclonal antibodies
- A clinical trial of different treatment combinations

AIDS-related primary central nervous system lymphoma: Treatment of AIDS-related primary central nervous system lymphoma is usually radiation therapy.

Chapter 63

Thymoma and Thymic Carcinoma

Thymoma and thymic carcinoma are diseases in which malignant (cancer) cells form on the outside surface of the thymus. The thymus, a small organ that lies in the upper chest under the breastbone, is part of the lymph system. It makes white blood cells, called lymphocytes, which protect the body against infections.

There are different types of tumors of the thymus. Thymomas and thymic carcinomas are rare tumors of the cells that are on the outside surface of the thymus. The tumor cells in a thymoma look similar to the normal cells of the thymus, grow slowly, and rarely spread beyond the thymus. On the other hand, the tumor cells in a thymic carcinoma look very different from the normal cells of the thymus, grow more quickly, and have usually spread to other parts of the body when the cancer is found. Thymic carcinoma is more difficult to treat than thymoma.

People with thymoma often have other diseases as well. These diseases may include myasthenia gravis, polymyositis, lupus erythematosus, rheumatoid arthritis, thyroiditis, Sjögren syndrome, and hypogammaglobulinemia.

Sometimes thymoma and thymic carcinoma do not cause symptoms. The cancer may be found during a routine chest x-ray. The following symptoms may be caused by thymoma, thymic carcinoma, or other conditions. A doctor should be consulted if any of the following problems occur:

PDQ® Cancer Information Summary. National Cancer Institute; Bethesda, MD. Thymoma and Thymic Carcinoma (PDQ®): Treatment - Patient. Updated 06/2005. Available at: http://cancer.gov. Accessed April 30, 2006.

- A cough that doesn't go away
- Chest pain
- Trouble breathing

The following tests and procedures may be used to detect (find) thymoma or thymic carcinoma:

Physical exam and history: An exam of the body to check general signs of health, including checking for signs of disease, such as lumps or anything else that seems unusual. A history of the patient's health habits and past illnesses and treatments will also be taken.

Chest x-ray: An x-ray of the organs and bones inside the chest. An x-ray is a type of energy beam that can go through the body and onto film, making a picture of areas inside the body.

CT scan (CAT scan): A procedure that makes a series of detailed pictures of areas inside the body, such as the chest, taken from different angles. The pictures are made by a computer linked to an x-ray machine. A dye may be injected into a vein or swallowed to help the organs or tissues show up more clearly. This procedure is also called computed tomography, computerized tomography, or computerized axial tomography.

MRI (magnetic resonance imaging): A procedure that uses a magnet, radio waves, and a computer to make a series of detailed pictures of areas inside the body, such as the chest. This procedure is also called nuclear magnetic resonance imaging (NMRI).

Prognosis

A biopsy of the tumor is done to diagnose the disease. The biopsy may be taken before or during surgery, using a thin needle to obtain the sample of cells (needle biopsy or fine-needle aspiration biopsy). A pathologist will view the sample under a microscope to check for cancer. If thymoma or thymic carcinoma is diagnosed, the pathologist will determine the type of cancer cell in the tumor. There may be more than one type of cancer cell in a thymoma. The surgeon will decide if all or part of the tumor can be removed by surgery. In some cases, lymph nodes and other tissues may be removed as well.

The prognosis (chance of recovery) and treatment options depend on the following:

- The stage of the cancer
- The type of cancer cell
- Whether the tumor can be removed completely by surgery
- The patient's general health
- Whether the cancer has just been diagnosed or has recurred (come back)

Stages of Thymoma and Thymic Carcinoma

Tests done to detect thymoma or thymic carcinoma are also used to stage the disease. Staging is the process used to find out if cancer has spread from the thymus to other parts of the body. The findings made during surgery and the results of tests and procedures are used to determine the stage of the disease. It is important to know the stage in order to plan treatment.

The following stages are used for thymoma:

Noninvasive thymoma (stage I): In stage I, cancer is found only within the thymus. All cancer cells are inside the capsule (sac) that surrounds the thymus.

Invasive thymoma (stage II, stage III, and stage IV): Invasive thymoma includes stage II, stage III, and stage IV.

- In stage II, cancer has spread through the capsule and into the fat around the thymus or into the lining of the chest cavity.
- In stage III, cancer has spread to nearby organs in the chest, including the lung, the sac around the heart, or large blood vessels that carry blood to the heart.
- Stage IV is divided into stage IVA and stage IVB, depending on where the cancer has spread.
  - In stage IVA, cancer has spread widely around the lungs and heart.
  - In stage IVB, cancer has spread to the blood or lymph system.

Thymic carcinomas have usually spread to other parts of the body when diagnosed.

The staging system used for thymomas is sometimes used for thymic carcinomas.

677

Recurrent thymoma and thymic carcinoma: Recurrent thymoma and thymic carcinoma is cancer that has recurred (come back) after it has been treated. The cancer may come back in the thymus or in other parts of the body. Thymic carcinomas commonly recur. Thymomas may recur after a long time. There is also an increased risk of having another type of cancer after having a thymoma. For these reasons, lifelong follow-up is needed.

Treatment Option Overview

Different types of treatments are available for patients with thymoma and thymic carcinoma. Some treatments are standard (the currently used treatment), and some are being tested in clinical trials. Before starting treatment, patients may want to think about taking part in a clinical trial. A treatment clinical trial is a research study meant to help improve current treatments or obtain information on new treatments for patients with cancer. When clinical trials show that a new treatment is better than the standard treatment, the new treatment may become the standard treatment.

Clinical trials are taking place in many parts of the country. Information about ongoing clinical trials is available from the National Cancer Institute website (http://www.cancer.gov). Choosing the most appropriate cancer treatment is a decision that ideally involves the patient, family, and health care team.

Three types of standard treatment are used:

Surgery: Surgery to remove the tumor is the most common treatment of thymoma.

Even if the doctor removes all the cancer that can be seen at the time of the surgery, some patients may be given radiation therapy after surgery to kill any cancer cells that are left. Treatment given after the surgery, to increase the chances of a cure, is called adjuvant therapy.

Radiation therapy: Radiation therapy is a cancer treatment that uses high-energy x-rays or other types of radiation to kill cancer cells. There are two types of radiation therapy. External radiation therapy uses a machine outside the body to send radiation toward the cancer. Internal radiation therapy uses a radioactive substance sealed in needles, seeds, wires, or catheters that are placed directly into or near the cancer. The way the radiation therapy is given depends on the type and stage of the cancer being treated.

Hormone therapy: Hormone therapy is a cancer treatment that removes hormones or blocks their action and stops cancer cells from growing. Hormones are substances produced by glands in the body and circulated in the bloodstream. Some hormones can cause certain cancers to grow. If tests show that the cancer cells have places where hormones can attach (receptors), drugs, surgery, or radiation therapy is used to reduce the production of hormones or block them from working.

Hormone therapy with drugs called corticosteroids may be used to treat thymoma or thymic carcinoma.

New Treatments

New types of treatment are being tested in clinical trials. These include chemotherapy. Chemotherapy is a cancer treatment that uses drugs to stop the growth of cancer cells, either by killing the cells or by stopping the cells from dividing. When chemotherapy is taken by mouth or injected into a vein or muscle, the drugs enter the bloodstream and can reach cancer cells throughout the body (systemic chemotherapy). When chemotherapy is placed directly into the spinal column, an organ, or a body cavity such as the abdomen, the drugs mainly affect cancer cells in those areas (regional chemotherapy). The way the chemotherapy is given depends on the type and stage of the cancer being treated.

Treatment Options for Thymoma and Thymic Carcinoma

Noninvasive thymoma and thymic carcinoma: Treatment of noninvasive thymoma and thymic carcinoma may include the following:

- Surgery to remove the tumor
- Radiation therapy

Invasive thymoma and thymic carcinoma: Treatment of invasive thymoma and thymic carcinoma that may be completely removed by surgery includes the following:

- Surgery followed by radiation therapy
- A clinical trial of other new treatments

Treatment of invasive thymoma and thymic carcinoma that cannot be removed completely by surgery includes the following:

- Surgery to remove part of the tumor, followed by radiation therapy with or without chemotherapy
- A clinical trial of chemotherapy using one or more anticancer drugs
- A clinical trial of chemotherapy before surgery, with or without radiation therapy
- A clinical trial of combination chemotherapy followed by radiation therapy
- A clinical trial of other new treatments

Recurrent thymoma and thymic carcinoma: Treatment of recurrent thymoma and thymic carcinoma may include the following:

- Surgery with or without radiation therapy
- Radiation therapy
- Hormone therapy
- A clinical trial of chemotherapy using one or more anticancer drugs
- A clinical trial of other new treatments

Chapter 64

Pituitary Tumors

Chapter Contents

Section 64.1

The Pituitary Gland

The pituitary gland is central to our well-being. It is the master gland of the entire body. It produces (secretes) many hormones that stimulate glands in the body to produce other hormones or to complete certain actions. A gland is an organ that makes hormones, substances which function as messengers and are carried to other parts of your body, where they have an effect or stimulate an action.

The pituitary gland makes many different hormones:

Prolactin: Prolactin stimulates milk production from the breasts after childbirth to enable nursing and can affect sex hormone levels from the ovaries in women and the testes in men.

Growth hormone or GH: GH stimulates growth in childhood and is important for maintaining a healthy body composition and well-being in adults. In adults it is important for maintaining muscle mass as well as bone mass. It also affects fat distribution in the body.

Adrenocorticotropin or ACTH: ACTH stimulates production of cortisol by the adrenal glands. Cortisol, a so-called "stress hormone" is vital to survival. It helps maintain blood pressure and blood glucose levels.

Thyroid-stimulating hormone or TSH: TSH stimulates the thyroid gland, which regulates the body's metabolism, energy, growth and development, and nervous system activity. This hormone also is vital to your survival.

Antidiuretic hormone or ADH: ADH, also called vasopressin, is stored in the back part of the pituitary gland and regulates water balance. If this hormone is not secreted properly, this can lead to a diabetes insipidus (different from diabetes mellitus which affects glucose) because your kidneys are not working well.

Luteinizing hormone or LH: LH regulates testosterone in men and estrogen in women.

Follicle-stimulating hormone or FSH: FSH promotes sperm production in men and stimulates the ovaries to enable ovulation in women. LH and FSH work together to cause normal function of the ovaries and testes.

Pituitary Tumors

The most frequent cause of pituitary disorders is pituitary tumors. The pituitary gland is made of several cell types. Each cell type releases one of the hormones mentioned above. Sometimes these cells grow too much or produce small growths.

These growths are called pituitary tumors, and they are fairly common in adults. These are not brain tumors and are not a form of cancer. Cancerous tumors of this sort are extremely rare. Pituitary tumors can interfere with the normal formation and release of hormones, however. In addition, some pituitary tumors make too much of the type of hormone produced by the pituitary cells forming the tumor.

Two types of tumors exist: secretory and non-secretory. Secretory tumors produce too much of a hormone. Non-secretory tumors cause problems because of their large size or because they interfere with normal function of the pituitary gland.

The problems caused by pituitary tumors fall into three categories:

1. **Hypersecretion:** Too much hormone is secreted into the body. This is usually caused by a secretory tumor. Common secretory tumors make too much prolactin. Other tumors make too much of the pituitary hormones which stimulate growth, the adrenal gland or the thyroid. Tumors making too much of the hormones stimulating the ovaries or testes are extremely rare.

2. **Hyposecretion:** Too little hormone is secreted into the body. This is usually caused by a non-secretory tumor, which interferes with the ability of the normal pituitary gland to make hormones. It can also be caused by a secretory tumor which is large. It can also result from therapy of a tumor with surgery or radiation treatment.

3. **Tumor mass effects:** As the tumor grows and presses against the normal pituitary gland or other areas in the brain, you may have headaches, vision problems, or hypo secretion. Tumor mass effects can be seen in any type of pituitary tumor that grows large enough. Injuries, certain medications, and other conditions can also affect the pituitary gland. Loss of normal pituitary function has been reported after major head trauma. The prolonged use of steroid medications such as prednisone can suppress levels of ACTH and result in adrenal insufficiency (a lack of cortisol production) if abruptly discontinued, which must be replaced until ACTH and adrenal function returns. A number of psychiatric medications can lead to an increase in prolactin levels.

If you think you have a problem with your pituitary gland, it is important that you see a pituitary specialist. An endocrinologist is an expert in hormone-related conditions, and some endocrinologists make the pituitary gland their specialty. You may be referred to other doctors if you need surgery or radiation treatments.

Section 64.2

Secretory Tumors

Prolactinoma

A prolactinoma is a tumor on the pituitary gland that produces too much prolactin (milk hormone). It is the most common secretory tumor (accounting for about 40% of pituitary tumors).

Symptoms of prolactinoma include the following:

- Changes in menstrual cycle/complete loss of periods
- Headaches
- Infertility

- Milk discharge from breasts in women (not related to giving birth) or men
- Vision disturbances
- Pain during intercourse/dryness in vagina
- Mood changes and depression
- Reduced sex drive
- Osteoporosis (because of inadequate function of the ovaries in women, leading to estrogen deficiency and inadequate function of the testes in men leading to testosterone deficiency)
- Inadequate function of the testes (in males) leading to impotence (inability to get or maintain an erection) or infertility

Treatment for Prolactinoma

About 80–90% of prolactinoma patients can be treated successfully with medication. The medication is a dopamine agonist drug. The use of a dopamine agonist should eliminate or reduce symptoms of a high prolactin level, return your prolactin levels to normal, help restore normal function to the pituitary, and usually reduce the tumor size.

This medication is taken in tablet form. Your doctor will monitor your prolactin levels and make adjustments if necessary depending on prolactin levels symptoms and tumor size. The most common side effects are nausea and dizziness. Sometimes drug treatment is not effective, so your doctor might recommend surgery. Radiation therapy is rarely used in the management of large tumors. Some patients with very small tumors, which are stable in size and do not have any associated symptoms, may be monitored carefully without treatment.

Acromegaly

Acromegaly is caused by the hypersecretion of growth hormone in adults. It can cause serious changes in the way you look as well as complications with your metabolism (the process, through which your body breaks down food, uses or stores food components, and eliminates waste products). It also affects the cardiac system, glucose metabolism, joints and bones; symptoms of acromegaly can come on slowly over time. A relative who has not seen you in a while might notice the changes that are part of this condition.

Acromegaly definitely puts you at risk for colon cancer. Your doctor should screen you for colon cancer and look for pre-cancerous colon polyps (growths). Because the risk is high for this type of cancer, you should have a colonoscopy regularly.

Symptoms of acromegaly include the following:

- Interrupted menstrual cycle
- Deepening of the voice
- Impotence (inability to get or maintain an erection)
- Oily skin or acne
- Coarser facial features (a noticeably large nose)
- Excessive sweating
- Teeth that are spreading out
- Enlarged hands, feet, head, nose, and jaw
- Enlarged tongue and sleep apnea (interrupted breathing while sleeping)
- Depression
- Skin tags (small growths of skin that might be dark)
- Memory loss/not being able to think as well
- Thicker flesh on the palms and feet
- High blood pressure
- Fatigue
- Headaches
- Carpal tunnel syndrome (pain in wrist and hands)
- Osteoarthritis
- Colon polyps (growths)
- Peripheral vision defects (inability to see well at the edges of your vision range)
- Reduced sex drive

Treatment of Acromegaly

The best way to treat acromegaly is by removing the tumor through surgery called transsphenoidal microsurgery. This is not brain surgery and does not involve drilling a hole or cutting through your skull. Instead, the surgery is performed through the sinus passages behind your nose. Removing or reducing the pituitary tumor that causes acromegaly will reduce growth hormone levels and relieve the pressure caused by the tumor mass. Rarely a craniotomy may be required to remove tumor that cannot be removed through a transsphenoidal method.

Your surgeon might not be able to remove the entire tumor. If that happens, your hormone levels will be tested. If there is still tumor left or your hormone levels are not yet normal, medicine or radiation therapy may be given.

The medication of choice is octreotide, which is given most often by a monthly intramuscular injection. This therapy sometimes is given to control overproduction of growth hormone as a sole therapy after non-curative surgery, or in patients who are not surgical candidates. It also may be given while you are waiting for radiation to be effective, something that can take years.

A new medication called pegvisomant has now been approved for acromegaly. Rather than suppressing growth hormone by the pituitary tumor, it works to inhibit the hormone from acting on the body. It is given by a daily subcutaneous injection.

Disappearance of symptoms varies. With treatment, some symptoms like sweating may disappear immediately. Hypertension or abnormal glucose, when due to excess GH may also quickly subside when GH levels become normal. Others, such as thicker tissue on your palms and feet, may take longer to reverse. If you have osteoarthritis, or bone changes, they may not go away.

Cushing Disease

Cushing disease is when a pituitary tumor is associated with hypersecretion of pituitary ACTH, which causes too much cortisol production by the adrenal glands. It is not very common but significant in that it affects as many as 4,000 people each year in the United States.

Symptoms for Cushing disease include the following:

- Easy bruising
- Muscle weakness
- Purple stretch marks
- Rapid and unexplained weight gain with a rounder face and abdomen often with thin legs or extremities
- Increased fat in your neck and above your collar bone and upper back
- Memory loss/not being able to think as well
- Menstrual cycle disorders

- Skin changes and red cheeks
- Osteoporosis
- Depression
- Mood and behavior disorders
- High blood sugar levels
- Hypertension

Treatment for Cushing Disease

Each person with Cushing disease needs his or her own treatment, which may mean a combination of medication, surgery, and radiation. The first line therapy is surgical and cure rates with an experienced neurosurgeon are over 90 percent. A patient will typically have trans-sphenoidal microsurgery (through the nasal sinuses).

Patients who are not cured but have proven pituitary Cushing usually have repeat surgery. When not effective, radiation therapy may treat any remaining tumor mass. Medication to block the adrenal glands is typically used while waiting for the radiation to have an effect. Rarely, the adrenal glands are removed. Your doctor may prescribe additional medication to treat high blood pressure, high glucose levels, or additional problems brought on by Cushing disease.

TSH-Secreting Tumor

A TSH-secreting tumor secretes too much thyroid stimulating hormone, which then causes the thyroid gland to make too much thyroid hormone (hyperthyroidism). These tumors are very rare.

Symptoms of a TSH-secreting tumor include the following:

- Heart palpitations
- Fast heart beat
- Irregular menstrual cycle
- Headaches
- Visual disturbances
- Difficulty sleeping
- More frequent bowel movements
- Inability to tolerate heat
- Excessive sweating
- Fatigue

- Weight loss
- Nervousness

Treatment for a TSH-Secreting Tumor:

The first treatment is usually transsphenoidal microsurgery. Unless the tumor is large, surgery alone can typically provide a complete cure. If so, you will need a long follow-up period with your doctor to be sure the treatment has worked.

If surgery doesn't remove the whole tumor, octreotide is an effective medication. Radiation therapy also may be prescribed. The radiation will destroy the remaining tumor, but the process is slow. Patients also may need additional medical therapy to lower TSH levels.

Section 64.3

Non-Secretory Tumors

"Pituitary: Non-Secretory Tumors," © 2004 The Hormone Foundation.
Reprinted with permission. For additional information, visit
www.hormone.org.

Nonfunctioning Adenoma

A nonfunctioning adenoma is a tumor that does not overproduce hormones, but causes problems because of its size and location in the pituitary. A nonfunctioning adenoma may cause headaches and vision problems. This type of tumor also may cause hyposecretion (not enough hormone production). These tumors often are found when doctors obtain an MRI after a head injury or another reason.

Symptoms of nonfunctioning adenomas fall into two categories:

1. Tumor mass effects:
   - Visual field disturbances, most commonly loss of peripheral vision (at the edges of your vision range)
   - Headaches
   - Abnormal control of eye movements

2. Hyposecretion effects:

- Loss of appetite
- Weight loss or weight gain
- Fatigue
- Irregular menstrual cycle
- Infertility
- Reduced sex drive
- Impotence (failure to get or maintain an erection)
- Inadequate function of the ovaries or testes
- Frequent urination during night
- Joint pains
- Dizziness
- Low blood pressure

Treatment for a Nonfunctioning Adenoma

The first therapy your doctor probably will employ is transsphenoidal microsurgery, especially if your vision is disturbed or you have compressed nerves around your brain, inside of your skull. After surgery, visual field problems improve in the majority of patients.

Hormone replacement may be necessary to restore normal hormone levels. If you have significant tumor remaining or the tumor regrows, you may need more surgery and/or radiation therapy.

Craniopharyngiomas and Rathke Cleft Cysts

Craniopharyngiomas and Rathke cleft cysts are tumors or lesions that are noncancerous growths that may be mistaken for a pituitary tumor on an MRI scan and can interfere with normal pituitary activities. They are common during childhood, but can grow and cause problems in adults. (Please note that cysts are not tumors)

Symptoms of craniopharyngiomas and Rathke cleft cysts are similar:

- Growth failure in children
- Delayed puberty in children
- Reduced or loss of sex drive
- Constipation

- Nausea
- Frequent urination
- Excessive thirst
- Obesity
- Headaches
- Menstrual irregularities/loss of menstrual cycle
- Milk discharge from breasts not related to childbirth
- Body temperature regulation problems
- Fatigue
- Increased drowsiness
- Dry skin
- Low blood pressure
- Visual disturbances
- Confusion
- Personality changes

Treatment for Craniopharyngiomas and Rathke Cleft Cysts

The primary treatment is surgery. The goal is to completely remove the tumor or cyst and preserve normal pituitary, brain, and visual function. If the mass located in the area of the pituitary, the surgery probably will be through your nasal sinuses (transsphenoidal). If the tumor is found above your pituitary, your surgeon may have to go in through the skull. If the tumor can't be completely removed, radiation treatment may be recommended.

Section 64.4

Treating Pituitary Tumors

"Pituitary: Treatment Options," © 2004 The Hormone Foundation.
Reprinted with permission. For additional information, visit
www.hormone.org.

Medications

Several types of medical therapy can help to relieve pituitary problems. Prolactinomas, for example, respond well to a dopamine agonist drug. If surgery does not remove the entire tumors, sometimes octreotide is used in patients with acromegaly or TSH-secreting tumors. Medication is used to lower high hormone levels or to shrink the tumor. Sometimes pegvisomant may be used to block the action of growth hormone. In many cases, medical therapy is combined with surgery or radiation treatment.

Hormone Therapy

Hormone replacement therapy is an important part of any treatment for a pituitary disorder. Hormones must be prescribed to meet your exact needs. Sometimes tumors cause a lack of hormone, which can lead to the symptoms you are having. Sometimes lack of hormone is caused by the treatment you have for pituitary tumors. Radiation therapy, for example, can lead to permanent loss of hormone secretion.

Some hormones are absolutely necessary for survival. These hormones must be replaced immediately. The replacement of cortisol is important, because this hormone regulates blood pressure and blood glucose levels. Cortisol replacement is common during tumor surgeries because it helps the body to handle stress.

TSH, or thyroid stimulating hormone, is also vital to survival, because it regulates the body's metabolism. If TSH secretion is low, you may also need to start thyroid hormone replacement.

ADH (vasopressin) needs immediate replacement, because it controls the body's water balance. If it is missing, this can cause excess thirst and urination, which is usually a temporary condition. (Please note that this is not the same as diabetes mellitus, a common confusion.)

Other hormones, such as estrogen and progesterone in women and testosterone in men also may need to be replaced. While they are not vital for survival, they help you to live a full and healthy life. In addition to reproductive effects, these hormones are important for many functions such as maintaining normal bone mass. It is important to remember that hormone replacement of estrogen and progesterone in young women, which is replacing hormones back to where they would be, of the pituitary works is not the same as post-menopausal hormone replacement. In the latter case, hormones are being given at a time in life when they are not normally made.

Some hormones may return to normal levels after treatment for a pituitary condition. In other cases, there may be some permanent loss of hormone function. You may need to take certain hormones for the rest of your life. Your doctor will work with you to monitor and adjust your hormone replacement therapy as needed. You should always take your hormone treatment as directed.

Surgery

The most common form of surgery to remove pituitary tumors is transsphenoidal microsurgery. A neurosurgeon approaches the pituitary tumor through the nose, in the sphenoid sinus cavity. Using this natural pathway the surgeon does not need to drill a hole in your skull. With a surgical microscope and special instruments, the surgeon can typically safely remove the tumor without damaging the surrounding pituitary gland.

This surgery is not very painful, and you won't have any outer scars. You may have a sore nose or what feels like a sinus headache. The biggest discomfort usually is from the padding inserted in the nose for 24 to 48 hours after surgery. However with newer techniques, packs are often not required at all. You will probably be in the hospital for two or three days. You should take it easy for a few weeks after the surgery, until your doctor says it is time to resume your usual activities, including exercise.

Radiation Treatments

To treat a pituitary tumor with radiation, doctors may use a variety of techniques depending on the size and location of the tumor. Conventional radiation covers a wide area in and around the tumor and is usually given daily for several weeks. A number of more focused "radiosurgery" therapies are also available and may be appropriate for your case including gamma knife and proton beam. These methods begin with an MRI scan to image your brain. The scan locates the precise location and size of the tumor. After the MRI, you go into a special treatment room. Using the points mapped from the MRI, several narrow beams of high-dose radiation are delivered to the exact tumor location. These beams are so precise that they can avoid the normal tissue surrounding the tumor. All radiation therapy works slowly and it may take from six months to several years for your condition to improve. This is why radiation therapy is typically used together with other therapies. It is important to have an evaluation for radiation therapy at a center with expertise in treating pituitary tumors.

Chapter 65

Adrenal Gland Cancers

Chapter Contents

Section 65.1

Pheochromocytoma

PDQ® Cancer Information Summary. National Cancer Institute; Bethesda, MD. Pheochromocytoma (PDQ®): Treatment - Patient. Updated 06/2003. Available at: http://cancer.gov. Accessed April 30, 2006.

What Is Pheochromocytoma?

Pheochromocytoma, a rare cancer, is a disease in which cancer (malignant) cells are found in special cells in the body called chromaffin cells. Most pheochromocytomas start inside the adrenal gland (the adrenal medulla) where most chromaffin cells are located. There are two adrenal glands, one above each kidney in the back of the upper abdomen. Cells in the adrenal glands make important hormones that help the body work properly. Usually pheochromocytoma affects only one adrenal gland. Pheochromocytoma may also start in other parts of the body, such as the area around the heart or bladder.

Most tumors that start in the chromaffin cells do not spread to other parts of the body and are not cancer. These are called benign tumors. If a tumor is found, the doctor will need to determine whether it is cancer or benign.

Pheochromocytomas often cause the adrenal glands to make too many hormones called catecholamines. The extra catecholamines cause high blood pressure (hypertension), which can cause headaches, sweating, pounding of the heart, pain in the chest, and a feeling of anxiety. High blood pressure that goes on for a long time without treatment can lead to heart disease, stroke, and other major health problems.

If there are symptoms, a doctor may order blood and urine tests to see if there are extra hormones in the body. A patient may also have a special nuclear medicine scan. A CT scan, an x-ray that uses a computer to make a picture of the inside of a part of the body or an MRI scan, which uses magnetic waves to make a picture of the abdomen, may also be done.

Pheochromocytoma is sometimes part of a condition called multiple endocrine neoplasia syndrome (MEN). People with MEN often have other cancers (such as thyroid cancer) and other hormonal problems.

The chance of recovery (prognosis) depends on how far the cancer has spread, and the patient's age and general health.

Stage Explanation

Once pheochromocytoma is found, more tests will be done to see how far the cancer has spread. This is called staging. A doctor needs to know the stage of the disease to plan treatment. The following stages are used for pheochromocytoma:

Localized benign pheochromocytoma: Tumor is found in only one area and has not spread to other tissues. Most pheochromocytomas do not spread to other parts of the body and are not cancer.

Regional pheochromocytoma: Cancer has spread to lymph nodes in the area or to other tissues around the original cancer. (Lymph nodes are small bean-shaped structures that are found throughout the body. They produce and store infection-fighting cells.)

Metastatic pheochromocytoma: The cancer has spread to other parts of the body.

Recurrent pheochromocytoma: Recurrent disease means that the cancer has come back (recurred) after it has been treated. It may come back in the area where it started or in another part of the body.

Treatment Option Overview

Surgery is the most common treatment of pheochromocytoma. A doctor may remove one or both adrenal glands in an operation called adrenalectomy. The doctor will look inside the abdomen to make sure all the cancer is removed. If the cancer has spread, lymph nodes or other tissues may also be taken out.

Chemotherapy uses drugs to kill cancer cells. Chemotherapy may be taken by pill, or it may be put into the body by a needle in the vein or muscle. Chemotherapy is called a systemic treatment because the drug enters the bloodstream, travels through the body, and can kill cancer cells throughout the body.

Radiation therapy uses high-energy x-rays to kill cancer cells and shrink tumors. Radiation comes from a machine outside the body (external radiation therapy).

Treatment by Stage

Treatments for pheochromocytoma depends on the stage of the disease, and the patient's age and overall health.

Localized benign pheochromocytoma: Treatment will probably be surgery to remove one or both adrenal glands (adrenalectomy). After surgery the doctor will order blood and urine tests to make sure hormone levels return to normal.

Regional pheochromocytoma: Treatment may be one of the following:

- Surgery to remove one or both adrenal glands (adrenalectomy) and as much of the cancer as possible. If cancer remains after surgery, drugs will be given to control high blood pressure.
- External radiation therapy to relieve symptoms (in rare cases)
- Chemotherapy

Metastatic pheochromocytoma: Treatment may be one of the following:

- Surgery to remove as much of the cancer as possible. If cancer remains after surgery, drugs will be given to control high blood pressure.
- External radiation therapy to relieve symptoms
- Chemotherapy

Recurrent pheochromocytoma: Treatment may be one of the following:

- Surgery to remove as much of the cancer as possible. If cancer remains after surgery, drugs will be given to control high blood pressure.
- External radiation therapy to relieve symptoms
- Chemotherapy

Section 65.2

Adrenocortical Carcinoma

PDQ® Cancer Information Summary. National Cancer Institute;
Bethesda, MD. Adrenocortical Carcinoma (PDQ®): Treatment - Patient.
Updated 07/2005. Available at: http://cancer.gov. Accessed May 11, 2006.

Cancer of the Adrenal Cortex

Cancer of the adrenal cortex, a rare cancer, is a disease in which cancer (malignant) cells are found in the adrenal cortex, which is the outside layer of the adrenal gland. Cancer of the adrenal cortex is also called adrenocortical carcinoma. There are two adrenal glands, one above each kidney in the back of the upper abdomen. The adrenal glands are also called the suprarenal glands. The inside layer of the adrenal gland is called the adrenal medulla. Cancer that starts in the adrenal medulla is called pheochromocytoma.

The cells in the adrenal cortex make important hormones that help the body work properly. When cells in the adrenal cortex become cancerous, they may make too much of one or more hormones, which can cause symptoms such as high blood pressure, weakening of the bones, or diabetes. If male or female hormones are affected, the body may go through changes such as a deepening of the voice, growing hair on the face, swelling of the sex organs, or swelling of the breasts. Cancers that make hormones are called functioning tumors. Many cancers of the adrenal cortex do not make extra hormones and are called nonfunctioning tumors.

A doctor should be seen if the following symptoms appear and won't go away:

- pain in the abdomen

- loss of weight without dieting

- weakness

If there is a functioning tumor, there may be symptoms or signs caused by too many hormones.

If there are symptoms, a doctor will order blood and urine tests to see whether the amounts of hormones in the body are normal. A doctor may also order a computed tomography scan of the abdomen, a special x-ray that uses a computer to make a picture of the inside of the abdomen. Other special x-rays may also be done to tell what kind of tumor is present.

The chance of recovery (prognosis) depends on how far the cancer has spread (stage) and on whether a doctor was able to surgically remove all of the cancer.

Stage Explanation

Once cancer of the adrenal cortex has been found, more tests will be done to see how far the cancer has spread. This is called staging. A doctor needs to know the stage of the cancer to plan treatment. The following stages are used for cancer of the adrenal cortex:

Stage I: The cancer is less than 5 centimeters (less than 2 inches) and has not spread into tissues around the adrenal gland.

Stage II: The cancer is more than 5 centimeters (greater than 2 inches) and has not spread into tissues around the adrenal gland.

Stage III: The cancer has spread into tissues around the adrenal gland or has spread to the lymph nodes around the adrenal gland. Lymph nodes are part of the lymph system and are small, bean shaped organs that make and store infection-fighting cells.

Stage IV: The cancer has spread to tissues or organs in the area and to lymph nodes around the adrenal cortex, or the cancer has spread to other parts of the body.

Recurrent: The cancer has come back (recurred) after it has been treated. It may come back in the adrenal cortex or in another part of the body.

Treatment Option Overview

A doctor may take out the adrenal gland in an operation called an adrenalectomy. Tissues around the adrenal glands that contain cancer may be removed. Lymph nodes in the area may also be removed (lymph node dissection).

Chemotherapy uses drugs to kill cancer cells. Chemotherapy may be taken by pill, or it may be put into the body by a needle in a vein or muscle. Chemotherapy is called a systemic treatment because the drug enters the bloodstream, travels through the body, and kills cancer cells throughout the body.

Radiation therapy uses high-energy x-rays to kill cancer cells and shrink tumors. Radiation for cancer of the adrenal cortex usually comes from a machine outside the body (external radiation therapy).

Besides treatment for cancer (chemotherapy, radiation therapy, or surgery), a patient may also receive therapy to prevent or treat symptoms caused by the extra hormones that are made by the cancer.

Treatment by Stage

Treatment depends on how far the cancer has spread, and a patient's age and overall health.

Standard treatment may be considered because of its effectiveness in past studies, or participation in a clinical trial may be considered. Not all patients are cured with standard therapy, and some standard treatments may have more side effects than are desired. For these reasons, clinical trials are designed to find better ways to treat cancer patients and are based on the most up-to-date information. Clinical trials are ongoing in some parts of the country for patients with cancer of the adrenal cortex.

Stage I adrenocortical carcinoma: Treatment will probably be surgery to remove the cancer.

Stage II adrenocortical carcinoma: Treatment will probably be surgery to remove the cancer. Clinical trials are testing new treatments.

Stage III adrenocortical carcinoma: Treatment may be one of the following:

- Surgery to remove the cancer. Lymph nodes in the area may also be removed (lymph node dissection)

- A clinical trial of radiation therapy

- A clinical trial of chemotherapy if the size of the tumor can be measured with x-rays or if the tumor is making hormones

Stage IV adrenocortical carcinoma: Treatment may be one of the following:

- Chemotherapy. Clinical trials are testing new drugs.

- Radiation therapy to bones where the cancer has spread

- Surgery to remove the cancer in places where it has spread

Recurrent adrenocortical carcinoma: Treatment depends on many factors, including where the cancer came back and what treatment has already been received. In some cases, surgery can be effective in decreasing the symptoms of the disease by removing some of the tumor. Clinical trials are testing new treatments.

Chapter 66

Thyroid Cancer

Chapter Contents

Section 66.1

Thyroid Nodules

What is a thyroid nodule?

The term thyroid nodule refers to any abnormal growth of thyroid
cells into a lump within the thyroid. Although the vast majority of
thyroid nodules are benign (noncancerous), a small proportion of thyroid nodules do contain thyroid cancer. Because of this possibility, the
evaluation of a thyroid nodule is aimed at discovering a potential thyroid cancer.

What are the symptoms of a thyroid nodule?

Most thyroid nodules do not cause any symptoms. Your doctor usually discovers them during a routine physical examination, or you
might notice a lump in your neck while looking in a mirror. If the
nodule is made up of thyroid cells that actively produce thyroid hormone without regard to the body's need, a patient may complain of
hyperthyroid symptoms. A few patients with thyroid nodules may
complain of pain in the neck, jaw, or ear. If the nodule is large enough,
it may cause difficulty swallowing or cause a "tickle in the throat" or
shortness of breath if it is pressing on the windpipe. Rarely, hoarseness can be caused if the nodule irritates a nerve to the voice box.

What causes a thyroid nodule?

The thyroid nodule is the most common endocrine problem in the
United States. The chances are 1 in 10 that you or someone you know
will develop a thyroid nodule. Although thyroid cancer is the most
important cause of the thyroid nodule, fortunately it occurs in less
than 10% of nodules. This means that about 9 of 10 nodules are benign (noncancerous). The most common types of noncancerous thyroid nodules are known as colloid nodules and follicular neoplasms.

If a nodule produces thyroid hormone without regard to the body's need, it is called an autonomous nodule, and it can occasionally lead to hyperthyroidism. If the nodule is filled with fluid or blood, it is called a thyroid cyst.

We do not know what causes most noncancerous thyroid nodules to form. A patient with hypothyroidism may also have a thyroid nodule, particularly if the cause is the inflammation known as Hashimoto thyroiditis. Sometimes a lack of iodine in the diet can cause a thyroid gland to produce nodules. Some autonomous nodules have a genetic defect that causes them to grow.

How is the thyroid nodule diagnosed?

Since most patients with thyroid nodules do not have symptoms, most nodules are discovered during an examination of the neck for another reason, such as during a routine physical examination or when you are sick with a cold or flu. Once the nodule is discovered, your doctor will try to determine whether the lump is the only problem with your thyroid or whether the entire thyroid gland has been affected by a more general condition such as hyperthyroidism or hypothyroidism. Your physician will feel the thyroid to see whether the entire gland is enlarged, whether there is a single nodule present, or whether there are many lumps or nodules in your thyroid. The initial laboratory tests may include blood tests to measure the amount of thyroid hormone (thyroxine, or T4) and thyroid-stimulating hormone (TSH) in your blood to determine whether your thyroid is functioning normally. Most patients with thyroid nodules will also have normal thyroid function tests.

Rarely is it possible to determine whether a thyroid nodule is cancerous by physical examination and blood tests alone, and so the evaluation of the thyroid nodule often includes specialized tests such as a thyroid fine needle biopsy, a thyroid scan, and/or a thyroid ultrasound.

Thyroid fine needle biopsy: A fine needle biopsy of a thyroid nodule may sound frightening, but the needle used is very small and a local anesthetic can be used. This simple procedure is done in the doctor's office. It does not require any special preparation (no fasting), and patients usually return home or to work after the biopsy without any ill effects. For a fine needle biopsy, your doctor will use a very thin needle to withdraw cells from the thyroid nodule. Ordinarily, several samples will be taken from different parts of the nodule to give your doctor the best chance of finding cancerous cells if a tumor is present. The cells are then examined under a microscope by a pathologist.

The report of a thyroid fine needle biopsy will usually indicate one of the following findings:

1. **The nodule is benign (noncancerous):** This result is obtained in 50% to 60% of biopsies and often indicates a colloid nodule. The risk of overlooking a cancer when the biopsy is benign is generally under 3 in 100 and is even lower when the biopsy is reviewed by an experienced pathologist at a major medical center. Generally, these nodules need not be removed, but another biopsy may be required in the future, especially if they get bigger.

2. **The nodule is malignant (cancerous):** This result is obtained in about 5% of biopsies and often indicates papillary cancer, one of the most common thyroid cancers. All of these nodules should be removed surgically, preferably by an experienced thyroid surgeon.

3. **The nodule is suspicious:** This result is obtained in about 10% of biopsies and indicates either a follicular adenoma (noncancerous) or a follicular cancer. Often, your doctor may want to obtain a thyroid scan to determine which nodules should be removed surgically.

4. **The biopsy is nondiagnostic or inadequate:** This result is obtained in up to 20% of biopsies and indicates that not enough cells were obtained to make a diagnosis. This is a common result if the nodule is a cyst. These nodules may be removed surgically or be re-evaluated with second fine needle biopsy, depending on the clinical judgment of your doctor.

Thyroid scan: The thyroid scan uses a small amount of a radioactive substance, usually radioactive iodine, to obtain a picture of the thyroid gland. Because thyroid cancer cells do not take up radioactive iodine as easily as normal thyroid cells do, this test is used to determine the likelihood that a thyroid nodule contains a cancer. If done as the first test, the thyroid scan is used to determine those patients who most need a biopsy. The scan usually gives the following results.

1. **The nodule is cold:** In other words, the nodule is not taking up radioactive iodine normally. This patient is referred for a fine needle biopsy of the nodule.

2. **The nodule is functioning:** Its uptake of radioactive iodine is similar to that of normal cells. A biopsy is not needed right away since the likelihood of cancer is very low.

3. **The nodule is hot:** Its uptake of radioactive iodine is greater than that of normal cells. The likelihood of cancer is extremely rare, and so biopsy is usually not necessary.

If the fine needle biopsy was done as the first test, then a scan is usually ordered to evaluate a suspicious biopsy result. In this case, patients with a "cold" nodule result should have their nodule removed. Patients with "functioning" or "hot" nodules on a scan and a suspicious biopsy can be watched, and surgery is not immediately necessary.

Thyroid ultrasound: The thyroid ultrasound uses high-frequency sound waves to obtain a picture of the thyroid. This very sensitive test can easily determine if a nodule is solid or cystic, and it can determine the precise size of the nodule. The thyroid ultrasound can be used to keep an eye on thyroid nodules that are not removed by surgery to determine if they are growing or shrinking. Some ultrasound characteristics of a nodule are more frequent in thyroid cancer than in noncancerous nodules. Even so, the thyroid ultrasound alone is rarely able to determine if a nodule is a thyroid cancer. The thyroid ultrasound also can be used to assist the placement of the needle within the nodule during a fine needle biopsy, especially if the nodule is hard to feel. Finally, the thyroid ultrasound can identify nodules that are very small and cannot be felt during a physical examination. The clinical importance of these very small nodules is uncertain; however, the ultrasound provides a means by which an accurate fine needle biopsy can be performed if your doctor thinks a biopsy is needed.

How are thyroid nodules treated?

All thyroid nodules that are found to contain a thyroid cancer, or that are highly suspicious of containing a cancer, should be removed surgically by an experienced thyroid surgeon. Most thyroid cancers are curable and rarely cause life-threatening problems. Any thyroid nodule not removed needs to be watched closely, with an examination of the nodule every 6 to 12 months. This follow-up may involve a physical examination by a doctor or a thyroid ultrasound or both. Occasionally, your doctor may want to try to shrink your nodule by treating you with thyroid hormone at doses slightly higher that your body needs (called suppression therapy). Whether you are on thyroid hormone suppression therapy or not, a repeat fine needle biopsy may be indicated if the nodule gets bigger. Also, even if the biopsy is benign, surgery may be recommended for removal of a nodule that is getting bigger.

Section 66.2

Papillary and Follicular Cancer of the Thyroid

The diagnosis of cancer is terrifying for most patients because it has become associated in our minds with pain and death. But, in fact, the outlook for patients with thyroid cancer is usually excellent because: 1) most thyroid cancer is easily curable with surgery, 2) it causes little pain or disability, and 3) novel and effective means of diagnosis and therapy are available for several kinds of thyroid cancer.

Thyroid cancer usually presents itself as a lump or nodule in the thyroid gland. However, it should be emphasized that most thyroid nodules (95% or more) are benign. Unfortunately, it may be difficult to distinguish a benign from a malignant nodule on the basis of history and physical examination, even with the help of laboratory tests including blood hormone levels and scans (images) of the thyroid gland. Therefore, biopsy of thyroid nodules (generally fine needle aspiration, FNA) provides the most valuable information in helping a physician to determine whether a surgical operation is necessary.

Occasionally, a thyroid cancer can present as a swollen lymph node in the neck, as hoarseness due to pressure from the tumor on the nerve to the voice box (recurrent laryngeal nerve), or as difficulty in swallowing or breathing due to a tumor obstructing the esophagus or windpipe. Rarely it presents as disease which has spread to another part of the body (metastatic disease).

What is well-differentiated thyroid cancer?

A cancer is a malignant tumor which grows in the body. A well-differentiated cancer is one which superficially looks like the normal parent tissue, in this case the thyroid gland. There are two types of well-differentiated thyroid cancer, papillary and follicular, both derived from the normal thyroid cell, the follicular cell.

Well-differentiated thyroid cancers account for about 90% of all thyroid malignancies and most are associated with an excellent outlook. Although we do not know exactly what causes these well-differentiated cancers to grow, we do know that they are more likely to develop in patients who have received x-ray treatments in childhood for enlarged tonsils, enlarged thymus glands, acne, and occasionally for other malignancies such as Hodgkin disease. An important epidemic of papillary carcinoma developed in the region surrounding Chernobyl after the nuclear power plant melt-down. Routine diagnostic x-rays (like chest x-rays, dental x-rays, or thyroid scans) do not cause such thyroid cancer.

What is papillary thyroid cancer?

A papilla is a nipple-like projection. Papillary cancers have multiple projections giving them a fern or frond-like appearance under the microscope. In addition the nuclei (central portion of the cells) are changed compared to normal thyroid cell nuclei. Tiny, microscopic areas of papillary cancer can be found in up to 10% of "normal" thyroid glands, when thyroid tissue is carefully examined with a microscope. The more carefully a pathologist looks for these tiny cancers, the more commonly they are found. These microscopic cancers seem to have no clinical importance and are more a curiosity than a disease. In other words, there does not seem to be a tendency for these small cancer-like growths to enlarge and become more serious malignant tumors.

On the other hand, when papillary cancer grows large enough to form a lump in the thyroid gland, we consider it clinically important, for it is likely to continue to enlarge and may spread elsewhere in the body. Papillary tumors make up about 70% to 80% of all thyroid cancers, and can occur at any age. There are only about 12,000 new cases of papillary cancer in the United States each year, but because these patients have such a long life expectancy, the Thyroid Foundation of America (TFA) estimates that one in a thousand people have or have had this form of cancer.

709

Papillary cancer tends to grow slowly and to spread by means of the lymphatic system to lymph glands in the neck. In fact, in about one third of the patients who undergo surgery for papillary cancer, the tumor has already spread to surrounding lymph glands (lymph node metastases). Fortunately, the generally excellent outlook is usually not altered by lymph gland metastases. Some clinicians believe that the presence of abnormal lymph nodes on both sides of the neck or abnormal lymph nodes in the chest area does worsen the prognosis.

The outlook or prognosis for patients with papillary thyroid carcinoma is determined by several features at the time of diagnosis. Many different staging systems have been used, without consensus among experts. Based on the Mayo Clinic system, the most favorable characteristic is a primary tumor confined to the thyroid itself (intrathyroidal). As noted above, the presence or absence of lymph gland involvement usually does not affect the prognosis. The 85% of patients with intrathyroidal papillary carcinoma have a 25 year mortality rate of 1%. This means that only 1 out of every 100 such patients will be dead of thyroid cancer 25 years later.

Since the outlook in patients with intrathyroidal primary tumors is so favorable, it is important that therapy not be more hazardous than the disease. Radical surgery is rarely indicated for this mild type of papillary cancer. Ten percent or more of patients with intrathyroidal papillary cancer will have a subsequent recurrence. Fortunately recurrences generally occur as enlarged lymph glands in the neck and are not life-threatening. Such recurrences are usually removed surgically.

The prognosis is not as good in patients where the cancer has grown through the thyroid into surrounding tissues (extrathyroidal). Specifically, this means spread through the fibrous capsule that surrounds the thyroid gland into the tissues of the neck. Lymph node involvement is not considered extrathyroidal spread. In a very small percentage of patients (about 5%), the cancer eventually spreads through the blood stream to distant sites, particularly the lungs and bones. These distant tumor sites (metastases) can often be treated with radioactive iodine but they are difficult to cure.

Young patients who have papillary thyroid cancer generally have an excellent prognosis (outlook). However, patients under the age of 20 have a higher risk of spread to the lungs and of local recurrence. The prognosis is also not as good in those older than age 50 and those with larger tumors (particularly greater than 3.5 to 4 cm. or 1.5 inches in diameter).

What is follicular thyroid cancer?

The normal thyroid gland is made up of sphere-shaped structures called follicles, which are lined by thyroid follicular cells. When a thyroid cancer resembles these normal structures, the cancer is called a follicular cancer. Follicular cancer makes up about 10% of all thyroid cancers in the United States, and tends to occur in somewhat older patients than papillary carcinoma.

Although follicular cancer of the thyroid is generally considered to be more aggressive than papillary cancer, this is not always true. Approximately one third of these patients have a minimally invasive follicular thyroid carcinoma. Since the follicular cells look just like normal thyroid cells, the diagnosis of cancer depends on finding these cells where they do not belong. Follicular carcinoma is considered minimally invasive when the cells grow through the lining (capsule) of the nodule or at most into a few blood vessels. The outcome is excellent in minimally invasive follicular carcinoma, particularly those diagnosed with capsular invasion alone. On the other hand, when the follicular cancer extensively invades blood vessels, the prognosis is worse and spread to distant sites including the lungs and bones is common. In general, the prognosis is better in younger patients than in those over 50 years of age.

What is the treatment of well-differentiated thyroid cancer?

The primary therapy for well differentiated thyroid cancer is surgical removal of the tumor, which also allows preliminary staging of the disease. When a skilled thyroid surgeon is available, a bilateral near total removal of the thyroid (thyroidectomy) should be performed for most patients with known papillary or follicular carcinoma. However, there are many patients, previously treated with removal of half of the thyroid gland (hemithyroidectomy) who continue to thrive without disease recurrence. A particular dilemma occurs when the diagnosis of a minimally invasive follicular carcinoma is made after final pathology review, usually days after surgery is completed. Preliminary pathological analysis (frozen section) generally cannot distinguish benign from malignant follicular tumors at the time of surgery. Therefore removal of only half of the thyroid is generally performed. When the final diagnosis is minimally invasive follicular carcinoma options include: additional surgery to remove the remaining half of the thyroid gland (completion thyroidectomy), radioactive iodine destruction (ablation) of the remaining half of the thyroid) or thyroid hormone therapy alone, if the diagnosis is made by capsular invasion alone. The advantages of each approach are still debated.

When thyroid cancer extensively invades local neck structures, aggressive surgery, including removal of part of the trachea (air passageway) or esophagus (food passageway) should be considered. These patients require radioactive iodine therapy and often external beam radiation as well.

It may trouble some patients to realize that there are no absolute rules for the management of these cancers. Although the general characteristics of tumor behavior are understood, in any particular patient the choice of treatment is best made by physicians skilled in the management of patients with thyroid cancer.

What is radioiodine therapy?

Once papillary or follicular cancer has spread through the blood stream into the surrounding tissues or to distant sites (especially lungs and bones), the usual therapy is to administer a radioactive form of iodine (I-131) to try to destroy the tumor. To understand this treatment, it is important to know the relationship between iodine and the thyroid gland.

The thyroid gland normally concentrates iodine from the bloodstream, and this process is stimulated by TSH (thyroid stimulating hormone) from the pituitary gland. The iodine is subsequently used to produce thyroid hormone (thyroxine, T4). Thyroid cancers or metastases from thyroid cancer concentrate only tiny amounts of iodine (or radioactive iodine) under normal conditions. However, when stimulated by high concentrations of TSH, papillary and follicular carcinoma and their metastases may be stimulated to concentrate significant amounts of iodine. This permits the delivery of a large radiation dose directly to the cancer, without damage to surrounding tissues. However, when the normal thyroid gland is present and producing normal amounts of thyroid hormone, the production of TSH by the pituitary remains relatively low. But if the entire thyroid gland is removed or destroyed, and the level of thyroid hormone is allowed to fall, the pituitary gland will increase TSH secretion dramatically. In turn, this will stimulate the thyroid cancer to concentrate radioactive iodine. To prepare for radioactive iodine therapy, patients must be off their thyroid hormone. TFA generally changes patients from levothyroxine (Levothroid, Levoxyl, Synthroid, Unithroid and others) (T4) to Cytomel (T3) for four weeks and then discontinue the Cytomel for two weeks prior to administering the scanning dose of radioiodine. Patients are generally asked to adhere to a low iodine diet for several weeks prior to such therapy.

For radioactive iodine therapy to successfully treat metastatic thyroid cancer serum TSH must be elevated, which generally requires removal or destruction of the entire thyroid gland. Once that has been accomplished patients with residual tumor in the neck or known distant metastases are scanned after receiving a small amount (scanning dose) of radioactive iodine (I-131, 2-10 millicuries or I-123, 1-2 millicuries), assuming the serum TSH concentration is greater than 25 microU/ml.

Patients then receive a therapeutic dose of I-131, usually 150 millicuries or more in an attempt to destroy the tumor, provided a significant amount of iodine is concentrated in the areas of the cancer. A repeat scan is often performed after the therapeutic dose; post-therapy scans identify additional sites of disease in approximately ten percent of patients.

In most states, treatment with large doses of radioactive iodine requires a one to several day hospitalization, until the amount of radioactivity in the body falls to levels which will not be hazardous to other people. However, this treatment has proved to be safe and well-tolerated, and may be curative in patients with well-differentiated thyroid cancer even after the tumor has spread to the lungs. The treatment is generally well tolerated, however, nausea, vomiting and pain in the salivary glands may occur. Salivary gland damage after this treatment may leave patients with a dry mouth.

Because of the safety and effectiveness of radioactive iodine in patients with more aggressive thyroid cancer, many physicians also use it routinely in patients with less aggressive papillary and follicular cancers. In this situation, radioactive iodine is used to destroy tiny remnants of thyroid tissue still present after surgery. This may improve the prognosis and makes it easier to monitor patients for tumor recurrence using a blood test for thyroglobulin. Whether radioactive iodine ablation improves the survival or recurrence rates in patients with favorable papillary carcinoma of the thyroid gland is still debated.

When surgery and radioactive iodine cannot check the growth of well-differentiated thyroid cancer, external radiation therapy to local tumor sites is often helpful. TFA continues to search for specific therapies when the tumor has spread widely and continues to grow. Current chemotherapy is rarely effective in this situation. Because lung metastases are often asymptomatic for years, when radioiodine is no longer effective, cautious observation is often recommended.

How are thyroid cancer patients followed?

Periodic follow-up examinations are essential for patients who have had surgery for papillary or follicular thyroid cancer, because recurrences sometimes occur many years after apparently successful surgery. These follow-up visits should include a careful history and physical examination with particular attention to the neck area.

Periodic measurement of the blood level of the protein thyroglobulin is also important.

This substance is produced and released by normal thyroid cells and also by well-differentiated thyroid cancer cells. The blood level of thyroglobulin is very low after total thyroid gland removal, and in most patients who are taking thyroid hormone after thyroid surgery. An elevated or rising level of thyroglobulin is a "tumor marker" which generally implies persistent or growing thyroid cancer, but does not necessarily imply a poor prognosis. A high thyroglobulin level found in a follow-up examination alerts the physician to the possibility that other tests may be needed to be sure the tumor is not recurring. Approximately 20 to 30% of thyroid cancer patients have interfering antibodies in their blood which prevent accurate thyroglobulin measurement. Thyroglobulin production is stimulated by TSH; the blood thyroglobulin concentration rises when TSH increases. Therefore a low serum thyroglobulin at the time of an elevated TSH is particularly reassuring.

How often should imaging and scanning be done?

Many different protocols have been suggested to follow patients with well-differentiated thyroid cancer. Generally the testing is modified based on the tumor stage. Patients with favorable papillary carcinomas with undetectable serum thyroglobulin concentrations need the fewest imaging tests. After radioactive iodine ablation of residual thyroid tissue, many endocrinologists and patients want the reassurance of a subsequent negative scan. Fortunately, a new method of radioiodine scanning is available for select patients, which does not require withdrawal of thyroid hormone. Patients receive injections of human TSH (made by genetic engineering) known as Thyrogen (recombinant human TSH, rhTSH) to raise their TSH concentrations. Radioiodine scanning and thyroglobulin measurements are performed. A negative post-Thyrogen scan and a serum thyroglobulin concentration less than 2 ng/ml after Thyrogen injections is very reassuring. Generally this scanning approach is restricted to patients who are expected to have a negative scan and who have a low serum thyroglobulin while on thyroid hormone therapy. In exceptional circumstances, radioactive iodine therapy can be performed after Thyrogen injections rather than after withdrawal of thyroid hormone.

Patients with persistent cancer need periodic rescanning and treatment with radioactive iodine. Currently, this is best done after withdrawing thyroid hormone. In some patients the radioiodine scan is negative but serum thyroglobulin is still high. Several approaches have been suggested. Generally doctors start with a thyroid ultrasound. If abnormal tissue or lymph nodes are found, additional surgery is generally indicated, sometimes after an ultrasound guided biopsy. If the ultrasound is negative, administration of larger doses of radioiodine with subsequent scanning may help localize the sites of disease. If these tests are negative, other scans and x-rays are necessary to localize the disease sites. These may include but are not limited to PET scanning, chest x-ray, CT or MRI, head CT or MRI, bone survey, CT or MRI of the spine, sestamibi, thallium or octreotide scanning. Whether serial neck ultrasounds should be performed in all patients with well-differentiated thyroid carcinoma is an unanswered question. However, TFA recommends ultrasounds in all patients with a history of locally invasive papillary thyroid carcinoma and in those with positive thyroglobulin antibodies where that tumor marker cannot be followed. You should feel comfortable asking the physician who is treating your tumor to discuss his or her choice of tests and treatments for your situation.

What about thyroid hormone treatment?

If the thyroid gland has been mostly or completely removed, thyroid hormone must be taken for the body to remain normal (euthyroid). Even if part of the thyroid remains, levothyroxine (Levothroid, Levoxyl, Synthroid, Unithroid and others) (T4) administration is an important therapy which lowers blood TSH concentration and seems to prevent tumor recurrence. Thyroid hormone should be administered in sufficient quantities to suppress TSH levels to subnormal values, except when medically contraindicated. Sensitive TSH measurements are necessary for monitoring TSH concentrations to confirm that the serum TSH is below normal or at the lower limits of normal in patients at low risk of cancer recurrence. Patients with more aggressive forms of papillary or follicular cancer should take larger doses of thyroxine in order to suppress TSH to undetectable levels.

715

Section 66.3

Anaplastic and Medullary Cancer of the Thyroid

Anaplastic or undifferentiated thyroid carcinoma makes up about 7% of all thyroid cancer. This tumor occurs in older patients, usually over sixty years of age. The tumor often originates in benign or low grade malignant tumors of the thyroid, even though the actual percentage of benign and low grade malignant tumors that progress to anaplastic carcinoma is extremely low. The change from a relatively slow growing to a rapidly growing tumor is usually caused by a mutation or change in a tumor suppressor gene known as p53. When present in its usual form, the p53 gene helps the body destroy newly formed abnormal tumor cells by inducing the cells to "commit suicide." When p53 is abnormal, tumor growth may proceed unchecked.

Anaplastic carcinoma usually starts as a rapidly enlarging lump in the neck, and is likely to cause local symptoms such as hoarseness, difficulty breathing or swallowing, or blockage of the large veins in the neck and chest. In contrast with papillary carcinoma, which is one of the slowest growing tumors in the body, anaplastic carcinoma is one of the most rapidly growing cancers. The diagnosis is usually suspected from the clinical situation and confirmed with a fine needle aspiration biopsy (FNA) or open biopsy. The role of surgery is controversial. TFA recommends radiation and chemotherapy, sometimes followed by surgery if the disease has not spread to distant sites. Others recommend surgery followed by radiation or chemotherapy. It is best to have a consultation with a medical oncologist (cancer specialist) to help plan therapy. The prognosis is generally but not invariably poor, as the tumor quickly spreads to distant sites.

Therapy and Follow-up

Surgery is the mainstay of therapy for medullary thyroid carcinoma. A bilateral near total thyroidectomy with dissection (removal) of surrounding lymph glands is mandatory. Because this tumor often starts on both sides of the thyroid gland, removal of only half of the thyroid is not recommended. Remember, when medullary thyroid cancer (MTC) is known or suspected, a pheochromocytoma should be excluded before surgery is performed to avoid sudden increases in blood pressure during the operation. The persistence of high serum calcitonin values after apparently successful surgery suggests that tumor is still present, but does not necessarily imply a poor prognosis. Obviously, a low or undetectable calcitonin value is a more favorable indicator.

Two additional tests may be helpful assessing the prognosis. Carcinoembryonic antigen (CEA) is a protein which is produced by many cancers including MTC. When postoperative CEA concentrations are very high, the prognosis is worse. Some institutions examine the DNA (genetic material) or calcitonin content of cells in the pathological specimen. The more abnormal the DNA content or the less calcitonin present, the worse the prognosis.

When calcitonin does not return to normal after surgery, residual tumor or metastatic tumor must be sought. A neck ultrasound is often helpful in localizing small abnormal lymph nodes which may harbor MTC. Some clinicians recommend extensive neck dissection to remove all possible abnormal nodes in the neck even when localization testing is negative. This lengthy operation may lower calcitonin to normal in a minority of patients. The ability to scan the body for residual MTC with the radioactively labeled chemical pentreotide is a major advance. However, in the TFA's experience when calcitonin values are only moderately elevated (< 1000 pg/ml) this scan is usually negative. In some patients, scanning with radioactively labeled anti-CEA antibodies or with PET scanning helps localize distant disease. When disease activity is not discovered, other tests including CT or MRI of the chest, abdomen and head, and a bone survey may be indicated. Whenever possible, surgery should be performed when new areas of MTC are discovered.

External radiation is recommended when the surgeon is unable to remove all the tumor in the neck and when painful bony metastases are present. The role of external radiation to the neck in selected patients with persistent calcitonin elevation is unresolved. Newer chemotherapy regimens are effective in a minority of patients. Aggressive radiotherapy using high dose radioisotope labeled anti-CEA antibodies may be effective but often requires bone marrow transplantation.

The ability to follow MTC by measuring the tumor marker calcitonin is both a boon and a curse. Persistent calcitonin elevations are often frustrating and frightening for patients. The calcitonin elevation suggests the presence of persistent tumor, but often the residual tumor cannot be located, or, if located, cannot be eradicated with our currently available therapies. It is extremely important to realize that calcitonin is a tumor marker (indicator), not a lethal substance. Some patients can lead perfectly normal lives for decades with markedly elevated calcitonin concentrations. In some patients with metastatic disease calcitonin and tumor mass change slowly or not at all. Unfortunately medullary carcinoma advances rapidly in some patients.

Medullary Thyroid Carcinoma

Medullary thyroid carcinoma (MTC) is relatively rare (about 3–5% of all thyroid cancer) and has several unique characteristics. Unlike other types of thyroid cancer, medullary carcinoma originates in the parafollicular cells of the thyroid gland. Parafollicular cells are not involved in making thyroid hormone. They are also known as C cells, because they produce calcitonin, a hormone which has poorly characterized effects on the skeleton. Almost all medullary cancers produce calcitonin. Thus, the presence of medullary carcinoma can be suspected on the basis of an elevated blood calcitonin level. The skill which a well-trained physician has is knowing to check a calcitonin blood level in a particular patient. Calcitonin is not routinely measured, even in patients with thyroid nodules, since the yield of such measurements is quite low. However the role of calcitonin measurements in patients with thyroid nodules is still debated.

Medullary carcinoma usually presents as a thyroid nodule or mass in the neck. Fine needle aspiration (FNA) biopsy may be difficult to interpret, but when the diagnosis of medullary thyroid carcinoma is considered, staining the biopsy material for calcitonin or measuring serum calcitonin is generally diagnostic. MTC is often misdiagnosed when a frozen section (preliminary pathological diagnosis) is analyzed at the time of surgery for a thyroid nodule. It is occasionally misdiagnosed as a very aggressive undifferentiated cancer and is sometimes confused with a typical follicular thyroid cancer. Positive tissue staining for calcitonin is diagnostic.

About twenty percent of patients with MTC have an inherited form of the disease. This means that once a patient is diagnosed as having MTC, it is essential that members of the patient's family be screened for MTC. All patients with thyroid nodules should be questioned about family members with thyroid cancer, particularly MTC.

The presence of MTC in both lobes of the thyroid gland may be an important clue pointing to the familial form of the disease. Although the cancer may appear to be confined to one lobe of the thyroid gland, it is important for the pathologist to examine the other lobe for increased numbers of C cells to be sure that the tumor is not present there as well.

There are three different types of hereditary MTC, two of which are associated with other endocrine gland tumors. The first kind is a condition called multiple endocrine neoplasia (or MEN) II a. Characteristics of MEN II a include: MTC, usually bilateral, pheochromocytomas (tumors of the adrenal gland which produce adrenaline and cause high blood pressure), and hyperparathyroidism (overactivity or tumors of the parathyroid glands which cause elevated serum calcium). Although MEN II a is relatively rare, its recognition is extremely important because it can be dangerous or even lethal to perform thyroid surgery when an unsuspected pheochromocytoma is present. When MTC is diagnosed on FNA, a twenty four hour urine collection for adrenaline and its metabolites or an appropriate blood test should be analyzed before surgery.

A rarer form of hereditary MTC is called multiple endocrine neoplasia II b (MEN II b) and includes MTC, pheochromocytomas, and a peculiar body shape, with long, thin legs, as well as multiple neuromas or nerve tumors on the lips, tongue, eyes, and in the intestinal tract.

The third variety of hereditary MTC is called familial MTC without other associated tumors. It is likely much more common than we realized.

All three of these diseases or syndromes are inherited in a dominant fashion. This means that on average, half of the children of a patient with this disease will also develop the disease.

Family screening is very important in patients with MTC. A major advance in this area occurred when the genetic basis was discovered for most patients with hereditary MTC. Mutations (changes) in a gene called RET have been identified in almost all patients with MEN II a and MEN II b and in about 85% of patients with familial MTC. It is likely that unrecognized mutations in this gene cause the disease in the remaining patients. Analysis of RET mutations is now available through several commercial laboratories. When a patient is found to have MTC, a RET analysis should be performed by analyzing the genetic material in blood cells after a simple bloodletting. If a RET mutation is found, all first degree relatives (parents, siblings, and children) should be screened by looking for the same mutation. When that RET mutation is discovered in a family member, surgery is generally recommended even when the thyroid gland appears normal. MTC or its precursor called C-cell hyperplasia will be found in 96% of patients who undergo preventative removal of the thyroid gland. Although the absence of a RET mutation in a patient with MTC is reassuring, a familial form of the disease is not completely excluded. In that situation the first degree blood relatives should have their calcitonin blood level tested. An elevated calcitonin level generally means that MTC or a premalignant precursor (C-cell hyperplasia) exists. When a member of a known hereditary but RET negative MTC family has a normal baseline calcitonin, further tests should be done to stimulate the release of calcitonin. While the calcitonin level of normal individuals will rise slightly after an intravenous injection of calcium or a chemical called pentagastrin, the calcitonin level of patients harboring MTC or C-cell hyperplasia will rise much higher. Pentagastrin is currently unavailable. Most patients with familial forms of MTC will have abnormal calcitonin blood measurements by age 35.

Most patients with MTC are diagnosed because: 1) a lump in the neck is discovered, or 2) as a result of a family screening program. Rarely, MTC can cause symptoms due to production of a variety of chemicals. Such patients may develop severe diarrhea or symptoms of excess cortisone production. Remarkably, many individuals with distant spread of MTC have no symptoms at all.

The prognosis of MTC is extremely variable. In many patients, the tumor behaves in a very indolent manner, while in others, the tumor is much more aggressive. The prognosis is usually excellent in patients with familial medullary carcinoma without other tumors and in MEN II a. The outlook is generally not as good in patients with MEN II b, while that for non-familial MTC falls somewhere in between.

The initial tumor stage influences the course of the disease. If the primary tumor is confined to the thyroid gland (intrathyroidal) the prognosis is usually excellent. When lymph nodes are positive the prognosis is not quite as good. When the tumor has grown through the wall of the thyroid into surrounding tissues (extrathyroidal), or spread through the blood to distant sites, the outlook is guarded.

Thyroid Lymphoma

A lymphoma is a cancer of the lymph glands or white blood cells called lymphocytes. Some lymphomas originate in the thyroid gland rather than in a lymph gland. Although thyroid lymphoma makes up only about 4% of all thyroid cancers, it has been increasing in frequency in recent decades. Most patients are middle-aged or older, but the disease can afflict younger people as well. The majority of patients with thyroid lymphoma have an underlying inflammation in the thyroid gland called Hashimoto thyroiditis. In Hashimoto thyroiditis the thyroid gland is filled with lymphocytes and the lymphoma presumably originates in those cells. It is worth emphasizing that while Hashimoto thyroiditis is very common, thyroid lymphoma is rare. The risk of a patient with Hashimoto developing a lymphoma is extremely low.

Thyroid lymphoma commonly presents as a rapidly enlarging neck mass. Hoarseness, difficulty swallowing, difficulty breathing and fever may be present. Lymphoma should be suspected in patients with known Hashimoto thyroiditis who develop an enlarging mass or goiter. Fine needle aspiration may be diagnostic of lymphoma, but when the diagnosis is uncertain a core needle or open surgical biopsy may be necessary.

The prognosis of thyroid lymphoma depends upon whether it is confined to the thyroid or has spread to other areas. Tumor staging with various scans is recommended to evaluate its spread to other parts of the body. This is usually done under the guidance of a medical oncologist. Therapy consists of external radiation, chemotherapy, or most commonly a combination of the two. Although surgery is usually performed for diagnostic purposes only, some physicians still recommend surgical excision for lymphoma confined to the thyroid gland. The prognosis is variable but frequently quite favorable.

Chapter 67

Parathyroid Cancer

Parathyroid cancer, a very rare cancer, is a disease in which cancer (malignant) cells are found in the tissues of the parathyroid gland. The parathyroid gland is at the base of the neck, near the thyroid gland. The parathyroid gland makes a hormone called parathyroid hormone (PTH), or parathormone, which helps the body store and use calcium.

Problems with the parathyroid gland are common and are usually not caused by cancer. The parathyroid gland may become overactive and make too much PTH, a condition called hyperparathyroidism. This causes too much calcium to be found in the blood. The extra PTH also takes calcium from the bones, which causes pain in the bones, kidney problems, and other types of problems. There are other conditions that can cause the parathyroid gland to make too much PTH. It is important for a doctor to determine what is causing the extra PTH. Very rarely, hyperparathyroidism is caused by cancer of the parathyroid gland, and too much PTH will be produced by the tumor. A rare inherited disorder of the parathyroid called familial isolated hyperparathyroidism may increase the risk of developing parathyroid cancer. A rare inherited disorder of the endocrine glands called multiple endocrine neoplasia 1 has also been linked with an increased risk of developing parathyroid cancer.

PDQ® Cancer Information Summary. National Cancer Institute; Bethesda, MD. Parathyroid Cancer (PDQ®): Treatment - Patient. Updated 07/2005. Available at: http://cancer.gov. Accessed June 23, 2006.

A doctor should be seen if there are the following symptoms: bone pain, a lump in the neck, pain in the upper part of the back, weak muscles, difficulty speaking, or vomiting.

If there are symptoms, the doctor will conduct a physical examination and feel for lumps in the throat. The doctor may also order blood tests and other tests to check for cancer or other types of tumors that may not be cancer (benign tumors).

The chance of recovery (prognosis) depends on whether the cancer is just in the parathyroid gland or has spread to other parts of the body (stage) and the patient's general health.

Stages of Parathyroid Cancer

Once parathyroid cancer is found, more tests will be done to find out if cancer cells have spread to other parts of the body. This is called staging. A doctor needs to know the stage of the disease to plan treatment. The following stages are used for parathyroid cancer.

Localized: The cancer is in the parathyroid gland and may or may not have spread into nearby tissues.

Metastatic: The cancer has spread beyond nearby tissues to lymph nodes in the area or to other parts of the body, such as the lungs, liver, bone, membrane around the heart, and pancreas.

Recurrent: Recurrent disease means that the cancer has come back (recurred) after it has been treated. It may come back in the original place or in another part of the body.

Treatment Option Overview

There are treatments for all patients with parathyroid cancer. Medical treatment to lower high blood levels of calcium caused by the disease is very important for all patients. In addition, three kinds of treatment are used:

1. Surgery (taking out the cancer)

2. Radiation therapy (using high-dose x-rays or other high-energy rays to kill cancer cells)

3. Chemotherapy (using anticancer drugs)

Surgery is the most effective treatment for parathyroid cancer. A doctor may remove the parathyroid gland (parathyroidectomy) and the half of the thyroid on the same side as the cancer (ipsilateral thyroidectomy). Nearby muscles, tissues and nerves may also be removed to prevent the cancer from spreading.

Radiation therapy uses high-energy x-rays to kill cancer cells and shrink tumors. Radiation may come from a machine outside the body (external radiation therapy) or from putting materials that produce radiation (radioisotopes) through thin plastic tubes in the area where the cancer cells are found (internal radiation therapy).

Chemotherapy uses drugs to kill cancer cells. Chemotherapy may be taken by pill, or it may be put into the body by a needle in the vein or muscle. Chemotherapy is called a systemic treatment because the drug enters the bloodstream, travels through the body, and can kill cancer cells outside the parathyroid gland.

Treatment by Stage

Treatment for parathyroid cancer depends on the type and stage of the disease and the patient's age and overall health.

Localized parathyroid cancer: Treatment may be one of the following:

- Surgery to remove the parathyroid gland (parathyroidectomy), the half of the thyroid on the same side as the cancer (ipsilateral thyroidectomy), and possibly other tissues around the thyroid. Medical treatment before surgery for high blood calcium levels and other complications of hyperparathyroidism is very important.

- Surgery followed by radiation therapy

- Radiation therapy

Metastatic parathyroid cancer: Parathyroid cancer which has spread beyond nearby tissues to areas such as the lungs may appear soon after surgery, or as much as 20 years later. Because parathyroid cancer tends to be slow-growing, some patients live for many years even after the cancer has spread.

Treatment may be one of the following:

- Surgery to remove the cancer from the places where it has spread

- Medicine to reduce the amount of calcium in the blood

- Surgery followed by radiation therapy
- Radiation therapy
- Chemotherapy

Recurrent parathyroid cancer: In about half of patients who have surgery for parathyroid cancer, the disease recurs (comes back), usually within 2 to 5 years. Because parathyroid cancer tends to be slow-growing, repeated surgeries to remove cancer which has come back can lower the level of parathyroid hormone and extend survival.
Treatment may be one of the following:

- Surgery to remove the cancer which has come back in the area of the thyroid or in other parts of the body
- Medicine to reduce the amount of calcium in the blood
- Surgery followed by radiation therapy
- Radiation therapy
- Chemotherapy

Chapter 68

Melanoma

Chapter Contents

Section 68.1

Understanding Melanoma

Excerpted from "What You Need to Know about™ Melanoma,"
National Cancer Institute, March 2003.

Melanoma is the most serious type of cancer of the skin. Each year
in the United States, more than 53,600 people learn they have melanoma. In some parts of the world, especially among Western countries,
melanoma is becoming more common every year. In the United States,
for example, the percentage of people who develop melanoma has more
than doubled in the past 30 years.

What is melanoma?

Melanoma is a type of skin cancer. It begins in cells in the skin called
melanocytes. To understand melanoma, it is helpful to know about the
skin and about melanocytes—what they do, how they grow, and what
happens when they become cancerous.

The skin: The skin is the body's largest organ. It protects against
heat, sunlight, injury, and infection. It helps regulate body temperature, stores water and fat, and produces vitamin D.

The skin has two main layers: the outer epidermis and the inner
dermis. The epidermis is mostly made up of flat, scalelike cells called
squamous cells. Round cells called basal cells lie under the squamous
cells in the epidermis. The lower part of the epidermis also contains
melanocytes.

The dermis contains blood vessels, lymph vessels, hair follicles, and
glands. Some of these glands produce sweat, which helps regulate body
temperature. Other glands produce sebum, an oily substance that
helps keep the skin from drying out. Sweat and sebum reach the skin's
surface through tiny openings called pores.

Melanocytes and moles: Melanocytes produce melanin, the pigment that gives skin its natural color. When skin is exposed to the sun,
melanocytes produce more pigment, causing the skin to tan, or darken.

728

Sometimes, clusters of melanocytes and surrounding tissue form noncancerous growths called moles. (Doctors call a mole a *nevus*; the plural is *nevi*.) Moles are very common. Most people have between 10 and 40 moles. Moles may be pink, tan, brown, or a color that is very close to the person's normal skin tone. People who have dark skin tend to have dark moles. Moles can be flat or raised. They are usually round or oval and smaller than a pencil eraser. They may be present at birth or may appear later on—usually before age 40. They tend to fade away in older people. When moles are surgically removed, they normally do not return.

Melanoma: Melanoma occurs when melanocytes (pigment cells) become malignant. Most pigment cells are in the skin; when melanoma starts in the skin, the disease is called cutaneous melanoma. Melanoma may also occur in the eye (ocular melanoma or intraocular melanoma). Rarely, melanoma may arise in the meninges, the digestive tract, lymph nodes, or other areas where melanocytes are found.

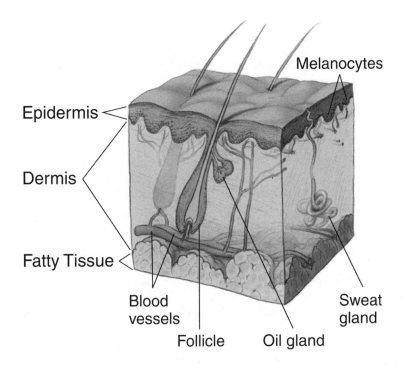

Figure 68.1. The skin has two main layers: the epidermis and the dermis.

Melanoma is one of the most common cancers. The chance of developing it increases with age, but this disease affects people of all ages. It can occur on any skin surface. In men, melanoma is often found on the trunk (the area between the shoulders and the hips) or the head and neck. In women, it often develops on the lower legs. Melanoma is rare in black people and others with dark skin. When it does develop in dark-skinned people, it tends to occur under the fingernails or toenails, or on the palms or soles.

When melanoma spreads, cancer cells may show up in nearby lymph nodes. Groups of lymph nodes are found throughout the body. Lymph nodes trap bacteria, cancer cells, or other harmful substances that may be in the lymphatic system. If the cancer has reached the lymph nodes, it may mean that cancer cells have spread to other parts of the body such as the liver, lungs, or brain. In such cases, the cancer cells in the new tumor are still melanoma cells, and the disease is called metastatic melanoma, not liver, lung, or brain cancer.

Who is at risk for melanoma?

No one knows the exact causes of melanoma. Doctors can seldom explain why one person gets melanoma and another does not. However, research has shown that people with certain risk factors are more likely than others to develop melanoma. A risk factor is anything that increases a person's chance of developing a disease. Still, many who do get this disease have no known risk factors. Studies have found the following risk factors for melanoma:

Dysplastic nevi: Dysplastic nevi are more likely than ordinary moles to become cancerous. Dysplastic nevi are common, and many people have a few of these abnormal moles. The risk of melanoma is greatest for people who have a large number of dysplastic nevi. The risk is especially high for people with a family history of both dysplastic nevi and melanoma.

Many (more than 50) ordinary moles: Having many moles increases the risk of developing melanoma.

Fair skin: Melanoma occurs more frequently in people who have fair skin that burns or freckles easily (these people also usually have red or blond hair and blue eyes) than in people with dark skin. White people get melanoma far more often than do black people, probably because light skin is more easily damaged by the sun.

Personal history of melanoma or skin cancer: People who have been treated for melanoma have a high risk of a second melanoma. Some people develop more than two melanomas. People who had one or more of the common skin cancers (basal cell carcinoma or squamous cell carcinoma) are at increased risk of melanoma.

Family history of melanoma: Melanoma sometimes runs in families. Having two or more close relatives who have had this disease is a risk factor. About 10 percent of all patients with melanoma have a family member with this disease. When melanoma runs in a family, all family members should be checked regularly by a doctor.

Weakened immune system: People whose immune system is weakened by certain cancers, by drugs given following organ transplantation, or by HIV are at increased risk of developing melanoma.

Severe, blistering sunburns: People who have had at least one severe, blistering sunburn as a child or teenager are at increased risk of melanoma. Because of this, doctors advise that parents protect children's skin from the sun. Such protection may reduce the risk of melanoma later in life. Sunburns in adulthood are also a risk factor for melanoma.

Ultraviolet (UV) radiation: Experts believe that much of the worldwide increase in melanoma is related to an increase in the amount of time people spend in the sun. This disease is also more common in people who live in areas that get large amounts of UV radiation from the sun. In the United States, for example, melanoma is more common in Texas than in Minnesota, where the sun is not as strong. UV radiation from the sun causes premature aging of the skin and skin damage that can lead to melanoma. Artificial sources of UV radiation, such as sunlamps and tanning booths, also can cause skin damage and increase the risk of melanoma. Doctors encourage people to limit their exposure to natural UV radiation and to avoid artificial sources.

Doctors recommend that people take steps to help prevent and reduce the risk of melanoma caused by UV radiation:

- Avoid exposure to the midday sun (from 10 AM to 4 PM) whenever possible. When your shadow is shorter than you are, remember to protect yourself from the sun.

- If you must be outside, wear long sleeves, long pants, and a hat with a wide brim.

- Protect yourself from UV radiation that can penetrate light clothing, windshields, and windows.

- Protect yourself from UV radiation reflected by sand, water, snow, and ice.

- Help protect your skin by using a lotion, cream, or gel that contains sunscreen. Many doctors believe sunscreens may help prevent melanoma, especially sunscreens that reflect, absorb, and/or scatter both types of ultraviolet radiation. These sunscreen products will be labeled with "broad-spectrum coverage." Sunscreens are rated in strength according to a sun protection factor (SPF). The higher the SPF, the more sunburn protection is provided. Sunscreens with an SPF value of 2 to 11 provide minimal protection against sunburns. Sunscreens with an SPF of 12 to 29 provide moderate protection. Those with an SPF of 30 or higher provide the most protection against sunburn.

- Wear sunglasses that have UV-absorbing lenses. The label should specify that the lenses block at least 99 percent of UVA and UVB radiation. Sunglasses can protect both the eyes and the skin around the eyes.

People who are concerned about developing melanoma should talk with their doctor about the disease, the symptoms to watch for, and an appropriate schedule for checkups. The doctor's advice will be based on the person's personal and family history, medical history, and other risk factors.

Section 68.2

Moles or Melanoma?

Excerpted from "What You Need to Know about™ Moles and
Dysplastic Nevi," National Cancer Institute, September 2002.

Moles are growths on the skin. Doctors call moles nevi (one mole
is a nevus). These growths occur when cells in the skin, called melanocytes, grow in a cluster with tissue surrounding them. Moles are
usually pink, tan, brown, or flesh-colored. Melanocytes are also spread
evenly throughout the skin and produce the pigment that gives skin
its natural color. When skin is exposed to the sun, melanocytes produce more pigment, causing the skin to tan, or darken.

Moles are very common. Most people have between 10 and 40 moles.
A person may develop new moles from time to time, usually until about
age 40. Moles can be flat or raised. They are usually round or oval and
no larger than a pencil eraser. Many moles begin as a small, flat spot
and slowly become larger in diameter and raised. Over many years, they
may flatten again, become flesh-colored, and go away.

Dysplastic Nevi

About one out of every ten people has at least one unusual (or atypical) mole that looks different from an ordinary mole. The medical term
for these unusual moles is dysplastic nevi. Doctors believe that dysplastic nevi are more likely than ordinary moles to develop into a type of
skin cancer called melanoma. Because of this, moles should be checked
regularly by a doctor or nurse specialist, especially if they look unusual;
grow larger; or change in color, outline, or in any other way.

Melanoma

Melanoma is one of the most serious types of skin cancer because
advanced melanomas have the ability to spread to other parts of the
body. Melanoma begins when melanocytes (pigment cells) gradually
become more abnormal and divide without control or order. These cells
can invade and destroy the normal cells around them. The abnormal

733

cells form a growth of malignant tissue (a cancerous tumor) on the surface of the skin. Melanoma can begin either in an existing mole or as a new growth on the skin. A doctor or nurse specialist can tell whether an abnormal-looking mole should be closely watched or should be removed and checked for melanoma cells. The purpose of routine skin exams is to identify and follow abnormal moles.

The removal of the entire mole or a sample of tissue for examination under a microscope is called a biopsy. If possible, it is best to remove moles by an excisional biopsy, rather than a shave biopsy.

If the biopsy results in a diagnosis of melanoma, the patient and the doctor should work together to make treatment decisions. In many cases, melanoma can be cured by minimal surgery if the tumor is discovered when it is thin (before it has grown downward from the skin surface) and before the cancer cells have begun to spread to other places in the body. However, if melanoma is not found early, the cancer cells can spread through the bloodstream and lymphatic system to form tumors in other parts of the body. Melanoma is much harder to control when it has spread. The spread of cancer is called metastasis.

Doctors and scientists believe that it is possible to prevent many melanomas and to detect most others early, when the disease is more likely to be cured with minimal surgery. In the past several decades, an increasing percentage of melanomas have been diagnosed at very early stages, when they are quite thin and unlikely to have spread. Learning about prevention and early detection, while important for everyone, is especially important for people who have an increased risk for melanoma. People who are at an increased risk include those who have dysplastic nevi or a very large number of ordinary moles.

Early Detection of Melanoma

Because melanoma usually begins on the surface of the skin, it often can be detected at an early stage with a total skin examination by a trained health care worker. Checking the skin regularly for any signs of the disease increases the chance of finding melanoma early. A monthly skin self-exam is very important for people who have any of the known risk factors, but doing skin self-exams routinely is a good idea for everyone. Here is how to do a skin self-exam:

- After a bath or shower, stand in front of a full-length mirror in a well-lighted room. Use a hand-held mirror to look at hard-to-see areas.

Melanoma

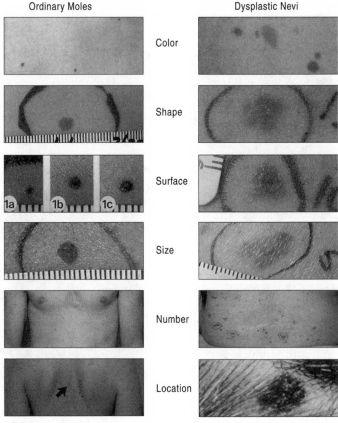

Ordinary Moles		Dysplastic Nevi
	Color	
	Shape	
	Surface	
	Size	
	Number	
	Location	

Color
Ordinary: Evenly tan or brown; all typical moles on one person tend to look similar.
Dysplastic: Mixture of tan, brown, and red/pink. A person's moles often look quite different from one another.

Shape
Ordinary: Round or oval, with a distinct edge that separates the mole from the rest of the skin.
Dysplastic: Have irregular, sometimes notched edges. May fade into the skin around it. The flat portion of the mole may be leve with the skin.

Surface
Ordinary: Begin as flat, smooth spots on skin (1a); may become raised (1b) and form a smooth bump (1c).
May have a smooth, slightly scaly, or rough, irregular, "pebbly" appearance.

Size
Ordinary: Usually less than 5 millimeters (about ¼ inch) across (size of a pencil eraser).
Dysplastic: Often larger than 5 millimeters (about ¼ inch) across and sometimes larger than 10 millimeters (about ½ inch).

Number
Ordinary: Between 10 and 40 typical moles may be present on an adult's body.
Dysplastic: May be present in large numbers (more than 100 on the same person). However, some people have only a few dysplastic nevi.

Location
Ordinary: Usually found above the waist on sun-exposed surfaces of the body. Scalp, breasts, and buttocks rarely have normal moles.
Dysplastic: May occur anywhere on the body but most frequently on the back and areas exposed to the sun. May also appear below the waist and on the scalp, breasts, and buttocks.

Figure 68.2. *Ordinary moles vs. dysplastic nevi.*

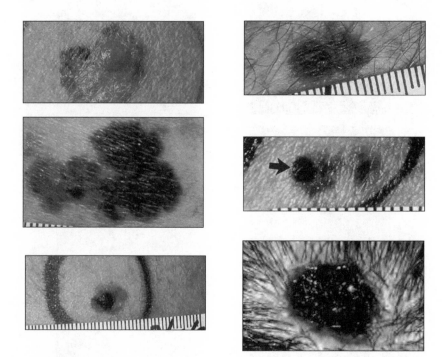

Large size
Most melanomas are at least 5 millimeters (about ¼ inch) across when they are found; many are much larger. An unusually large mole may be melanoma.

Many colors
A mixture of tan, brown, white, pink, red, gray, blue, and especially black in a mole suggests melanoma.

Irregular border
If a mole has an edge that is irregular or notched, it may be melanoma.

Abnormal surface
If a mole is scaly, flaky, oozing, or bleeding, has an open sore that does not heal, or has a hard lump in it, it may be melanoma.

Unusual sensation
If a mole itches or is painful or tender, melanoma may be present.

Abnormal skin around mole
If color from the mole spreads into the skin around it or if this skin becomes red or loses its color (becomes white or gray), melanoma may be present.

Figure 68.3. Pictures of melanoma.

- Begin with the face and scalp and work downward, checking the head, neck, shoulders, back, chest, and so on. Be sure to check the front, back, and sides of the arms and legs. Also, check the groin, the palms, the fingernails, the soles of the feet, the toenails, and the area between the toes.

- Be sure to check the hard-to-see areas of the body, such as the scalp and neck. A friend or relative may be able to help inspect these areas. Use a comb or a blow dryer to help move hair so you can see the scalp and neck better.

- Be aware of where your moles are and how they look. By checking your skin regularly, you will become familiar with what your moles look like. Look for any signs of change, particularly a new black mole or a change in outline, shape, size, color (especially a new black area), or feel of an existing mole. Also, note any new, unusual, or "ugly-looking" moles. If your doctor has taken photos of your skin, compare these pictures with the way your skin looks on self-examination.

- Check moles carefully during times of hormone changes, such as adolescence, pregnancy, and menopause. As hormone levels change, moles may change.

- It may be helpful to record the dates of your skin exams and to write notes about the way your skin looks. If you find anything unusual, see your doctor right away. Remember, the earlier a melanoma is found, the better the chance for a cure.

In addition to doing routine skin self-exams, people should have their skin checked regularly by a doctor or nurse specialist. A doctor can do a skin exam during visits for regular checkups. People who think they have dysplastic nevi should point them out to the doctor. It is also important to tell the doctor about any new, changing, or "ugly-looking" moles.

Sometimes it is necessary to see a specialist. A dermatologist (skin doctor) is likely to have the most training in diseases of the skin. Some plastic surgeons, general surgeons, oncologists, internists, and family doctors also have a special interest and training in moles and melanoma.

A doctor may want to watch a slightly abnormal mole closely to see whether it changes over time. Pictures taken at one visit may be compared with the appearance of the mole at the next visit. Sometimes a doctor decides that a mole should be removed so that the tissue can be examined under a microscope. The removal of a mole, called a biopsy, is usually done in the doctor's office using a local anesthetic. It generally takes only a few minutes. The patient may require stitches, and a small scar will remain after healing. A pathologist examines the tissue under a microscope to see whether the melanocytes are normal, dysplastic, or cancerous.

Because most moles, including most dysplastic nevi, do not develop into melanoma, removing all of them is not necessary. A doctor can recommend when and when not to remove moles. Usually, only moles that look like melanoma, those that change, or those that are both new and look abnormal need to be removed.

Section 68.3

Treating Melanoma

Excerpted from: PDQ® Cancer Information Summary. National Cancer Institute; Bethesda, MD. Melanoma (PDQ®): Treatment - Patient. Updated 12/2004. Available at: http://cancer.gov. Accessed April 30, 2006.

Stages of Melanoma

After melanoma has been diagnosed, tests are done to find out if cancer cells have spread within the skin or to other parts of the body. The process used to find out whether cancer has spread within the skin or to other parts of the body is called staging. The information gathered from the staging process determines the stage of the disease. It is important to know the stage in order to plan treatment. The following tests and procedures may be used in the staging process:

- **Wide local excision:** A surgical procedure to remove some of the normal tissue surrounding the area where melanoma was found, to check for cancer cells.

- **Lymph node mapping and sentinel lymph node biopsy:** Procedures in which a radioactive substance and/or blue dye is injected near the tumor. The substance or dye flows through lymph ducts to the sentinel node or nodes (the first lymph node or nodes where cancer cells are likely to have spread). The surgeon removes only the nodes with the radioactive substance or dye. A pathologist then checks the sentinel lymph nodes for cancer cells. If no cancer cells are detected, it may not be necessary to remove additional nodes.

- **Chest x-ray:** An x-ray of the organs and bones inside the chest. An x-ray is a type of energy beam that can go through the body and onto film, making a picture of areas inside the body.

- **CT scan (CAT scan):** A procedure that makes a series of detailed pictures of areas inside the body, taken from different angles. The pictures are made by a computer linked to an x-ray machine. A dye may be injected into a vein or swallowed to help the organs or tissues show up more clearly. This procedure is also called computed tomography, computerized tomography, or computerized axial tomography. For melanoma, pictures may be taken of the chest, abdomen, and pelvis.

- **MRI (magnetic resonance imaging):** A procedure that uses a magnet, radio waves, and a computer to make a series of detailed pictures of areas inside the body. This procedure is also called nuclear magnetic resonance imaging (NMRI).

- **PET (positron emission tomography) scan:** A procedure to find malignant tumor cells in the body. A small amount of radionuclide glucose (sugar) is injected into a vein. The PET scanner rotates around the body and makes a picture of where glucose is being used in the body. Malignant tumor cells show up brighter in the picture because they are more active and take up more glucose than normal cells.

- **Laboratory tests:** Medical procedures that test samples of tissue, blood, urine, or other substances in the body. These tests help to diagnose disease, plan and check treatment, or monitor the disease over time.

The results of these tests are viewed together with the results of the tumor biopsy to determine the melanoma stage. The following stages are used for melanoma:

Stage 0: In stage 0, melanoma is found only in the epidermis (outer layer of the skin). Stage 0 is also called melanoma in situ.

Stage I: Stage I is divided into stages IA and IB.

- **Stage IA:** In stage IA, the tumor is not more than 1 millimeter thick, with no ulceration. The tumor is in the epidermis and upper layer of the dermis.

- **Stage IB:** In stage IB, the tumor is either not more than 1 millimeter thick, with ulceration, and may have spread into the dermis or the tissues below the skin; or 1 to 2 millimeters thick, with no ulceration.

Stage II: Stage II is divided into stages IIA, IIB, and IIC.

- **Stage IIA:** In stage IIA, the tumor is either 1 to 2 millimeters thick, with ulceration; or 2 to 4 millimeters thick, with no ulceration.

- **Stage IIB:** In stage IIB, the tumor is either 2 to 4 millimeters thick, with ulceration; or more than 4 millimeters thick, with no ulceration.

- **Stage IIC:** In stage IIC, the tumor is more than 4 millimeters thick, with ulceration.

Stage III: In stage III, the tumor may be any thickness, with or without ulceration, and:

- has spread to 1 or more lymph nodes; or

- has spread into the nearby lymph system but not into nearby lymph nodes; or

- has spread to lymph nodes that are matted (not moveable); or

- satellite tumors (additional tumor growths within 2 centimeters of the original tumor) are present and nearby lymph nodes are involved.

Stage IV: In stage IV, the tumor may be any thickness, with or without ulceration, may have spread to 1 or more nearby lymph nodes, and has spread to other places in the body.

Recurrent: Recurrent melanoma is cancer that has recurred (come back) after it has been treated. The cancer may come back in the original site or in other parts of the body, such as the lungs or liver.

Treatment Option Overview

Different types of treatment are available for patients with melanoma. Some treatments are standard (the currently used treatment), and some are being tested in clinical trials. Before starting treatment, patients may want to think about taking part in a clinical trial. A treatment clinical trial is a research study meant to help improve current treatments or obtain information on new treatments for patients with cancer. When clinical trials show that a new treatment is better than the standard treatment, the new treatment may become the standard treatment.

Clinical trials are taking place in many parts of the country. Information about ongoing clinical trials is available from the National Cancer Institute website (http://www.cancer.gov). Choosing the most appropriate cancer treatment is a decision that ideally involves the patient, family, and health care team.

Four types of standard treatment are used:

Surgery: Surgery to remove the tumor is the primary treatment of all stages of melanoma. The doctor may remove the tumor using the following operations:

- **Local excision and wide local excision:** Taking out the melanoma and some of the normal tissue around it, with or without removal of lymph nodes.

- **Lymphadenectomy:** A surgical procedure in which the lymph nodes are removed and examined to see whether they contain cancer.

- **Sentinel lymph node biopsy:** The removal of the sentinel lymph node (the first lymph node the cancer is likely to spread to from the tumor) during surgery. A radioactive substance and/or blue dye is injected near the tumor. The substance or dye flows through the lymph ducts to the lymph nodes. The first lymph node to receive the substance or dye is removed for biopsy. A pathologist views the tissue under a microscope to look for cancer cells. If cancer cells are not found, it may not be necessary to remove more lymph nodes.

Skin grafting (taking skin from another part of the body to replace the skin that is removed) may be done to cover the wound caused by surgery.

Even if the doctor removes all the melanoma that can be seen at the time of the operation, some patients may be offered chemotherapy after surgery to kill any cancer cells that are left. Chemotherapy given after surgery, to increase the chances of a cure, is called adjuvant therapy.

Chemotherapy: Chemotherapy is a cancer treatment that uses drugs to stop the growth of cancer cells, either by killing the cells or by stopping the cells from dividing. When chemotherapy is taken by mouth or injected into a vein or muscle, the drugs enter the bloodstream and can reach cancer cells throughout the body (systemic chemotherapy). When chemotherapy is placed directly into the spinal column, an organ, or a body cavity such as the abdomen, the drugs mainly affect cancer cells in those areas (regional chemotherapy). The way the chemotherapy is given depends on the type and stage of the cancer being treated.

In treating melanoma, chemotherapy drugs may be given as a hyperthermic isolated limb perfusion. This technique sends anticancer drugs directly to the arm or leg in which the cancer is located. The flow of blood to and from the limb is temporarily stopped with a tourniquet, and a warm solution containing anticancer drugs is put directly into the blood of the limb. This allows the patient to receive a high dose of drugs in the area where the cancer occurred.

Radiation therapy: Radiation therapy is a cancer treatment that uses high-energy x-rays or other types of radiation to kill cancer cells. There are two types of radiation therapy. External radiation therapy uses a machine outside the body to send radiation toward the cancer. Internal radiation therapy uses a radioactive substance sealed in needles, seeds, wires, or catheters that are placed directly into or near the cancer. The way the radiation therapy is given depends on the type and stage of the cancer being treated.

Biologic therapy: Biologic therapy is a treatment that uses the patient's immune system to fight cancer. Substances made by the body or made in a laboratory are used to boost, direct, or restore the body's natural defenses against cancer. This type of cancer treatment is also called biotherapy or immunotherapy.

New Treatments: Other types of treatment are being tested in clinical trials. These include chemoimmunotherapy. Chemoimmunotherapy is the use of anticancer drugs combined with biologic therapy to boost the immune system to kill cancer cells.

Treatment Options by Stage

Stage 0: Treatment of stage 0 melanoma is usually surgery to remove the tumor and a small amount of normal tissue around it.

Stage I: Treatment of stage I melanoma may include the following:

- Surgery to remove the tumor and some of the normal tissue around it

- A clinical trial of surgery to remove the tumor and some of the normal tissue around it, with or without lymph node mapping and selective lymphadenectomy

- A clinical trial of new techniques to detect cancer cells in the lymph nodes

- A clinical trial of lymphadenectomy with or without adjuvant therapy

Stage II: Treatment of stage II melanoma may include the following:

- Surgery to remove the tumor and some of the normal tissue around it, followed by removal of nearby lymph nodes

- Lymph node mapping and sentinel lymph node biopsy, followed by surgery to remove the tumor and some of the normal tissue around it. If cancer is found in the sentinel lymph node, a second surgical procedure can be performed to remove additional nearby lymph nodes

- Surgery followed by high-dose biologic therapy

- A clinical trial of adjuvant chemotherapy and/or biologic therapy, or immunotherapy

- A clinical trial of new techniques to detect cancer cells in the lymph nodes

Stage III: Treatment of stage III melanoma may include the following:

- Surgery to remove the tumor and some of the normal tissue around it

- Surgery to remove the tumor with skin grafting to cover the wound caused by surgery

- Surgery followed by biologic therapy

- A clinical trial of surgery followed by chemotherapy and/or biologic therapy

- A clinical trial of biologic therapy

- A clinical trial comparing surgery alone to surgery with biologic therapy

- A clinical trial of chemoimmunotherapy or biologic therapy

- A clinical trial of hyperthermic isolated limb perfusion using chemotherapy and biologic therapy

- A clinical trial of biologic therapy and radiation therapy

Stage IV: Treatment of stage IV melanoma may include the following:

- Surgery or radiation therapy as palliative therapy to relieve symptoms and improve quality of life

- Chemotherapy and/or biologic therapy

- A clinical trial of new chemotherapy and/or biologic therapy, or vaccine therapy

- A clinical trial of radiation therapy as palliative therapy to relieve symptoms and improve quality of life

- A clinical trial of surgery to remove all known cancer

Treatment Options for Recurrent Melanoma: Treatment of recurrent melanoma may include the following:

- Surgery to remove the tumor

- Radiation therapy as palliative therapy to relieve symptoms and improve quality of life

- Palliative treatment with biologic therapy

- Hyperthermic isolated limb perfusion

- A clinical trial of biologic therapy and/or chemotherapy as palliative therapy to relieve symptoms and improve quality of life

Chapter 69

Non-Melanoma
Skin Cancers

Chapter Contents

Section 69.1

Actinic Keratosis: A Common Precancer

From "Actinic Keratosis: What You Should Know About This Common Precancer," an undated document; reprinted with permission from the Skin Cancer Foundation, http://www.skincancer.org. Accessed April 18, 2006.

You have surely seen an actinic keratosis. The name may be unfamiliar, but the appearance is commonplace. Anyone who spends time in the sun runs a high risk of developing one or more.

What is it?

An actinic keratosis (AK), also known as a solar keratosis, is a small crusty, scaly, or crumbly bump or horn that arises on the skin surface. The base may be light or dark, tan, pink, red, or a combination of these. Or, it may be the same color as your skin. The scale or crust is horny, dry, and rough, and is often recognized by touch rather than sight. Occasionally it itches or produces a pricking or tender sensation. It can also become inflamed and surrounded by redness. In rare instances, actinic keratoses can bleed.

The skin abnormality or lesion develops slowly and usually reaches a size from an eighth to a quarter of an inch (2 mm to 4 mm) but can sometimes be as large as one inch. Early on, it may disappear only to reappear later. You will often see several AKs at a time. An AK is most likely to appear on the face, lips, ears, scalp, neck, backs of the hands and forearms, shoulders and back—the parts of the body most often exposed to sunshine. The growths may be flat and pink or raised and rough.

Why is it dangerous?

AK can be the first step in the development of skin cancer. It is thus a precursor of cancer or a precancer.

If treated early, almost all AKs can be eliminated without becoming skin cancers. But untreated, about two to five percent may progress to squamous cell carcinoma (SCC), the second most common form of skin cancer. In fact, some scientists now believe that AK is the earliest form of SCC. Although SCCs are usually not life-threatening when detected and treated in the early stages, they can grow large and invade the surrounding tissues. On rare occasions, they metastasize or spread to the internal organs.

Another form of AK, actinic cheilitis, develops on the lips and may evolve into a type of SCC that can spread rapidly to other parts of the body.

If you have AKs, it indicates that you have sustained sun damage and could develop any kind of skin cancer—not just squamous cell carcinoma. The more keratoses that you have, the greater the chance that one or more may turn into skin cancer. People may also have up to 10 times as many subclinical (invisible) lesions as visible, surface lesions.

Actinic keratosis is skin cancer's warning signal. Heed that signal.

Where does AK develop and what does it look like?

Common forms of AK include the following:

- **Back of hand:** Scattered, thickened red, scaly patches.
- **Cheek and ear:** Multiple crusted lesions, ranging in color from red to brown.
- **Forehead and bald scalp:** Small red bumps and small tan crusts.
- **Lower lip:** Fissures filled with dried blood and large keratosis covered with horny scale.

Examine your skin regularly for any lesions that look like AK. If you ever spot these or any other suspicious or changing growths, see your doctor promptly.

What is the cause?

Chronic sun exposure is the cause of almost all AKs. Sun damage to the skin accumulates over time, so that even a brief exposure adds to the lifetime total. The likelihood of developing AK is highest in regions near the equator. However, regardless of climate, everyone is exposed to the sun. About 80 percent of solar ultraviolet (UV) rays can pass through clouds. These rays can also bounce off sand, snow, and other reflective surfaces, giving you extra exposure.

AKs can appear on skin that has been frequently exposed to artificial sources of UV light (such as tanning devices). More rarely, they may be caused by extensive exposure to x-rays or specific industrial chemicals.

Who is at greatest risk?

People who have fair skin, blonde or red hair, and/or blue, green, or gray eyes are at greatest risk. Because their skin has little protective pigment, they are most susceptible to sunburn. But even darker-skinned people can develop AKs if exposed to the sun without protection.

Individuals whose immune systems are weakened as a result of cancer chemotherapy, AIDS, or organ transplantation are also at higher risk.

How common is it?

AK is the most common type of precancerous skin lesion. Older people are more likely than younger ones to develop these lesions, because cumulative sun exposure increases with the years. Some experts believe that the majority of people who live to the age of 80 will have AKs. However, a considerable amount of our lifetime sun exposure occurs before age 20. Thus, AKs also appear in people in their early twenties who have spent too much time in the sun with little or no protection.

How is it treated?

There are many effective methods for eliminating AKs. All cause a certain amount of reddening, and some may cause scarring, while other approaches are less likely to do so. You and your doctor should decide together the best course of treatment, based on the nature of the lesion and your age and health.

Cryosurgery: The most common treatment for AK, it is especially effective when a limited number of lesions exist. Liquid nitrogen is applied to the growths with a spray device or cotton-tipped applicator to freeze them. They subsequently shrink or become crusted and fall off, without requiring any cutting or anesthesia. Some temporary redness and swelling may occur after treatment, and in dark-skinned patients, some pigment may be lost.

Curettage and desiccation: This is a valuable procedure for lesions suspected to be early cancers. To test for malignancy, the physician takes a biopsy specimen, either by shaving off the top of the lesion with a scalpel or scraping it off with a curette. Then the curette is used to remove the base of the lesion. Bleeding is stopped with an electrocautery needle, and local anesthesia is required.

Topical medications: Medicated creams and solutions are especially useful in removing both visible and invisible AKs when the lesions are numerous. The patient applies the medication according to a schedule worked out by the physician. The doctor will also regularly check progress. After treatment, some discomfort may result from skin breakdown, but the risk of scarring is minimal.

5-fluorouracil (5-FU) cream or solution, in concentrations from 0.5 to 5 percent, is the most widely used topical treatment for AK. It works well on the face, ears, and neck. Some redness, swelling, and crusting may occur.

Another preparation, imiquimod cream, is used for multiple keratoses. It causes cells to produce interferon, a chemical that destroys cancerous and precancerous cells.

An alternative treatment, a gel combining hyaluronic acid and the anti-inflammatory drug diclofenac, also may prove effective.

Chemical peeling: This method makes use of trichloroacetic acid (TCA) or a similar agent applied directly to the skin. The top skin layers slough off, usually replaced within seven days by new epidermis (the skin's outermost layer). This technique requires local anesthesia and can cause temporary discoloration and irritation.

Laser surgery: A carbon dioxide or erbium YAG laser is focused onto the lesion, removing epidermis and different amounts of deeper skin. This finely controlled treatment is an option for lesions in small or narrow areas; it can be effective for keratoses on the face and scalp, as well as actinic cheilitis on the lips. Laser surgery is useful for people with bleeding disorders and is also used as a secondary therapy when other techniques are unsuccessful. However, local anesthesia is usually necessary, and some scarring and pigment loss can occur.

Photodynamic therapy (PDT): PDT may be used to treat lesions on the face and scalp. Topical 5-aminolevulinic acid (5-ALA) is applied to the lesions by the physician. Within the next 24 hours, the medicated areas are exposed to strong light, which activates the 5-ALA. The treatment selectively destroys actinic keratoses, causing little damage to surrounding normal skin, although some swelling and redness often occur.

Section 69.2

Basal Cell Carcinoma

From "About Basal Cell Carcinoma," an undated document; reprinted with permission from the Skin Cancer Foundation, http://www.skincancer.org. Accessed April 18, 2006.

The Most Common Skin Cancer

Basal cell carcinoma is the most common form of skin cancer, affecting 800,000 Americans each year. In fact, it is the most common of all cancers. One out of every three new cancers is a skin cancer, and the vast majority are basal cell carcinomas, often referred to by the abbreviation, BCC. These cancers arise in the basal cells, which are at the bottom of the epidermis (outer skin layer). Until recently, those most often affected were older people, particularly men who had worked outdoors. Although the number of new cases has increased sharply each year in the last few decades, the average age of onset of the disease has steadily decreased. More women are getting BCCs than in the past; nonetheless, men still outnumber them greatly.

Chronic exposure to sunlight is the cause of almost all basal cell carcinomas, which occur most frequently on exposed parts of the body—the face, ears, neck, scalp, shoulders, and back. Rarely, however, tumors develop on non-exposed areas. In a few cases, contact with arsenic, exposure to radiation, and complications of burns, scars, vaccinations, or even tattoos are contributing factors.

Anyone with a history of frequent sun exposure can develop BCC. But people who have fair skin, blonde or red hair, and blue, green, or gray eyes are at highest risk. Those whose occupations require long hours outdoors or who spend extensive leisure time in the sun are in particular jeopardy.

What to Look For

The five most typical characteristics of basal cell carcinoma are described below. Frequently, two or more features are present in one tumor. In addition, basal cell carcinoma sometimes resembles non-cancerous skin conditions such as psoriasis or eczema. Only a trained physician, usually a specialist in diseases of the skin, can decide for sure. Learn the signs of basal cell carcinoma, and examine your skin regularly— once a month, or more often if you are at high risk. Be sure to include the scalp, backs of ears, neck, and other hard-to-see areas. (A full-length mirror and a hand-held mirror can be very useful). If you observe any of the warning signs or some other change in your skin, consult your physician immediately. The Skin Cancer Foundation advises people to have a total-body skin exam by a dermatologist at regular intervals. The physician will suggest the correct time frame for follow-up visits, depending on your specific risk factors, such as skin type and history of sun exposure.

The Five Warning Signs of Basal Cell Carcinoma

- An open sore that bleeds, oozes, or crusts and remains open for three or more weeks. A persistent, non-healing sore is a very common sign of an early basal cell carcinoma.

- A reddish patch or irritated area, frequently occurring on the chest, shoulders, arms, or legs. Sometimes the patch crusts. It may also itch or hurt. At other times, it persists with no noticeable discomfort.

- A shiny bump, or nodule, that is pearly or translucent and is often pink, red, or white. The bump can also be tan, black, or brown, especially in dark-haired people, and can be confused with a mole.

- A pink growth with a slightly elevated rolled border and a crusted indentation in the center. As the growth slowly enlarges, tiny blood vessels may develop on the surface.

- A scar-like area which is white, yellow, or waxy, and often has poorly defined borders. The skin itself appears shiny and taut. This warning sign can indicate the presence of an aggressive tumor.

Treatment Options

If skin cancer is suspected, a biopsy must be taken and examined microscopically. If the diagnosis is confirmed, there are many treatment options from which to choose.

Topical medications: In addition to being used to treat actinic keratosis (AK), the most common skin precancer, imiquimod and 5-FU

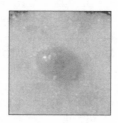

*Small, smooth, shiny, pale,
or waxy lump*

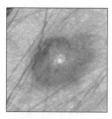

Firm, red lump

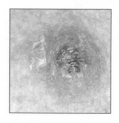

*Sore or lump that
bleeds or develops a
crust or a scab*

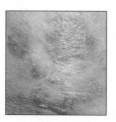

*Flat red spot that is rough,
dry, or scaly and may be-
come itchy or tender*

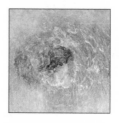

*Red or brown patch that is
rough and scaly*

Figure 69.1. *A change on the skin is the most common sign of skin cancer (Source: This image is from "What You Need to Know About™ Skin Cancer," National Cancer Institute, 2005.)*

are also approved for the treatment of superficial basal cell carcinoma (sBCC).

Curettage and electrodesiccation: The growth is scraped off with a curette and the tumor site desiccated with an electrocautery needle. The procedure is typically repeated a few times to help assure that all cancer cells are eliminated. Local anesthesia is required.

Excisional surgery: Along with the above procedure, this is one of the most common treatments for BCCs and SCCs. Using a scalpel, the physician removes the entire growth along with a surrounding border of apparently normal skin as a safety margin. The incision is closed, and the growth is sent to the laboratory to verify that all cancerous cells have been removed.

Radiation: X-ray beams are directed at the tumor. Total destruction usually requires several treatments a week for a few weeks. This is ideal for tumors that are hard to manage surgically and for elderly patients who are in poor health.

Mohs micrographic surgery: The physician removes the visible tumor with a curette or scalpel and then removes very thin layers of the remaining surrounding skin one layer at a time. Each layer is checked under a microscope, and the procedure is repeated until the last layer viewed is cancer-free. This technique has the highest cure rate and can save the greatest amount of healthy tissue. It is often used for tumors that have recurred or are in hard-to-treat places such as the head, neck, hands, and feet.

Cryosurgery: Liquid nitrogen is applied to the growths with a cotton-tipped applicator or spray device. This freezes them without requiring any cutting or anesthesia. They subsequently blister or become crusted and fall off. The procedure may be repeated to ensure total destruction of malignant cells. Some temporary redness and swelling can occur. In some patients, pigment may be lost.

Laser surgery: The skin's outer layer and variable amounts of deeper skin are removed using a carbon dioxide or erbium YAG laser. Lasers give the physician good control over the depth of tissue removed, much like chemical peels. Lasers are also used as a secondary therapy when topical medications or other techniques are unsuccessful. However, local anesthesia may be required. The risks of scarring and pigment loss are slightly greater than with other techniques.

Photodynamic therapy (PDT): PDT can be especially useful for lesions on the face and scalp, and when patients have multiple BCCs. Topical 5-aminolevulinic acid (5-ALA) is applied to the lesions at the physician's office. As soon as an hour later, those medicated areas can be activated by a strong light. This treatment selectively destroys BCCs while causing minimal damage to surrounding normal tissue. Some redness and swelling can result from this newer therapy.

Section 69.3

Squamous Cell Carcinoma

From "About Squamous Cell," an undated document; reprinted with permission from the Skin Cancer Foundation, http://www.skincancer.org. Accessed April 18, 2006.

Squamous cell carcinoma (SCC), the second most common skin cancer after basal cell carcinoma, afflicts more than 200,000 Americans each year. It arises from the epidermis and resembles the squamous cells that comprise most of the upper layers of skin. SCCs may occur on all areas of the body including the mucous membranes, but are most common in areas exposed to the sun.

Although SCCs usually remain confined to the epidermis for some time, they eventually penetrate the underlying tissues if not treated. When this happens, they can be disfiguring. In a small percentage of cases, they spread (metastasize) to distant tissues and organs and can become fatal. SCCs that metastasize most often arise on sites of chronic inflammatory skin conditions or on the mucous membranes or lips.

Causes and Risk Factors

Chronic exposure to sunlight causes most cases of squamous cell carcinoma. That is why tumors appear most frequently on sun-exposed parts of the body: the face, neck, bald scalp, hands, shoulders, arms, and back. The rim of the ear and the lower lip are especially vulnerable to the development of these cancers.

Squamous cell carcinomas may also occur where skin has suffered certain kinds of injury: burns, scars, long-standing sores, sites previously exposed to x-rays or certain chemicals (such as arsenic and petroleum by-products). In addition, chronic skin inflammation or medical conditions that suppress the immune system over an extended period of time may encourage development of squamous cell carcinoma.

Occasionally, squamous cell carcinoma arises spontaneously on what appears to be normal, healthy, undamaged skin. Some researchers believe that a tendency to develop this cancer may be inherited.

Anyone with a substantial history of sun exposure can develop squamous cell carcinoma. But people who have fair skin, light hair, and blue, green, or gray eyes are at highest risk. Those whose occupations require long hours outdoors or who spend extensive leisure time in the sun are in particular jeopardy.

Dark-skinned individuals of African descent are far less likely than fair-skinned individuals to develop skin cancer. More than two thirds of the skin cancers that individuals of African descent develop are SCCs, usually arising on the sites of preexisting inflammatory skin conditions or burn injuries. Although dark-skinned individuals of any background are less likely than fair-skinned individuals to develop skin cancer, it is still essential for them to practice sun protection.

Precancerous Conditions

Certain precursor conditions, some of which result from extensive sun damage, are worth noting. They are sometimes associated with the later development of SCC. They include the following:

- **Actinic, or solar, keratosis:** Actinic keratoses are rough, scaly, slightly raised growths that range in color from brown to red and may be up to one inch in diameter. They appear most often in older people. Some experts believe that actinic keratosis is the earliest form of SCC. Actinic cheilitis is a type of actinic keratosis occurring on the lips. It causes them to become dry, cracked, scaly, and pale or white. It mainly affects the lower lip, which typically receives more sun exposure than the upper lip.

- **Leukoplakia:** These white patches or plaques on the tongue or inside of the mouth, arising in the mucous membranes, have the potential to develop into SCC. They are caused by sources of chronic irritation, including smoking or other tobacco use, and rough teeth or rough edges on dentures and fillings. Leukoplakia on the lips are mainly caused by sun damage.

- **Bowen disease:** This is generally considered to be a superficial SCC that has not yet spread. It appears as a persistent red-brown, scaly patch which may resemble psoriasis or eczema. If untreated, it may invade deeper structures.

Regardless of appearance, any change in a preexisting skin growth, or the development of a new growth or open sore that fails to heal, should prompt an immediate visit to a physician. If it is a precursor condition, early treatment will prevent it from developing into SCC. Often, all that is needed is a simple surgical procedure or application of a topical chemotherapeutic agent.

Squamous cell carcinomas occur most frequently on areas of the body that have been exposed to the sun for prolonged periods. Usually, the skin in these areas reveals telltale signs of sun damage, such as wrinkling, changes in pigmentation, and loss of elasticity.

Warning Signs of Squamous Cell Carcinoma

- A wart-like growth that crusts and occasionally bleeds

- A persistent, scaly red patch with irregular borders that sometimes crusts or bleeds

- An open sore that bleeds and crusts and persists for weeks

- An elevated growth with a central depression that occasionally bleeds. A growth of this type may rapidly increase in size.

- A persistent, scaly red patch with irregular borders that sometimes crusts or bleeds

- An open sore that bleeds and crusts and persists for weeks

Treatment Options

After a physician's examination, a biopsy will be performed to confirm the diagnosis of SCC. This involves removing a piece of the affected tissue and examining it under a microscope. If tumor cells are present, treatment (usually surgery) is required. Fortunately, there are several effective ways to eradicate SCC. The choice of treatment is based on the type, size, location, and depth of penetration of the tumor, as well as the patient's age and general state of health.

Treatment can almost always be performed on an outpatient basis in a physician's office or at a clinic. A local anesthetic is used during most procedures. Pain or discomfort is usually minimal with most techniques, and there is rarely much pain afterwards.

- **Curettage and electrodesiccation:** As with AKs, the growth is scraped off with a curette and the tumor site desiccated with an electrocautery needle. But when treating BCCs or SCCs, the procedure is typically repeated a few times to help assure that all cancer cells are eliminated. Local anesthesia is required.

- **Excisional surgery:** Along with the above procedure, this is one of the most common treatments for BCCs and SCCs. Using a scalpel, the physician removes the entire growth along with a surrounding border of apparently normal skin as a safety margin. The incision is closed, and the growth is sent to the laboratory to verify that all cancerous cells have been removed.

- **Radiation:** X-ray beams are directed at the tumor. Total destruction usually requires several treatments a week for a few weeks. This is ideal for tumors that are hard to manage surgically and for elderly patients who are in poor health.

- **Mohs micrographic surgery:** The physician removes the visible tumor with a curette or scalpel and then removes very thin layers of the remaining surrounding skin one layer at a time. Each layer is checked under a microscope, and the procedure is repeated until the last layer viewed is cancer-free. This technique has the highest cure rate and can save the greatest amount of healthy tissue. It is often used for tumors that have recurred or are in hard-to-treat places such as the head, neck, hands, and feet.

- **Imiquimod:** U.S. Food and Drug Administration (FDA)–approved for the treatment of genital warts, this topical cream is a promising new treatment for actinic keratoses and Bowen disease. It causes cells to produce interferon, a chemical that attacks cancerous and precancerous cells.

Section 69.4

Merkel Cell Carcinoma

Excerpted from: PDQ® Cancer Information Summary. National Cancer
Institute; Bethesda, MD. Merkel Cell Carcinoma (PDQ®): Treatment -
Patient. Updated 03/2006. Available at: http://cancer.gov. Accessed April
30, 2006.

Merkel cell carcinoma is a very rare disease in which malignant
(cancer) cells form in the skin. Merkel cells are hormone-making cells
found in the top layer of the skin. These cells are very close to the nerve
endings that receive the sensation of touch. Merkel cell carcinoma,
also called neuroendocrine carcinoma, is a very rare type of skin cancer that develops when Merkel cells grow out of control. Merkel cell
carcinoma starts most often in areas of skin exposed to the sun, such
as the head, neck, arms, and legs.

Merkel cell carcinoma tends to grow quickly and to metastasize
(spread) at an early stage. It spreads first to nearby lymph nodes and
then may spread to the liver, bone, lungs, brain, or other parts of the body.

Sun exposure and having a weak immune system can affect the risk
of developing Merkel cell carcinoma. Risk factors include the following:

- Being exposed to a lot of natural sunlight

- Being exposed to artificial sunlight, such as during treatment
  for psoriasis

- Having an immune system weakened by disease, such as HIV
  infection

- Taking drugs that make the immune system less active, such as
  after an organ transplant

- Having a history of other types of skin cancer, such as basal cell
  or squamous cell cancer

- Being older than 70 years, male, or white

Merkel cell carcinoma usually appears on sun-exposed skin as a
single painless lump that is fast-growing, firm and dome-shaped or

raised, and red or violet in color. This and other changes in the skin may be caused by Merkel cell carcinoma. Other conditions may cause the same symptoms. A doctor should be consulted if changes in the skin are seen.

Tests and procedures that examine the skin are used to detect (find) and diagnose Merkel cell carcinoma. The following tests and procedures may be used:

- **Physical exam and history:** An exam of the body to check general signs of health, including checking for signs of disease, such as lumps or anything else that seems unusual. A history of the patient's health habits and past illnesses and treatments will also be taken.

- **Full-body skin exam:** A doctor or nurse checks the skin for bumps or spots that look abnormal in color, size, shape, or texture. The size, shape, and texture of the lymph nodes will also be checked.

- **Biopsy:** The removal of cells or tissues so they can be viewed under a microscope by a pathologist to check for signs of cancer. To diagnose Merkel cell carcinoma, cells are treated with a special stain and viewed with an electron microscope.

Certain factors affect prognosis (chance of recovery) and treatment options. The prognosis (chance of recovery) and treatment options depend on the following:

- The stage of the cancer (the size of the tumor and whether it has spread to the lymph nodes or other parts of the body)

- Where the cancer is in the body

- Whether the cancer has just been diagnosed or has recurred (come back)

- The patient's age and general health

Prognosis also depends on how deeply the tumor has grown into the skin.

Stages of Merkel Cell Carcinoma

After Merkel cell carcinoma has been diagnosed, tests are done to find out if cancer cells have spread to other parts of the body. The

759

process used to find out if cancer has spread to other parts of the body is called staging. The information gathered from the staging process determines the stage of the disease. It is important to know the stage in order to plan treatment. The following tests and procedures may be used in the staging process:

- **Complete blood count (CBC):** A procedure in which a sample of blood is drawn and checked for the following: the number of red blood cells, white blood cells, and platelets; the amount of hemoglobin (the protein that carries oxygen) in the red blood cells; and the portion of the blood sample made up of red blood cells

- **Lymph node biopsy:** The removal of all or part of a lymph node. A pathologist views the tissue under a microscope to look for cancer cells.

- **Liver function test:** A blood test to measure the blood levels of certain substances released by the liver. A high or low level of certain substances can be a sign of disease in the liver.

- **CT scan (CAT scan):** A procedure that makes a series of detailed pictures of areas inside the body, taken from different angles. The pictures are made by a computer linked to an x-ray machine. A dye may be injected into a vein or swallowed to help the organs or tissues show up more clearly. This procedure is also called computed tomography, computerized tomography, or computerized axial tomography. CT scanning of the head and neck may be used to detect Merkel cell carcinoma that has spread to the lymph nodes.

- **Octreotide scan:** A type of radionuclide scan used to find carcinomas and other types of tumors. A small amount of radioactive octreotide (a hormone that attaches to carcinoid tumors) is injected into a vein and travels through the bloodstream. The radioactive octreotide attaches to the tumor and a special camera that detects radioactivity is used to show where the tumor cells are in the body.

The following stages are used for Merkel cell carcinoma:

Stage IA: In stage IA, the cancer is 2 centimeters or smaller in diameter and has not spread to lymph nodes or other parts of the body.

Stage IB: In stage IB, the cancer is larger than 2 centimeters in diameter and has not spread to lymph nodes or other parts of the body.

Stage II: In stage II, the cancer may be any size and has spread to nearby lymph nodes, but has not spread to other parts of the body.

Stage III: In stage III, the cancer may be any size and has spread beyond nearby lymph nodes to other parts of the body.

Recurrent: Recurrent Merkel cell carcinoma is cancer that has recurred (come back) after it has been treated. The cancer may come back in the skin, lymph nodes, or other parts of the body. It is common for Merkel cell carcinoma to recur.

Treatment Option Overview

Different types of treatments are available for patients with Merkel cell carcinoma. Some treatments are standard (the currently used treatment), and some are being tested in clinical trials. Before starting treatment, patients may want to think about taking part in a clinical trial. A treatment clinical trial is a research study meant to help improve current treatments or obtain information on new treatments for patients with cancer. When clinical trials show that a new treatment is better than the standard treatment, the new treatment may become the standard treatment.

Clinical trials are taking place in many parts of the country. Information about ongoing clinical trials is available from the National Cancer Institute website (http://www.cancer.gov). Choosing the most appropriate cancer treatment is a decision that ideally involves the patient, family, and health care team.

Three types of standard treatment are used:

Surgery: One or more of the following surgical procedures may be used to treat Merkel cell carcinoma:

- **Wide local excision:** The cancer is cut from the skin along with some of the healthy tissue around it.

- **Mohs micrographic surgery:** Individual layers of cancerous tissue are removed and examined under a microscope one at a time until no more cancer cells are seen. This type of surgery removes as little normal tissue as possible and is often used to remove skin cancer on the face.

- **Sentinel lymph node biopsy:** The removal of the sentinel lymph node (the first lymph node the cancer is likely to spread to from the tumor) during surgery. A radioactive substance and/or blue dye is injected near the tumor. The substance or dye flows through the lymph ducts to the lymph nodes. The first lymph node to receive the substance or dye is removed for biopsy. A pathologist views the tissue under a microscope to look for cancer cells. If cancer cells are not found, it may not be necessary to remove more lymph nodes.

- **Lymph node dissection:** A surgical procedure in which the lymph nodes are removed and examined to see whether they contain cancer. For a regional lymph node dissection, some of the lymph nodes in the tumor area are removed; for a radical lymph node dissection, most or all of the lymph nodes in the tumor area are removed. This procedure is also called lymphadenectomy.

Even if the doctor removes all the cancer that can be seen at the time of the surgery, some patients may be given chemotherapy or radiation therapy after surgery to kill any cancer cells that are left. Treatment given after the surgery, to increase the chances of a cure, is called adjuvant therapy.

Radiation therapy: Radiation therapy is a cancer treatment that uses high-energy x-rays or other types of radiation to kill cancer cells. There are two types of radiation therapy. External radiation therapy uses a machine outside the body to send radiation toward the cancer. Internal radiation therapy uses a radioactive substance sealed in needles, seeds, wires, or catheters that are placed directly into or near the cancer. The way the radiation therapy is given depends on the type and stage of the cancer being treated.

Chemotherapy: Chemotherapy is a cancer treatment that uses drugs to stop the growth of cancer cells, either by killing the cells or by stopping the cells from dividing. When chemotherapy is taken by mouth or injected into a vein or muscle, the drugs enter the bloodstream and can reach cancer cells throughout the body (systemic chemotherapy). When chemotherapy is placed directly into the spinal column, an organ, or a body cavity such as the abdomen, the drugs mainly affect cancer cells in those areas (regional chemotherapy). The way the chemotherapy is given depends on the type and stage of the cancer being treated.

Treatment Options by Stage

Stage I: Treatment of stage I Merkel cell carcinoma may include the following:

- Surgery (wide local excision; Mohs micrographic surgery; sentinel lymph node biopsy; lymph node dissection)
- Radiation therapy after surgery

Stage II: Treatment of stage II Merkel cell carcinoma may include the following:

- Surgery (wide local excision and lymph node dissection)
- Radiation therapy after surgery
- Chemotherapy

Stage III: Treatment of stage III Merkel cell carcinoma is usually chemotherapy.

Recurrent Merkel cell carcinoma: Treatment of recurrent Merkel cell carcinoma may include the following:

- Surgery (sentinel lymph node biopsy or lymph node dissection) with or without radiation therapy
- Radiation therapy after surgery
- Chemotherapy

Chapter 70

Bone Sarcomas

Chapter Contents

Section 70.1

Information about Bone Sarcomas

"General Information/Classification of Bone Sarcomas," reprinted with permission from www.bonecancer.org, Orthopedic Oncology - New York University Medical Center © 2002 James C. Wittig, M.D.

Cells and Cancer

The human body is made up of various organ systems, such as the musculoskeletal system (bones and muscles), respiratory system (lungs), cardiovascular system (heart and blood vessels), gastrointestinal system, integumentary system (skin), nervous system (brain, spinal cord and nerves), urinary system (kidneys, bladder). Each system is made up of individual organs that function together to make the system work. Each organ is made up of tissues, such as muscle, nerves, connective tissue, bone, and epithelial tissue. Tissues combine to make organs. Each individual tissue is made up of specific types of cells.

The cell is the smallest building block of the body. The body is made up of billions of cells. The cell contains genetic material in its nucleus (the brain of the cell) that determines the function and characteristics of the cell and, therefore, of the body and person. The genetic material tells the cell when to grow, divide, and replicate. As cells age, they eventually die and are replaced by other cells that divide to replenish the aging cells.

Occasionally, an alteration occurs in a cell's genetic material or some other alteration occurs in the cell, and the cell begins to grow, divide, and replicate itself uncontrollably. The body's immune system may detect this and destroy the abnormal cells. If the body does not detect this abnormality, then the cell continues to divide and form a tumor.

A tumor refers to an abnormal growth in the body. Tumors are made up of abnormal cells that are uncontrollably dividing and replicating themselves. Tumors can be classified as benign or malignant (cancerous). Depending upon the type of cell that the tumor is derived from, a malignant tumor can be classified as a sarcoma or a carcinoma. Malignant tumors can also be considered primary or secondary. In terms of bone tumors, a primary bone tumor arises directly from a particular bone. Secondary bone tumors are tumors that involve the bone but have traveled from a cancer in another part of the body. Primary malignant bone tumors are sarcomas. Secondary bone tumors are called metastatic bone tumors or metastatic bone cancers, and most are carcinomas that have traveled from other primary tumors such as breast cancer, lung cancer, prostate cancer, kidney cancer, thyroid cancer, and gastrointestinal cancer. For instance, when breast cancer spreads to the bone, the breast cancer is the primary cancer and the breast cancer that is in the bone is a secondary cancer or a metastatic cancer.

Benign tumors are not considered cancers. They do not have the ability to spread throughout the body. They generally cause problems or destruction in the bone that they arise from. Benign tumors can also cause additional problems if they grow near critical organs. When they arise from the bone they can cause extensive destruction of the bone.

Malignant tumors are cancers. Malignant tumors have the ability to spread throughout the rest of the body. For instance, a malignant bone tumor can spread (metastasize) to the lungs. The tumor in the lung looks exactly like the bone tumor under a microscope. The patient is not considered to have lung cancer but to have a metastatic bone cancer. Malignant tumors also cause destruction in the bone or adjacent tissue that they arise from, in addition to spreading throughout the body.

Sarcomas vs. Carcinomas

A sarcoma is a specific type of malignant tumor. It is derived from a particular type of cell referred to as a pluripotential mesenchymal cell. Under normal situations, mesenchymal cells in the body form the bones, muscles, cartilage, connective tissue, blood vessels, blood cells, and nerves. Pluripotential means that the cell has the ability to differentiate or grow along different pathways and form these various types of tissues.

Under cancerous conditions, the mesenchymal cells that form a sarcoma can grow along a specific pathway and form tissue that looks like bone, cartilage, muscle, connective tissue, or blood vessels. Thus, you can have a bone sarcoma (malignant tumor of bone made up of mesenchymal cells) that is actually producing bone. The name given to this type of tumor is osteosarcoma (*osteo* means bone; thus osteosarcoma is a bone forming sarcoma). A patient can have a malignant bone tumor that produces cartilage. This is called a chondrosarcoma (*chondro* means cartilage).

Malignant tumors that arise directly from bone are called sarcomas. Sarcoma is Greek for "fleshy" or "fish-flesh." The name was given to these types of tumors because of their appearance. They have a fleshy appearance when cut open and examined.

Carcinomas are distinctly different from sarcomas. They are derived from cells that look like epithelial cells or glandular cells. These cells do not form bone, muscle, nerve, etc. They do not have this ability. If a carcinoma is growing from a bone, it has usually come from a primary cancer in another part of the body. It is always considered cancerous and malignant because it has spread from another body part or another cancer. Breast cancer, lung cancer, kidney cancer, prostate cancer, thyroid cancer, and gastrointestinal cancer are the most common carcinomas that travel, or metastasize, to bone. They can result in extensive destruction of the bone and can cause the bone to break/fracture. In some areas such as the pelvis and scapula, they can form large tumors that can involve the major nerves and blood vessels to the extremities. This is a serious situation. It can lead to uncontrollable pain and death of the arm or extremity. The tumor in the bone is the same type of tumor as the primary carcinoma. For instance, if breast cancer has spread to the bone, the tumor in the bone is exactly the same as the breast cancer under the microscope. This is considered metastatic breast cancer to the bone.

Sarcomas are rare cancers and constitute about 1% of all cancers. Carcinomas are much more common and make up the majority of the remaining cancers that occur yearly.

Bone Tumors and Sarcomas

Bone tumors and sarcomas are rare types of tumors. Bone sarcomas constitute about 1% of all types of cancers that occur in the United States each year. The most common type of bone sarcoma is an osteosarcoma, of which, approximately 600 occur in the United States each year. Bone sarcomas can affect all age groups and particular types have a predilection for specific age groups. For instance, osteosarcoma and Ewing sarcoma typically occur during the teenage years or early 20s. Chondrosarcoma affects older adults. Overall, there is no strong sex predilection. For the most part, they occur equally as common in males and females, except for a few certain types of bone sarcomas or bone tumors.

In reality, nobody knows what causes a sarcoma or a benign bone tumor. Because of the rarity of these tumors it has been difficult to perform extensive research on these types of tumors. Some tumors are related to genetic alterations that can actually be identified with special laboratory tests. There are also some rare genetic syndromes such as neurofibromatosis in which patients are predisposed to sarcomas. Radiation, a commonly employed treatment for certain cancers, can also cause bone sarcomas. Bone sarcomas can arise in the presence of Paget disease. Certain chemicals have been loosely linked to sarcomas. There are predisposing factors for some carcinomas, such as cigarette smoking and lung cancer. There is a familial or genetic link for breast cancer as well as it being linked to the female sex (males have breast tissue also).

Grading Sarcomas

Sarcomas are graded by pathologists. When the pathologist views a biopsy specimen or the final tumor under the microscope, he assigns a grade to the tumor. The grade is based on particular characteristics of the cells that compose the tumor. The grade reflects the degree of malignancy of the sarcoma. The degree of malignancy reflects the potential for the tumor to come back locally (local recurrence) and spread to other parts (metastasize).

Sarcomas can be divided into low, intermediate, and high grade tumors. Low grade tumors grow slowly and have very little chance of spreading to other areas of the body. High grade tumors grow rapidly and have a high likelihood of spreading to other body parts, particularly the lungs. Usually, high grade sarcomas have already spread microscopically to other parts of the body by the time the tumor is noticed by the patient. The behavior of intermediate grade tumors falls somewhere in between low and high grade tumors.

Treating Sarcomas

The grade of the tumor helps determine the type of treatment. Higher grade tumors are generally treated with more aggressive surgery. High grade tumors respond to chemotherapy and low grade tumors do not respond to chemotherapy. High grade tumors tend to respond better to radiation in comparison to low grade tumors. Thus chemotherapy is usually only used for treating high grade tumors with rare exceptions.

Chemotherapy

Chemotherapy is the administration of certain toxic drugs in an attempt to kill cancer cells and cure patients of their cancer, shrink tumors to facilitate surgical resection, or prolong a patient's life. Chemotherapy is typically administered for high grade bone sarcomas. It is usually given before surgery (this is called preoperative chemotherapy, neoadjuvant chemotherapy, or induction chemotherapy) to try to kill the tumor before taking it out.

The terms induction chemotherapy and neoadjuvant chemotherapy refer to giving the chemotherapy before surgery. Giving chemotherapy before surgery makes it easier to remove the tumor and makes it less likely for the tumor to come back in the area where it was removed. At the same time, any microscopic tumor cells that have spread throughout the body are killed. Certain tumors may shrink dramatically following chemotherapy which makes the surgery easier. Less normal tissue is removed.

Preoperative chemotherapy also permits doctors to examine the response that the tumor had to the chemotherapy which helps estimate the patient's prognosis (it helps estimate the response of the microscopic tumor cells that have already spread).

Preoperative or induction chemotherapy is largely responsible for the present day ability to save 90%–95% of limbs with high grade sarcomas instead of performing amputations. Amputations for high grade bone sarcomas are rarely performed nowadays.

For high grade bone sarcomas, chemotherapy is also usually given postoperatively. When it is given postoperatively, it is referred to as adjuvant chemotherapy. The same chemotherapy agents are used before and after surgery. The purpose of chemotherapy is to kill any tumor cells that have spread throughout the body that can grow and kill the patient. By killing or eradicating these cells, the patient can be cured of the cancer.

The entire chemotherapy regimen may require six months to 12 months to complete. Some chemotherapy agents require a hospital admission for a few days in order to administer the medications. The following chemotherapy drugs may be used in the treatment of sarcomas:

- Adriamycin (doxorubicin)

- ifosfamide

- cisplatin

- high dose methotrexate
- cyclophosphamide
- vincristine
- actinomycin-D
- etoposide

There are complications that are specific to each type of medication. These complications should be thoroughly discussed with the medical oncologist. Some of the general complications or side effects include: hair loss, nausea and vomiting, mucositis, myelosuppression/decrease in the blood counts (neutropenia, which refers to a drop in white blood cells; anemia, which refers to drop in red blood cells; or thrombocytopenia, which refers to a drop in platelets), cardiac dysfunction, hearing loss, kidney failure, and neuropathy.

Many of these side effects and complications can be minimized with specific medications. Prior to initiating chemotherapy several blood tests will be ordered along with a hearing test and an echocardiogram (assesses the function of the heart). Blood tests will be required frequently throughout the course of the chemotherapy regimen to follow kidney function and blood counts.

A special intravenous line will be placed (Port-A-Cath or Groshong) that can stay in place for prolonged periods. This line is directed into the large veins that empty into the cardiopulmonary circulation. It is necessary to place these lines so the chemotherapy can be administered directly into the large veins. Infusion of chemotherapy agents into small veins causes destruction of the small veins. Additionally some agents may spill under the skin and cause skin damage.

The patient and family members must be aware that these ports can get infected when the patient's white blood cell count drops. Any fever that develops during chemotherapy must be reported to the oncologist. The patient will be admitted, cultures of blood obtained (along with a chest x-ray), and a urinalysis done to check for bacteria. The patient will be started immediately on intravenous antibiotics.

If a line gets infected postoperatively in a patient who has had a prosthetic replacement, the line should be removed. Bacteria can live for long periods on the part of the line that is in the venous system. Intravenous antibiotics may not eradicate the bacteria, and the bacteria can spread to the prosthesis and cause a severe limb-threatening infection that requires additional surgery and is difficult to cure without removing the prosthesis.

Radiation Therapy

Radiation is a form of energy that is used to destroy tumors or microscopic tumor cells. It can be administered in several ways. The most common way is by an external beam. This is referred to as external beam radiation. It is used only in special circumstances when treating bone sarcomas. It is most commonly used when the tumor can not be removed surgically (when the tumor is unresectable) or when it can only be removed partially (an unresectable or partially resectable tumor rarely occurs; however, it most commonly occurs around the spine, pelvis, and sacrum). In the case when the tumor can only be partially removed, radiation may be used to destroy the residual tumor cells. Rarely, radiation may be prescribed for some benign tumors, only under special circumstances. In general, a doctor may choose to refrain from using radiation for benign tumors except for very extreme and unusual circumstances because of the risk that the radiation may turn the benign tumor into a malignant tumor (also known as malignant degeneration).

Whenever radiation is prescribed, the benefits of radiation must be weighed against the risks. The complications include stiffness and scarring, burns, muscle contractures, chronic swelling and lymphedema, muscle atrophy, muscle weakness, hair loss in the exposed area, skin burns, radiation induced cancers of bone and soft tissue, malignant degeneration of benign tumors, nerve damage, nerve pain, and nerve paralysis. Radiation induced changes and damage continue to progress with time and compound year after year. The severity of these complications varies according to the dose of radiation administered and varies between patients.

Most patients experience minor radiation induced changes or complications. Precautions are taken to minimize these complications. Physical therapy is required during and after radiation. Specific exercises should be continued for the rest of the patient's life. The entire course of radiation depends upon the dose that is administered. Typically three to four weeks of treatment is required. The patient goes for the treatment daily, five days per week.

Radiation can also be delivered to the wound by catheters that are planted in the wound at the time of surgery. This is referred to as brachytherapy. Some doctors do not prefer to use brachytherapy because of the high wound complication rates that occur with its use. Additionally, some believe it does not reliably deliver the radiation to all areas of the surgical bed where it is needed. For these reasons, external beam radiation delivered postoperatively may be preferred.

The required field is most reliably treated and since the radiation is administered when the wound is healed, wound complications are rarely an issue.

Surgery

Nowadays, almost all high grade bone sarcomas (malignancies; cancers) are treated with limb sparing surgery. (Limb sparing surgery refers to surgically removing the tumor without amputating the extremity). The bone that the tumor came from usually requires removal along with the joint that is next to the tumor. Once the tumor, bone, and joint are removed, the defect (bone and joint) must be restored with a metallic endoprosthetic replacement or some alternative means of restoring the resected bone. Approximately, 95% of high grade bone sarcomas can be treated with limb sparing surgery.

Amputations are rarely performed for primary tumors. If you have a bone sarcoma and you are told that you need an amputation, you should seek an additional opinion. The success of limb sparing surgery can be attributed largely to: the development of effective preoperative and postoperative chemotherapy protocols (kills the tumor and any residual cells which prevents the tumor from coming back after it is removed); advances and increasing experience with complex surgical techniques; the development of durable, mechanically sound and highly functional, metallic endoprosthetic bone and joint replacements; and advances in imaging studies such as computed tomography (CT) scans and magnetic resonance imaging (MRI) scans which allow the surgeon to more accurately plan the surgery.

Almost all benign bone tumors (not cancerous) are treated less aggressively than the malignant bone tumors because they have less chance of coming back after being treated and they do not spread to other body parts. They are rarely ever treated with an amputation. Less complicated surgery is usually performed. Rarely must the bone and joint be resected (removed in entirety). Depending upon the type of tumor, the tumor can usually be curetted (scooped out of the bone). A high speed drill is used to shave the cavity walls until they appear normal. This is referred to as a resectional curettage. Liquid nitrogen (cryosurgery) may be used to freeze the tumor cavity and kill any residual microscopic tumor cells depending upon the type of tumor and its propensity to come back after curetting it; it is therefore used primarily in the treatment of benign aggressive tumors. Cryosurgery minimizes the risk of the tumor coming back. After curetting the tumor there is a bony defect (a hole in the bone) that can usually be fixed with methylmethacrylate (bone cement; the hole is filled with bone cement) and bone graft. Metallic rods, plates, and screws may utilized to prevent the bone from fracturing (breaking).

Metastatic carcinoma to bone (metastatic cancer) is treated surgically if there is risk that the bone is going to fracture (break), if the bone has already fractured through the tumor, if there is a large soft tissue component ready to invade adjacent nerves, blood vessels, the chest, or other critical structures, or if the bone tumor represents the only site of metastatic disease (isolated site of metastatic disease). In instances where the tumor represents the only site of disease, the tumor may be treated surgically to remove all gross disease which may cure the patient or may make chemotherapy or immunotherapy protocols more effective. Radiation or other more conservative measures are often utilized if the patient does not meet these criteria or if the patient is too ill to undergo surgery. Surgery for metastatic carcinomas usually consists of stabilizing the bone with a rod and cement or with a long stem joint replacement. Occasionally the tumor will be removed with the bone and joint and the bone and joint will require a metallic endoprosthetic replacement with cement. In general, the operation that is chosen is the procedure that is most reliable with least chance of complications or failure. It should be the procedure that will relieve the patient's pain and restore function most rapidly and reliably. Radiation may be prescribed postoperatively.

Surgical Methods

Several different surgical methods are used to treat bone tumors. The type of method that is chosen depends on the type of tumor, the grade of the tumor, the size of the tumor, and the tumor's inherent ability to come back after it is removed. The types of surgical procedures can be divided into several broad categories:

Curettage and cryosurgery: A curettage refers to scooping the tumor out of the bone. This leaves a cavity in the bone (much like a cavity of a tooth). The sides of the cavity are scraped with hand curettes (instruments that look like small deep spoons with sharp edges) and typically shaved with a high speed drill (like a dental drill). The high speed drill removes additional microscopic tumor cells. A curettage is typically performed for benign tumors and metastatic tumors (carcinomas).

Cryosurgery refers to freezing the tumor cavity to subzero temperatures with liquid nitrogen in order to kill residual microscopic tumor cells after the curettage and burr drilling. A curettage, alone, may be performed for benign tumors that have small to no risk of returning after the curettage. Curettage and cryosurgery is performed for benign aggressive tumors (for example, giant cell tumor)—tumors that have a significant risk of coming back after a curettage alone. If these tumors come back they cause more bony destruction and become more difficult to cure.

Once the tumor is removed, a hole in the bone exists that must be restored to prevent the bone from breaking and to allow function to return. The hole is usually filled with cement or a combination of cement and bone graft (bone from the patient's own pelvic bone). Metal rods, screws, and plates may be placed to give additional support to prevent a fracture after surgery. Stabilization procedures are usually performed for metastatic carcinomas. The tumor is usually curetted and packed with cement. Cryosurgery may be used and the bone is stabilized with a metal rod, screws, or plates to fix or prevent any fractures from occurring, facilitate nursing care, restore function, and relieve pain. Radiation may be prescribed postoperatively.

Limb sparing surgery: A limb sparing surgery is also called a resection. Resections are usually performed for malignant tumors and very large benign aggressive tumors that have destroyed almost the entire bone. A radical resection is typically performed for high grade tumors. Limb sparing surgery can be performed for approximately 95% of malignant bone tumors. With a resection, the tumor is removed with the bone (or part of the bone) and usually the adjacent joint.

The bone and joint must be restored. This part of the procedure is called a reconstruction. Usually a metal prosthesis (replica of the bone and joint) is used to restore (reconstruct) the bony and joint deficiency. Metal prostheses restore the patient to good function rapidly and are associated with few short term complications (for example, infections) so that chemotherapy can be resumed promptly after surgery (few complications to delay chemotherapy if the type of tumor being treated requires chemotherapy). Ninety to 99% of prostheses last 10 years depending upon the anatomic site in which they are placed.

Amputation: An amputation refers to removal of the entire extremity without replacing it. There are several different types of amputations. The name given to the type of amputation depends upon how much of the limb is removed. Some special names given to amputations are as follows:

- **Transmetatarsal amputation:** removing the forefoot by cutting through the metatarsals

- **Chopart amputation:** amputation through the midfoot closer to the ankle

- **Ankle disarticulation:** amputation through the ankle joint (between the tibia/fibula and the talus)

- **Syme amputation:** removal through the lower tibia

- **Below the knee amputation (BKA):** amputation through the tibia and fibula (through the leg bones) usually approximately 6–8 inches below the knee

- **Above the knee amputation (AKA):** amputation through the thigh bone

- **Hip disarticulation:** Removal of the entire leg by cutting through the hip joint (between the femoral head and the acetabulum)

- **Hemipelvectomy:** removal of the entire lower extremity including the same side of the pelvis

- **Extended hemipelvectomy:** removal of the entire lower extremity including the same side of the pelvis and the sacrum on the same side

- **Ray amputation:** removal of a digit including a portion of the hand

- **Shoulder disarticulation:** removal of the upper extremity (entire arm) by cutting through the shoulder joint (between the humeral head and the glenoid)

- **Forequarter amputation:** removal of the entire upper extremity including the shoulder and scapula

Summarizing the Differences between Sarcomas and Carcinomas

Sarcomas and carcinomas are types of malignant tumors that can affect bones. They are derived from different types of cells. Sarcomas are derived from mesodermal (mesenchymal cells) and carcinomas are derived from epithelial types of cells. Sarcomas and carcinomas grow and spread differently.

Sarcomas grow like "ball-like" masses and tend to push adjacent structures like arteries, nerves, veins away. They compress adjacent muscles into a pseudocapsule that contains microscopic projections of the tumor referred to as satellite nodules. The local growth of sarcomas like a ball enables resection in most instances. Sarcomas tend to arise primarily (directly) from bone as opposed to spreading to bone from another site. Sarcomas spread most commonly to the lungs. They can also spread to other bones (that is, arise from a bone and spread to other bones) and to the liver. These are the most common sites of spread. Sarcomas rarely spread to lymph nodes.

Carcinomas grow in an infiltrative manner and grow through infiltration or invasion of adjacent structures. They more easily invade adjacent nerves, blood vessels, and muscles. They do not form a pseudocapsular layer and therefore it is difficult to determine its exact anatomic extent during surgery. This makes it more difficult to remove entirely with surgery. Carcinomas spread to lymph nodes, lungs, bones, and many other organs depending on the type of carcinoma. Carcinomas involve bone secondarily, that is by spreading from another site, such as the breast, to the bone. A patient can have the primary site removed and treated (for example, the breast cancer removed) and years later develop a bone tumor/metastasis from the old breast cancer.

Section 70.2

Osteosarcoma

"Childhood Cancer: Osteosarcoma," was provided by KidsHealth, one of the largest resources online for medically reviewed health information written for parents, kids, and teens. For more articles like this one, visit www.KidsHealth.org, or www.TeensHealth.org. © 2005 The Nemours Foundation.

Osteosarcoma is the most common type of bone cancer, and the sixth most common type of cancer in children. Although other types of cancer can eventually spread to parts of the skeleton, osteosarcoma is one of the few that actually begin in bones and sometimes spread (or metastasize) elsewhere.

Because osteosarcoma usually develops from osteoblasts (the cells that make growing bone), it most commonly affects teens who are experiencing a growth spurt. Boys are more likely to have osteosarcoma than girls, and most cases of osteosarcoma involve the knee.

Most osteosarcomas arise from random and unpredictable errors in the DNA of growing bone cells during times of intense bone growth. There currently isn't an effective way to prevent this type of cancer. But with the proper diagnosis and treatment, most kids with osteosarcoma do recover.

Risk for Childhood Osteosarcoma

Osteosarcoma is most often seen in teenage boys, and evidence shows that teens who are taller than average have an added risk for developing the disease.

Kids who have inherited one of the rare cancer syndromes also are at higher risk for osteosarcoma. These syndromes include retinoblastoma (a malignant tumor that develops in the retina, usually in children younger than age 2) and Li-Fraumeni syndrome (a kind of inherited genetic mutation). Because exposure to radiation is another trigger for DNA mutations, children who have received radiation treatments for a prior episode of cancer are also at increased risk for osteosarcoma.

Symptoms of Osteosarcoma

The most common symptoms of osteosarcoma are pain and swelling in a child's leg or arm. It occurs most often in the longer bones of the body—such as above or below the knee or in the upper arm near the shoulder. Pain may be worse during exercise or at night, and a lump or swelling may develop in the affected area up to several weeks after the pain starts. In osteosarcoma of the leg, the child may also develop an unexplained limp. In some cases, the first sign of the disease is a broken arm or leg, because the cancer has weakened the bone to make it vulnerable to a break.

If your child or teen has any of the above symptoms, it's important to see a doctor.

Diagnosing Osteosarcoma

To diagnose osteosarcoma, your child's doctor will likely perform a physical exam, obtain a detailed medical history, and order x-rays to detect any changes in bone structure. The doctor will probably order a bone biopsy to obtain a sample of the tumor for examination in the lab.

The doctor may also order a computed tomography (CT) scan of the affected area, which will find the best area to biopsy and show whether the osteosarcoma has spread from the bone into nearby muscles and fat. Magnetic resonance imaging (MRI) is also often used.

Sometimes the doctor does a needle biopsy, using a long hollow needle to take a sample of the tumor. A local anesthesia is typically used in the area that's being biopsied. Alternatively, the doctor may order an open biopsy, in which a portion of the tumor is removed in the operating room by a surgeon while the child is under general anesthesia.

If a diagnosis of osteosarcoma is made, the doctor will order CT scans of your child's chest, as well as a bone scan and, sometimes, additional MRI studies. These will show if the cancer has spread to any part of the body beyond the original tumor. These tests will be repeated after treatment starts to determine how well it is working and whether the cancer is continuing to spread.

Treating Osteosarcoma

Treatment of osteosarcoma in children includes surgery (to remove cancerous cells or tumors) and chemotherapy (the use of medical drugs to kill cancer cells). Surgery often can effectively remove bone cancer, while chemotherapy can help eliminate remaining cancer cells in the body.

Surgical treatment: Surgical treatments for osteosarcoma consist of either amputation or limb-salvage surgery.

Currently, most teens with osteosarcomas involving an arm or leg can be treated with limb-salvage surgery rather than amputation. In limb-salvage surgery, only the osteosarcoma is removed, leaving a gap in the bone that is filled by a bone graft, which is usually taken from the patient's own pelvis (hipbone).

If the cancer has spread to the nerves and blood vessels surrounding the original tumor on the bone, amputation (removing part of a limb along with the osteosarcoma) is often the only choice.

When osteosarcoma has spread to the lungs or elsewhere, surgery may also be performed to remove tumors in these distant locations.

Chemotherapy: Chemotherapy is usually given both before and after surgery. It eliminates small pockets of cancer cells in the body, even those too small to appear on medical scans. A child or teen with osteosarcoma is given the chemotherapy drugs intravenously (through a vein) or orally (by mouth). The drugs enter the bloodstream and work to kill cancer in parts of the body where the disease has spread, such as the lungs or other organs.

Short-Term and Long-Term Side Effects

Amputation carries its own short-term and long-term side effects. It usually takes at least three to six months until a young person learns to use a prosthetic (artificial) leg or arm, and this is just the beginning of long-term psychological and social rehabilitation.

Many of the medications used in chemotherapy also carry the risk of both short-term and long-term problems. Short-term effects include anemia, abnormal bleeding, and increased risk of infection due to destruction of the bone marrow, as well as kidney damage and menstrual irregularities. Some drugs carry a risk of bladder inflammation and bleeding into the urine, hearing loss, and liver damage. Others may cause heart and skin problems. Years after chemotherapy for osteosarcoma, patients have an increased risk of developing other cancers.

Chances for a Cure

Recent studies have reported that survival rates of 60% to 80% are possible for osteosarcoma that hasn't spread beyond the tumor, depending on the success of chemotherapy.

Osteosarcoma that has spread cannot always be treated as success-fully. Also, a child whose osteosarcoma is located in an arm or leg gen-erally has a better prognosis than one whose disease involves the ribs, shoulder blades, spine, or hipbones.

New Treatments

Treatments are being developed and researched with new chemo-therapy drugs. Other research is focused on the role certain growth factors may play in the development of osteosarcoma. This research may be used to develop new medications to slow these growth factors as a way to treat the cancer.

For osteosarcomas that cannot be removed surgically, studies are now underway to test treatments that use new combinations of che-motherapy and localized, high-dose radiation.

Section 70.3

Ewing Sarcoma

From PDQ® Cancer Information Summary. National Cancer Institute; Bethesda, MD. Ewing's Family of Tumors (PDQ®): Treatment - Patient. Updated 02/2006. Available at: http://cancer.gov. Accessed April 30, 2006.

The Ewing family of tumors include: Ewing tumor of bone, extra-osseous Ewing (tumor growing outside of the bone), primitive neuro-ectodermal tumor (PNET; also known as peripheral neuroepithelioma), and Askin tumor (PNET of the chest wall). These tumors are rare diseases in which cancer (malignant) cells are found in the bone and soft tissues. Ewing family of tumors most frequently occurs in teen-agers.

If a patient has symptoms (such as pain, stiffness, or tenderness in the bone) the doctor may order x-rays and other tests. The doctor may also cut out a piece of tissue from the affected area. This is called a biopsy. The tissue will be looked at under a microscope to see if there are any cancer cells. This test may be done in the hospital.

The chance of recovery (prognosis) and choice of treatment depend on the location, size, and stage of the cancer (how far the cancer has spread), how the cancer cells react to the treatment, and the patient's age and general health.

Stages of the Ewing Family of Tumors

Once one of the Ewing family of tumors has been found, more tests will be done to find out if cancer cells have spread to other parts of the body. This is called staging. At present, there is no formal staging system for the Ewing family of tumors. Instead, most patients are grouped depending on whether cancer is found in only one part of the body (localized disease) or whether cancer has spread from one part of the body to another (metastatic disease). Extraosseous Ewing has been grouped using the rhabdomyosarcoma staging system because they are both soft tissue tumors. Your doctor needs to know where the cancer is located and how far the disease has spread to plan treatment. The following groups are used for the Ewing family of tumors.

- **Localized:** The cancer cells have not been shown to have spread beyond the bone in which the cancer began or are found only in the bone and nearby tissues.

- **Metastatic:** The cancer cells have spread from the bone in which the cancer began to other parts of the body. The cancer most often spreads to the lung, other bones, and bone marrow (the spongy tissue inside of the large bones of your body that makes red blood cells). Spread of cancer to the lymph nodes (small bean-shaped structures found throughout your body which produce and store infection-fighting cells) or the central nervous system (brain and spinal cord) is less common.

- **Recurrent:** Recurrent disease means that the cancer has come back (recurred) after it has been treated. It may come back in the tissues where it first started or it may come back in another part of the body.

Treatment Option Overview

It is important for patients to be evaluated by several specialists as early as possible so that treatment may be coordinated effectively from the beginning. These specialists may include: a radiologist, chemotherapist, pathologist, surgeon, or orthopedic oncologist, and a radiation oncologist. Before treatment decisions are made patients will probably be required to undergo several diagnostic tests including tissue sampling, x-rays, magnetic resonance imaging (MRI) scans, and computed tomography (CT) scans.

There are treatments for all patients with one of the Ewing family of tumors. Three kinds of treatment are used:

- **Surgery:** Surgery may be used in certain cases to try to remove the cancer and some of the tissue around it. Surgery may also be used to remove any tumor that is left after chemotherapy or radiation therapy.

- **Radiation:** Radiation therapy uses x-rays or other high-energy rays to kill cancer cells and shrink tumors. Radiation for the Ewing family of tumors usually comes from a machine outside the body (external radiation therapy). Clinical trials are evaluating radiation given inside the body during surgery (intraoperative radiation therapy).

- **Chemotherapy:** Chemotherapy uses drugs to kill cancer cells. Chemotherapy may be taken by pill, or it may be put into the body by a needle in a vein or muscle. Chemotherapy is called a systemic treatment because the drug enters the blood stream, travels through the body, and can kill cancer cells throughout the body. When more than one drug is given to kill tumor cells, the treatment is called combination chemotherapy. Treatment for the Ewing family of tumors may include surgery or radiation to remove or shrink the tumor as much as possible, followed by chemotherapy to kill any cancer cells that remain in the body.

A supplement to the treatment options listed above is myeloablative therapy with stem cell support. Myeloablative therapy is a very intense regimen of chemotherapy designed to destroy all cells that divide rapidly. These cells include some blood cells and hair cells, as well as malignant (cancer) cells. Stem cells are self-renewing cells that create all of the other various types of blood cells. Stem cell support involves enriching the stem cells to increase the number of these important cells circulating in the blood after the chemotherapy has been given to kill the remaining tumor cells.

Treatment for the Ewing family of tumors depends on where the cancer is located, how far the cancer has spread, the stage of the disease, and the age and general health of the patient.

A patient may receive treatment that is considered standard based on its effectiveness in a number of patients in past studies or may choose to go into a clinical trial. Not all patients are cured with standard therapy and some standard treatments may have more side effects than are desired. For these reasons, clinical trials are designed to find better ways to treat cancer patients and are based on the most up-to-date information. Clinical trials for the Ewing family of tumors are ongoing in many parts of the country. If you want more information, call the Cancer Information Service at 800-4-CANCER (800-422-6237); TTY at 800-332-8615.

Treatment Options by Stage

Treatment for localized tumors of the Ewing family may be one of the following:

- A clinical trial of chemotherapy followed by radiation therapy

- Combination chemotherapy followed by surgery with or without radiation therapy

- A clinical trial of intensified chemotherapy

- A randomized trial of post-surgical chemotherapy with or without stem cell transplant

Treatment for metastatic tumors of the Ewing family may be one of the following:

- Combination chemotherapy followed by radiation therapy and/or surgery

- High-dose chemotherapy with or without radiation therapy plus additional stem cell support

- A clinical trial of intensive chemotherapy with multiple chemotherapy drug combinations

For recurrent tumors of the Ewing family, treatment depends on where the cancer recurred, how the cancer was treated before, as well as individual patient factors. Chemotherapy may be used for patients who did not receive previous chemotherapy. Radiation treatment may be given to reduce symptoms. Surgery may be used to remove tumors that have spread to the lungs or other organs. Clinical trials are testing new treatments.

Chapter 71

Soft Tissue Sarcomas

Chapter Contents

Section 71.1

Questions and Answers about Soft Tissue Sarcomas

"Soft Tissue Sarcomas: Questions and Answers,"
National Cancer Institute fact sheet updated on May 6, 2002.

What is soft tissue?

The term soft tissue refers to tissues that connect, support, or surround other structures and organs of the body. Soft tissue includes muscles, tendons (bands of fiber that connect muscles to bones), fibrous tissues, fat, blood vessels, nerves, and synovial tissues (tissues around joints).

What are soft tissue sarcomas?

Malignant (cancerous) tumors that develop in soft tissue are called sarcomas, a term that comes from a Greek word meaning "fleshy growth." There are many different kinds of soft tissue sarcomas. They are grouped together because they share certain microscopic characteristics, produce similar symptoms, and are generally treated in similar ways. (Bone tumors, osteosarcomas, are also called sarcomas, but are in a separate category because they have different clinical and microscopic characteristics and are treated differently.)

Sarcomas can invade surrounding tissue and can metastasize (spread) to other organs of the body, forming secondary tumors. The cells of secondary tumors are similar to those of the primary (original) cancer. Secondary tumors are referred to as "metastatic soft tissue sarcoma" because they are part of the same cancer and are not a new disease.

Some tumors of the soft tissue are benign (noncancerous). These tumors do not spread and are rarely life-threatening. However, benign tumors can crowd nearby organs and cause symptoms or interfere with normal body functions.

What are the possible causes of soft tissue sarcomas?

Scientists do not fully understand why some people develop sarcomas while the vast majority do not. However, by identifying common characteristics in groups with unusually high occurrence rates, researchers have been able to single out some factors that may play a role in causing soft tissue sarcomas.

Studies suggest that workers who are exposed to phenoxyacetic acid in herbicides and chlorophenols in wood preservatives may have an increased risk of developing soft tissue sarcomas. An unusual percentage of patients with a rare blood vessel tumor, angiosarcoma of the liver, have been exposed to vinyl chloride in their work. This substance is used in the manufacture of certain plastics.

In the early 1900s, when scientists were just discovering the potential uses of radiation to treat disease, little was known about safe dosage levels and precise methods of delivery. At that time, radiation was used to treat a variety of noncancerous medical problems, including enlargement of the tonsils, adenoids, and thymus gland. Later, researchers found that high doses of radiation caused soft tissue sarcomas in some patients. Because of this risk, radiation treatment for cancer is now planned to ensure that the maximum dosage of radiation is delivered to diseased tissue while surrounding healthy tissue is protected as much as possible.

Researchers believe that a retrovirus plays an indirect role in the development of Kaposi sarcoma, a rare cancer of the cells that line blood vessels in the skin and mucus membranes. Kaposi sarcoma often occurs in patients with AIDS (acquired immune deficiency syndrome). AIDS-related Kaposi sarcoma, however, has different characteristics and is treated differently than typical soft tissue sarcomas.

Studies have focused on genetic alterations that may lead to the development of soft tissue sarcomas. Scientists have also found a small number of families in which more than one member in the same generation has developed sarcoma. There have also been reports of a few families in which relatives of children with sarcoma have developed other forms of cancer at an unusually high rate. Sarcomas in these family clusters, which represent a very small fraction of all cases, may be related to a rare inherited genetic alteration.

Certain inherited diseases are associated with an increased risk of developing soft tissue sarcomas. For example, people with Li-Fraumeni syndrome (associated with alterations in the p53 gene) or von Recklinghausen disease (also called neurofibromatosis, and associated with alterations in the NF1 gene) are at an increased risk of developing soft tissue sarcomas.

Where do soft tissue sarcomas develop?

Soft tissue sarcomas can arise almost anywhere in the body. About 50 percent occur in the extremities (the arms, legs, hands, or feet), 40 percent occur in the trunk (chest, back, hips, shoulders, and abdomen), and 10 percent occur in the head and neck.

How often do soft tissue sarcomas occur?

Soft tissue sarcomas are relatively uncommon cancers. They account for less than 1 percent of all new cancer cases each year. In 2000, there will be an estimated 8,100 new cases of soft tissue sarcoma in the United States. Approximately 850 to 900 of these cases will occur among children and adolescents under age 20.

What are the symptoms of soft tissue sarcomas?

In their early stages, soft tissue sarcomas usually do not cause symptoms. Because soft tissue is relatively elastic, tumors can grow rather large, pushing aside normal tissue, before they are felt or cause any problems. The first noticeable symptom is usually a painless lump or swelling. As the tumor grows, it may cause other symptoms, such as pain or soreness, as it presses against nearby nerves and muscles.

How are soft tissue sarcomas diagnosed?

The only reliable way to determine whether a soft tissue tumor is benign or malignant is through a surgical biopsy. Therefore, all soft tissue lumps that persist or grow should be biopsied. During this procedure, a doctor makes an incision or uses a special needle to remove a sample of tumor tissue. A pathologist examines the tissue under a microscope. If cancer is present, the pathologist can usually determine the type of cancer and its grade. The grade of the tumor is determined by how abnormal the cancer cells appear when examined under a microscope. The grade predicts the probable growth rate of the tumor and its tendency to spread. Low-grade sarcomas, although cancerous, are unlikely to metastasize. High-grade sarcomas are more likely to spread to other parts of the body.

How are soft tissue sarcomas treated?

In general, treatment for soft tissue sarcomas depends on the stage of the cancer. The stage of the sarcoma is based on the size and grade of the tumor, and whether the cancer has spread to the lymph nodes or other parts of the body (metastasized). Treatment options for soft tissue sarcomas include surgery, radiation therapy, and chemotherapy.

- Surgery is the most common treatment for soft tissue sarcomas. If possible, the doctor may remove the cancer and a safe margin of the healthy tissue around it. Depending on the size and location of the sarcoma, it may occasionally be necessary to remove all or part of an arm or leg (amputation). However, the need for amputation rarely arises; no more than 10 percent to 15 percent of individuals with sarcoma undergo amputation. In most cases, limb-sparing surgery is an option to avoid amputating the arm

Table 71.1: Major Types of Soft Tissue Sarcomas in Adults

Tissue of Origin	Type of Cancer	Usual Location in the Body
Fibrous tissue	Fibrosarcoma	Arms, legs, trunk
	Malignant fibrous histiocytoma	Legs
Fat	Liposarcoma	Arms, legs, trunk
Muscle		
Striated muscle	Rhabdomyosarcoma	Arms, legs
Smooth muscle	Leiomyosarcoma	Uterus, digestive tract
Blood vessels	Hemangiosarcoma	Arms, legs, trunk
	Kaposi sarcoma	Legs, trunk
Lymph vessels	Lymphangiosarcoma	Arms
Synovial tissue (linings of joint cavities, tendon sheaths)	Synovial sarcoma	Legs
Peripheral nerves	Neurofibrosarcoma	Arms, legs, trunk
Cartilage and bone-forming tissue	Extraskeletal chondrosarcoma	Legs
	Extraskeletal osteosarcoma	Legs, trunk (not involving the bone)

or leg. In limb-sparing surgery, as much of the tumor is removed as possible, and radiation therapy or chemotherapy are given either before the surgery to shrink the tumor or after surgery to kill the remaining cancer cells.

Table 71.2: Major Types of Soft Tissue Sarcomas in Children

Tissue of Origin	Type of Cancer	Usual Location in the Body	Most Common Ages
Muscle			
Striated muscle	Rhabdomyosarcoma		
	Embryonal	Head and neck, genitourinary tract	Infant–4
	Alveolar	Arms, legs, head, and neck	Infant–19
Smooth muscle	Leiomyosarcoma	Trunk	15–19
Fibrous tissue	Fibrosarcoma	Arms and legs	15–19
	Malignant fibrous histiocytoma	Legs	15–19
	Dermatofibrosarcoma	Trunk	15–19
Fat	Liposarcoma	Arms and Legs	15–19
Blood vessels	Infantile hemangioma-pericytoma	Arms, legs, trunk, head, and neck	Infant–4
Synovial tissue (linings of joint cavities, tendon sheaths)	Synovial sarcoma	Legs, arms, and trunk	15–19
Peripheral nerves	Malignant peripheral nerve sheath tumors (also called neurofibrosarcomas, malignant schwannomas, and neurogenic sarcomas)	Arms, legs, and trunk	15–19
Muscular nerves	Alveolar soft part sarcoma	Arms and legs	Infant–19
Cartilage and bone-forming tissue	Extraskeletal myxoid chondrosarcoma	Legs	10–14
	Extraskeletal mesenchymal	Legs	10–14

- Radiation therapy (treatment with high-dose x-rays) may be used either before surgery to shrink tumors or after surgery to kill any cancer cells that may have been left behind.

- Chemotherapy (treatment with anticancer drugs) may be used with radiation therapy either before or after surgery to try to shrink the tumor or kill any remaining cancer cells. If the cancer has spread to other areas of the body, chemotherapy may be used to shrink tumors and reduce the pain and discomfort they cause, but is unlikely to eradicate the disease. The use of chemotherapy to prevent the spread of soft tissue sarcomas has not been proven to be effective. Patients with soft tissue sarcomas usually receive chemotherapy intravenously (injected into a blood vessel).

Doctors are conducting clinical trials in the hope of finding new, more effective treatments for soft tissue sarcomas, and better ways to use current treatments. Clinical trials are in progress at hospitals and cancer centers around the country. Clinical trials are an important part of the development of new methods of treatment. Before a new treatment can be recommended for general use, doctors conduct clinical trials to find out whether the treatment is safe for patients and effective against the disease.

Patients who are interested in learning more about participating in clinical trials can call the National Cancer Institute (NCI')s Cancer Information Service (800-4-CANCER) or access NCI's Cancer.gov website at http://www.cancer.gov/clinical_trials.

Section 71.2

Synovial Sarcoma

"Synovial Sarcoma: Questions and Answers,"
National Cancer Institute fact sheet, reviewed June 29, 2005.

What is synovial sarcoma?

Synovial sarcoma is a type of soft tissue sarcoma. Soft tissue sarcomas are cancers of the muscle, fat, fibrous tissue, blood vessels, or other supporting tissue of the body, including synovial tissue. Synovial tissue lines the cavities of joints, such as the knee or elbow, tendons (tissues that connect muscle to bone), and bursae (fluid-filled, cushioning sacs in the spaces between tendons, ligaments, and bones). Although synovial sarcoma does not have a clearly defined cause, genetic factors are believed to influence the development of this disease.

How often does synovial sarcoma occur?

Synovial sarcoma is rare. It accounts for between 5 and 10 percent of the approximately 10,000 new soft tissue sarcomas reported each year.[1] Synovial sarcoma occurs mostly in young adults, with a median age of 26.5.[1] Approximately 30 percent of patients with synovial sarcoma are younger than 20. This disease occurs more often in men than in women.[1]

Where does synovial sarcoma develop?

About 50 percent of synovial sarcomas develop in the legs, especially the knees. The second most common location is the arms.[2] Less frequently, the disease develops in the trunk, head and neck region, or the abdomen.[1,2] It is common for synovial cancer to recur (come back), usually within the first two years after treatment. Half of the cases of synovial sarcoma metastasize (spread to other areas of the body) to the lungs, lymph nodes, or bone marrow.[1]

What are the symptoms of synovial sarcoma?

Synovial sarcoma is a slow-growing tumor. Because it grows slowly, a person may not have or notice symptoms for some time, resulting in a delay in diagnosis. The most common symptoms of synovial sarcoma are swelling or a mass that may be tender or painful.[1] The tumor may limit range of motion or press against nerves and cause numbness. The symptoms of synovial sarcoma can be mistaken for those of inflammation of the joints, the bursae, or synovial tissue. These noncancerous conditions are called arthritis, bursitis, and synovitis, respectively.

How is synovial sarcoma diagnosed?

The doctor may use the following procedures and tests to diagnose synovial sarcoma:

- **Biopsy:** Tissue is removed for examination under a microscope.

- **Immunohistochemical analysis:** Tumor tissue is tested for certain antigen and antibody interactions common to synovial sarcoma.

- **Ultrastructural findings:** The tissue is examined using an ultramicroscope and electron microscope.

- **Genetic testing:** Tissue is tested for a specific chromosome abnormality common to synovial sarcoma.

How is synovial sarcoma treated?

The type of treatment depends on the age of the patient, the location of the tumor, its size, its grade (how abnormal the cancer cells look under a microscope and how likely the tumor will quickly grow and spread), and the extent of the disease. The most common treatment is surgery to remove the entire tumor with negative margins (no cancer cells are found at the edge or border of the tissue removed during surgery). If the first surgery does not obtain negative tissue margins, a second surgery may be needed.

The patient may also receive radiation therapy before or after surgery to control the tumor or decrease the chance of recurrence (cancer coming back). The use of intraoperative radiation therapy (radiation aimed directly at the tumor during surgery) and brachytherapy (radioactive material sealed in needles, wires, seeds, or catheters, and placed directly into or near a tumor) are under study.

Patients may also receive chemotherapy alone or in combination with radiation therapy.

Are clinical trials (research studies) available? Where can people get more information about clinical trials?

Yes. Participation in clinical trials is an important treatment option for many people with synovial sarcoma. Studies are in progress to determine the effectiveness of biological therapies (treatment to stimulate or restore the ability of the immune system to fight cancer), including monoclonal antibodies, and chemotherapy with hyperthermia (kills tumor cells by heating them to several degrees above body temperature).

People interested in taking part in a clinical trial should talk with their doctor. Information about clinical trials is available from the National Cancer Institute (NCI)'s Cancer Information Service (CIS) at 800-4-CANCER and in the NCI booklet "Taking Part in Clinical Trials: What Cancer Patients Need To Know," which can be found at http://www.cancer.gov/publications on the internet. This booklet describes how research studies are carried out and explains their possible benefits and risks. Further information about clinical trials is available at http://www.cancer.gov/clinicaltrials on the NCI website. The website offers detailed information about specific ongoing studies by linking to PDQ®, the NCI's cancer information database. The CIS also provides information from PDQ.

Selected References

1. Zeitouni N, Cheney RT, Oseroff AR. Unusual cutaneous malignancies. In: Williams CJ, Krikorian JG, Green MR, Raghavan D, editors. *Textbook of Uncommon Cancers*. 2nd ed. New York: John Wiley & Sons, 1999.

2. Brennan M, Singer S, Maki R, O'Sullivan B. Sarcomas of the soft tissue and bone. In: DeVita VT Jr., Hellman S, Rosenberg SA, editors. Cancer: *Principles and Practice of Oncology*. Vol. 2. 7th ed. Philadelphia: Lippincott Williams & Wilkins, 2004.

Section 71.3

Rhabdomyosarcoma and Non-Rhabdomyosarcoma Soft Tissue Sarcoma

"Rhabdomyosarcoma for the Pediatric Patient," and "Non-Rhabdomyosarcoma Soft Tissue Sarcoma for the Pediatric Patient," are reprinted with permission from The University of Texas M.D. Anderson Cancer Center. © 2004 M.D. Anderson Cancer Center.

Rhabdomyosarcoma for the Pediatric Patient

What is rhabdomyosarcoma?

Rhabdomyosarcoma is a cancer that develops from muscle cells or other soft tissue cells. It can arise in many different areas of the body. The most common sites are the head and neck, bladder, prostate gland, arms, legs, and vagina. Other less common sites are the chest, abdomen, genital area, and anal area.

Rhabdomyosarcoma accounts for more than half of all the soft tissue sarcomas diagnosed in children. Most children are diagnosed younger than 9 years of age, but rhabdomyosarcoma can occur at any age. It is slightly more common in males than in females.

What are the symptoms of rhabdomyosarcoma?

The symptoms of rhabdomyosarcoma depend upon the location of the tumor. For example if the tumor is located in the head or neck, there may be swelling around the eye or a lump in the neck. Tumors of the nose and sinus may cause a nasal voice, blockage of the airway, nosebleeds, and difficulty swallowing. If the tumor is located in the arm or leg there may be a tender or enlarged area in the muscle. Tumors in the bladder may cause bloody urine or difficulty in urination.

How is rhabdomyosarcoma diagnosed and treated?

If your child has symptoms of rhabdomyosarcoma, his or her doctor may order several diagnostic tests including a biopsy of the tumor,

795

x-rays, a computed tomography (CT) scan, a skeletal survey, bone scans and bone marrow aspiration and biopsy. These tests will help to determine the size and location of the tumor and whether it has spread to another part of the body. This is called staging. It is important to know the stage of the disease to plan treatment.

Rhabdomyosarcoma is a very aggressive tumor and must be treated aggressively. Three types of treatment are used, most often in combination with each other: surgery, chemotherapy, and radiation therapy. Bone marrow transplantation is a treatment that some have recommended for recurrent rhabdomyosarcoma, but its effectiveness is not established at this time. Instead, different combinations of drugs, surgery, and possibly radiation therapy can be used.

Non-Rhabdomyosarcoma Soft Tissue: Sarcoma for the Pediatric Patient

What is non-rhabdomyosarcoma soft tissue sarcoma?

Childhood soft tissue sarcoma is a disease in which cancer cells begin growing in soft tissue. The soft tissues include muscles, tendons (bands of fiber that connect muscles to bones), fibrous (connective) tissues, fat, blood vessels, nerves, and synovial tissues (tissues around joints). Soft tissues connect, support, and surround other body parts and organs.

Soft tissue sarcomas are rare in children and adolescents. When they occur they are most commonly found in the trunk, arms, and legs. Soft tissue sarcomas are more likely to develop in children who have specific genetic or infectious conditions or who have previously received radiation therapy.

Soft tissue sarcomas are classified according to the type of soft tissue they originate from. The types of soft tissue sarcoma include the following:

- Desmoid tumor
- Liposarcoma
- Hemangiopericytoma
- Extraskeletal osteosarcoma
- Clear cell sarcoma
- Fibrosarcoma
- Leiomyosarcoma

- Synovial sarcoma
- Extraskeletal chondrosarcoma
- Epithelioid sarcoma
- Malignant fibrous histiocytoma
- Angiosarcoma
- Malignant schwannoma
- Alveolar soft part sarcoma

What are the symptoms of non-rhabdomyosarcoma soft tissue sarcoma?

The first symptom of soft tissue sarcoma may be a solid mass or lump. If the mass interferes with a function of the body it may cause other symptoms. Soft tissue sarcoma rarely causes fever or weight loss.

How is non-rhabdomyosarcoma soft tissue sarcoma diagnosed and treated?

If a patient has symptoms of a soft tissue sarcoma, the doctor may order a biopsy, x-rays, and other tests to find out if the cancer cells have spread to other parts of the body. This is called staging. It is important to know the stage of the disease to plan treatment.

Treatment options are based on whether the cancer has spread, the amount of tumor left after surgery, and whether the child has reached full growth. Surgery, radiation, and chemotherapy are all treatment options, either alone or in combination.

Section 71.4

Angiosarcomas

What are angiosarcomas?

Angiosarcomas are uncommon malignant tumors (cancers) that arise from the cells that are normally used to make up the walls of the blood or lymphatic vessels. Hemangiosarcomas start in blood vessel walls and lymphangiosarcomas start in lymph vessel walls.

Angiosarcomas may occur in any organ of the body but are more frequently found in skin and soft tissue. They can also originate in the liver, breast, spleen, bone, or heart.

What causes angiosarcomas?

The cause of angiosarcomas is usually unknown. The tumours may develop as a complication of a pre-existing condition. Certain patient groups may be at greater risk of developing angiosarcomas, these include the following:

- Patients with chronic lymphoedema (accumulation of lymph fluid in the arms) whom have undergone a radical mastectomy for breast cancer (removal of breast and all lymph nodes under the arm)

- Radiotherapy patients (especially those who have been exposed to radiation emitting contrast agent Thorotrast—this agent is no longer used but angiosarcomas have occurred in people decades after exposure)

- Patients with foreign material (such as Dacron, shrapnel, steel, and plastic) in the body

- Patients exposed to environmental agents such as sprays containing arsenic and vinyl chloride in the plastic industry

What are the signs and symptoms of angiosarcomas?

The signs and symptoms of angiosarcomas differ according to the location of the tumor. Often symptoms of the disease are not apparent until the tumor is well advanced.

Soft Tissue

- Rapidly growing tumor in the extremities or abdomen
- Abdominal tumours may grow to large sizes before being detected as the abdomen can accommodate tumours
- Hemorrhage, anemia, hematoma, gastrointestinal bleeding
- Adjacent lymph nodes enlarged

Skin

- Enlarging bruise, a blue-black nodule, or unhealed ulceration
- Lesions may bleed and be painful
- Angiosarcomas occurring on the head and neck in elderly people are one of the most common forms of cutaneous angiosarcoma

Bone

- Tumours may grow on multiple bones of the same extremity
- Pain and tenderness of the affected area is common
- Swelling and increased size of the affected limb may be present

Breast

- Rapidly enlarging palpable mass without tenderness
- Often there is no pain
- Tumours often grow deep within breast tissue and cause diffuse breast enlargement with associated bluish skin discoloration

Other Organs

- Hepatic—non-specific symptoms such as fatigue, weight loss, right upper quadrant pain
- Lung—chest pain, bloody sputum, weight loss, cough, difficulty breathing

Cutaneous Angiosarcomas

This is the most common form of angiosarcoma not associated with chronic lymphoedema. The disease is primarily located on the head and neck of elderly persons and is also known as Wilson-Jones angiosarcoma, senile angiosarcoma or malignant angioendothelioma.

Clinical features of this form of angiosarcoma are the following:

- Lesions most commonly appear on the scalp or upper forehead.

- In the early stages of disease lesions may be singular or multifocal, slow spreading patches of livid or dusky red color, somewhat like an ill-defined bruise.

- Lesions may develop into elevated nodules or plaques that may bleed and ulcerate.

- Lesions grow rapidly and spread, making margins difficult to define.

What is the treatment of angiosarcomas?

Treatment of angiosarcomas is dependent on the location of the angiosarcoma and the extent of the tumor. Treatment includes chemotherapy, surgery, radiotherapy, or a combination of these treatment modalities.

The optimum treatment of cutaneous angiosarcomas has not been defined. These angiosarcomas are difficult to treat because of their multifocal nature and extensive spread pattern. Radical surgery and postoperative radiotherapy is generally used but tumor recurrence is common after treatment. Despite aggressive treatment, prognosis is poor in patients with cutaneous angiosarcomas.

Chapter 72

Kaposi Sarcoma

Kaposi sarcoma (KS) is a disease in which cancer (malignant) cells are found in the tissues under the skin or mucous membranes that line the mouth, nose, and anus. KS causes red or purple patches (lesions) on the skin and/or mucous membranes and spreads to other organs in the body, such as the lungs, liver, or intestinal tract.

Until the early 1980's, Kaposi sarcoma was a very rare disease that was found mainly in older men, patients who had organ transplants, or African men. With the acquired immune deficiency syndrome (AIDS) epidemic in the early 1980's, doctors began to notice more cases of Kaposi sarcoma in Africa and in gay men with AIDS. Kaposi sarcoma usually spreads more quickly in these patients.

If there are signs of KS, a doctor will examine the skin and lymph nodes carefully (lymph nodes are small bean-shaped structures that are found throughout the body; they produce and store infection-fighting cells). The doctor also may order other tests to see if the patient has other diseases.

The chance of recovery (prognosis) depends on what type of Kaposi sarcoma the patient has, the patient's age and general health, and whether or not the patient has AIDS.

PDQ® Cancer Information Summary. National Cancer Institute; Bethesda, MD. Kaposi's Sarcoma (PDQ®): Treatment - Patient. Updated 03/2006. Available at: http://cancer.gov. Accessed April 30, 2006.

Stages of Kaposi Sarcoma

There is no accepted staging system for Kaposi sarcoma. Patients are grouped depending on which type of Kaposi sarcoma they have. There are three types of Kaposi sarcoma:

Classic: Classic Kaposi sarcoma usually occurs in older men of Jewish, Italian, or Mediterranean heritage. This type of Kaposi sarcoma progresses slowly, sometimes over 10 to 15 years. As the disease gets worse, the lower legs may swell and the blood may not be able to flow properly. After some time, the disease may spread to other organs. Many patients with classic Kaposi sarcoma may develop another type of cancer later on in their lives.

Immunosuppressive treatment related: Kaposi sarcoma may occur in people who are taking drugs to make their immune systems weaker (immunosuppressants). The immune system helps the body fight off infection. People who have had an organ transplant (such as a liver or kidney transplant) have to take drugs to prevent their immune system from attacking the new organ.

Epidemic: Kaposi sarcoma in patients who have acquired immune deficiency syndrome (AIDS) is called epidemic Kaposi sarcoma. AIDS is caused by a virus called the human immunodeficiency virus (HIV), which attacks and weakens the immune system. Infections and other diseases can then invade the body, and the immune system cannot fight against them. Kaposi sarcoma in people with AIDS usually spreads more quickly than other kinds of Kaposi sarcoma and often is found in many parts of the body.

Recurrent: Recurrent disease means that the Kaposi sarcoma has come back (recurred) after it has been treated. It may come back in the area where it first started or in another part of the body.

Treatment Option Overview

There are treatments for all patients with Kaposi sarcoma. Four kinds of treatment are used:

- Surgery (taking out the cancer)
- Chemotherapy (using drugs to kill cancer cells)
- Radiation therapy (using high-dose x-rays to kill cancer cells)

- Biological therapy (using the body's immune system to fight cancer)

Radiation therapy is a common treatment of Kaposi sarcoma. Radiation therapy uses high-dose x-rays or other high-energy rays to kill cancer cells and shrink tumors. Radiation for Kaposi sarcoma comes from a machine outside the body (external-beam radiation therapy).

Surgery means taking out the cancer. A doctor may remove the cancer using one of the following:

- Local excision cuts out the lesion and some of the tissue around it.

- Electrodesiccation and curettage burns the lesion and removes it with a sharp instrument.

- Cryotherapy freezes the tumor and kills it.

Chemotherapy uses drugs to kill cancer cells. Chemotherapy may be taken by pill, or it may be put into the body by a needle in a vein or muscle. Chemotherapy is called a systemic treatment because the drug enters the bloodstream, travels through the body, and can kill cancer cells outside the original site. Chemotherapy for Kaposi sarcoma also may be injected into the lesion (intralesional chemotherapy).

Biological therapy tries to get the body to fight the cancer. It uses materials made by the body or made in a laboratory to boost, direct, or restore the body's natural defenses against disease. Biological therapy is sometimes called biological response modifier (BRM) therapy or immunotherapy.

For the treatment of epidemic Kaposi sarcoma, a type of biological therapy called highly active antiretroviral therapy (HAART) is used alone, or with other therapies. HAART combines several antiretroviral drugs that target HIV (which is a retrovirus). These drugs help block the virus from multiplying in the body and lower the risk of epidemic Kaposi sarcoma.

Treatment by Stage

Standard treatment may be considered because of its effectiveness in patients in past studies, or participation in a clinical trial may be considered. Not all patients are cured with standard therapy and some standard treatments may have more side effects than are desired. For these reasons, clinical trials are designed to find better ways to treat cancer patients and are based on the most up-to-date information. Clinical trials are ongoing in most parts of the country for most stages of Kaposi sarcoma. To learn more about clinical trials, call the Cancer Information Service at 800-4-CANCER (800-422-6237); TTY at 800-332-8615.

Classic Kaposi sarcoma: Treatment may be one of the following:

- Radiation therapy
- Local excision
- Systemic or intralesional chemotherapy
- Chemotherapy plus radiation therapy

Immunosuppressive treatment related Kaposi sarcoma: Depending on the patient's condition, the cancer may be controlled if immunosuppressive drugs are stopped. If the patient cannot stop taking these drugs or if this does not work, treatment may be one of the following:

- Radiation therapy
- A clinical trial of chemotherapy

Epidemic Kaposi sarcoma: Treatment may be one of the following:

- Surgery (local excision, electrodesiccation and curettage, or cryotherapy) with or without radiation therapy
- Systemic chemotherapy. Clinical trials are testing new drugs and drug combinations
- Biological therapy
- A clinical trial evaluating new treatments

Recurrent Kaposi sarcoma: Treatment of recurrent Kaposi sarcoma depends on the type of Kaposi sarcoma, and the patient's general health and response to earlier treatments. The patient may want to take part in a clinical trial.

Chapter 73

Metastatic Cancer: How and Where a Cancer Spreads

How a Cancer Spreads

The main reason cancer can be difficult to cure is that it can spread to another part of the body from where it started. The cancer that is growing where it started in the body is called the primary cancer. The place a cancer spreads to and starts growing is called the secondary cancer or metastasis.

In order to spread, some cells from the primary cancer must break away, travel to another part of the body and start growing there. Cancer cells do not stick together as well as normal cells. They also may produce substances that stimulate them to move. But how do cancer cells travel through the body?

There are three main ways a cancer spreads:

- Local spread
- Through the blood circulation
- Through the lymphatic system

Local spread: The cancer grows directly into nearby body tissues.

Spread through the blood stream: In order to spread, the cancer cell must first become detached from the primary tumor. It must

This chapter includes "How a Cancer Spreads" and "Where a Cancer Spreads" reprinted with permission of CancerHelp UK, the patient information website of Cancer Research UK. www.cancerhelp.org.uk. © 2006 Cancer Research UK.

then burrow through the wall of a blood vessel to get into the blood stream.

When it is in the blood stream, it will be swept along by the circulating blood until it gets stuck somewhere, usually in a very small blood vessel called a capillary.

Then it must burrow through the wall of the capillary and into the tissue of the organ it finds itself in. There it must start to multiply to grow a new tumor.

This is a complicated journey. Most cancer cells do not survive it. Probably, out of many thousands of cancer cells that reach the circulation only one will survive to form a secondary cancer or metastasis. Some are probably killed off by the white blood cells. Others may die because they are battered around by the fast flowing blood. Some researchers believe that, although cancer cells are capable of surviving on their own, they cannot do this for long. They need to re-attach quite quickly in order to live.

Cancer cells in the circulation may try to stick to platelets to form clumps to provide themselves with some protection. This may also help them to be filtered out in the next capillary network they come across and move into the tissues to start a secondary tumor.

Spread through the lymphatic system: The way a cancer spreads through the lymphatic system is very similar to the way it spreads through the blood stream. The cancer cell must become detached from the primary tumor. Then it will travel along with the circulating lymph until it gets stuck in the small channels inside a lymph node and begins to grow a secondary cancer.

Why Cancers Spread Where They Do

Whether it is in the blood or the lymph, the spreading cancer cell stops at the first place it gets stuck. In the blood stream, this is often the first capillary network it comes across. The blood flow from most body organs goes next through the capillaries in the lungs. So not surprisingly, the lungs are a very common site of cancer spread.

The blood from the organs of the digestive system goes through the capillaries of the liver before going back to the heart and then to the lungs. So it is common for digestive system cancers to spread to the liver. In fact, the liver is the second commonest site of cancer spread.

Some cancers show unexpected patterns of spread. For example prostate cancer often spreads to the bones. Scientists are still investigating why this happens.

During cancer surgery, it is routine for the surgeon to remove the main lymph nodes that drain the organ where the cancer is. For example, the surgeon operating to remove a breast cancer will remove at least some of the lymph nodes from under the arm. These are the first lymph nodes through which lymph draining from the breast flows. The surgeon does this because the first lymph nodes draining an organ are the most likely ones to contain cancer cells.

Micrometastases

Micrometastases are metastases (cancer spread) that are too small to be seen. If there are individual cells, or even small areas of growing cells elsewhere in the body, there is no scan that is detailed enough to spot them.

For a few tumors, there are blood tests that detect proteins released by the cancer cells. These may detect metastases too small to show up on a scan. But for most cancers, there is no blood test that can say whether a cancer has spread or not.

For most cancers the doctor can only say whether it is likely or not that a patient has micrometastases. This "best guess" may be based on:

- Previous experience of many other patients treated in the same way. Doctors naturally collect and publish this information to help each other.

- Whether cancer cells are found in the blood vessels in the lump of tumor removed during surgery (for example, in testicular cancer). If they are found then cancer cells are more likely to have reached the blood stream and spread to somewhere else in the body.

- The grade of the cancer. The higher the grade, the more aggressive the cancer. So the more likely it is that cells have spread.

- Whether lymph nodes that were removed at operation contained cancer cells (for example, in breast cancer or colorectal cancer). This is direct evidence that cancer cells have broken away from the original cancer. But there is no way of knowing whether any have spread further.

This information is important. If the doctor thinks it is probable that there are micrometastases, he or she may offer further treatment with chemotherapy, radiotherapy, or hormone therapy. This is called adjuvant treatment. The aim is to kill the cancer deposits before they grow big enough to be seen on a scan.

Some doctors say to their patients that it is "belt and braces" treatment. In other words, the treatment is to try to make sure the cancer does not come back. No one can know for sure if all the cancer cells have been destroyed when someone has finished treatment. It is this uncertainty that can make cancer difficult to cope with for many people, even if they seem to have been successfully treated.

Where a Cancer Spreads

Cancers can really spread just about anywhere. But most cancers tend to spread most often to one or two places.

The treatment for cancer that has spread (secondary cancer) depends on where the cancer started in the body (the primary cancer), so it is difficult to generalize in this section. Where particular treatments are used for cancer that has spread is mentioned below.

The lungs: The lungs are the most common organ for cancers to spread to. This is because the blood from most parts of the body flows back to the heart and then to the lungs before it goes to any other organ. Cancer cells that have found their way into the blood stream can get stuck in the tiny capillaries of the lungs.

Cancer that has spread to the lungs may not cause any symptoms or may cause the following symptoms:

- A cough that doesn't go away

- Shortness of breath

- Chest infections

- Fluid build up between the chest wall and the lung causing a pleural effusion, which in turn causes shortness of breath, chest aching, discomfort, and heaviness

Fluid builds up because cancer cells are irritating the pleura. The pleura are the two sheets of tissue that cover the lungs. The irritated tissues make extra fluid and this collects between them. There may also be cancer cells in the pleural space that stop the extra fluid draining away. The lungs inflate as we breathe in. This fluid build up gets in their way and stops them from inflating properly.

Doctors can drain the fluid by putting in a needle. This is often called a pleural tap. But unless they can stop the fluid from collecting, it will build up again.

808

The liver: Many cancers spread to the liver. The cancers of the digestive system are most likely to spread to the liver because the blood from the digestive system circulates through the liver before it goes back to the heart. Cancer that has spread to the liver can cause the following symptoms:

* Lack of energy

* Feeling generally unwell

* Feeling sick

* Lack of appetite

* Discomfort on the right side of the body under the rib cage

* Jaundice

* Fluid build up in the abdomen (ascites)

Jaundice is the medical name for a build up of bile salts in the blood. This makes the skin and whites of the eyes turn yellow. It can also cause the skin to become itchy. The urine often looks very dark and bowel motions can look pale.

Ascites can happen for a number of reasons. It does not always mean cancer has spread to the liver. Cancer cells may have spread to the lining of the abdomen. This irritates the lining and causes it to make extra fluid, which builds up in the abdominal cavity.

There are a number of ways cancer in the liver can cause ascites. Cancer may be blocking the normal blood flow through the liver causing a back pressure of fluid. The healthy liver makes proteins that circulate in the blood. The proteins help to keep fluid in the blood and stop it from leaking out into the tissues.

If the liver is damaged, it may not be making enough of these proteins and so fluid tends to leak out and collect in the abdomen or in other parts of the body, such as the feet and ankles. Doctors can drain excess fluid from inside the abdomen by putting in a needle. But unless they can stop the fluid from collecting, it will build up again.

The lymph nodes: It is very common for cancer cells to travel from the site of the original cancer to the nearest lymph nodes. This is because there is a natural circulation of tissue fluid from the organs through the lymphatic system. This is not the same as having a cancer of the lymphatic system, such as Hodgkin lymphoma or non-Hodgkin lymphoma.

Surgeons will often remove the nearest lymph nodes when they are operating for a primary cancer. Some cancers, such as testicular cancer often spread to the lymph nodes. So your doctor may want you to have preventative treatment, such as radiotherapy to particular lymph nodes.

Cancer that has spread to the lymph nodes may cause them to swell up. The swollen lymph nodes are easy to see if they are near the surface of the body, for example in the neck or under the arm. But if the nodes are deep in the body, they can only be seen on a scan.

Cancer in the lymph nodes may not cause any symptoms. But sometimes, the swollen lymph nodes can block the circulation of tissue fluid. This can cause swelling in the part of the body affected. For example, swollen lymph nodes in the armpit, or groin can cause swelling in the arm or leg on the same side of the body. This swelling is called lymphoedema.

The bones: Some cancers quite often spread to the bones, for example prostate cancer, breast cancer, and lung cancer.

The most common effects of secondary cancer in the bones are the following:

* Pain in the affected bones

* Weakness in the affected bones

* Raised calcium levels in the blood

Pain is caused because the cancer cells are multiplying in the bone and pressing on nerves. The growing cancer can weaken the bone by damaging its normal structure. This may mean it is more likely to break. You may hear this called pathological fracture. Sometimes these fractures are fixed during an operation to put in a metal pin or attach a metal plate to strengthen the bone.

If you have a bone that has become weakened like this, your doctor will probably suggest you have some radiotherapy. Radiotherapy kills off the cancer cells and the bone begins to strengthen itself.

Calcium can be released by damaged bone. If high calcium levels build up in the blood you may experience the following symptoms:

* Feel sick

* Feel tired, drowsy, or muddled

* Become constipated

* Feel very thirsty

If the calcium levels become very high they can cause irritability and confusion, and eventually unconsciousness. Drug treatment is available for high calcium levels.

The brain: It is not that common for cancers to spread to the brain, but it does happen. Lung cancer and breast cancer can both spread to the brain. So can colon (bowel) cancer, kidney cancer, and melanoma.

Some types of lung cancer are quite likely to spread to the brain, so your doctor may want you to have preventative radiotherapy treatment to the brain for these types of cancer.

The most common symptoms from cancer that has spread to the brain are the following:

- Headaches
- Feeling sick

These symptoms are caused because the cancer growing in the brain is taking up space. The space for the brain is limited by the skull so the growing cancer causes an increase in pressure inside the skull. This is called raised intracranial pressure. Other symptoms depend on where in the brain the cancer is growing and the size of the tumor or tumors. Small secondary brain tumors may not cause very many symptoms at all. Symptoms of secondary cancer in the brain can include the following:

- Weakness in an arm, leg, or on one side of the body
- Changes in behavior or moodiness
- Fits
- Confusion
- Drowsiness
- Vertigo

Secondary cancer in the brain can sometimes be treated, usually with radiotherapy (although this will depend on the type of cancer you have). Steroids are often prescribed to reduce the swelling in the brain and so reduce raised intracranial pressure. Steroids can often make a big improvement in symptoms.

The skin: Sometimes cancer cells can start growing in the skin. This is not the same as having skin cancer, melanoma, or cutaneous

T cell lymphoma (a type of lymphoma that affects the skin). The secondary cancer may start to grow on or near an operation scar where the primary cancer was removed. Sometimes secondary skin cancers can grow in other parts of the body.

A secondary skin cancer looks like a pink or red raised lump (a bit like a boil). Skin nodules can be treated. It is important to tell your doctor if you think you have one, because if it is not treated, it may become ulcerated.

Chapter 74

Cancer of Unknown Primary Origin

Carcinoma of unknown primary (CUP) is a disease in which cancer (malignant) cells are found somewhere in the body, but the place where they first started growing (the origin or primary site) cannot be found. This occurs in about 2%–4% of cancer patients.

Actually, CUP can be described as a group of different types of cancer all of which have become known by the place or places in the body where the cancer has spread (metastasized) from another part of the body. Because all of these diseases are not alike, chance of recovery (prognosis) and choice of treatment may be different for each patient.

If CUP is suspected, a doctor will order several tests, one of which may be a biopsy. This means a small piece of tissue is cut from the tumor and looked at under a microscope. The doctor may also do a complete history and physical examination, and order chest x-rays along with blood, urine, and stool tests. A cancer can be called CUP when the doctor cannot tell from the test results where the cancer began.

The pattern of how CUP has spread may also give the doctor information to help determine where it started. For example, lung metastases are more common when cancer begins above the diaphragm (the thin muscle under the lungs that helps the breathing process). Most large studies have shown that CUP often starts in the lungs or pancreas. Less often, it may start in the colon, rectum, breast, or prostate.

PDQ® Cancer Information Summary. National Cancer Institute; Bethesda, MD. Carcinoma of Unknown Primary (PDQ®): Treatment - Patient. Updated 06/2005. Available at: http://cancer.gov. Accessed April 30, 2006.

An important part of trying to find out where the cancer started is to see how the cancer cells look under a microscope (histology). Other special tests may also be done that help the doctor find out where the cancer started and choose the best type of treatment.

Stages of Carcinoma of Unknown Primary

When cancer is diagnosed, more tests are usually done to find out if cancer cells have spread to other parts of the body. This is called staging. But, when CUP is diagnosed, the number and type of tests done may be different for each patient. The treatment options in this chapter are based on whether the cancer has just been found (newly diagnosed) or the cancer has come back after it has been treated (recurrent).

The treatment options are also based on where the cancer is found or what it looks like. A doctor may find that the cancer fits into one of the following groups:

- **Cancer in the cervical lymph nodes:** Cancer in the small, bean-shaped organs that make and store infection-fighting cells (lymph nodes) in the neck area

- **Poorly differentiated carcinomas:** The cancer cells look very different from normal cells

- **Metastatic melanoma to a single nodal site:** Cancer of the cells that color the skin (melanocytes) that has spread to lymph nodes in only one part of the body

- **Isolated axillary metastasis:** Cancer that has spread only to lymph nodes in the area of the armpits

- **Inguinal node metastasis:** Cancer that has spread to lymph nodes in the groin area

- **Multiple involvement:** Cancer that has spread to several different areas of the body

Treatment Option Overview

Many different treatments are used either alone or in combination to treat CUP. Some of the treatments that are used include the following:

- Surgery (taking out the cancer in an operation)

814

- Radiation therapy (using high-dose x-rays to kill cancer cells)
- Chemotherapy (using drugs to kill cancer cells)
- Hormone therapy (using hormones to stop the cancer cells from growing)

Surgery is a common treatment for CUP. A doctor may remove the cancer and some of the healthy tissue around it. Different operations are used depending on where the cancer is found. If the cancer has spread to lymph nodes, the lymph nodes may be removed (lymph node dissection). If the nodes involved are in the groin, this operation is called a superficial groin dissection. If the cancer has spread to lymph nodes and also to some surrounding areas, the doctor may have to remove a larger portion of tissue around the nodes. When muscles, nerves, and other tissue in the neck are removed, this is called a radical neck dissection.

Radiation therapy uses x-rays or other high-energy rays to kill cancer cells and shrink tumors. Radiation may be used alone or before or after surgery.

Chemotherapy uses drugs to kill cancer cells. Chemotherapy may be taken by mouth or it may be put into the body by a needle in a vein or muscle. Chemotherapy is called a systemic treatment because the drugs enter the bloodstream, travel through the body, and can kill cancer cells throughout the body. Chemotherapy may be used alone or after surgery. Therapy given after an operation when there are no cancer cells that can be seen is called adjuvant therapy.

Hormone therapy is used to stop the hormones in the body that help cancer cells grow. This may be done by using drugs that change the way hormones work or by surgery that takes out organs that make hormones, such as the testicles (orchiectomy).

Treatment by Stage

Treatment of CUP depends on where the doctor thinks the cancer started, what the cancer cells look like under a microscope, and other factors. Surgery and tests may be done to find where the cancer started.

Standard treatment may be considered because of its effectiveness in patients in past studies, or participation in a clinical trial may be considered. Not all patients are cured with standard therapy and some standard treatments may have more side effects than are desired. For these reasons, clinical trials are designed to find better ways to treat cancer patients and are based on the most up-to-date information. Clinical trials are ongoing in most parts of the country for CUP. To learn more about clinical trials, call the Cancer Information Service at 800-4-CANCER (800-422-6237); TTY at 800-332-8615.

Newly diagnosed carcinoma of unknown primary: If the cancer is in the neck area (cervical lymph nodes), treatment may be one of the following:

- Surgery to remove the tonsils (tonsillectomy)
- Radiation therapy
- Radiation therapy followed by surgery
- Neck surgery (radical neck dissection)
- Neck surgery followed by radiation therapy

If the cancer is a poorly differentiated carcinoma (the cancer cells look very different than normal cells), the treatment will probably be chemotherapy. Surgery or radiation therapy has also been used for patients with neuroendocrine (nervous system and hormonal system) cancer.

If the cancer is peritoneal adenocarcinomatosis (the tumor is in the lining inside the abdomen), the treatment will probably be chemotherapy.

If the cancer is an isolated axillary nodal metastasis, it is likely that the cancer started in the lung or breast. If female, a mammogram (an x-ray picture of the breast) will be used to check for breast cancer. After tests to check for lung and breast cancer, the treatment may be one of the following:

- Surgery to remove the lymph nodes with or without surgery to remove the breast (mastectomy) or radiation therapy to the breast
- Treatment as described above plus chemotherapy that is used for breast cancer

If the cancer is in the inguinal nodes, the treatment may be one of the following:

- Surgery to remove the cancer
- Groin surgery (superficial groin dissection)

- Surgery to remove some of the tumor (biopsy) with or without radiation therapy, surgery to remove the lymph nodes, or chemotherapy

If the cancer is melanoma that has spread to a single nodal site, the treatment will probably be surgery to remove the lymph nodes.

If there is cancer in several different areas of the body and the doctor thinks that the origin of the cancer is one for which there is standard systemic therapy, then that therapy should be given. The following are examples:

- Hormone therapy for prostate cancer

- Chemotherapy or hormone therapy for breast cancer

- Chemotherapy for ovarian cancer

If the source of the cancer cannot be found, then the best treatment may not be known. Patients may want to consider taking part in a clinical trial.

Recurrent carcinoma of unknown primary: Treatment of recurrent CUP depends on the type of cancer, what treatment was received before, the part of the body where the cancer has come back, and other factors. A patient may want to consider taking part in a clinical trial.

Part Three

Understanding Cancer Treatments

Chapter 75

Chemotherapy

Chapter Contents

Section 75.1

What Is Chemotherapy?

Excerpted from "Chemotherapy and You: A Guide to Self-Help
During Cancer Treatment," National Cancer Institute, June 1999;
accessed November 22, 2006.

Chemotherapy is the treatment of cancer with drugs that can destroy cancer cells. These drugs often are called "anticancer" drugs.

How does chemotherapy work?

Normal cells grow and die in a controlled way. When cancer occurs, cells in the body that are not normal keep dividing and forming more cells without control. Anticancer drugs destroy cancer cells by stopping them from growing or multiplying. Healthy cells can also be harmed, especially those that divide quickly. Harm to healthy cells is what causes side effects. These cells usually repair themselves after chemotherapy.

Because some drugs work better together than alone, two or more drugs are often given at the same time. This is called combination chemotherapy.

Other types of drugs may be used to treat your cancer. These may include certain drugs that can block the effect of your body's hormones. Or doctors may use biological therapy, which is treatment with substances that boost the body's own immune system against cancer. Your body usually makes these substances in small amounts to fight cancer and other diseases. These substances can be made in the laboratory and given to patients to destroy cancer cells or change the way the body reacts to a tumor. They may also help the body repair or make new cells destroyed by chemotherapy.

What can chemotherapy do?

Depending on the type of cancer and how advanced it is, chemotherapy can be used for different goals:

- **To cure the cancer:** Cancer is considered cured when the patient remains free of evidence of cancer cells.

- **To control the cancer:** This is done by keeping the cancer from spreading; slowing the cancer's growth; and killing cancer cells that may have spread to other parts of the body from the original tumor.

- **To relieve symptoms that the cancer may cause:** Relieving symptoms such as pain can help patients live more comfortably.

Is chemotherapy used with other treatments?

Sometimes chemotherapy is the only treatment a patient receives. More often, however, chemotherapy is used in addition to surgery, radiation therapy, and/or biological therapy to do the following:

- Shrink a tumor before surgery or radiation therapy. This is called neoadjuvant therapy.

- Help destroy any cancer cells that may remain after surgery and/or radiation therapy. This is called adjuvant chemotherapy.

- Make radiation therapy and biological therapy work better.

- Help destroy cancer if it recurs or has spread to other parts of the body from the original tumor.

What should I ask my doctor about chemotherapy?

- Why do I need chemotherapy?
- What are the benefits of chemotherapy?
- What are the risks of chemotherapy?
- Are there any other possible treatment methods for my type of cancer?
- What is the standard care for my type of cancer?
- Are there any clinical trials for my type of cancer?

What should I ask my doctor about my cancer treatments?

- How many treatments will I be given?
- What drug or drugs will I be taking?
- How will the drugs be given?
- Where will I get my treatment?
- How long will each treatment last?

What should I ask my doctor about side effects?

- What are the possible side effects of the chemotherapy? When are side effects likely to occur?

- What side effects are more likely to be related to my type of cancer?

- Are there any side effects that I should report right away?

- What can I do to relieve the side effects?

- What are the short-term side effects that may occur?

- What are the long-term side effects that may occur?

- How serious are the side effects likely to be?

- How long will the side effects last?

- What can I do to relieve or lessen the side effects?

- When should I call the doctor or nurse about side effects?

- How do I contact a health professional after hours, and when should I call?

- What can I do to feel better emotionally while trying to cope with the side effects?

Hints for Talking with Your Doctor: These tips might help you keep track of the information you learn during visits with your doctor:

- Bring a friend or family member to sit with you while you talk with your doctor. This person can help you understand what your doctor says during your visit and help refresh your memory afterward.

- Ask your doctor for printed information that is available on your cancer and treatment.

- You, or the person who goes with you, may want to take notes during your appointment.

- Ask your doctor to slow down when you need more time to write.

- You may want to ask if you can use a tape recorder during your visit. Take notes from the tape after the visit is finished. That way, you can review your conversation later as many times as you wish.

Section 75.2

What to Expect during Chemotherapy

Excerpted from "Chemotherapy and You: A Guide to Self-Help
During Cancer Treatment," National Cancer Institute, June 1999;
accessed November 22, 2006.

Some people with cancer want to know every detail about their condition and their treatment. Others prefer only general information. The choice of how much information to seek is yours, but there are questions that every person getting chemotherapy should ask.

This list is just a start. Always feel free to ask your doctor, nurse, and pharmacist as many questions as you want. If you do not understand their answers, keep asking until you do. Remember, there is no such thing as a "stupid" question, especially about cancer or your treatment. To make sure you get all the answers you want, you may find it helpful to draw up a list of questions before each doctor's appointment. Some people keep a "running list" and jot down each new question as it occurs to them.

Where will I get chemotherapy?

Chemotherapy can be given in many different places: at home, a doctor's office, a clinic, a hospital's outpatient department, or as an "inpatient" in a hospital. The choice of where you get chemotherapy depends on which drug or drugs you are getting, your insurance, and sometimes your own and your doctor's wishes. Most patients receive their treatment as an "outpatient" and are not hospitalized. Sometimes, a patient starting chemotherapy may need to stay at the hospital for a short time so that the medicine's effects can be watched closely and any needed changes can be made.

How often and for how long will I get chemotherapy?

How often and how long you get chemotherapy depends on the following:

- The kind of cancer you have

- The goals of the treatment
- The drugs that are used
- How your body responds to them

You may get treatment every day, every week, or every month. Chemotherapy is often given in cycles that include treatment periods alternated with rest periods. Rest periods give your body a chance to build healthy new cells and regain its strength. Ask your health care provider to tell you how long and how often you may expect to get treatment.

Sticking with your treatment schedule is very important for the drugs to work right. Schedules may need to be changed for holidays and other reasons. If you miss a treatment session or skip a dose of the drug, contact your doctor.

Sometimes, your doctor may need to delay a treatment based on the results of certain blood tests. Your doctor will let you know what to do during this time and when to start your treatment again.

How is chemotherapy given?

Chemotherapy can be given in several different ways: intravenously (through a vein), by mouth, through an injection (shot), or applied on the skin.

By vein (intravenous, or IV, treatment): Chemotherapy is most often given intravenously (IV), through a vein. Usually a thin needle is inserted into a vein on the hand or lower arm at the beginning of each treatment session and is removed at the end of the session. If you feel coolness, burning, or other unusual sensation in the area of the needle stick when the IV is started, tell your doctor or nurse. Also report any pain, burning, skin redness, swelling, or discomfort that occurs during or after an IV treatment.

Chemotherapy can also be delivered by IV through catheters, ports, and pumps. A catheter is a soft, thin, flexible tube that is placed in a large vein in the body and remains there as long as it is needed. Patients who need to have many IV treatments often have a catheter, so a needle does not have to be used each time. Drugs can be given and blood samples can be drawn through this catheter. Sometimes the catheter is attached to a port—a small round plastic or metal disc placed under the skin. The port can be used for as long as it is needed. A pump, which is used to control how fast the drug goes into a catheter or port, is sometimes used. There are two types of pumps. An external pump remains outside the body. Most are portable; they allow a person to move around while the pump is being used. An internal pump is placed inside the body during surgery, usually right under the skin. Pumps contain a small storage area for the drug and allow people to go about their normal activities. Catheters, ports, and pumps cause no pain if they are properly placed and cared for, although a person is aware they are there.

Catheters are usually placed in a large vein, most commonly in your chest, called a central venous catheter. A peripherally inserted central catheter (PICC) is inserted into a vein in the arm. Catheters can also be placed in an artery or other locations in your body, such as:

- intrathecal (delivers drugs into the spinal fluid);
- intracavitary (IC) catheter (placed in the abdomen, pelvis, or chest).

By mouth (orally): The drug is given in pill, capsule, or liquid form. You swallow the drug, just as you do many other medicines.

By injection: A needle and syringe are used to give the drug in one of several ways:

- intramuscularly, or IM (into a muscle)
- subcutaneously, or SQ or SC (under the skin)
- intralesionally, or IL (directly into a cancerous area in the skin)

Topically: The drug is applied on the surface of the skin.

How will I feel during chemotherapy?

Most people receiving chemotherapy find that they tire easily, but many feel well enough to continue to lead active lives. Each person and treatment is different, so it is not always possible to tell exactly how you will react. Your general state of health, the type and extent of cancer you have, and the kind of drugs you are receiving can all affect how well you feel.

You may want to have someone available to drive you to and from treatment if, for example, you are taking medicine for nausea or vomiting that could make you tired. You may also feel especially tired from the chemotherapy as early as one day after a treatment and for several days. It may help to schedule your treatment when you can take off the day of and the day after your treatment. If you have young children, you may want to schedule the treatment when you have someone to help at home the day of and at least the day after your treatment. Ask your doctor when your greatest fatigue or other side effects are likely to occur.

Most people can continue working while receiving chemotherapy. However, you may need to change your work schedule for a while if your chemotherapy makes you feel very tired or have other side effects. Talk with your employer about your needs and wishes. You may be able to agree on a part-time schedule, find an area for a short nap during the day, or perhaps you can do some of your work at home.

Under Federal and state laws, some employers may be required to let you work a flexible schedule to meet your treatment needs. To find out about your on-the-job protections, check with a social worker, or your congressional or state representative.

How will I know if my chemotherapy is working?

Your doctor and nurse will use several ways to see how well your treatments are working. You may have physical exams and tests often. Always feel free to ask your doctor about the test results and what they show about your progress.

Tests and exams can tell a lot about how chemotherapy is working; however, side effects tell very little. Sometimes people think that if they have no side effects, the drugs are not working, or, if they do have side effects, the drugs are working well. But side effects vary so much from person to person, and from drug to drug, that side effects are not a sign of whether the treatment is working or not.

Section 75.3

Coping with the Side Effects of Chemotherapy

Excerpted from "Chemotherapy and You: A Guide to Self-Help
During Cancer Treatment," National Cancer Institute, June 1999;
accessed November 22, 2006.

What causes side effects?

Because cancer cells may grow and divide more rapidly than normal cells, many anticancer drugs are made to kill growing cells. But certain normal, healthy cells also multiply quickly, and chemotherapy can affect these cells, too. This damage to normal cells causes side effects. The fast-growing, normal cells most likely to be affected are blood cells forming in the bone marrow and cells in the digestive tract (mouth, stomach, intestines, esophagus), reproductive system (sexual organs), and hair follicles. Some anticancer drugs may affect cells of vital organs, such as the heart, kidney, bladder, lungs, and nervous system.

You may have none of these side effects or just a few. The kinds of side effects you have and how severe they are, depend on the type and dose of chemotherapy you get and how your body reacts. Before starting chemotherapy, your doctor will discuss the side effects that you are most likely to get with the drugs you will be receiving. Before starting the treatment, you will be asked to sign a consent form. You should be given all the facts about treatment including the drugs you will be given and their side effects before you sign the consent form.

How long do side effects last?

Normal cells usually recover when chemotherapy is over, so most side effects gradually go away after treatment ends, and the healthy cells have a chance to grow normally. The time it takes to get over side effects depends on many things, including your overall health and the kind of chemotherapy you have been taking.

Most people have no serious long-term problems from chemotherapy. However, on some occasions, chemotherapy can cause permanent changes or damage to the heart, lungs, nerves, kidneys, reproductive or other organs. And certain types of chemotherapy may have delayed effects, such as a second cancer, that show up many years later. Ask your doctor about the chances of any serious, long-term effects that can result from the treatment you are receiving (but remember to balance your concerns with the immediate threat of your cancer).

Great progress has been made in preventing and treating some of chemotherapy's common as well as rare serious side effects. Many new drugs and treatment methods destroy cancer more effectively while doing less harm to the body's healthy cells.

The side effects of chemotherapy can be unpleasant, but they must be measured against the treatment's ability to destroy cancer. Medicines can help prevent some side effects such as nausea. Sometimes people receiving chemotherapy become discouraged about the length of time their treatment is taking or the side effects they are having. If that happens to you, talk to your doctor or nurse. They may be able to suggest ways to make side effects easier to deal with or reduce them.

Fatigue

Fatigue, feeling tired and lacking energy, is the most common symptom reported by cancer patients. The exact cause is not always known. It can be due to your disease, chemotherapy, radiation, surgery, low blood counts, lack of sleep, pain, stress, poor appetite, along with many other factors.

Fatigue from cancer feels different from fatigue of everyday life. Fatigue caused by chemotherapy can appear suddenly. Patients with cancer have described it as a total lack of energy and have used words such as 'worn out,' 'drained,' and 'wiped out' to describe their fatigue. And rest does not always relieve it. Not everyone feels the same kind of fatigue. You may not feel tired while someone else does or your fatigue may not last as long as someone else's does. It can last days, weeks, or months. But severe fatigue does go away gradually as the tumor responds to treatment.

How can I cope with fatigue?

- Plan your day so that you have time to rest.
- Take short naps or breaks, rather than one long rest period.
- Save your energy for the most important things.
- Try easier or shorter versions of activities you enjoy.

- Take short walks or do light exercise if possible. You may find this helps with fatigue.

- Talk to your health care provider about ways to save your energy and treat your fatigue.

- Try activities such as meditation, prayer, yoga, guided imagery, visualization, etc. You may find that these help with fatigue.

- Eat as well as you can and drink plenty of fluids. Eat small amounts at a time, if that is helpful.

- Join a support group. Sharing your feelings with others can ease the burden of fatigue. You can learn how others deal with their fatigue. Your health care provider can put you in touch with a support group in your area.

- Limit the amount of caffeine and alcohol you drink.

- Allow others to do some things for you that you usually do.

- Keep a diary of how you feel each day. This will help you plan your daily activities.

- Report any changes in energy level to your doctor or nurse.

Nausea and Vomiting

Many patients fear that they will have nausea and vomiting while receiving chemotherapy. But new drugs have made these side effects far less common and, when they do occur, much less severe. These powerful antiemetic or antinausea drugs can prevent or lessen nausea and vomiting in most patients. Different drugs work for different people, and you may need more than one drug to get relief. Do not give up. Continue to work with your doctor and nurse to find the drug or drugs that work best for you. Also, be sure to tell your doctor or nurse if you are very nauseated or have vomited for more than a day, or if your vomiting is so bad that you cannot keep liquids down.

What can I do if I have nausea and vomiting?

- Drink liquids at least an hour before or after mealtime, instead of with your meals. Drink frequently and drink small amounts.

- Eat and drink slowly.

- Eat small meals throughout the day, instead of one, two, or three large meals.

- Eat foods cold or at room temperature so you won't be bothered by strong smells.

- Chew your food well for easier digestion.

- If nausea is a problem in the morning, try eating dry foods like cereal, toast, or crackers before getting up. (Do not try this if you have mouth or throat sores or are troubled by a lack of saliva.)

- Drink cool, clear, unsweetened fruit juices, such as apple or grape juice or light-colored sodas such as ginger ale that have lost their fizz and do not have caffeine.

- Suck on mints, or tart candies. (Do not use tart candies if you have mouth or throat sores.)

- Prepare and freeze meals in advance for days when you do not feel like cooking.

- Wear loose-fitting clothes.

- Breathe deeply and slowly when you feel nauseated.

- Distract yourself by chatting with friends or family members, listening to music, or watching a movie or TV show.

- Use relaxation techniques.

- Try to avoid odors that bother you, such as cooking smells, smoke, or perfume.

- Avoid sweet, fried, or fatty foods.

- Rest but do not lie flat for at least 2 hours after you finish a meal.

- Avoid eating for at least a few hours before treatment if nausea usually occurs during chemotherapy.

- Eat a light meal before treatment.

Pain

Chemotherapy drugs can cause some side effects that are painful. The drugs can damage nerves, leading to burning, numbness, tingling or shooting pain, most often in the fingers or toes. Some drugs can also cause mouth sores, headaches, muscle pains, and stomach pains.

Not everyone with cancer or who receives chemotherapy experiences pain from the disease or its treatment. But if you do, it can be relieved. The first step to take is to talk with your doctor, nurse, and pharmacist about your pain. They need to know as many details about your pain as possible. You may want to describe your pain to your family and friends. They can help you talk to your caregivers about your pain, especially if you are too tired or in too much pain to talk to them yourself.

You need to tell your doctor, nurse, and pharmacist, and family or friends the following information about your pain:

- Where you feel pain

- What it feels like—sharp, dull, throbbing, steady

- How strong the pain feels

- How long it lasts

- What eases the pain, what makes the pain worse

- What medicines you are taking for the pain and how much relief you get from them

Using a pain scale is helpful in describing how much pain you are feeling. Try to assign a number from 0 to 10 to your pain level. If you have no pain, use a 0. As the numbers get higher, they stand for pain that is getting worse. A 10 means the pain is as bad as it can be. You may wish to use your own pain scale using numbers from 0 to 5 or even 0 to 100. Be sure to let others know what pain scale you are using and use the same scale each time, for example, "My pain is 7 on a scale of 0 to 10."

The goal of pain control is to prevent pain that can be prevented, and treat the pain that can't. To do this:

- If you have persistent or chronic pain, take your pain medicine on a regular schedule (by the clock).

- Do not skip doses of your scheduled pain medicine. If you wait to take pain medicine until you feel pain, it is harder to control.

- Try using relaxation exercises at the same time you take medicine for the pain. This may help to lessen tension, reduce anxiety, and manage pain.

- Some people with chronic or persistent pain that is usually controlled by medicine can have breakthrough pain. This occurs when moderate to severe pain "breaks through" or is felt for a short time. If you experience this pain, use a short-acting medicine ordered by your doctor. Don't wait for the pain to get worse. If you do, it may be harder to control.

There are many different medicines and methods available to control cancer pain. You should expect your doctor to seek all the information and resources necessary to make you as comfortable as possible. If you are in pain and your doctor has no further suggestions, ask to see a pain specialist or have your doctor consult with a pain specialist. A pain specialist may be an oncologist, anesthesiologist, neurologist, neurosurgeon, other doctor, nurse, or pharmacist.

Hair Loss

Hair loss (alopecia) is a common side effect of chemotherapy, but not all drugs cause hair loss. Your doctor can tell you if hair loss might occur with the drug or drugs you are taking. When hair loss does occur, the hair may become thinner or fall out entirely. Hair loss can occur on all parts of the body, including the head, face, arms and legs, underarms, and pubic area. The hair usually grows back after the treatments are over. Some people even start to get their hair back while they are still having treatments. Sometimes, hair may grow back a different color or texture.

Hair loss does not always happen right away. It may begin several weeks after the first treatment or after a few treatments. Many people say their head becomes sensitive before losing hair. Hair may fall out gradually or in clumps. Any hair that is still growing may become dull and dry.

How can I care for my scalp and hair during chemotherapy?

- Use a mild shampoo.
- Use a soft hair brush.
- Use low heat when drying your hair.
- Have your hair cut short. A shorter style will make your hair look thicker and fuller. It also will make hair loss easier to manage if it occurs.
- Use a sun screen, sun block, hat, or scarf to protect your scalp from the sun if you lose hair on your head.
- Avoid brush rollers to set your hair.
- Avoid dying, perming, or relaxing your hair.

Some people who lose all or most of their hair choose to wear turbans, scarves, caps, wigs, or hair pieces. Others leave their head uncovered. Still others switch back and forth, depending on whether they are in public or at home with friends and family members. There are no "right" or "wrong" choices; do whatever feels comfortable for you.

If you choose to cover your head:

- Get your wig or hairpiece before you lose a lot of hair. That way, you can match your current hair style and color. You may be able to buy a wig or hairpiece at a specialty shop just for cancer patients. Someone may even come to your home to help you. You also can buy a wig or hair piece through a catalog or by phone.

- You may also consider borrowing a wig or hairpiece, rather than buying one. Check with the nurse or social work department at your hospital about resources for free wigs in your community.

- Take your wig to your hairdresser or the shop where it was purchased for styling and cutting to frame your face.

- Some health insurance policies cover the cost of a hairpiece needed because of cancer treatment. It is also a tax-deductible expense. Be sure to check your policy and ask your doctor for a "prescription."

Losing hair from your head, face, or body can be hard to accept. Feeling angry or depressed is common and perfectly all right. At the same time, keep in mind that it is a temporary side effect. Talking about your feelings can help. If possible, share your thoughts with someone who has had a similar experience.

Anemia

Chemotherapy can reduce the bone marrow's ability to make red blood cells, which carry oxygen to all parts of your body. When there are too few red blood cells, body tissues do not get enough oxygen to do their work. This condition is called anemia. Anemia can make you feel short of breath, very weak, and tired. Call your doctor if you have any of these symptoms:

- Fatigue (feeling very weak and tired)
- Dizziness or feeling faint
- Shortness of breath
- Feeling as if your heart is "pounding" or beating very fast

Your doctor will check your blood cell count often during your treatment. She or he may also prescribe a medicine that can boost the growth of your red blood cells. Discuss this with your doctor if you become anemic often. If your red count falls too low, you may need a blood transfusion or a medicine called erythropoietin to raise the number of red blood cells in your body.

Things you can do if you are anemic:

- **Get plenty of rest:** Sleep more at night and take naps during the day if you can.

- **Limit your activities:** Do only the things that are essential or most important to you.

- **Ask for help when you need it:** Ask family and friends to pitch in with things like child care, shopping, housework, or driving.

- **Eat a well-balanced diet.**

- **When sitting, get up slowly:** When lying down, sit first and then stand. This will help prevent dizziness.

Central Nervous System Problems

Chemotherapy can interfere with certain functions in your central nervous system (brain) causing tiredness, confusion, and depression. These feelings will go away once the chemotherapy dose is lowered or you finish chemotherapy. Call your doctor if these symptoms occur.

Infection

Chemotherapy can make you more likely to get infections. This happens because most anticancer drugs affect the bone marrow, making it harder to make white blood cells (WBCs), the cells that fight many types of infections. Your doctor will check your blood cell count often while you are getting chemotherapy. There are medicines that help speed the recovery of white blood cells, shortening the time when the white blood count is very low. These medicines are called colony stimulating factors (CSF). Raising the white blood cell count greatly lowers the risk of serious infection.

Most infections come from bacteria normally found on your skin and in your mouth, intestines and genital tract. Sometimes, the cause of an infection may not be known. Even if you take extra care, you still may get an infection. But there are some things you can do.

How can I help prevent infections?

- Wash your hands often during the day. Be sure to wash them before you eat, after you use the bathroom, and after touching animals.

- Clean your rectal area gently but thoroughly after each bowel movement. Ask your doctor or nurse for advice if the area becomes irritated or if you have hemorrhoids. Also, check with your doctor before using enemas or suppositories.

- Stay away from people who have illnesses you can catch, such as a cold, the flu, measles, or chicken pox.

- Try to avoid crowds. For example, go shopping or to the movies when the stores or theaters are least likely to be busy.

- Stay away from children who recently have received "live virus" vaccines such as chicken pox and oral polio, since they may be contagious to people with a low blood cell count. Call your doctor or local health department if you have any questions.

- Do not cut or tear the cuticles of your nails.

- Be careful not to cut or nick yourself when using scissors, needles, or knives.

- Maintain good mouth care.

- Do not squeeze or scratch pimples.

- Take a warm (not hot) bath, shower, or sponge bath every day. Pat your skin dry using a light touch. Do not rub too hard.

- Use lotion or oil to soften and heal your skin if it becomes dry and cracked.

- Clean cuts and scrapes right away and daily until healed with warm water, soap, and an antiseptic.

- Avoid contact with animal litter boxes and waste, bird cages, and fish tanks.

- Avoid standing water, for example, bird baths, flower vases, or humidifiers.

- Wear protective gloves when gardening or cleaning up after others, especially small children.

- Do not get any immunizations, such as flu or pneumonia shots, without checking with your doctor first.

- Do not eat raw fish, seafood, meat, or eggs.

- Use an electric shaver instead of a razor to prevent breaks or cuts in your skin.

What are the symptoms of infection?

Call your doctor right away if you have any of these symptoms:

- Fever over 100° F or 38° C

- Chills, especially shaking chills

- Sweating

- Loose bowel movements

- Frequent urgency to urinate or a burning feeling when you urinate

- A severe cough or sore throat

- Unusual vaginal discharge or itching

- Redness, swelling, or tenderness, especially around a wound, sore, ostomy, pimple, rectal area or catheter site

- Sinus pain or pressure

- Earaches, headaches, or stiff neck

- Blisters on the lips or skin

- Mouth sores

Report any signs of infection to your doctor right away, even if it is in the middle of the night. This is especially important when your white blood cell count is low. If you have a fever, do not take aspirin, acetaminophen, or any other medicine to bring your temperature down without checking with your doctor first.

Blood Clotting Problems

Anticancer drugs can affect the bone marrow's ability to make platelets, the blood cells that help stop bleeding by making your blood clot. If your blood does not have enough platelets, you may bleed or bruise more easily than usual, even without an injury.

Call your doctor if you have any of these symptoms:

- unexpected bruising

- small, red spots under the skin
- reddish or pinkish urine
- black or bloody bowel movements
- bleeding from your gums or nose
- vaginal bleeding that is new or lasts longer than a regular period
- headaches or changes in vision
- warm to hot feeling of an arm or leg

Your doctor will check your platelet count often while you are having chemotherapy. If your platelet count falls too low, the doctor may give you a platelet transfusion to build up the count. There are also medicines called colony stimulating factors that help increase your platelets.

How can I help prevent problems if my platelet count is low?

- Check with your doctor or nurse before taking any vitamins, herbal remedies, including all over-the-counter medicines. Many of these products contain aspirin, which can affect platelets.
- Before drinking any alcoholic beverages, check with your doctor.
- Use a very soft toothbrush to clean your teeth.
- When cleaning your nose blow gently into a soft tissue.
- Take extra care not to cut or nick yourself when using scissors, needles, knives, or tools.
- Be careful not to burn yourself when ironing or cooking.
- Avoid contact sports and other activities that might result in injury.
- Ask your doctor if you should avoid sexual activity.
- Use an electric shaver instead of a razor.

Mouth, Gum, and Throat Problems

Good oral care is important during cancer treatment. Some anticancer drugs can cause sores in the mouth and throat, a condition called stomatitis or mucositis. Anticancer drugs also can make these tissues dry and irritated or cause them to bleed. Patients who have not been eating well since beginning chemotherapy are more likely to get mouth sores.

839

In addition to being painful, mouth sores can become infected by the many germs that live in the mouth. Every step should be taken to prevent infections, because they can be hard to fight during chemotherapy and can lead to serious problems.

How can I keep my mouth, gums, and throat healthy?

- Talk to your doctor about seeing your dentist at least several weeks before you start chemotherapy. You may need to have your teeth cleaned and to take care of any problems such as cavities, gum abscesses, gum disease, or poorly fitting dentures. Ask your dentist to show you the best ways to brush and floss your teeth during chemotherapy. Chemotherapy can make you more likely to get cavities, so your dentist may suggest using a fluoride rinse or gel each day to help prevent decay.

- Brush your teeth and gums after every meal. Use a soft tooth-brush and a gentle touch. Brushing too hard can damage soft mouth tissues. Ask your doctor, nurse, or dentist to suggest a special toothbrush and/or toothpaste if your gums are very sensitive. Rinse with warm salt water after meals and before bedtime.

- Rinse your toothbrush well after each use and store it in a dry place.

- Avoid mouthwashes that contain any amount of alcohol. Ask your doctor or nurse to suggest a mild or medicated mouthwash that you might use. For example, mouthwash with sodium bicarbonate (baking soda) is non-irritating.

If you develop sores in your mouth, tell your doctor or nurse. You may need medicine to treat the sores.

How can I cope with mouth sores?

- Ask your doctor if there is anything you can apply directly to the sores or to prescribe a medicine you can use to ease the pain.

- Eat foods cold or at room temperature. Hot and warm foods can irritate a tender mouth and throat.

- Eat soft, soothing foods, such as ice cream, milkshakes, baby food, soft fruits (bananas and applesauce), mashed potatoes, cooked cereals, soft-boiled or scrambled eggs, yogurt, cottage cheese, macaroni and cheese, custards, puddings, and gelatin.

You also can puree cooked foods in the blender to make them smoother and easier to eat.

- Avoid irritating, acidic foods and juices, such as tomato and citrus (orange, grapefruit, and lemon); spicy or salty foods; and rough or coarse foods such as raw vegetables, granola, popcorn, and toast.

How can I cope with mouth dryness?

- Ask your doctor if you should use an artificial saliva product to moisten your mouth.
- Drink plenty of liquids.
- Ask your doctor if you can suck on ice chips, popsicles, or sugarless hard candy. You can also chew sugarless gum. (Sorbitol, a sugar substitute that is in many sugar-free foods, can cause diarrhea in many people. If diarrhea is a problem for you, check the labels of sugar-free foods before you buy them and limit your use of them.)
- Moisten dry foods with butter, margarine, gravy, sauces, or broth.
- Dunk crisp, dry foods in mild liquids.
- Eat soft and pureed foods.
- Use lip balm or petroleum jelly if your lips become dry.
- Carry a water bottle with you to sip from often.

Diarrhea

When chemotherapy affects the cells lining the intestine, it can cause diarrhea (watery or loose stools). If you have diarrhea that continues for more than 24 hours, or if you have pain and cramping along with the diarrhea, call your doctor. In severe cases, the doctor may prescribe a medicine to control the diarrhea. If diarrhea persists, you may need intravenous (IV) fluids to replace the water and nutrients you have lost. Often these fluids are given as an outpatient and do not require hospitalization. Do not take any over-the-counter medicines for diarrhea without asking your doctor.

How can I help control diarrhea?

- Drink plenty of fluids. This will help replace those you have lost through diarrhea. Mild, clear liquids, such as water, clear broth, sports drinks such as Gatorade, or ginger ale, are best. If these drinks make you more thirsty or nauseous, try diluting them with water. Drink slowly and make sure drinks are at room temperature. Let carbonated drinks lose their fizz before you drink them.

- Eat small amounts of food throughout the day instead of three large meals. Unless your doctor has told you otherwise, eat potassium-rich foods. Diarrhea can cause you to lose this important mineral. Bananas, oranges, potatoes, and peach and apricot nectars are good sources of potassium.

- Ask your doctor if you should try a clear liquid diet to give your bowels time to rest. A clear liquid diet does not provide all the nutrients you need, so do not follow one for more than three to five days.

- Eat low-fiber foods. Low-fiber foods include white bread, white rice or noodles, creamed cereals, ripe bananas, canned or cooked fruit without skins, cottage cheese, yogurt without seeds, eggs, mashed or baked potatoes without the skin, pureed vegetables, chicken, or turkey without the skin, and fish.

- Avoid high-fiber foods, which can lead to diarrhea and cramping. High-fiber foods include whole grain breads and cereals, raw vegetables, beans, nuts, seeds, popcorn, and fresh and dried fruit.

- Avoid hot or very cold liquids, which can make diarrhea worse.

- Avoid coffee, tea with caffeine, alcohol, and sweets. Stay away from fried, greasy, or highly spiced foods, too. They are irritating and can cause diarrhea and cramping.

- Avoid milk and milk products, including ice cream, if they make your diarrhea worse.

Constipation

Some anticancer medicines, pain medicines, and other medicines can cause constipation. It can also occur if you are less active or if your diet lacks enough fluid or fiber. If you have not had a bowel movement for more than a day or two, call your doctor, who may suggest taking a laxative or stool softener. Do not take these measures without checking with your doctor, especially if your white blood cell count or platelets are low.

What can I do about constipation?

- Drink plenty of fluids to help loosen the bowels. If you do not have mouth sores, try warm and hot fluids, including water, which work especially well.

- Check with your doctor to see if you can increase the fiber in your diet (there are certain kinds of cancer and certain side effects you may have for which a high-fiber diet is not recommended). High fiber foods include bran, whole-wheat breads and cereals, raw or cooked vegetables, fresh and dried fruit, nuts, and popcorn.

- Get some exercise every day. Go for a walk or you may want to try a more structured exercise program. Talk to your doctor about the amount and type of exercise that is right for you.

Nerve and Muscle Effects

Sometimes anticancer drugs can cause problems with your body's nerves. One example of a condition affecting the nervous system is peripheral neuropathy, where you feel a tingling, burning, weakness, or numbness or pain in the hands and/or feet. Some drugs can also affect the muscles, making them weak, tired, or sore.

Sometimes, these nerve and muscle side effects, though annoying, may not be serious. In other cases, nerve and muscle symptoms may be serious and need medical attention. Be sure to report any nerve or muscle symptoms to your doctor. Most of the time, these symptoms will get better; however, it may take up to a year after your treatment ends.

Some nerve and muscle-related symptoms include the following:

- tingling
- burning
- weakness or numbness in the hands and/or feet
- pain when walking
- weak, sore, tired or achy muscles
- loss of balance
- clumsiness
- difficulty picking up objects and buttoning clothing
- shaking or trembling
- walking problems

- jaw pain
- hearing loss
- stomach pain
- constipation

How can I cope with nerve and muscle problems?

- If your fingers are numb, be very careful when grasping objects that are sharp, hot, or otherwise dangerous.

- If your sense of balance or muscle strength is affected, avoid falls by moving carefully, using handrails when going up or down stairs, and using bath mats in the bathtub or shower.

- Always wear shoes with rubber soles (if possible).

- Ask your doctor for pain medicine.

Effects on Skin and Nails

You may have minor skin problems while you are having chemotherapy, such as redness, rashes, itching, peeling, dryness, acne, and increased sensitivity to the sun. Certain anticancer drugs, when given intravenously, may cause the skin all along the vein to darken, especially in people who have very dark skin. Some people use makeup to cover the area, but this can take a lot of time if several veins are affected. The darkened areas will fade a few months after treatment ends.

Your nails may also become darkened, yellow, brittle, or cracked. They also may develop vertical lines or bands.

While most of these problems are not serious and you can take care of them yourself, a few need immediate attention. Certain drugs given intravenously (IV) can cause serious and permanent tissue damage if they leak out of the vein. Tell your doctor or nurse right away if you feel any burning or pain when you are getting IV drugs. These symptoms do not always mean there is a problem, but they must always be checked at once. Don't hesitate to call your doctor about even the less serious symptoms.

Some symptoms may mean you are having an allergic reaction that may need to be treated at once. Call your doctor or nurse right away if you experience the following:

- you develop sudden or severe itching

- your skin breaks out in a rash or hives
- you have wheezing or any other trouble breathing

How can I cope with skin and nail problems?

Acne

- Try to keep your face clean and dry.
- Ask your doctor or nurse if you can use over-the-counter medicated creams or soaps.

Itching and Dryness

- Apply corn starch as you would a dusting powder.
- To help avoid dryness, take quick showers or sponge baths. Do not take long, hot baths. Use a moisturizing soap.
- Apply cream and lotion while your skin is still moist.
- Avoid perfume, cologne, or aftershave lotion that contains alcohol.
- Use a colloid oatmeal bath or diphenhydramine for generalized pruritus.

Nail Problems

- You can buy nail-strengthening products in a drug store. Be aware that these products may bother your skin and nails.
- Protect your nails by wearing gloves when washing dishes, gardening, or doing other work around the house.
- Be sure to let your doctor know if you have redness, pain, or changes around the cuticles.

Sunlight Sensitivity

- Avoid direct sunlight as much as possible, especially between 10 a.m. and 4 p.m. when the sun's rays are the strongest.
- Use a sun screen lotion with a skin protection factor (SPF) of 15 or higher to protect against sun damage. A product such as zinc oxide, sold over the counter, can block the sun's rays completely.
- Use a lip balm with a sun protection factor.

845

- Wear long-sleeve cotton shirts, pants and hats with a wide brim (particularly if you are having hair loss), to block the sun.

- Even people with dark skin need to protect themselves from the sun during chemotherapy.

Radiation Recall

Some people who have had radiation therapy develop "radiation recall" during their chemotherapy. During or shortly after certain anticancer drugs are given, the skin over an area that had received radiation turns red—a shade anywhere from light to very bright. The skin may blister and peel. This reaction may last hours or even days. Report radiation recall reactions to your doctor or nurse. You can soothe the itching and burning by taking the following steps:

- Placing a cool, wet compress over the affected area

- Wearing soft, non-irritating fabrics. Women who have radiation for breast cancer following lumpectomy often find cotton bras the most comfortable.

Kidney and Bladder Effects

Some anticancer drugs can irritate the bladder or cause temporary or permanent damage to the bladder or kidneys. If you are taking one or more of these drugs, your doctor may ask you to collect a 24-hour urine sample. A blood sample may also be obtained before you begin chemotherapy to check your kidney function. Some anticancer drugs cause the urine to change color (orange, red, green, or yellow) or take on a strong or medicine-like odor for 24–72 hours. Check with your doctor to see if the drugs you are taking may have any of these effects.

Always drink plenty of fluids to ensure good urine flow and help prevent problems. This is very important if you are taking drugs that affect the kidney and bladder. Water, juice, soft drinks, broth, ice cream, soup, popsicles, and gelatin are all considered fluids.

Tell your doctor if you have any of these symptoms:

- Pain or burning when you urinate (pass your water)

- Frequent urination

- Not being able to urinate

- A feeling that you must urinate right away ("urgency")

- Reddish or bloody urine
- Fever
- Chills, especially shaking chills

Flu-Like Symptoms

Some people feel as though they have the flu for a few hours to a few days after chemotherapy. This may be especially true if you are receiving chemotherapy in combination with biological therapy. Flu-like symptoms—muscle and joint aches, headache, tiredness, nausea, slight fever (usually less than 100° F), chills, and poor appetite—may last from one to three days. An infection or the cancer itself can also cause these symptoms. Check with your doctor if you have flu-like symptoms.

Fluid Retention

Your body may retain fluid when you are having chemotherapy. This may be due to hormonal changes from your therapy, to the drugs themselves, or to your cancer. Check with your doctor or nurse if you notice swelling or puffiness in your face, hands, feet, or abdomen. You may need to avoid table salt and foods that have a lot of salt. If the problem is severe, your doctor may prescribe a diuretic, medicine to help your body get rid of excess fluids.

Effects on Sexual Organs

Chemotherapy may—but does not always—affect sexual organs (testis in men, vagina and ovaries in women) and functioning in both men and women. The side effects that might occur depend on the drugs used and the person's age and general health.

How does chemotherapy affect men?

Chemotherapy drugs may lower the number of sperm cells and reduce their ability to move. These changes can result in infertility, which may be temporary or permanent. Infertility affects a man's ability to father a child, but not a man's ability to have sexual intercourse. Other possible effects of these drugs are problems with getting or keeping an erection and damage to the chromosomes, which could lead to birth defects.

What can men do?

- Before starting treatment, talk to your doctor about the possibility of sperm banking—a procedure that freezes sperm for future use—if infertility may be a problem. Ask about the cost of sperm banking.

- Use birth control with your partner during treatment. Ask your doctor how long you need to use birth control.

- Use a condom during sexual intercourse for the first 48 hours after the last dose of chemotherapy because some of the chemotherapy may end up in the sperm.

- Ask your doctor if the chemotherapy will likely affect your ability to father a child. If so, will the effects be temporary or permanent?

How does chemotherapy affect women?

Effects on the ovaries. Anticancer drugs can affect the ovaries and reduce the amount of hormones they produce. Some women find that their menstrual periods become irregular or stop completely while having chemotherapy. Related side effects may be temporary or permanent.

- **Infertility:** Damage to the ovaries may result in infertility, the inability to become pregnant. The infertility can be either temporary or permanent. Whether infertility occurs, and how long it lasts, depends on many factors, including the type of drug, the dosage given, and the woman's age.

- **Menopause:** A woman's age and the drugs and dosages used will determine whether she experiences menopause while on chemotherapy. Chemotherapy may also cause menopause-like symptoms such as hot flashes and dry vaginal tissues. These tissue changes can make intercourse uncomfortable and can make a woman more prone to bladder and/or vaginal infections. Any infection should be treated right away. Menopause may be temporary or permanent.

What can women do for hot flashes?

- Dress in layers
- Avoid caffeine and alcohol

- Exercise
- Try meditation or other relaxation methods

How can women relieve vaginal symptoms and prevent infection?

- Use a water or mineral oil-based vaginal lubricant at the time of intercourse.
- There are products that can be used to stop vaginal dryness. Ask your pharmacist about vaginal gels that can be applied to the vagina.
- Avoid using petroleum jelly, which is difficult for the body to get rid of and increases the risk of infection.
- Wear cotton underwear and pantyhose with a ventilated cotton lining.
- Avoid wearing tight slacks or shorts.
- Ask your doctor about prescribing a vaginal cream or suppository to reduce the chances of infection.
- Ask your doctor about using a vaginal dilator if painful intercourse continues.

Is pregnancy possible during chemotherapy?

Although pregnancy may be possible during chemotherapy, it still is not advisable because some anticancer drugs may cause birth defects. Doctors advise women of childbearing age, from the teens through the end of menopause, to use some method of birth control throughout their treatment, such as condoms, spermicidal agents, diaphragms or birth control pills. Birth control pills may not be appropriate for some women, such as those with breast cancer. Ask your doctor about these contraceptive options.

If a woman is pregnant when her cancer is discovered, it may be possible to delay chemotherapy until after the baby is born. For a woman who needs treatment sooner, the possible effects of chemotherapy on the fetus need to be evaluated.

How does chemotherapy affect feelings about sexuality?

Sexual feelings and attitudes vary among people during chemotherapy. Some people find that they feel closer than ever to their partners and have an increased desire for sexual activity. Others experience little or no change in their sexual desire and energy level. Still others find that their sexual interest declines because of the physical and emotional stresses of having cancer and getting chemotherapy. These stresses may include the following:

- worries about changes in appearance
- anxiety about health, family, or finances
- side effects of treatment, including fatigue, and hormonal changes

A partner's concerns or fears also can affect the sexual relationship. Some may worry that physical intimacy will harm the person who has cancer. Others may fear that they might "catch" the cancer or be affected by the drugs. Both you and your partner should feel free to discuss sexual concerns with your doctor, nurse, social worker, or other counselor who can give you the information and the reassurance you need.

You and your partner also should try to share your feelings with each other. If talking to each other about sex, cancer, or both, is hard, you may want to speak to a counselor who can help you talk more openly. People who can help include psychiatrists, psychologists, social workers, marriage counselors, sex therapists, and members of the clergy.

If you were comfortable with and enjoyed sexual relations before starting chemotherapy, chances are you will still find pleasure in physical intimacy during your treatment. You may discover, however, that intimacy changes during treatment. Hugging, touching, holding, and cuddling may become more important, while sexual intercourse may become less important. Remember that what was true before you started chemotherapy remains true now: There is no one "right" way to express your sexuality. You and your partner should decide together what gives both of you pleasure.

Chapter 76

Radiation Therapy

Chapter Contents

Section 76.1

Questions and Answers about Radiation Therapy

From "Radiation Therapy for Cancer: Questions and Answers,"
National Cancer Institute, August 25, 2004.

What is radiation therapy?

Radiation therapy (also called radiotherapy, x-ray therapy, or irradiation) is the use of a certain type of energy (called ionizing radiation) to kill cancer cells and shrink tumors. Radiation therapy injures or destroys cells in the area being treated (the "target tissue") by damaging their genetic material, making it impossible for these cells to continue to grow and divide. Although radiation damages both cancer cells and normal cells, most normal cells can recover from the effects of radiation and function properly. The goal of radiation therapy is to damage as many cancer cells as possible, while limiting harm to nearby healthy tissue.

There are different types of radiation and different ways to deliver the radiation. For example, certain types of radiation can penetrate more deeply into the body than can others. In addition, some types of radiation can be very finely controlled to treat only a small area (an inch of tissue, for example) without damaging nearby tissues and organs. Other types of radiation are better for treating larger areas.

In some cases, the goal of radiation treatment is the complete destruction of an entire tumor. In other cases, the aim is to shrink a tumor and relieve symptoms. In either case, doctors plan treatment to spare as much healthy tissue as possible.

About half of all cancer patients receive some type of radiation therapy. Radiation therapy may be used alone or in combination with other cancer treatments, such as chemotherapy or surgery. In some cases, a patient may receive more than one type of radiation therapy.

When is radiation therapy used?

Radiation therapy may be used to treat almost every type of solid tumor, including cancers of the brain, breast, cervix, larynx, lung, pancreas, prostate, skin, spine, stomach, uterus, or soft tissue sarcomas. Radiation can also be used to treat leukemia and lymphoma (cancers of the blood-forming cells and lymphatic system, respectively). Radiation dose to each site depends on a number of factors, including the type of cancer and whether there are tissues and organs nearby that may be damaged by radiation.

For some types of cancer, radiation may be given to areas that do not have evidence of cancer. This is done to prevent cancer cells from growing in the area receiving the radiation. This technique is called prophylactic radiation therapy.

Radiation therapy also can be given to help reduce symptoms such as pain from cancer that has spread to the bones or other parts of the body. This is called palliative radiation therapy.

What is the difference between external radiation therapy, internal radiation therapy (brachytherapy), and systemic radiation therapy? When are these types used?

Radiation may come from a machine outside the body (external radiation), may be placed inside the body (internal radiation), or may use unsealed radioactive materials that go throughout the body (systemic radiation therapy). The type of radiation to be given depends on the type of cancer, its location, how far into the body the radiation will need to go, the patient's general health and medical history, whether the patient will have other types of cancer treatment, and other factors.

Most people who receive radiation therapy for cancer have external radiation. Some patients have both external and internal or systemic radiation therapy, either one after the other or at the same time.

External radiation: External radiation therapy usually is given on an outpatient basis; most patients do not need to stay in the hospital. External radiation therapy is used to treat most types of cancer, including cancer of the bladder, brain, breast, cervix, larynx, lung, prostate, and vagina. In addition, external radiation may be used to relieve pain or ease other problems when cancer spreads to other parts of the body from the primary site.

Intraoperative radiation therapy (IORT) is a form of external radiation that is given during surgery. IORT is used to treat localized cancers that cannot be completely removed or that have a high risk of recurring (coming back) in nearby tissues. After all or most of the cancer is removed, one large, high-energy dose of radiation is aimed directly at the tumor site during surgery (nearby healthy tissue is protected with special shields). The patient stays in the hospital to recover from the surgery. IORT may be used in the treatment of thyroid and colorectal cancers, gynecological cancers, cancer of the small intestine, and cancer of the pancreas. It is also being studied in clinical trials (research studies) to treat some types of brain tumors and pelvic sarcomas in adults.

Prophylactic cranial irradiation (PCI) is external radiation given to the brain when the primary cancer (for example, small cell lung cancer) has a high risk of spreading to the brain.

Internal radiation: Internal radiation therapy (also called brachytherapy) uses radiation that is placed very close to or inside the tumor. The radiation source is usually sealed in a small holder called an implant. Implants may be in the form of thin wires, plastic tubes called catheters, ribbons, capsules, or seeds. The implant is put directly into the body. Internal radiation therapy may require a hospital stay. Internal radiation is usually delivered in one of two ways; both methods use sealed implants.

Interstitial radiation therapy is inserted into tissue at or near the tumor site. It is used to treat tumors of the head and neck, prostate, cervix, ovary, breast, and perianal and pelvic regions. Some women treated with external radiation for breast cancer receive a "booster dose" of radiation that may use interstitial radiation or external radiation.

Intracavitary or intraluminal radiation therapy is inserted into the body with an applicator. It is commonly used in the treatment of uterine cancer. Researchers are also studying these types of internal radiation therapy for other cancers, including breast, bronchial, cervical, gallbladder, oral, rectal, tracheal, uterine, and vaginal.

Systemic radiation: Systemic radiation therapy uses radioactive materials such as iodine 131 and strontium 89. The materials may be taken by mouth or injected into the body. Systemic radiation therapy is sometimes used to treat cancer of the thyroid and adult non-Hodgkin lymphoma. Researchers are investigating agents to treat other types of cancer.

Will radiation therapy make the patient radioactive?

Cancer patients receiving radiation therapy are often concerned that the treatment will make them radioactive. The answer to this question depends on the type of radiation therapy being given.

External radiation therapy will not make the patient radioactive. Patients do not need to avoid being around other people because of the treatment.

Internal radiation therapy (interstitial, intracavitary, or intraluminal) that involves sealed implants emits radioactivity, so a stay in the hospital may be needed. Certain precautions are taken to protect hospital staff and visitors. The sealed sources deliver most of their radiation mainly around the area of the implant, so while the area around the implant is radioactive, the patient's whole body is not radioactive.

Systemic radiation therapy uses unsealed radioactive materials that travel throughout the body. Some of this radioactive material will leave the body through saliva, sweat, and urine before the radioactivity decays, making these fluids radioactive. Therefore, certain precautions are sometimes used for people who come in close contact with the patient. The patient's doctor or nurse will provide information if these special precautions are needed.

What are stereotactic radiosurgery and stereotactic radiotherapy?

Stereotactic (or stereotaxic) radiosurgery uses a large dose of radiation to destroy tumor tissue in the brain. The procedure does not involve actual surgery. The patient's head is placed in a special frame, which is attached to the patient' skull. The frame is used to aim high-dose radiation beams directly at the tumor inside the patient's head. The dose and area receiving the radiation are coordinated very precisely. Most nearby tissues are not damaged by this procedure.

Stereotactic radiosurgery can be done in one of three ways. The most common technique uses a linear accelerator to administer high-energy photon radiation to the tumor (called "LINAC-based stereotactic radiosurgery"). The gamma knife, the second most common technique, uses cobalt 60 to deliver radiation. The third technique uses heavy charged particle beams (such as protons and helium ions) to deliver stereotactic radiation to the tumor.

Stereotactic radiosurgery is mostly used in the treatment of small benign and malignant brain tumors (including meningiomas, acoustic neuromas, and pituitary cancer). It can also be used to treat other conditions (for example, Parkinson disease and epilepsy). In addition, stereotactic radiosurgery can be used to treat metastatic brain tumors (cancer that has spread to the brain from another part of the body) either alone or along with whole-brain radiation therapy. (Whole-brain radiation therapy is a form of external radiation therapy that treats the entire brain with radiation).

Stereotactic radiotherapy uses essentially the same approach as stereotactic radiosurgery to deliver radiation to the target tissue. However, stereotactic radiotherapy uses multiple small fractions of radiation as opposed to one large dose. Giving multiple smaller doses may improve outcomes and minimize side effects. Stereotactic radiotherapy is used to treat tumors in the brain as well as other parts of the body.

Clinical trials are under way to study the effectiveness of stereotactic radiosurgery and stereotactic radiotherapy alone and in combination with other types of radiation therapy.

Who plans and delivers the radiation treatment to the patient?

Many health care providers help to plan and deliver radiation treatment to the patient. The radiation therapy team includes the radiation oncologist, a doctor who specializes in using radiation to treat cancer; the dosimetrist, who determines the proper radiation dose; the radiation physicist, who makes sure that the machine delivers the right amount of radiation to the correct site in the body; and the radiation therapist, who gives the radiation treatment. Often, radiation treatment is only one part of the patient's total therapy. Combined modality therapy, the use of radiation with drug therapy, is commonly used.

The radiation oncologist also works with the medical or pediatric oncologist, surgeon, radiologist (a doctor who specializes in creating and interpreting pictures of areas inside the body), pathologist (a doctor who identifies diseases by studying cells and tissues under a microscope), and others to plan the patient's total course of therapy. A close working relationship between the radiation oncologist, medical or pediatric oncologist, surgeon, radiologist, and pathologist is important in planning the total therapy.

Section 76.2

What to Expect during Radiation Therapy

Excerpted from "Radiation Therapy and You: A Guide to Self-Help During Cancer Treatment," National Cancer Institute, September 22, 1999, accessed November 24, 2006.

Questions and Answers about External Radiation Therapy

How does the doctor plan my treatment?

The high energy rays used for radiation therapy can come from a variety of sources. Your doctor may choose to use x-rays, an electron beam, or cobalt-60 gamma rays. Some cancer treatment centers have special equipment that produces beams of protons or neutrons for radiation therapy. The type of radiation your doctor decides to use depends on what kind of cancer you have and how far into your body the radiation should go. High-energy radiation is used to treat many types of cancer. Low-energy x-rays are used to treat some kinds of skin diseases.

After a physical exam and a review of your medical history, the doctor plans your treatment. In a process called simulation, you will be asked to lie very still on an examining table while the radiation therapist uses a special x-ray machine to define your treatment port or field. This is the exact place on your body where the radiation will be aimed. Depending on the location of your cancer, you may have more than one treatment port.

Simulation may also involve CT scans or other imaging studies to plan how to direct the radiation. Depending on the type of treatment you will be receiving, body molds or other devices that keep you from moving during treatment (immobilization devices) may be made at this time. They will be used each time you have treatment to be sure that you are positioned correctly. Simulation may take from a half hour to about two hours.

The radiation therapist often will mark the treatment port on your skin with tattoos or tiny dots of colored, permanent ink. It's important that the radiation be targeted at the same area each time. If the dots appear to be fading, tell your radiation therapist who will darken them so that they can be seen easily.

Once simulation has been done, your doctor will meet with the radiation physicist and the dosimetrist. Based on the results of your medical history, lab tests, x-rays, other treatments you may have had, and the location and kind of cancer you have, they will decide how much radiation is needed, what kind of machine to use to deliver it, and how many treatments you should have.

After you have started the treatments, your doctor and the other members of your health care team will follow your progress by checking your response to treatment and how you are feeling at least once a week. When necessary, your doctor may revise the treatment plan by changing the radiation dose or the number and length of your remaining radiation sessions.

Your nurse will be available daily to discuss your concerns and answer any questions you may have. Be sure to tell your nurse if you are having any side effects or if you notice any unusual symptoms.

How long does the treatment take?

For most types of cancer, radiation therapy usually is given five days a week for six or seven weeks. (When radiation is used for palliative care, the course of treatment is shorter, usually two to three weeks.) The total dose of radiation and the number of treatments you need will depend on the size, location, and kind of cancer you have, your general health, and other medical treatments you may be receiving.

Using many small doses of daily radiation rather than a few large doses helps protect normal body tissues in the treatment area. Weekend rest breaks allow normal cells to recover.

It's very important that you have all of your scheduled treatments to get the most benefit from your therapy. Missing or delaying treatments can lessen the effectiveness of your radiation treatment.

What happens during the treatment visits?

Before each treatment, you may need to change into a hospital gown or robe. It's best to wear clothing that is easy to take off and put on again.

In the treatment room, the radiation therapist will use the marks on your skin to locate the treatment area and to position you correctly. You may sit in a special chair or lie down on a treatment table. For each external radiation therapy session, you will be in the treatment room about 15 to 30 minutes, but you will be getting radiation for only about 1 to 5 minutes of that time. Receiving external radiation treatments is painless, just like having an x-ray taken. You will not hear, see, or smell the radiation.

The radiation therapist may put special shields (or blocks) between the machine and certain parts of your body to help protect normal tissues and organs. There might also be plastic or plaster forms that help you stay in exactly the right place. You need to remain very still during the treatment so that the radiation reaches only the area where it's needed and the same area is treated each time. You don't have to hold your breath—just breathe normally.

The radiation therapist will leave the treatment room before your treatment begins. The radiation machine is controlled from a nearby area. You will be watched on a television screen or through a window in the control room. Although you may feel alone, keep in mind that the therapist can see and hear you and even talk with you using an intercom in the treatment room. If you should feel ill or very uncomfortable during the treatment, tell your therapist at once. The machine can be stopped at any time.

The machines used for radiation treatments are very large, and they make noises as they move around your body to aim at the treatment area from different angles. Their size and motion may be frightening at first. Remember that the machines are being moved and controlled by your radiation therapist. They are checked constantly to be sure they're working right. If you have concerns about anything that happens in the treatment room, discuss these concerns with the radiation therapist.

What is hyperfractionated radiation therapy?

Radiation is usually given once daily in a dose that is based on the type and location of the tumor. In hyperfractionated radiation therapy, the daily dose is divided into smaller doses that are given more than once a day. The treatments usually are separated by four to six hours. Doctors are studying hyperfractionated therapy to learn if it is equal to, or perhaps more effective than, once-a-day therapy and whether there are fewer long-term side effects. Early results of treatment studies of some kinds of tumors are encouraging, and hyperfractionated therapy is becoming a more common way to give radiation treatments for some types of cancer.

What is intraoperative radiation?

Intraoperative radiation combines surgery and radiation therapy. The surgeon first removes as much of the tumor as possible. Before the surgery is completed, a large dose of radiation is given directly to the tumor bed (the area from which the tumor has been removed) and nearby areas where cancer cells might have spread. Sometimes intraoperative radiation is used in addition to external radiation therapy. This gives the cancer cells a larger amount of radiation than would be possible using external radiation alone.

What can I do to take care of myself during therapy?

Each patient's body responds to radiation therapy in its own way. That's why your doctor must plan, and sometimes adjust, your treatment. In addition, your doctor or nurse will give you suggestions for caring for yourself at home that are specific for your treatment and the possible side effects.

Nearly all cancer patients receiving radiation therapy need to take special care of themselves to protect their health and to help the treatment succeed.

- Before starting treatment, be sure your doctor knows about any medicines you are taking and if you have any allergies. Do not start taking any medicine (whether prescription or over-the-counter) during your radiation therapy without first telling your doctor or nurse.

- Fatigue is common during radiation therapy. Your body will use a lot of extra energy over the course of your treatment, and you may feel very tired. Be sure to get plenty of rest and sleep as often as you feel the need. It's common for fatigue to last for four to six weeks after your treatment has been completed.

- Good nutrition is very important. Try to eat a balanced diet that will prevent weight loss.

- Check with your doctor before taking vitamin supplements or herbal preparations during treatment.

- Avoid wearing tight clothes such as girdles or close-fitting collars over the treatment area. Be extra kind to your skin in the treatment area:

  - Ask your doctor or nurse if you may use soaps, lotions, deodorants, sun blocks, medicines, perfumes, cosmetics, talcum powder, or other substances in the treated area.

  - Wear loose, soft cotton clothing over the treated area.

  - Do not wear starched or stiff clothing over the treated area.

- Do not scratch, rub, or scrub treated skin.

- Do not use adhesive tape on treated skin. If bandaging is necessary, use paper tape and apply it outside of the treatment area. Your nurse can help you place dressings so that you can avoid irritating the treated area.

- Do not apply heat or cold (heating pad, ice pack, etc.) to the treated area. Use only lukewarm water for bathing the area.

- Use an electric shaver if you must shave the treated area but only after checking with your doctor or nurse. Do not use a preshave lotion or hair removal products on the treated area.

- Protect the treatment area from the sun. Do not apply sunscreens just before a radiation treatment. If possible, cover treated skin (with light clothing) before going outside. Ask your doctor if you should use a sunscreen or a sunblocking product. If so, select one with a protection factor of at least 15 and reapply it often. Ask your doctor or nurse how long after your treatments are completed you should continue to protect the treated skin from sunlight.

- If you have questions, ask your doctor or nurse. They are the only ones who can properly advise you about your treatment, its side effects, home care, and any other medical concerns you may have.

Questions and Answers about Internal Radiation Therapy

When is internal radiation therapy used?

Your doctor may decide that a high dose of radiation given to a small area of your body is the best way to treat your cancer. Internal radiation therapy allows the doctor to give a higher total dose of radiation in a shorter time than is possible with external treatment.

Internal radiation therapy places the radiation source as close as possible to the cancer cells. Instead of using a large radiation machine, the radioactive material, sealed in a thin wire, catheter, or tube (implant), is placed directly into the affected tissue. This method of treatment concentrates the radiation on the cancer cells and lessens radiation damage to some of the normal tissue near the cancer. Some of the radioactive substances used for internal radiation treatment include cesium, iridium, iodine, phosphorus, and palladium.

Internal radiation therapy may be used for cancers of the head and neck, breast, uterus, thyroid, cervix, and prostate. Your doctor may suggest using both internal and external radiation therapy.

In this chapter, "internal radiation treatment" refers to implant radiation. Health professionals prefer to use the term "brachytherapy" for implant radiation therapy. You may hear your doctor or nurse use the terms, interstitial radiation or intracavitary radiation; each is a form of internal radiation therapy. Sometimes radioactive implants are called "capsules" or "seeds."

How is the implant placed in the body?

The type of implant and the method of placing it depend on the size and location of the cancer. Implants may be put right into the tumor (interstitial radiation), in special applicators inside a body cavity (intracavitary radiation) or passage (intraluminal radiation), on the surface of a tumor, or in the area from which the tumor has been removed. Implants may be removed after a short time or left in place permanently. If they are to be left in place, the radioactive substance used will lose radiation quickly and become non-radioactive in a short time.

When interstitial radiation is given, the radiation source is placed in the tumor in catheters, seeds, or capsules. When intracavitary radiation is used, a container or applicator of radioactive material is placed in a body cavity such as the uterus. In surface brachytherapy the radioactive source is sealed in a small holder and placed in or against the tumor. In intraluminal brachytherapy the radioactive source is placed in a body lumen or tube, such as the bronchus or esophagus.

Internal radiation also may be given by injecting a solution of radioactive substance into the bloodstream or a body cavity. This form of radiation therapy may be called unsealed internal radiation therapy.

For most types of implants, you will need to be in the hospital. You will be given general or local anesthesia so that you will not feel any pain when the doctor places the holder for the radioactive material in your body. In many hospitals, the radioactive material is placed in its holder or applicator after you return to your room so that other patients, staff, and visitors are not exposed to radiation.

How are other people protected from radiation while the implant is in place?

Sometimes the radiation source in your implant sends its high energy rays outside your body. To protect others while you are having implant therapy, the hospital will have you stay in a private room. Although the nurses and other people caring for you will not be able to spend a long time in your room, they will give you all of the care you need. You should call for a nurse when you need one, but keep in mind that the nurse will work quickly and speak to you from the doorway more often than from your bedside. In most cases, your urine and stool will contain no radioactivity unless you are having unsealed internal radiation therapy.

There also will be limits on visitors while your implant is in place. Children younger than 18 or pregnant women should not visit patients who are having internal radiation therapy. Be sure to tell your visitors to ask the hospital staff for any special instructions before they come into your room. Visitors should sit at least 6 feet from your bed and the radiation oncology staff will determine how long your visitors may stay. The time can vary from 30 minutes to several hours per day. In some hospitals a rolling lead shield is placed beside the bed and kept between the patient and visitors or staff members.

What are the side effects of internal radiation therapy?

The side effects of implant therapy depend on the area being treated. You are not likely to have severe pain or feel ill during implant therapy. However, if an applicator is holding your implant in place, it may be somewhat uncomfortable. If you need it, the doctor will order medicine to help you relax or to relieve pain. If general anesthesia was used while your implant was put in place, you may feel drowsy, weak, or nauseated but these effects do not last long. If necessary, medications can be ordered to relieve nausea. Be sure to tell the nurse about any symptoms that concern you.

How long does the implant stay in place?

Your doctor will decide the amount of time that an implant is to be left in place. It depends on the dose (amount) of radioactivity needed for effective treatment. Your treatment schedule will depend on the type of cancer, where it is located, your general health, and other cancer treatments you have had. Depending on where the implant is placed, you may have to keep it from shifting by staying in bed and lying fairly still.

Temporary implants may be either low dose-rate (LDR) or high dose-rate (HDR). Low dose-rate implants are left in place for several days; high dose-rate implants are removed after a few minutes.

For some cancer sites, the implant is left in place permanently. If your implant is permanent, you may need to stay in your hospital room away from other people for a few days while the radiation is most active. The implant becomes less radioactive each day; by the time you are ready to go home, the radiation in your body will be much weaker. Your doctor will advise you if there are any special precautions you need to use at home.

What happens after the implant is removed?

Usually, an anesthetic is not needed when the doctor removes a temporary implant. Most can be taken out right in the patient's hospital room. Once the implant is removed, there is no radioactivity in your body. The hospital staff and your visitors will no longer have to limit the time they stay with you.

Your doctor will tell you if you need to limit your activities after you leave the hospital. Most patients are allowed to do as much as they feel like doing. You may need some extra sleep or rest breaks during your days at home, but you should feel stronger quickly.

The area that has been treated with an implant may be sore or sensitive for some time. If any particular activity such as sports or sexual intercourse cause irritation in the treatment area, your doctor may suggest that you limit these activities for a while.

What is remote brachytherapy?

In remote brachytherapy, a computer sends the radioactive source through a tube to a catheter that has been placed near the tumor by the patient's doctor. The procedure is directed by the brachytherapy team, who watch the patient on closed-circuit television and communicate with the patient using an intercom. The radioactivity remains at the tumor for only a few minutes. In some cases, several remote treatments may be required and the catheter may stay in place between treatments.

Remote brachytherapy may be used for low dose-rate (LDR) treatments in an inpatient setting. High dose-rate (HDR) remote brachytherapy allows a person to have internal radiation therapy in an outpatient setting. High dose-rate treatments take only a few minutes. Because no radioactive material is left in the body, the patient can return home after the treatment. Remote brachytherapy has been used to treat cancers of the cervix, breast, lung, pancreas, prostate, and esophagus.

Section 76.3

Managing the Side Effects of Radiation Therapy

Excerpted from "Radiation Therapy and You: A Guide to Self-Help During Cancer Treatment," National Cancer Institute, September 22, 1999, accessed November 24, 2006.

Are the side effects of radiation treatment the same for everyone?

The side effects of radiation treatment vary from patient to patient. Side effects may be acute or chronic. Acute side effects are sometimes referred to as "early side effects." They occur soon after the treatment begins and usually are gone within a few weeks of finishing therapy. Chronic side effects, sometimes called "late side effects," may take months or years to develop and usually are permanent.

The most common early side effects of radiation therapy are fatigue and skin changes. They can result from radiation to any treatment site. Other side effects are related to treatment of specific areas. For example, temporary or permanent hair loss may be a side effect of radiation treatment to the head. Appetite can be altered if treatment affects the mouth, stomach, or intestine.

Fortunately, most side effects will go away in time. In the meantime, there are ways to reduce discomfort. If you have a side effect that is especially severe, the doctor may prescribe a break in your treatments or change your treatment in some way.

What causes fatigue?

Most people begin to feel tired after a few weeks of radiation therapy. During radiation therapy, the body uses a lot of energy for healing. You also may be tired because of stress related to your illness, daily trips for treatment, and the effects of radiation on normal cells. Feelings of weakness or weariness will go away gradually after your treatment has been completed.

You can help yourself during radiation therapy by not trying to do too much. If you do feel tired, limit your activities and use your leisure time in a restful way. Save your energy for doing the things that you feel are most important. Do not feel that you have to do everything you normally do. Try to get more sleep at night, and plan your day so that you have time to rest if you need it. Several short naps or breaks may be more helpful than a long rest period.

Sometimes, light exercise such as walking may combat fatigue. Talk with your doctor or nurse about how much exercise you may do while you are having therapy. Talking with other cancer patients in a support group may also help you learn how to deal with fatigue.

If you have a full-time job, you may want to try to continue to work your normal schedule. However, some patients prefer to take time off while they're receiving radiation therapy; others work a reduced number of hours. Speak frankly with your employer about your needs and wishes during this time. A part-time schedule may be possible or perhaps you can do some work at home. Ask your doctor's office or the radiation therapy department to help by trying to schedule treatments with your workday in mind.

Whether you're going to work or not, it's a good idea to ask family members or friends to help with daily chores, shopping, child care, housework, or driving. Neighbors may be able to help by picking up groceries for you when they do their own shopping. You also could ask someone to drive you to and from your treatment visits to help conserve your energy.

How are skin problems treated?

You may notice that your skin in the treatment area is red or irritated. It may look as if it is sunburned, or tanned. After a few weeks your skin may be very dry from the therapy. Ask your doctor or nurse for advice on how to relieve itching or discomfort.

With some kinds of radiation therapy, treated skin may develop a "moist reaction," especially in areas where there are skin folds. When this happens, the skin is wet and it may become very sore. It's important to notify your doctor or nurse if your skin develops a moist reaction. They can give you suggestions on how to care for these areas and prevent them from becoming infected. Other tips on skin care can be found in the section on external radiation therapy.

During radiation therapy you will need to be very gentle with the skin in the treatment area. The following suggestions may be helpful:

- Avoid irritating treated skin.

- When you wash, use only lukewarm water and mild soap; pat dry.

- Do not wear tight clothing over the area.

- Do not rub, scrub, or scratch the skin in the treatment area.

- Avoid putting anything that is hot or cold, such as heating pads or ice packs, on your treated skin.

- Ask your doctor or nurse to recommend skin care products that will not cause skin irritation. Do not use any powders, creams, perfumes, deodorants, body oils, ointments, lotions, or home remedies in the treatment area while you're being treated and for several weeks afterward unless approved by your doctor or nurse.

- Do not apply any skin lotions within two hours of a treatment.

- Avoid exposing the radiated area to the sun during treatment. If you expect to be in the sun for more than a few minutes you will need to be very careful. Wear protective clothing (such as a hat with a broad brim and a shirt with long sleeves) and use a sunscreen. Ask your doctor or nurse about using sunblocking lotions. After your treatment is over, ask your doctor or nurse how long you should continue to take extra precautions in the sun.

The majority of skin reactions to radiation therapy go away a few weeks after treatment is completed. In some cases, though, the treated skin will remain slightly darker than it was before and it may continue to be more sensitive to sun exposure.

What can be done about hair loss?

Radiation therapy can cause hair loss, also known as alopecia, but only in the area being treated. For example, if you are receiving treatment to your hip, you will not lose the hair from your head. Radiation of your head may cause you to lose some or all of the hair on your scalp. Many patients find that their hair grows back again after the treatments are finished. The amount of hair that grows back will depend on how much and what kind of radiation you receive. You may notice that your hair has a slightly different texture or color when it grows back. Other types of cancer treatment, such as chemotherapy, also can affect how your hair grows back.

Although your scalp may be tender after the hair is lost, it's a good idea to cover your head with a hat, turban, or scarf. You should wear a protective cap or scarf when you're in the sun or outdoors in cold weather. If you prefer a wig or toupee, be sure the lining does not irritate your scalp. The cost of a hairpiece that you need because of cancer treatment is a tax-deductible expense and may be covered in part by your health insurance. If you plan to buy a wig, it's a good idea to select it early in your treatment if you want to match the color and style to your own hair.

How are side effects on the blood managed?

Radiation therapy can cause low levels of white blood cells and platelets. These blood cells normally help your body fight infection and prevent bleeding. If large areas of active bone marrow are treated, your red blood cell count may be low as well. If your blood tests show these side effects, your doctor may wait until your blood counts increase to continue treatments. Your doctor will check your blood counts regularly and change your treatment schedule if it is necessary.

Will eating be a problem?

Sometimes radiation treatment causes loss of appetite and interferes with eating, digesting, and absorbing food. Try to eat enough to help damaged tissues rebuild themselves. It is not unusual to lose one or two pounds a week during radiation therapy. You will be weighed weekly to monitor your weight.

It is very important to eat a balanced diet. You may find it helpful to eat small meals often and to try to eat a variety of different foods. Your doctor or nurse can tell you whether you should eat a special diet, and a dietitian will have some ideas that will help you maintain your weight.

The list below suggests ways to perk up your appetite when it's poor and to make the most of it when you do feel like eating.

- Eat when you are hungry, even if it is not mealtime.

- Eat several small meals during the day rather than three large ones.

- Use soft lighting, quiet music, brightly colored table settings, or whatever helps you feel good while eating.

- Vary your diet and try new recipes. If you enjoy company while eating, try to have meals with family or friends. It may be helpful to have the radio or television on while you eat.

- Ask your doctor or nurse whether you can have a glass of wine or beer with your meal to increase your appetite. Keep in mind that, in some cases, alcohol may not be allowed because it could worsen the side effects of treatment. This may be especially true if you are receiving radiation therapy for cancer of the head, neck, or upper chest area including the esophagus.

- Keep simple meals in the freezer to use when you feel hungry.

- If other people offer to cook for you, let them. Don't be shy about telling them what you'd like to eat.

- Keep healthy snacks close by for nibbling when you get the urge.

- If you live alone, you might want to arrange for "Meals on Wheels" to bring food to you. Ask your doctor, nurse, social worker, or local social service agencies about "Meals on Wheels." This service is available in most large communities.

If you are able to eat only small amounts of food, you can increase the calories per serving by:

- Adding butter or margarine.

- Mixing canned cream soups with milk or half-and-half rather than water.

- Drinking eggnog, milkshakes, or prepared liquid supplements between meals.

- Adding cream sauce or melted cheese to your favorite vegetables.

Some people find they can drink large amounts of liquids even when they don't feel like eating solid foods. If this is the case for you, try to get the most from each glassful by making drinks enriched with powdered milk, yogurt, honey, or prepared liquid supplements.

Will radiation therapy affect me emotionally?

Nearly all patients being treated for cancer report feeling emotionally upset at different times during their therapy. It's not unusual to feel anxious, depressed, afraid, angry, frustrated, alone, or helpless. Radiation therapy may affect your emotions indirectly through fatigue or changes in hormone balance, but the treatment itself is not a direct cause of mental distress.

You may find that it's helpful to talk about your feelings with a close friend, family member, chaplain, nurse, social worker, or psychologist with whom you feel at ease. You may want to ask your doctor or nurse about meditation or relaxation exercises that might help you unwind and feel calmer.

Nationwide support programs can help cancer patients to meet others who share common problems and concerns. Some medical centers have formed peer support groups so that patients can meet to discuss their feelings and inspire each other.

There are several helpful books, tapes, and videos on dealing with the emotional effects of having cancer. The National Cancer Institute's Cancer Information Service (800-4-CANCER) can direct you to reading matter and other resources in your area for emotional support.

What side effects occur with radiation therapy to the head and neck?

Some people who receive radiation to the head and neck experience redness, irritation, and sores in the mouth; a dry mouth or thickened saliva; difficulty in swallowing; changes in taste; or nausea. Try not to let these symptoms keep you from eating.

Other problems that may occur during treatment to the head and neck are a loss of taste, which may diminish appetite and affect nutrition, and earaches (caused by hardening of ear wax). You may notice some swelling or drooping of the skin under your chin as well as changes in the skin texture. Your jaw may also feel stiff and you may be unable to open your mouth as wide as before treatment. Jaw exercises may help ease this problem. Report all side effects to your doctor or nurse and ask what you should do about them.

If you are receiving radiation therapy to the head or neck, you need to take especially good care of your teeth, gums, mouth, and throat. Side effects from treatment to these areas commonly involve the mouth, which may be sore and dry. Here are a few tips that may help you manage mouth problems:

- Avoid spices and coarse foods such as raw vegetables, dry crackers, and nuts.

- Remember that acidic foods and liquids can cause mouth and throat irritation.

- Don't smoke, chew tobacco, or drink alcohol.

- Stay away from sugary snacks because they can promote tooth decay.

- Clean your mouth and teeth often, using the method your dentist or doctor recommends.

- Use only alcohol-free mouthwash; many commercial mouthwashes contain alcohol which has a drying effect on mouth tissues.

Mouth care: Radiation treatment for head and neck cancer can increase your chances of getting cavities in your teeth. Mouth care designed to prevent problems will be a very important part of your treatment. Before starting radiation therapy, make an appointment for a complete dental/oral checkup. Ask your dentist and radiation oncologist to consult before your radiation treatments begin.

Your dentist probably will want to see you often during your radiation therapy to help you care for your mouth and teeth. This is a good way to reduce the risk of tooth decay and help you deal with possible problems such as soreness of the tissues in your mouth. It's important that you follow the dentist's advice while you're receiving radiation therapy. Most likely, your dentist will suggest that you take the following precautions:

- Clean your teeth and gums thoroughly with a soft brush at least four times a day (after meals and at bedtime).

- Use a fluoride toothpaste that contains no abrasives.

- Floss gently between teeth daily if you flossed regularly before your illness. Use waxed, non-shredding dental floss.

- Rinse your mouth gently and frequently with a salt and baking soda solution especially after you brush. Use ½ teaspoon of salt and ½ teaspoon of baking soda in a large glass of warm water. Follow with a plain water rinse.

- Apply fluoride regularly as prescribed by your dentist.

Your dentist can explain how to mix the salt and baking soda mouthwash and how to use the fluoride treatment method that best suits your needs. You can probably get printed instructions for proper dental care at the dentist's office. If dry mouth continues after your treatment is complete, you will need to continue the mouth care recommended during treatment. Always share your dentist's instructions with your radiation nurse.

Dealing with mouth or throat problems: Soreness in your mouth or throat may appear in the second or third week of external radiation therapy and it will most likely have disappeared within a month or so after your treatments have ended. You may have trouble swallowing during this time because your mouth feels dry. Your doctor or dentist can prescribe medicine for mouth discomfort and tell you about methods to relieve other mouth problems during and following your radiation therapy. If you wear dentures you may notice that they no longer fit well. This occurs if the radiation causes your gums to swell. You may need to stop wearing your dentures until your radiation therapy is over. It's important not to risk denture-induced gum sores because they may become infected and heal slowly.

Your salivary glands may produce less saliva than usual, making your mouth feel dry. Unfortunately dry mouth may continue to be a problem even after treatment is over. You may be given medication to help lessen this side effect. It's helpful to sip cool drinks throughout the day. Although many radiation therapy patients have said that drinking carbonated beverages helps relieve dry mouth, water probably is your best choice. In the morning, fill a large container with ice, add water, and carry it with you during the day so that you can take frequent sips. Keep a glass of cool water at your bedside at night, too. Sugar-free candy or gum also may help; be careful about overuse of these products as they can cause diarrhea in some people. Avoid tobacco and alcoholic drinks because they tend to dry and irritate your mouth tissues. Moisten food with gravies and sauces to make eating easier. If these measures are not enough, ask your dentist, radiation oncologist, or nurse about products that either replace or stimulate your own saliva. Artificial saliva and medication to increase saliva production are available.

Tips on eating: You may find that it's difficult or painful to swallow. Some patients say that they feel as if something is stuck in their throat. Soreness or dryness in your mouth or throat can also make it hard to eat. The section on eating problems may be helpful. In addition, some of the following tips may help to make eating more comfortable:

- Choose foods that taste good to you and are easy to eat.

- Try changing the consistency of foods by adding fluids and using sauces and gravies to make them softer.

- Avoid highly spiced foods and textures that are dry and rough, such as crackers.

- Eat small meals, and eat more frequently than usual.

- Cut your food into small, bite-sized pieces.

- Ask your doctor for special liquid medicines to reduce the pain in your throat so that you can eat and swallow more easily.

- Ask your doctor about liquid food supplements that are easier to swallow than solids. They can help you get enough calories each day to avoid losing weight.

- If you are being treated for lung cancer, it's important to keep mucus and other secretions thin and manageable; drinking extra fluids can help.

- If familiar foods no longer taste good, try new foods and use different methods of food preparation.

What side effects occur with radiation therapy to the chest?

Radiation treatment to the chest may cause several changes. For example, you may find that it is hard to swallow or that swallowing hurts. You may develop a cough or a fever. You may notice that when you cough the amount and color of the mucus is different. Shortness of breath is also common. Be sure to let your treatment team know right away if you have any of these symptoms. Remember that your doctor and nurse have seen these changes in many radiation patients and they know how to help you deal with them.

Are there side effects with radiation therapy for breast cancer?

The most common side effects with radiation therapy for breast cancer are fatigue and skin changes. However there may be other side effects as well. If you notice that your shoulder feels stiff, ask your doctor or nurse about exercises to keep your arm moving freely. Other side effects include breast or nipple soreness, swelling from fluid buildup in the treated area, and skin reddening or tanning. Except for tanning which may take up to six months to fade, these side effects will most likely disappear in four to six weeks.

If you are being treated for breast cancer and you are having radiation therapy after a lumpectomy or mastectomy, it's a good idea to go without your bra whenever possible or, if this makes you more uncomfortable, wear a soft cotton bra without underwires. This will help reduce skin irritation in the treatment area.

What side effects occur with radiation therapy to the stomach and abdomen?

If you are having radiation treatment to the stomach or some portion of the abdomen, you may have an upset stomach, nausea, or diarrhea. Your doctor can prescribe medicines to relieve these problems. Do not take any medications for these symptoms unless you first check with your doctor or nurse.

Managing nausea: It's not unusual to feel queasy for a few hours right after radiation treatment to the stomach or abdomen. Some patients find that they have less nausea if they have their treatment with an empty stomach. Others report that eating a light meal one to two hours before treatment lessens queasiness. You may find that nausea is less of a problem if you wait one to two hours after your treatment before you eat. If this problem persists, ask your doctor to prescribe a medicine (an antiemetic to prevent nausea. If antiemetics are prescribed, take them within the hour before treatment or when your doctor or nurse suggests, even if you sometimes feel that they are not needed.

If your stomach feels upset just before every treatment, the queasiness or nausea may be caused by anxiety and concerns about cancer treatment. Try having a bland snack such as toast or crackers and apple juice before your appointment. It may also help to try to unwind before your treatment. Reading a book, writing a letter, or working a crossword puzzle may help you relax.

Here are some other tips to help an unsettled stomach:

- Stick to any special diet that your doctor, nurse, or dietitian gives you.

- Eat small meals.

- Eat often and try to eat and drink slowly.

- Avoid foods that are fried or are high in fat.

- Drink cool liquids between meals.

- Eat foods that have only a mild aroma and can be served cool or at room temperature.

- For severe nausea and vomiting, try a clear liquid diet (broth and clear juices) or bland foods that are easy to digest, such as dry toast and gelatin.

Diarrhea: Diarrhea may begin in the third or fourth week of radiation therapy to the abdomen or pelvis. You may be able to prevent diarrhea by eating a low fiber diet when you start therapy: avoid foods such as raw fruits and vegetables, beans, cabbage, and whole grain breads and cereals. Your doctor or nurse may suggest other changes to your diet, prescribe antidiarrhea medicine, or give you special instructions to help with the problem. Tell the doctor or nurse if these changes fail to control your diarrhea. The following changes in your diet may help:

- Try a clear liquid diet (water, weak tea, apple juice, clear broth, plain gelatin) as soon as diarrhea starts or when you feel that it's going to start.

- Ask your doctor or nurse to advise you about liquids that won't make your diarrhea worse. Weak tea and clear broth are frequent suggestions.

- Avoid foods that are high in fiber or can cause cramps or a gassy feeling such as raw fruits and vegetables, coffee and other beverages that contain caffeine, beans, cabbage, whole grain breads and cereals, sweets, and spicy foods.

- Eat frequent small meals.

- If milk and milk products irritate your digestive system, avoid them or use lactose-free dairy products.

- Continue a diet that is low in fat and fiber and lactose-free for 2 weeks after you have finished your radiation therapy. Gradually re-introduce other foods. You may want to start with small amounts of low-fiber foods such as rice, bananas, applesauce, mashed potatoes, low-fat cottage cheese, and dry toast.

- Be sure your diet includes foods that are high in potassium (bananas, potatoes, apricots), an important mineral that you may lose through diarrhea.

Diet planning is very important for patients who are having radiation treatment of the stomach and abdomen. Try to pack the highest possible food value into every meal and snack so that you will be eating enough calories and vital nutrients. Remember that nausea, vomiting, and diarrhea are likely to disappear once your treatment is over.

What side effects occur with radiation therapy to the pelvis?

If you are having radiation therapy to any part of the pelvis (the area between your hips), you might have some of the digestive problems already described. You also may have bladder irritation which can cause discomfort or frequent urination. Drinking a lot of fluid can help relieve some of this discomfort. Avoid caffeine and carbonated beverages. Your doctor also can prescribe some medicine to help relieve these problems.

The effects of radiation therapy on sexual and reproductive functions depend on which organs are in the radiation treatment area. Some of the more common side effects do not last long after treatment is finished. Others may be long-term or permanent. Before your treatment begins, ask your doctor about possible side effects and how long they might last.

Depending on the radiation dose, women having radiation therapy in the pelvic area may stop menstruating and have other symptoms of menopause such as vaginal itching, burning, and dryness. You should report these symptoms to your doctor or nurse, who can suggest treatment.

Effects on fertility: Scientists are still studying how radiation treatment affects fertility. If you are a woman in your childbearing years, it's important to discuss birth control and fertility issues with your doctor. You should not become pregnant during radiation therapy because radiation treatment during pregnancy may injure the fetus, especially in the first three months. If you are pregnant before your therapy begins, be sure to tell your doctor so that the fetus can be protected from radiation, if possible.

Radiation therapy to the area that includes the testes can reduce both the number of sperm and their effectiveness. This does not mean that conception cannot occur, however. Ask your doctor or nurse about effective measures to prevent pregnancy while you are having radiation. If you have any concerns about fertility, be sure to discuss them with your doctor. For example, if you want to have children, you may be concerned about reduced fertility after your cancer treatment is completed. Your doctor can help you get information about the option of banking your sperm before treatment.

Sexual relations: With most types of radiation therapy, neither men nor women are likely to notice any change in their ability to enjoy sex.

Both sexes, however, may notice a decrease in their level of desire. This is more likely to be due to the stress of having cancer than to the effects of radiation therapy. Once the treatment ends, sexual desire is likely to return to previous levels.

During radiation treatment to the pelvis, some women are advised not to have intercourse. Others may find that intercourse is uncomfortable or painful. Within a few weeks after treatment ends, these symptoms usually disappear. If shrinking of vaginal tissues occurs as a side effect of radiation therapy, your doctor or nurse can explain how to use a dilator, a device that gently stretches the tissues of the vagina.

If you have questions or concerns about sexual activity during and after cancer treatment, discuss them with your nurse or doctor. Ask them to recommend booklets that may be helpful.

Chapter 77

Bone Marrow and Peripheral Blood Stem Cell Transplantation

What are bone marrow and hematopoietic stem cells?

Bone marrow is the soft, sponge-like material found inside bones. It contains immature cells known as hematopoietic or blood-forming stem cells. (Hematopoietic stem cells are different from embryonic stem cells. Embryonic stem cells can develop into every type of cell in the body.) Hematopoietic stem cells divide to form more blood-forming stem cells, or they mature into one of three types of blood cells: white blood cells, which fight infection; red blood cells, which carry oxygen; and platelets, which help the blood to clot. Most hematopoietic stem cells are found in the bone marrow, but some cells, called peripheral blood stem cells (PBSCs), are found in the bloodstream. Blood in the umbilical cord also contains hematopoietic stem cells. Cells from any of these sources can be used in transplants.

What are bone marrow transplantation and peripheral blood stem cell transplantation?

Bone marrow transplantation (BMT) and peripheral blood stem cell transplantation (PBSCT) are procedures that restore stem cells that have been destroyed by high doses of chemotherapy and/or radiation therapy. There are three types of transplants:

"Bone Marrow Transplantation and Peripheral Blood Stem Cell Transplantation: Questions and Answers," National Cancer Institute, August 31, 2004.

879

- In autologous transplants, patients receive their own stem cells.

- In syngeneic transplants, patients receive stem cells from their identical twin.

- In allogeneic transplants, patients receive stem cells from their brother, sister, or parent. A person who is not related to the patient (an unrelated donor) also may be used.

Why are BMT and PBSCT used in cancer treatment?

One reason BMT and PBSCT are used in cancer treatment is to make it possible for patients to receive very high doses of chemotherapy and/or radiation therapy. To understand more about why BMT and PBSCT are used, it is helpful to understand how chemotherapy and radiation therapy work.

Chemotherapy and radiation therapy generally affect cells that divide rapidly. They are used to treat cancer because cancer cells divide more often than most healthy cells. However, because bone marrow cells also divide frequently, high-dose treatments can severely damage or destroy the patient's bone marrow. Without healthy bone marrow, the patient is no longer able to make the blood cells needed to carry oxygen, fight infection, and prevent bleeding. BMT and PBSCT replace stem cells that were destroyed by treatment. The healthy, transplanted stem cells can restore the bone marrow's ability to produce the blood cells the patient needs.

In some types of leukemia, the graft-versus-tumor (GVT) effect that occurs after allogeneic BMT and PBSCT is crucial to the effectiveness of the treatment. GVT occurs when white blood cells from the donor (the graft) identify the cancer cells that remain in the patient's body after the chemotherapy and/or radiation therapy (the tumor) as foreign and attack them.

What types of cancer use BMT and PBSCT?

BMT and PBSCT are most commonly used in the treatment of leukemia and lymphoma. They are most effective when the leukemia or lymphoma is in remission (the signs and symptoms of cancer have disappeared). BMT and PBSCT are also used to treat other cancers such as neuroblastoma (cancer that arises in immature nerve cells and affects mostly infants and children) and multiple myeloma. Researchers are evaluating BMT and PBSCT in clinical trials (research studies) for the treatment of various types of cancer.

How are the donor's stem cells matched to the patient's stem cells in allogeneic or syngeneic transplantation?

To minimize potential side effects, doctors most often use transplanted stem cells that match the patient's own stem cells as closely as possible. People have different sets of proteins, called human leukocyte-associated (HLA) antigens, on the surface of their cells. The set of proteins, called the HLA type, is identified by a special blood test.

In most cases, the success of allogeneic transplantation depends in part on how well the HLA antigens of the donor's stem cells match those of the recipient's stem cells. The higher the number of matching HLA antigens, the greater the chance that the patient's body will accept the donor's stem cells. In general, patients are less likely to develop a complication known as graft-versus-host disease (GVHD) if the stem cells of the donor and patient are closely matched.

Close relatives, especially brothers and sisters, are more likely than unrelated people to be HLA-matched. However, only 25 to 35 percent of patients have an HLA-matched sibling. The chances of obtaining HLA-matched stem cells from an unrelated donor are slightly better, approximately 50 percent. Among unrelated donors, HLA-matching is greatly improved when the donor and recipient have the same ethnic and racial background. Although the number of donors is increasing overall, individuals from certain ethnic and racial groups still have a lower chance of finding a matching donor. Large volunteer donor registries can assist in finding an appropriate unrelated donor.

Because identical twins have the same genes, they have the same set of HLA antigens. As a result, the patient's body will accept a transplant from an identical twin. However, identical twins represent a small number of all births, so syngeneic transplantation is rare.

How is bone marrow obtained for transplantation?

The stem cells used in BMT come from the liquid center of the bone, called the marrow. In general, the procedure for obtaining bone marrow, which is called "harvesting," is similar for all three types of BMTs (autologous, syngeneic, and allogeneic). The donor is given either general anesthesia, which puts the person to sleep during the procedure, or regional anesthesia, which causes loss of feeling below the waist. Needles are inserted through the skin over the pelvic (hip) bone or, in rare cases, the sternum (breastbone), and into the bone marrow to draw the marrow out of the bone. Harvesting the marrow takes about an hour.

The harvested bone marrow is then processed to remove blood and bone fragments. Harvested bone marrow can be combined with a preservative and frozen to keep the stem cells alive until they are needed. This technique is known as cryopreservation. Stem cells can be cryopreserved for many years.

How are PBSCs obtained for transplantation?

The stem cells used in PBSCT come from the bloodstream. A process called apheresis or leukapheresis is used to obtain PBSCs for transplantation. For four or five days before apheresis, the donor may be given a medication to increase the number of stem cells released into the bloodstream. In apheresis, blood is removed through a large vein in the arm or a central venous catheter (a flexible tube that is placed in a large vein in the neck, chest, or groin area). The blood goes through a machine that removes the stem cells. The blood is then returned to the donor and the collected cells are stored. Apheresis typically takes four to six hours. The stem cells are then frozen until they are given to the recipient.

How are umbilical cord stem cells obtained for transplantation?

Stem cells also may be retrieved from umbilical cord blood. For this to occur, the mother must contact a cord blood bank before the baby's birth. The cord blood bank may request that she complete a questionnaire and give a small blood sample.

Cord blood banks may be public or commercial. Public cord blood banks accept donations of cord blood and may provide the donated stem cells to another matched individual in their network. In contrast, commercial cord blood banks will store the cord blood for the family, in case it is needed later for the child or another family member.

After the baby is born and the umbilical cord has been cut, blood is retrieved from the umbilical cord and placenta. This process poses minimal health risk to the mother or the child. If the mother agrees, the umbilical cord blood is processed and frozen for storage by the cord blood bank. Only a small amount of blood can be retrieved from the umbilical cord and placenta, so the collected stem cells are typically used for children or small adults.

Are any risks associated with donating bone marrow?

Because only a small amount of bone marrow is removed, donating usually does not pose any significant problems for the donor. The most serious risk associated with donating bone marrow involves the use of anesthesia during the procedure.

The area where the bone marrow was taken out may feel stiff or sore for a few days, and the donor may feel tired. Within a few weeks, the donor's body replaces the donated marrow; however, the time required for a donor to recover varies. Some people are back to their usual routine within two or three days, while others may take up to three to four weeks to fully recover their strength.

Are any risks associated with donating PBSCs?

Apheresis usually causes minimal discomfort. During apheresis, the person may feel lightheadedness, chills, numbness around the lips, and cramping in the hands. Unlike bone marrow donation, PBSC donation does not require anesthesia. The medication that is given to stimulate the release of stem cells from the marrow into the bloodstream may cause bone and muscle aches, headaches, fatigue, nausea, vomiting, and/or difficulty sleeping. These side effects generally stop within two to three days of the last dose of the medication.

How does the patient receive the stem cells during the transplant?

After being treated with high-dose anticancer drugs and/or radiation, the patient receives the stem cells through an intravenous (IV) line just like a blood transfusion. This part of the transplant takes one to five hours.

Are any special measures taken when the cancer patient is also the donor (autologous transplant)?

The stem cells used for autologous transplantation must be relatively free of cancer cells. The harvested cells can sometimes be treated before transplantation in a process known as "purging" to get rid of cancer cells. This process can remove some cancer cells from the harvested cells and minimize the chance that cancer will come back. Because purging may damage some healthy stem cells, more cells are obtained from the patient before the transplant so that enough healthy stem cells will remain after purging.

What happens after the stem cells have been transplanted to the patient?

After entering the bloodstream, the stem cells travel to the bone marrow, where they begin to produce new white blood cells, red blood cells, and platelets in a process known as "engraftment." Engraftment usually occurs within about two to four weeks after transplantation. Doctors monitor it by checking blood counts on a frequent basis. However, complete recovery of immune function takes much longer—up to several months for autologous transplant recipients and one to two years for patients receiving allogeneic or syngeneic transplants. Doctors evaluate the results of various blood tests to confirm that new blood cells are being produced and that the cancer has not returned. Bone marrow aspiration (the removal of a small sample of bone marrow through a needle for examination under a microscope) can also help doctors determine how well the new marrow is working.

What are the possible side effects of BMT and PBSCT?

The major risk of both treatments is an increased susceptibility to infection and bleeding as a result of the high-dose cancer treatment. Doctors may give the patient antibiotics to prevent or treat infection. They may also give the patient transfusions of platelets to prevent bleeding and red blood cells to treat anemia. Patients who undergo BMT and PBSCT may experience short-term side effects such as nausea, vomiting, fatigue, loss of appetite, mouth sores, hair loss, and skin reactions.

Potential long-term risks include complications of the pretransplant chemotherapy and radiation therapy, such as infertility (the inability to produce children); cataracts (clouding of the lens of the eye, which causes loss of vision); secondary (new) cancers; and damage to the liver, kidneys, lungs, and/or heart.

With allogeneic transplants, a complication known as graft-versus-host disease (GVHD) sometimes develops. GVHD occurs when white blood cells from the donor (the graft) identify cells in the patient's body (the host) as foreign and attack them. The most commonly damaged organs are the skin, liver, and intestines. This complication can develop within a few weeks of the transplant (acute GVHD) or much later (chronic GVHD). To prevent this complication, the patient may receive medications that suppress the immune system. Additionally, the donated stem cells can be treated to remove the white blood cells that cause GVHD in a process called "T-cell depletion." If GVHD develops, it can be very serious and is treated with steroids or other immunosuppressive agents. GVHD can be difficult to treat, but some studies suggest that patients with leukemia who develop GVHD are less likely to have the cancer come back. Clinical trials are being conducted to find ways to prevent and treat GVHD.

The likelihood and severity of complications are specific to the patient's treatment and should be discussed with the patient's doctor.

What is a "mini-transplant"?

A "mini-transplant" (also called a non-myeloablative or reduced-intensity transplant) is a type of allogeneic transplant. This approach is being studied in clinical trials for the treatment of several types of cancer, including leukemia, lymphoma, multiple myeloma, and other cancers of the blood.

A mini-transplant uses lower, less toxic doses of chemotherapy and/ or radiation to prepare the patient for an allogeneic transplant. The use of lower doses of anticancer drugs and radiation eliminates some, but not all, of the patient's bone marrow. It also reduces the number of cancer cells and suppresses the patient's immune system to prevent rejection of the transplant.

Unlike traditional BMT or PBSCT, cells from both the donor and the patient may exist in the patient's body for some time after a mini-transplant. Once the cells from the donor begin to engraft, they may cause the graft-versus-tumor (GVT) effect and work to destroy the cancer cells that were not eliminated by the anticancer drugs and/or radiation. To boost the GVT effect, the patient may be given an injection of their donor's white blood cells. This procedure is called a "donor lymphocyte infusion.

What is a "tandem transplant"?

A "tandem transplant" is a type of autologous transplant. This method is being studied in clinical trials for the treatment of several types of cancer, including multiple myeloma and germ cell cancer. During a tandem transplant, a patient receives two sequential courses of high-dose chemotherapy with stem cell transplant. Typically, the two courses are given several weeks to several months apart. Researchers hope that this method can prevent the cancer from recurring (coming back) at a later time.

How do patients cover the cost of BMT or PBSCT?

Advances in treatment methods, including the use of PBSCT, have reduced the amount of time many patients must spend in the hospital by speeding recovery. This shorter recovery time has brought about a reduction in cost. However, because BMT and PBSCT are complicated technical procedures, they are very expensive. Many health insurance companies cover some of the costs of transplantation for certain types of cancer. Insurers may also cover a portion of the costs if special care is required when the patient returns home.

There are options for relieving the financial burden associated with BMT and PBSCT. A hospital social worker is a valuable resource in planning for these financial needs. Federal Government programs and local service organizations may also be able to help.

The National Cancer Institute's (NCI) Cancer Information Service (CIS) can provide patients and their families with additional information about sources of financial assistance.

What are the costs of donating bone marrow, PBSCs, or umbilical cord blood?

Persons willing to donate bone marrow or PBSCs must have a sample of blood drawn to determine their HLA type. This blood test usually costs $65 to $96. The donor may be asked to pay for this blood test, or the donor center may cover part of the cost. Community groups and other organizations may also provide financial assistance. Once a donor is identified as a match for a patient, all of the costs pertaining to the retrieval of bone marrow or PBSCs is covered by the patient or the patient's medical insurance.

A woman can donate her baby's umbilical cord blood to public cord blood banks at no charge. However, commercial blood banks do charge varying fees to store umbilical cord blood for the private use of the patient or his or her family.

Where can people get more information about potential donors and transplant centers?

The National Marrow Donor Program® (NMDP), a federally funded nonprofit organization, was created to improve the effectiveness of the search for donors. The NMDP maintains an international registry of volunteers willing to be donors for all sources of blood stem cells used in transplantation: bone marrow, peripheral blood, and umbilical cord blood.

The NMDP website contains a list of participating transplant centers at http://www.marrow.org/NMDP/transplant_centers.html on the internet. The list includes descriptions of the centers as well as their transplant experience, survival statistics, research interests, pretransplant costs, and contact information.

National Marrow Donor Program
3001 Broadway Street, NE, Suite 500
Minneapolis, MN 55413-1753
Toll-Free: 800-627-7692 (800-MARROW-2)
Office of Patient Advocacy: 888-999-6743
Phone: 612-627-5800
Website: http://www.marrow.org

Where can people get more information about clinical trials of BMT and PBSCT?

Clinical trials that include BMT and PBSCT are a treatment option for some patients. Information about ongoing clinical trials is available from NCI's Cancer Information Service, or from the NCI's website at http://www.cancer.gov/clinicaltrials.

Chapter 78

Cryosurgery in Cancer Treatment

What is cryosurgery?

Cryosurgery (also called cryotherapy) is the use of extreme cold produced by liquid nitrogen (or argon gas) to destroy abnormal tissue. Cryosurgery is used to treat external tumors, such as those on the skin. For external tumors, liquid nitrogen is applied directly to the cancer cells with a cotton swab or spraying device.

Cryosurgery is also used to treat tumors inside the body (internal tumors and tumors in the bone). For internal tumors, liquid nitrogen or argon gas is circulated through a hollow instrument called a cryoprobe, which is placed in contact with the tumor. The doctor uses ultrasound or magnetic resonance imaging (MRI) to guide the cryoprobe and monitor the freezing of the cells, thus limiting damage to nearby healthy tissue. (In ultrasound, sound waves are bounced off organs and other tissues to create a picture called a sonogram.) A ball of ice crystals forms around the probe, freezing nearby cells. Sometimes more than one probe is used to deliver the liquid nitrogen to various parts of the tumor. The probes may be put into the tumor during surgery or through the skin (percutaneously). After cryosurgery, the frozen tissue thaws and is either naturally absorbed by the body (for internal tumors), or it dissolves and forms a scab (for external tumors).

"Cryosurgery in Cancer Treatment: Questions And Answers," National Cancer Institute, September 10, 2003.

What types of cancer can be treated with cryosurgery?

Cryosurgery is used to treat several types of cancer, and some precancerous or noncancerous conditions. In addition to prostate and liver tumors, cryosurgery can be an effective treatment for the following:

- Retinoblastoma (a childhood cancer that affects the retina of the eye). Doctors have found that cryosurgery is most effective when the tumor is small and only in certain parts of the retina.

- Early-stage skin cancers (both basal cell and squamous cell carcinomas)

- Precancerous skin growths known as actinic keratosis

- Precancerous conditions of the cervix known as cervical intraepithelial neoplasia (abnormal cell changes in the cervix that can develop into cervical cancer)

- Cryosurgery is also used to treat some types of low-grade cancerous and noncancerous tumors of the bone. It may reduce the risk of joint damage when compared with more extensive surgery, and help lessen the need for amputation. The treatment is also used to treat AIDS-related Kaposi sarcoma when the skin lesions are small and localized.

Researchers are evaluating cryosurgery as a treatment for a number of cancers, including breast, colon, and kidney cancer. They are also exploring cryotherapy in combination with other cancer treatments, such as hormone therapy, chemotherapy, radiation therapy, or surgery.

In what situations can cryosurgery be used to treat prostate cancer? What are the side effects?

Cryosurgery can be used to treat men who have early-stage prostate cancer that is confined to the prostate gland. It is less well established than standard prostatectomy and various types of radiation therapy. Long-term outcomes are not known. Because it is effective only in small areas, cryosurgery is not used to treat prostate cancer that has spread outside the gland, or to distant parts of the body.

Some advantages of cryosurgery are that the procedure can be repeated, and it can be used to treat men who cannot have surgery or radiation therapy because of their age or other medical problems.

Cryosurgery for the prostate gland can cause side effects. These side effects may occur more often in men who have had radiation to the prostate.

- Cryosurgery may obstruct urine flow or cause incontinence (lack of control over urine flow); often, these side effects are temporary.

- Many men become impotent (loss of sexual function).

- In some cases, the surgery has caused injury to the rectum.

In what situations can cryosurgery be used to treat primary liver cancer or liver metastases (cancer that has spread to the liver from another part of the body)? What are the side effects?

Cryosurgery may be used to treat primary liver cancer that has not spread. It is used especially if surgery is not possible due to factors such as other medical conditions. The treatment also may be used for cancer that has spread to the liver from another site (such as the colon or rectum). In some cases, chemotherapy and/or radiation therapy may be given before or after cryosurgery. Cryosurgery in the liver may cause damage to the bile ducts and/or major blood vessels, which can lead to hemorrhage (heavy bleeding) or infection.

Does cryosurgery have any complications or side effects?

Cryosurgery does have side effects, although they may be less severe than those associated with surgery or radiation therapy. The effects depend on the location of the tumor. Cryosurgery for cervical intraepithelial neoplasia has not been shown to affect a woman's fertility, but it can cause cramping, pain, or bleeding. When used to treat skin cancer (including Kaposi sarcoma), cryosurgery may cause scarring and swelling; if nerves are damaged, loss of sensation may occur, and, rarely, it may cause a loss of pigmentation and loss of hair in the treated area. When used to treat tumors of the bone, cryosurgery may lead to the destruction of nearby bone tissue and result in fractures, but these effects may not be seen for some time after the initial treatment and can often be delayed with other treatments. In rare cases, cryosurgery may interact badly with certain types of chemotherapy. Although the side effects of surgery may be less severe than those associated with conventional surgery or radiation, more studies are needed to determine the long-term effects.

What are the advantages of cryosurgery?

Cryosurgery offers advantages over other methods of cancer treatment. It is less invasive than surgery, involving only a small incision or insertion of the cryoprobe through the skin. Consequently, pain, bleeding, and other complications of surgery are minimized. Cryosurgery is less expensive than other treatments and requires shorter recovery time and a shorter hospital stay, or no hospital stay at all. Sometimes cryosurgery can be done using only local anesthesia.

Because physicians can focus cryosurgical treatment on a limited area, they can avoid the destruction of nearby healthy tissue. The treatment can be safely repeated and may be used along with standard treatments such as surgery, chemotherapy, hormone therapy, and radiation. Cryosurgery may offer an option for treating cancers that are considered inoperable or that do not respond to standard treatments. Furthermore, it can be used for patients who are not good candidates for conventional surgery because of their age or other medical conditions.

What are the disadvantages of cryosurgery?

The major disadvantage of cryosurgery is the uncertainty surrounding its long-term effectiveness. While cryosurgery may be effective in treating tumors the physician can see by using imaging tests (tests that produce pictures of areas inside the body), it can miss microscopic cancer spread. Furthermore, because the effectiveness of the technique is still being assessed, insurance coverage issues may arise.

What does the future hold for cryosurgery?

Additional studies are needed to determine the effectiveness of cryosurgery in controlling cancer and improving survival. Data from these studies will allow physicians to compare cryosurgery with standard treatment options such as surgery, chemotherapy, and radiation. Moreover, physicians continue to examine the possibility of using cryosurgery in combination with other treatments.

Where is cryosurgery currently available?

Cryosurgery is widely available in gynecologists' offices for the treatment of cervical neoplasias. A limited number of hospitals and cancer centers throughout the country currently have skilled doctors and the necessary technology to perform cryosurgery for other non-cancerous, precancerous, and cancerous conditions. Individuals can consult with their doctors or contact hospitals and cancer centers in their area to find out where cryosurgery is being used.

Chapter 79

Laser Therapy in Cancer Treatment

What is laser light?

The term "laser" stands for light amplification by stimulated emission of radiation. Ordinary light, such as that from a light bulb, has many wavelengths and spreads in all directions. Laser light, on the other hand, has a specific wavelength. It is focused in a narrow beam and creates a very high-intensity light. This powerful beam of light may be used to cut through steel or to shape diamonds. Because lasers can focus very accurately on tiny areas, they can also be used for very precise surgical work or for cutting through tissue (in place of a scalpel).

What is laser therapy, and how is it used in cancer treatment?

Laser therapy uses high-intensity light to treat cancer and other illnesses. Lasers can be used to shrink or destroy tumors. Lasers are most commonly used to treat superficial cancers (cancers on the surface of the body or the lining of internal organs) such as basal cell skin cancer and the very early stages of some cancers, such as cervical, penile, vaginal, vulvar, and non-small cell lung cancer.

Lasers also may be used to relieve certain symptoms of cancer, such as bleeding or obstruction. For example, lasers can be used to shrink

"Lasers in Cancer Treatment: Questions and Answers," National Cancer Institute, August 10, 2004.

or destroy a tumor that is blocking a patient's trachea (windpipe) or esophagus. Lasers also can be used to remove colon polyps or tumors that are blocking the colon or stomach.

Laser therapy can be used alone, but most often it is combined with other treatments, such as surgery, chemotherapy, or radiation therapy. In addition, lasers can seal nerve endings to reduce pain after surgery and seal lymph vessels to reduce swelling and limit the spread of tumor cells.

How is laser therapy given to the patient?

Laser therapy is often given through a flexible endoscope (a thin, lighted tube used to look at tissues inside the body). The endoscope is fitted with optical fibers (thin fibers that transmit light). It is inserted through an opening in the body, such as the mouth, nose, anus, or vagina. Laser light is then precisely aimed to cut or destroy a tumor.

Laser-induced interstitial thermotherapy (LITT) (or interstitial laser photocoagulation) also uses lasers to treat some cancers. LITT is similar to a cancer treatment called hyperthermia, which uses heat to shrink tumors by damaging or killing cancer cells. During LITT, an optical fiber is inserted into a tumor. Laser light at the tip of the fiber raises the temperature of the tumor cells and damages or destroys them. LITT is sometimes used to shrink tumors in the liver.

Photodynamic therapy (PDT) is another type of cancer treatment that uses lasers. In PDT, a certain drug, called a photosensitizer or photosensitizing agent, is injected into a patient and absorbed by cells all over the patient's body. After a couple of days, the agent is found mostly in cancer cells. Laser light is then used to activate the agent and destroy cancer cells. Because the photosensitizer makes the skin and eyes sensitive to light for approximately six weeks, patients are advised to avoid direct sunlight and bright indoor light during that time.

What types of lasers are used in cancer treatment?

Three types of lasers are used to treat cancer: carbon dioxide (CO_2) lasers, argon lasers, and neodymium: yttrium-aluminum-garnet (Nd:YAG) lasers. Each of these can shrink or destroy tumors and can be used with endoscopes. CO_2 and argon lasers can cut the skin's surface without going into deeper layers. Thus, they can be used to remove superficial cancers, such as skin cancer. In contrast, the Nd:YAG laser is more commonly applied through an endoscope to treat internal organs, such as the uterus, esophagus, and colon. Nd:YAG laser light can also travel through optical fibers into specific areas of the body during LITT. Argon lasers are often used to activate the drugs used in PDT.

What are the advantages of laser therapy?

Lasers are more precise than standard surgical tools (scalpels), so they do less damage to normal tissues. As a result, patients usually have less pain, bleeding, swelling, and scarring. With laser therapy, operations are usually shorter. In fact, laser therapy can often be done on an outpatient basis. It takes less time for patients to heal after laser surgery, and they are less likely to get infections. Patients should consult with their health care provider about whether laser therapy is appropriate for them.

What are the disadvantages of laser therapy?

Laser therapy also has several limitations. Surgeons must have specialized training before they can do laser therapy, and strict safety precautions must be followed. Also, laser therapy is expensive and requires bulky equipment. In addition, the effects of laser therapy may not last long, so doctors may have to repeat the treatment for a patient to get the full benefit.

What does the future hold for laser therapy?

In clinical trials (research studies), doctors are using lasers to treat cancers of the brain and prostate, among others. To learn more about clinical trials, call the National Cancer Institute (NCI)'s Cancer Information Service at the telephone number listed below or visit the clinical trials page of the NCI's website at http://www.cancer.gov/clinicaltrials on the internet.

Chapter 80

Biological Therapies for Cancer

What is biological therapy?

Biological therapy (sometimes called immunotherapy, biotherapy, or biological response modifier therapy) is a relatively new addition to the family of cancer treatments that also includes surgery, chemotherapy, and radiation therapy. Biological therapies use the body's immune system, either directly or indirectly, to fight cancer or to lessen the side effects that may be caused by some cancer treatments.

What is the immune system and what are its components?

The immune system is a complex network of cells and organs that work together to defend the body against attacks by "foreign" or "nonself" invaders. This network is one of the body's main defenses against infection and disease. The immune system works against diseases, including cancer, in a variety of ways. For example, the immune system may recognize the difference between healthy cells and cancer cells in the body and works to eliminate cancerous cells. However, the immune system does not always recognize cancer cells as "foreign." Also, cancer may develop when the immune system breaks down or does not function adequately. Biological therapies are designed to repair, stimulate, or enhance the immune system's responses.

Immune system cells include the following:

"Biological Therapies for Cancer: Questions and Answers," National Cancer Institute, April 12, 2006.

- Lymphocytes are a type of white blood cell found in the blood and many other parts of the body. Types of lymphocytes include B cells, T cells, and natural killer cells.

  B cells (B lymphocytes) mature into plasma cells that secrete proteins called antibodies (immunoglobulins). Antibodies recognize and attach to foreign substances known as antigens, fitting together much the way a key fits a lock. Each type of B cell makes one specific antibody, which recognizes one specific antigen.

  T cells (T lymphocytes) work primarily by producing proteins called cytokines. Cytokines allow immune system cells to communicate with each other and include lymphokines, interferons, interleukins, and colony-stimulating factors. Some T cells, called cytotoxic T cells, release pore-forming proteins that directly attack infected, foreign, or cancerous cells. Other T cells, called helper T cells, regulate the immune response by releasing cytokines to signal other immune system defenders.

  Natural killer cells (NK cells) produce powerful cytokines and pore-forming proteins that bind to and kill many foreign invaders, infected cells, and tumor cells. Unlike cytotoxic T cells, they are poised to attack quickly, upon their first encounter with their targets.

- Phagocytes are white blood cells that can swallow and digest microscopic organisms and particles in a process known as phagocytosis. There are several types of phagocytes, including monocytes, which circulate in the blood, and macrophages, which are located in tissues throughout the body.

What are biological response modifiers, and how can they be used to treat cancer?

Some antibodies, cytokines, and other immune system substances can be produced in the laboratory for use in cancer treatment. These substances are often called biological response modifiers (BRMs). They alter the interaction between the body's immune defenses and cancer cells to boost, direct, or restore the body's ability to fight the disease. BRMs include interferons, interleukins, colony-stimulating factors, monoclonal antibodies, vaccines, gene therapy, and nonspecific immunomodulating agents. Each of these BRMs are described in the following questions.

Researchers continue to discover new BRMs, to learn more about how they function, and to develop ways to use them in cancer therapy. Biological therapies may be used to:

- Stop, control, or suppress processes that permit cancer growth.

- Make cancer cells more recognizable and, therefore, more susceptible to destruction by the immune system.

- Boost the killing power of immune system cells, such as T cells, NK cells, and macrophages.

- Alter the growth patterns of cancer cells to promote behavior like that of healthy cells.

- Block or reverse the process that changes a normal cell or a precancerous cell into a cancerous cell.

- Enhance the body's ability to repair or replace normal cells damaged or destroyed by other forms of cancer treatment, such as chemotherapy or radiation.

- Prevent cancer cells from spreading to other parts of the body.

Some BRMs are a standard part of treatment for certain types of cancer, while others are being studied in clinical trials (research studies). BRMs are being used alone or in combination with each other. They are also being used with other treatments, such as radiation therapy and chemotherapy.

What are interferons?

Interferons (IFNs) are types of cytokines that occur naturally in the body. They were the first cytokines produced in the laboratory for use as BRMs. There are three major types of interferons—interferon alpha, interferon beta, and interferon gamma; interferon alpha is the type most widely used in cancer treatment.

Researchers have found that interferons can improve the way a cancer patient's immune system acts against cancer cells. In addition, interferons may act directly on cancer cells by slowing their growth or promoting their development into cells with more normal behavior. Researchers believe that some interferons may also stimulate NK cells, T cells, and macrophages, boosting the immune system's anticancer function.

The U.S. Food and Drug Administration (FDA) has approved the use of interferon alpha for the treatment of certain types of cancer, including hairy cell leukemia, melanoma, chronic myeloid leukemia, and AIDS-related Kaposi sarcoma. Studies have shown that interferon alpha may also be effective in treating other cancers such as kidney cancer and non-Hodgkin lymphoma. Researchers are exploring combinations of interferon alpha and other BRMs or chemotherapy in clinical trials to treat a number of cancers.

What are interleukins?

Like interferons, interleukins (ILs) are cytokines that occur naturally in the body and can be made in the laboratory. Many interleukins have been identified; interleukin-2 (IL-2 or aldesleukin) has been the most widely studied in cancer treatment. IL-2 stimulates the growth and activity of many immune cells, such as lymphocytes, that can destroy cancer cells. The FDA has approved IL-2 for the treatment of metastatic kidney cancer and metastatic melanoma.

Researchers continue to study the benefits of interleukins to treat a number of other cancers, including leukemia, lymphoma, and cancers of the brain, colorectal, ovarian, breast, and prostate cancers.

What are colony-stimulating factors?

Colony-stimulating factors (CSFs) (sometimes called hematopoietic growth factors) usually do not directly affect tumor cells; rather, they encourage bone marrow stem cells to divide and develop into white blood cells, platelets, and red blood cells. Bone marrow is critical to the body's immune system because it is the source of all blood cells.

Stimulation of the immune system by CSFs may benefit patients undergoing cancer treatment. Because anticancer drugs can damage the body's ability to make white blood cells, red blood cells, and platelets, patients receiving anticancer drugs have an increased risk of developing infections, becoming anemic, and bleeding more easily. By using CSFs to stimulate blood cell production, doctors can increase the doses of anticancer drugs without increasing the risk of infection or the need for transfusion with blood products. As a result, researchers have found CSFs particularly useful when combined with high-dose chemotherapy.

Some examples of CSFs and their use in cancer therapy are as follows:

- G-CSF (filgrastim) and GM-CSF (sargramostim) can increase the number of white blood cells, thereby reducing the risk of infection in patients receiving chemotherapy. G-CSF and GM-CSF can also stimulate the production of stem cells in preparation for stem cell or bone marrow transplants.

• Erythropoietin (epoetin) can increase the number of red blood cells and reduce the need for red blood cell transfusions in patients receiving chemotherapy.

• Interleukin-11 (oprelvekin) helps the body make platelets and can reduce the need for platelet transfusions in patients receiving chemotherapy.

Researchers are studying CSFs in clinical trials to treat a large variety of cancers, including lymphoma, leukemia, multiple myeloma, melanoma, and cancers of the brain, lung, esophagus, breast, uterus, ovary, prostate, kidney, colon, and rectum.

What are monoclonal antibodies?

Researchers are evaluating the effectiveness of certain antibodies made in the laboratory called monoclonal antibodies (MOABs or MoABs). These antibodies are produced by a single type of cell and are specific for a particular antigen. Researchers are examining ways to create MOABs specific to the antigens found on the surface of various cancer cells.

To create MOABs, scientists first inject human cancer cells into mice. In response, the mouse immune system makes antibodies against these cancer cells. The scientists then remove the mouse plasma cells that produce antibodies, and fuse them with laboratory-grown cells to create "hybrid" cells called hybridomas. Hybridomas can indefinitely produce large quantities of these pure antibodies, or MOABs.

MOABs may be used in cancer treatment in a number of ways:

• MOABs that react with specific types of cancer may enhance a patient's immune response to the cancer.

• MOABs can be programmed to act against cell growth factors, thus interfering with the growth of cancer cells.

• MOABs may be linked to anticancer drugs, radioisotopes (radioactive substances), other BRMs, or other toxins. When the antibodies latch onto cancer cells, they deliver these poisons directly to the tumor, helping to destroy it.

MOABs carrying radioisotopes may also prove useful in diagnosing certain cancers, such as colorectal, ovarian, and prostate.

Rituxan® (rituximab) and Herceptin® (trastuzumab) are examples of MOABs that have been approved by the FDA. Rituxan is used for the treatment of non-Hodgkin lymphoma. Herceptin is used to treat metastatic breast cancer in patients with tumors that produce excess amounts of a protein called HER-2. In clinical trials, researchers are testing MOABs to treat lymphoma, leukemia, melanoma, and cancers of the brain, breast, lung, kidney, colon, rectum, ovary, prostate, and other areas.

What are cancer vaccines?

Cancer vaccines are another form of biological therapy currently under study. Vaccines for infectious diseases, such as measles, mumps, and tetanus, are injected into a person before the disease develops. These vaccines are effective because they expose the body's immune cells to weakened forms of antigens that are present on the surface of the infectious agent. This exposure causes the immune system to increase production of plasma cells that make antibodies specific to the infectious agent. The immune system also increases production of T cells that recognize the infectious agent. These activated immune cells remember the exposure, so that the next time the agent enters the body, the immune system is already prepared to respond and stop the infection.

Researchers are developing vaccines that may encourage the patient's immune system to recognize cancer cells. Cancer vaccines are designed to treat existing cancers (therapeutic vaccines) or to prevent the development of cancer (prophylactic vaccines). Therapeutic vaccines are injected in a person after cancer is diagnosed. These vaccines may stop the growth of existing tumors, prevent cancer from recurring, or eliminate cancer cells not killed by prior treatments. Cancer vaccines given when the tumor is small may be able to eradicate the cancer. On the other hand, prophylactic vaccines are given to healthy individuals before cancer develops. These vaccines are designed to stimulate the immune system to attack viruses that can cause cancer. By targeting these cancer-causing viruses, doctors hope to prevent the development of certain cancers.

Early cancer vaccine clinical trials involved mainly patients with melanoma. Therapeutic vaccines are also being studied in the treatment of many other types of cancer, including lymphoma, leukemia, and cancers of the brain, breast, lung, kidney, ovary, prostate, pancreas, colon, and rectum. Researchers are also studying prophylactic vaccines to prevent cancers of the cervix and liver. Moreover, scientists are investigating ways that cancer vaccines can be used in combination with other BRMs.

What is gene therapy?

Gene therapy is an experimental treatment that involves introducing genetic material into a person's cells to fight disease. Researchers are studying gene therapy methods that can improve a patient's immune response to cancer. For example, a gene may be inserted into an immune cell to enhance its ability to recognize and attack cancer cells. In another approach, scientists inject cancer cells with genes that cause the cancer cells to produce cytokines and stimulate the immune system. A number of clinical trials are currently studying gene therapy and its potential application to the biological treatment of cancer.

What are nonspecific immunomodulating agents?

Nonspecific immunomodulating agents are substances that stimulate or indirectly augment the immune system. Often, these agents target key immune system cells and cause secondary responses such as increased production of cytokines and immunoglobulins. Two nonspecific immunomodulating agents used in cancer treatment are bacillus Calmette-Guerin (BCG) and levamisole.

BCG, which has been widely used as a tuberculosis vaccine, is used in the treatment of superficial bladder cancer following surgery. BCG may work by stimulating an inflammatory, and possibly an immune, response. A solution of BCG is instilled in the bladder and stays there for about two hours before the patient is allowed to empty the bladder by urinating. This treatment is usually performed once a week for six weeks.

Levamisole is sometimes used along with fluorouracil (5-FU) chemotherapy in the treatment of stage III (Dukes C) colon cancer following surgery. Levamisole may act to restore depressed immune function.

Do biological therapies have any side effects?

Like other forms of cancer treatment, biological therapies can cause a number of side effects, which can vary widely from agent to agent and patient to patient. Rashes or swelling may develop at the site where the BRMs are injected. Several BRMs, including interferons and interleukins, may cause flu-like symptoms including fever, chills, nausea, vomiting, and appetite loss. Fatigue is another common side effect of some BRMs. Blood pressure may also be affected. The side effects of IL-2 can often be severe, depending on the dosage given. Patients need to be closely monitored during treatment with high doses of IL-2. Side effects of CSFs may include bone pain, fatigue, fever, and appetite loss. The side effects of MOABs vary, and serious allergic reactions may occur. Cancer vaccines can cause muscle aches and fever.

Where can a person get more information about clinical trials?

Information about ongoing clinical trials involving these and other biological therapies is available from the Cancer Information Service or the clinical trials page of the National Cancer Institute website at http://www.cancer.gov/clinicaltrials.

Chapter 81

Photodynamic Therapy for Cancer

What is photodynamic therapy?

Photodynamic therapy (PDT) is a treatment that uses a drug, called a photosensitizer or photosensitizing agent, and a particular type of light. When photosensitizers are exposed to a specific wavelength of light, they produce a form of oxygen that kills nearby cells.[1, 2, 3]

Each photosensitizer is activated by light of a specific wavelength.[3, 4] This wavelength determines how far the light can travel into the body.[3, 5] Thus, doctors use specific photosensitizers and wavelengths of light to treat different areas of the body with PDT.

How is PDT used to treat cancer?

In the first step of PDT for cancer treatment, a photosensitizing agent is injected into the bloodstream. The agent is absorbed by cells all over the body, but stays in cancer cells longer than it does in normal cells. Approximately 24 to 72 hours after injection,[1] when most of the agent has left normal cells but remains in cancer cells, the tumor is exposed to light. The photosensitizer in the tumor absorbs the light and produces an active form of oxygen that destroys nearby cancer cells.[1, 2, 3]

"Photodynamic Therapy for Cancer: Questions and Answers," National Cancer Institute, May 12, 2004.

In addition to directly killing cancer cells, PDT appears to shrink or destroy tumors in two other ways.[1, 2, 3, 4] The photosensitizer can damage blood vessels in the tumor, thereby preventing the cancer from receiving necessary nutrients. In addition, PDT may activate the immune system to attack the tumor cells.

The light used for PDT can come from a laser or other sources of light.[2, 5] Laser light can be directed through fiber optic cables (thin fibers that transmit light) to deliver light to areas inside the body.[2] For example, a fiber optic cable can be inserted through an endoscope (a thin, lighted tube used to look at tissues inside the body) into the lungs or esophagus to treat cancer in these organs. Other light sources include light-emitting diodes (LEDs), which may be used for surface tumors, such as skin cancer.[5]

PDT is usually performed as an outpatient procedure.[6] PDT may also be repeated and may be used with other therapies, such as surgery, radiation, or chemotherapy.[2]

What types of cancer are currently treated with PDT?

To date, the U.S. Food and Drug Administration (FDA) has approved the photosensitizing agent called porfimer sodium, or Photofrin®, for use in PDT to treat or relieve the symptoms of esophageal cancer and non-small cell lung cancer.[7] Porfimer sodium is approved to relieve symptoms of esophageal cancer when the cancer obstructs the esophagus or when the cancer cannot be satisfactorily treated with laser therapy alone. Porfimer sodium is used to treat non-small cell lung cancer in patients for whom the usual treatments are not appropriate, and to relieve symptoms in patients with non-small cell lung cancer that obstructs the airways. In 2003, the FDA approved porfimer sodium for the treatment of precancerous lesions in patients with Barrett esophagus (a condition that can lead to esophageal cancer).[8]

What are the limitations of PDT?

The light needed to activate most photosensitizers cannot pass through more than about one-third of an inch of tissue (one centimeter). For this reason, PDT is usually used to treat tumors on or just under the skin or on the lining of internal organs or cavities.[3] PDT is also less effective in treating large tumors, because the light cannot pass far into these tumors.[2, 3, 6] PDT is a local treatment and generally cannot be used to treat cancer that has spread (metastasized).[6]

Does PDT have any complications or side effects?

Porfimer sodium makes the skin and eyes sensitive to light for approximately six weeks after treatment.[1,3,6] Thus, patients are advised to avoid direct sunlight and bright indoor light for at least six weeks.

Photosensitizers tend to build up in tumors and the activating light is focused on the tumor. As a result, damage to healthy tissue is minimal. However, PDT can cause burns, swelling, pain, and scarring in nearby healthy tissue.[3] Other side effects of PDT are related to the area that is treated. They can include coughing, trouble swallowing, stomach pain, painful breathing, or shortness of breath; these side effects are usually temporary.

What does the future hold for PDT?

Researchers continue to study ways to improve the effectiveness of PDT and expand it to other cancers. Clinical trials (research studies) are under way to evaluate the use of PDT for cancers of the brain, skin, prostate, cervix, and peritoneal cavity (the space in the abdomen that contains the intestines, stomach, and liver). Other research is focused on the development of photosensitizers that are more powerful,[1] more specifically target cancer cells,[1,3,5] and are activated by light that can penetrate tissue and treat deep or large tumors.[2] Researchers are also investigating ways to improve equipment[1] and the delivery of the activating light.[5]

Selected References

1. Dolmans DEJGJ, Fukumura D, Jain RK. Photodynamic therapy for cancer. *Nature Reviews Cancer* 2003;3(5):380–387.

2. Wilson BC. Photodynamic therapy for cancer: Principles. *Canadian Journal of Gastroenterology* 2002;16(6):393–396.

3. Vrouenraets MB, Visser GWM, Snow GB, van Dongen GAMS. Basic principles, applications in oncology and improved selectivity of photodynamic therapy. *Anticancer Research* 2003;23: 505–522.

4. Dougherty TJ, Gomer CJ, Henderson BW, et al. Photodynamic therapy. *Journal of the National Cancer Institute* 1998;90(12): 889–905.

5. Dickson EFG, Goyan RL, Pottier RH. New directions in photo-dynamic therapy. *Cellular and Molecular Biology* 2003;48(8): 939–954.

6. Capella MAM, Capella LS. A light in multidrug resistance: Photodynamic treatment of multidrug-resistant tumors. *Journal of Biomedical Science* 2003;10:361–366.

7. U.S. Food and Drug Administration (December 2003). *Approved claims for palliative line therapy.* Retrieved December 29, 2003, from: http://www.accessdata.fda.gov/scripts/cder/ onctools/linelist.cfm?line=Palliative.

8. U.S. Food and Drug Administration (August 2003). *FDA approves photofrin for treatment of pre-cancerous lesions in Barrett's esophagus.* Retrieved December 29, 2003, from: http:// www.fda.gov/bbs/topics/ANSWERS/2003/ANS01246.html.

Chapter 82

Targeted Cancer Therapies

What are targeted cancer therapies?

Targeted cancer therapies use drugs that block the growth and spread of cancer. They interfere with specific molecules involved in carcinogenesis (the process by which normal cells become cancer cells) and tumor growth. Because scientists call these molecules "molecular targets," these therapies are sometimes called "molecular-targeted drugs," "molecularly targeted therapies," or other similar names. By focusing on molecular and cellular changes that are specific to cancer, targeted cancer therapies may be more effective than current treatments and less harmful to normal cells.

Most targeted cancer therapies are in preclinical testing (research with animals), but some are in clinical trials (research studies with people), or have been approved by the U.S. Food and Drug Administration (FDA). Targeted cancer therapies are being studied for use alone, in combination with each other, and in combination with other cancer treatments, such as chemotherapy.

What are some of the cellular changes that lead to cancer?

Normally, cells grow and divide to form new cells as the body needs them. When cells grow old, they die, and new cells take their place. Sometimes this orderly process goes wrong. New cells form when the

"Targeted Cancer Therapies: Questions and Answers," National Cancer Institute, April 27, 2004.

body does not need them, and old cells do not die when they should. These extra cells can form a mass of tissue called a growth or tumor. The cells in malignant (cancerous) tumors are abnormal and divide without control or order. They can invade and damage nearby tissues and organs. Also, cancer cells can break away from a malignant tumor and spread to other parts of the body.

Normal cell growth and division are largely under the control of a network of chemical and molecular signals that give instructions to cells. Genetic alterations (changes) can disrupt the signaling process so that cells no longer grow and divide normally, or no longer die when they should. Alterations in two types of genes can contribute to the cancer process. Proto-oncogenes are normal genes that are involved in cell growth and division. Changes in these genes lead to the development of oncogenes, which can promote or allow excessive and continuous cell growth and division. Tumor suppressor genes are normal genes that slow down cell growth and division. When a tumor suppressor gene does not work properly, cells may be unable to stop growing and dividing, which leads to tumor growth.

To use the metaphor of a car, the presence of an oncogene is like having a gas pedal that is stuck to the floorboard, causing cells to continually grow and divide. Tumor suppressor genes act like a brake pedal. The loss of a functioning tumor suppressor gene is like having a brake pedal that does not work properly, allowing cells to continually grow and divide.

Genetic changes that are not corrected by the cell can lead to the production of abnormal proteins. Normally, proteins interact with each other as a kind of relay team to carry out the work of the cell. For example, when molecules called growth factors (GFs) attach to their corresponding growth factor receptors (GFRs) on the surface of the cell, a process carried out by proteins signals the cell to divide. Damaged proteins may not respond to normal signals, may over-respond to normal signals, or otherwise fail to carry out their normal functions. Cancer develops when abnormal proteins inside a cell cause it to reproduce excessively and allow that cell to live longer than normal cells.

How do targeted cancer therapies work?

Targeted cancer therapies interfere with cancer cell growth and division in different ways and at various points during the development, growth, and spread of cancer. Many of these therapies focus on proteins that are involved in the signaling process. By blocking the signals that tell cancer cells to grow and divide uncontrollably, targeted cancer therapies can help to stop the growth and division of cancer cells.

What are some types of targeted cancer therapies?

Targeted cancer therapies include several types of drugs. Some examples are listed below:

- "Small-molecule" drugs block specific enzymes and GFRs involved in cancer cell growth. These drugs are also called signal-transduction inhibitors. Gleevec® (STI–571 or imatinib mesylate) is a small-molecule drug approved by the FDA to treat gastrointestinal stromal tumor (a rare cancer of the gastrointestinal tract) and certain kinds of chronic myeloid leukemia.[1,2] Gleevec targets abnormal proteins, or enzymes, that form inside cancer cells and stimulate uncontrolled growth. Iressa® (ZD1839 or gefitinib) is approved by the FDA to treat advanced non-small cell lung cancer. This drug targets the epidermal growth factor receptor (EGFR), which is overproduced by many types of cancer cells. Other small-molecule drugs are being studied in clinical trials in the United States.

- "Apoptosis-inducing" drugs cause cancer cells to undergo apoptosis (cell death) by interfering with proteins involved in the process. Velcade® (bortezomib) is approved by the FDA to treat multiple myeloma that has not responded to other treatments.[3] Velcade causes cancer cells to die by blocking enzymes called proteasomes, which help to regulate cell function and growth. Another apoptosis-inducing drug called Genasense™ (oblimersen), which is only available in clinical trials, is being studied to treat leukemia, non-Hodgkin lymphoma, and solid tumors. Genasense blocks the production of a protein known as BCL-2, which promotes the survival of tumor cells. By blocking BCL-2, Genasense leaves the cancer cells more vulnerable to anticancer drugs.

- Monoclonal antibodies, cancer vaccines, angiogenesis inhibitors, and gene therapy are considered by some to be targeted therapies because they interfere with the growth of cancer cells.

What impact will targeted therapies have on cancer treatment?

Targeted cancer therapies will give doctors a better way to tailor cancer treatment. Eventually, treatments may be individualized based

911

on the unique set of molecular targets produced by the patient's tumor. Targeted cancer therapies also hold the promise of being more selective, thus harming fewer normal cells, reducing side effects, and improving the quality of life.

What are some resources for more information?

The National Cancer Institute (NCI)'s Molecular Targets Development Program (MTDP) is working to identify and evaluate molecular targets that may be candidates for drug development. As part of the NCI's Center for Cancer Research, the MTDP provides research support for NCI-designated, high-priority drug discovery, development, and research focused on specific molecular targets, pathways, or processes. The MTDP's website is http://home.ncifcrf.gov/mtdp.

Information about clinical trials is available from the Cancer Information Service (CIS). Information specialists at the CIS use PDQ®, the NCI's cancer information database, to identify and provide detailed information about specific ongoing clinical trials. PDQ includes all NCI-funded clinical trials and some studies conducted by independent investigators at hospitals and medical centers in the United States and other countries around the world.

People also have the option of searching for clinical trials on their own. The clinical trials page of the NCI's website (located at http://www.cancer.gov/clinicaltrials) provides information about clinical trials and links to PDQ.

Selected References

1. Demetri GD, von Mehren M, Blanke CD, et al. Efficacy and safety of imatinib mesylate in advanced gastrointestinal stromal tumors. *New England Journal of Medicine* 2002; 347(7): 472–480.

2. Kantarjian H, Sawyers C, Hochhaus A, et al. Hematologic and cytogenetic responses to imatinib mesylate in chronic myelogenous leukemia. *New England Journal of Medicine* 2002; 346(9):645–652.

3. Richardson PG, Barlogie B, Berenson J, et al. A phase 2 study of bortezomib in relapsed, refractory myeloma. *New England Journal of Medicine* 2003; 348(26):2609–2617.

Chapter 83

Proton Therapy

How Proton Treatment Works

There is a significant difference between standard (x-ray) radiation treatment and proton therapy. If given in sufficient doses, x-ray radiation techniques will control many cancers. But, because of the physician's inability to adequately conform the irradiation pattern to the cancer, healthy tissues may receive a similar dose and can be damaged. Consequently, a less-than-desired dose is frequently used to reduce damage to healthy tissues and avoid unwanted side effects. The power of protons is that higher doses of radiation can be used to control and manage cancer while significantly reducing damage to healthy tissue and vital organs.

Understanding how protons work provides patients and physicians with an insight into this mainstream treatment modality. Essentially, protons are a superior form of radiation therapy. Fundamentally, all tissues are made up of molecules with atoms as their building blocks. In the center of every atom is the nucleus. Orbiting the nucleus of the atom are negatively charged electrons.

This chapter includes text from "How Proton Treatment Works," © 1990 National Association for Proton Therapy, and questions and answers from "Proton Therapy—A Mainstream Option for the Treatment of Cancerous and Non-Cancerous Tumors," © 2006 National Association for Proton Therapy. Both documents are reprinted with permission from http://www.proton-therapy.org. This chapter was reviewed for currency in December 2006 by David A. Cooke, M.D.

When energized charged particles, such as protons or other forms of radiation, pass near orbiting electrons, the positive charge of the protons attracts the negatively charged electrons, pulling them out of their orbits. This is called ionization; it changes the characteristics of the atom and consequentially the character of the molecule within which the atom resides. This crucial change is the basis for the beneficial aspects of all forms of radiation therapy. Because of ionization, the radiation damages molecules within the cells, especially the DNA or genetic material. Damaging the DNA destroys specific cell functions, particularly the ability to divide or proliferate. Enzymes develop with the cells and attempt to rebuild the injured areas of the DNA; however, if damage from the radiation is too extensive, the enzymes fail to adequately repair the injury. While both normal and cancerous cells go through this repair process, a cancer cell's ability to repair molecular injury is frequently inferior. As a result, cancer cells sustain more permanent damage and subsequent cell death than occurs in the normal cell population. This permits selective destruction of bad cells growing among good cells.

Both standard x-ray therapy and proton beams work on the principle of selective cell destruction. The major advantage of proton treatment over conventional radiation, however, is that the energy distribution of protons can be directed and deposited in tissue volumes designated by the physicians in a three-dimensional pattern from each beam used. This capability provides greater control and precision and, therefore, superior management of treatment. Radiation therapy requires that conventional x-rays be delivered into the body in total doses sufficient to assure that enough ionization events occur to damage all the cancer cells. The conventional x-rays lack of charge and mass, however, results in most of their energy from a single conventional x-ray beam being deposited in normal tissues near the body's surface, as well as undesirable energy deposition beyond the cancer site. This undesirable pattern of energy placement can result in unnecessary damage to healthy tissues, often preventing physicians from using sufficient radiation to control the cancer.

Protons, on the other hand, are energized to specific velocities. These energies determine how deeply in the body protons will deposit their maximum energy. As the protons move through the body, they slow down, causing increased interaction with orbiting electrons.

Maximum interaction with electrons occurs as the protons approach their targeted stopping point. Thus, maximum energy is released within the designated cancer volume. The surrounding healthy cells receive significantly less injury than the cells in the designated volume.

As a result of protons' dose-distribution characteristics, the radiation oncologist can increase the dose to the tumor while reducing the dose to surrounding normal tissues. This allows the dose to be increased beyond that which less-conformal radiation will allow. The overall affects lead to the potential for fewer harmful side effects, more direct impact on the tumor, and increased tumor control.

The patient feels nothing during treatment. The minimized normal-tissue injury results in the potential for fewer effects following treatment, such as nausea, vomiting, or diarrhea. The patients experiences a better quality of life during and after proton treatment.

Questions and Answers about Proton Therapy

How does proton therapy work in relation to other mainstream radiation therapy and chemotherapy?

Proton therapy is the most precise and advanced form of radiation treatment today. It primarily radiates the tumor site, leaving surrounding healthy tissue and organs intact. Conventional x-ray radiation often radiates healthy tissue in its path and surrounding the tumor site. Chemotherapy moves throughout the entire body, unlike radiation and surgery which are considered "site specific" treatments.

What are the side effects from proton therapy?

There are minimal to no side effects, compared to conventional forms of radiation. Proton therapy is generally much more easily tolerated than standard radiation therapy.

What kinds of tumors are best treated by proton therapy?

Proton therapy is best for tumors that are localized and have not spread to distant areas of the body.

How would I know if proton therapy is the appropriate treatment option for myself or a loved one?

Do your homework. Learn as much as possible about all the treatment options available for your condition. Ask lots of questions and discuss them thoroughly with your doctors.

Can proton therapy be used in conjunction with other forms of cancer treatment?

Yes. Depending on the case, proton therapy may be used in combination with traditional radiation, chemotherapy and/or as a follow-up to surgery.

My doctor never mentioned proton therapy as a cancer treatment option. How long has proton therapy been in use for medical purposes?

Most radiation oncologists do know about proton therapy, but have had little experience working with proton beam radiation technology. This makes it more difficult to advise patients.

Proton therapy was first proposed in 1954, but it was available only for limited experimental use. There were no hospital-based proton treatment facilities in the world until the Proton Treatment Center at Loma Linda University Medical Center opened for patients in 1990. Today, the benefits of proton therapy have expanded beyond Loma Linda's southern, California location into other regions of the United States. The following centers are all now treating patients: in the northeast, Massachusetts General Hospital's proton center in Boston; in the midwest, Indiana University's Midwest Proton Radiotherapy Institute (MPRI); in Texas, M.D. Anderson Cancer Center's Proton Therapy Center (Houston); and in the south, the University of Florida's Proton Therapy Institute (Jacksonville). Future proton centers in development include Hampton University (Virginia) and the University of Pennsylvania Medical Center (Philadelphia).

How long does proton therapy take? How soon will I know if the treatment is successful?

Proton therapy can take anywhere from one day to seven weeks depending on the tumor site. The length of treatment time will also decrease over time as heavier doses begin to increase. With most cancer cases, success is determined if the cancer does not re-occur within five years after treatment.

Does proton therapy cost more than conventional forms of cancer treatment? Is it covered by most insurance plans?

Nearly all insurance providers nationwide cover proton therapy as does the U.S. medicare program. Proton therapy costs more than conventional radiation, but generally less than surgery.

Why is proton therapy so limited in its availability?

Proton therapy was been limited to research labs until 1990. Like most new technologies, developing a proton facility is costly. Building a new proton center can cost between $150–200 million. However, many universities and medical centers across the country are looking into providing proton therapy as part of their cancer treatment options.

Chapter 84

Complementary and Alternative Medicine (CAM) in Cancer Treatment

You have many choices to make before, during, and after your cancer treatment. One choice you may be thinking about is complementary and alternative medicine. We call this CAM, for short.

Reasons People with Cancer Choose CAM

People with cancer may use CAM to:

- help cope with the side effects of cancer treatments, such as nausea, pain, and fatigue;
- comfort themselves and ease the worries of cancer treatment and related stress;
- feel that they are doing something more to help with their own care;
- try to treat or cure their cancer.

It's natural to want to fight your cancer in any way you can. There is a lot of information available, and new methods for treating cancer are always being tested, so it may be hard to know where to start.

This chapter may help you understand what you find and make it easier to decide whether CAM is right for you. Many people try CAM

"Thinking about Complementary and Alternative Medicine," National Cancer Institute, June 8, 2005.

therapies during cancer care. CAM does not work for everyone, but some methods may help you manage stress, nausea, pain, or other symptoms or side effects.

The most important message of this chapter is to talk to your doctor before you try anything new. This will help ensure that nothing gets in the way of your cancer treatment.

What Is CAM?

CAM is any medical system, practice, or product that is not thought of as standard care. Standard medical care is care that is based on scientific evidence. For cancer, it includes chemotherapy, radiation, biological therapy, and surgery.

Complementary medicine: Complementary medicine is used along with standard medical treatments. One example is using acupuncture to help with side effects of cancer treatment.

Alternative medicine: Alternative medicine is used in place of standard medical treatments. One example is using a special diet to treat cancer instead of a method that a cancer specialist (an oncologist) suggests.

Integrative medicine: Integrative medicine is a total approach to care that involves the patient's mind, body, and spirit. It combines standard medicine with the CAM practices that have shown the most promise. For example, some people learn to use relaxation as a way to reduce stress during chemotherapy.

Types of Complementary and Alternative Medicine (CAM)

We are learning about CAM therapies every day, but there is still more to learn. Consumers may use the terms "natural," "holistic," "home remedy," or "Eastern medicine" to refer to CAM. However, experts use five categories to describe it. These are listed below with a few examples for each.

Mind-body medicines: These are based on the belief that your mind is able to affect your body. Some examples are:

• **Meditation:** Focused breathing or repetition of words or phrases to quiet the mind;

- **Biofeedback:** Using simple machines, the patient learns how to affect certain body functions that are normally out of one's awareness (such as heart rate);

- **Hypnosis:** A state of relaxed and focused attention in which the patient concentrates on a certain feeling, idea, or suggestion to aid in healing;

- **Yoga:** Systems of stretches and poses, with special attention given to breathing;

- **Imagery:** Imagining scenes, pictures, or experiences to help the body heal;

- **Creative outlets:** Such as art, music, or dance.

Biologically based practices: This type of CAM uses things found in nature. This includes dietary supplements and herbal products. Vitamins, herbs, foods, and special diets are some examples

A note about nutrition: It's common for people with cancer to have questions about different foods to eat during treatment. Yet it's important to know that there is no one food or special diet that has been proven to control cancer. Too much of any one food is not helpful, and may even be harmful. Because of nutrition needs you may have, it's best to talk with the doctor in charge of your treatment about the foods you should be eating.

Manipulative and body-based practices: These are based on working with one or more parts of the body. Some examples include the following:

- **Massage:** Manipulation of tissues with hands or special tools

- **Chiropractic care:** A type of manipulation of the joints and skeletal system

- **Reflexology:** Using pressure points in the hands or feet to affect other parts of the body

Energy medicine: Energy medicine involves the belief that the body has energy fields that can be used for healing and wellness. Therapists use pressure or move the body by placing their hands in or through these fields. Here are some examples:

- **Tai chi:** Involves slow, gentle movements with a focus on the breath and concentration

- **Reiki:** Balancing energy either from a distance or by placing hands on or near the patient

- **Therapeutic touch:** Moving hands over energy fields of the body

Whole medical systems: These are healing systems and beliefs that have evolved over time in different cultures and parts of the world. The following are some examples:

- **Ayurvedic medicine:** A system from India emphasizing balance among body, mind, and spirit

- **Chinese medicine:** Based on the view that health is a balance in the body of two forces called yin and yang. Acupuncture is a common practice in Chinese medicine that involves stimulating specific points on the body to promote health or to lessen disease symptoms and treatment side effects.

- **Homeopathy:** Uses very small doses of substances to trigger the body to heal itself

- **Naturopathic medicine:** Uses different methods that help the body naturally heal itself

Talk with Your Doctor Before You Use CAM

Some people with cancer are afraid that their doctor won't understand or approve of the use of CAM. But doctors know that people with cancer want to take an active part in their care. They want the best for their patients and often are willing to work with them.

Talk to your doctor to make sure that all aspects of your cancer care work together. This is important because things that seem safe, such as certain foods or pills, may interfere with your cancer treatment.

What questions should I ask my doctor about CAM?

What types of CAM might:

- Help me cope, reduce my stress, and feel better?

- Help me feel less tired?

- Help me deal with cancer symptoms, such as pain, or side effects of treatment, such as nausea?

If I decide to try a CAM therapy:

- Will it interfere with my treatment or medicines?
- Can you help me understand these articles I found about CAM?
- Can you suggest a CAM practitioner for me to talk to?
- Will you work with my CAM practitioner?

A Natural Product Does Not Mean a Safe Product

Here are some important facts about dietary supplements such as herbs and vitamins:

- *They may affect how well other medicines work in your body:* Herbs and some plant-based products may keep medicines from doing what they are supposed to do. These medicines can be ones your doctor prescribes for you, or even ones you buy off the shelf at the store. For example, the herb St. John's wort, which some people with cancer use for depression, may cause certain anti-cancer drugs not to work as well as they should.

- *Herbal supplements can act like drugs in your body:* They may be harmful when taken by themselves, with other substances, or in large doses. For example, some studies have shown that kava, an herb that has been used to help with stress and anxiety, may cause liver damage.

- *Vitamins can also take strong action in your body:* For example, high doses of vitamins, even vitamin C, may affect how chemotherapy and radiation work. Too much of any vitamin is not safe—even in a healthy person.

Tell your doctor if you are taking any dietary supplements, no matter how safe you think they are. This is very important. Even though there are ads or claims that something has been used for years, they do not prove that it is safe or effective. It is still important to be careful.

Supplements do not have to be approved by the federal government before being sold to the public. Also, a prescription is not needed to buy them. Therefore, it's up to consumers to decide what is best for them.

Choose Practitioners with Care

CAM practitioners are people who have training in the therapies listed previously. Choosing one should be done with the same care as choosing a doctor. Here are some things to remember when choosing a practitioner:

- Ask your doctor or nurse to suggest someone or speak with someone who knows about CAM.

- Ask whether someone at your cancer center or doctor's office can help you find a CAM practitioner. There may be a social worker or physical therapist who can help you.

- Ask whether your hospital keeps lists of centers or has staff who can suggest people.

- Contact CAM professional organizations to get names of practitioners who are certified. This means that they have proper training in their field.

- Contact local health and wellness organizations.

- Ask about each practitioner's training and experience.

- Ask whether the practitioner has a license to practice in your state. If you want to confirm the answer, ask what organization gives out the licenses. Then, you may choose to follow up with a phone call.

- Call your health care plan to see if it covers this therapy.

What general questions should I ask the CAM practitioner?

- What types of CAM do you practice?
- What are your training and qualifications?
- Do you see other patients with my type of cancer?
- Will you work with my doctor?

What questions about the therapy should I ask the CAM practitioner?

- How can this help me?
- Do you know of studies that prove it helps?
- What are the risks and side effects?
- Will this interfere with my cancer treatment?
- How long will I be on the therapy?

- What will it cost?
- Do you have information that I can read about it?
- Are there any reasons why I should not use it?

What other questions should I ask myself?

- Do I feel comfortable with this person?
- Do I like how the office looks and feels?
- Do I like the staff?
- Does this person support standard cancer treatments?
- How far am I willing to travel for treatment?
- Is it easy to get an appointment?
- Are the hours good for me?
- Will insurance cover the cost of CAM?

Call your health plan or insurer to see whether they cover CAM therapies. Many are not covered.

Getting Information from Trusted Sources

Government Agencies

There is a lot of information on CAM, so it's important to go to sources you can trust. Good places to start are the government agencies listed at the end of this chapter. They offer lots of information about CAM that might be helpful to you. They may also know of universities or hospitals that have CAM resources.

Be careful of products advertised by people or companies that:

- Make claims that they have a "cure";
- Do not give specific information about how well their product works;
- Make claims only about positive results that have few side effects;
- Say they have clinical studies, but provide no proof or copies of the studies.

Just remember, if it sounds too good to be true, it probably is.

925

Websites

Patients and families have been able to find answers to many of their questions about CAM on the internet. Many websites are good resources for CAM information. However, some may be unreliable or misleading.

Questions to ask about a website:

• Who runs and pays for the site?

• Does it list any credentials?

• Does it represent an organization that is well-known and respected?

• What is the purpose of the site, and who is it for?

• Is the site selling or promoting something?

• Where does the information come from?

• Is the information based on facts or only on someone's feelings or opinions?

• How is the information chosen? Is there a review board or is the content reviewed by experts?

• How current is the information?

• Does the site tell when it was last updated?

• How does the site choose which other sites to link you to?

Books

A number of books have been written about different CAM therapies. Some books are better than others and contain trustworthy content, while others do not.

If you go to the library and ask the staff for suggestions. Or if you live near a college or university, there may be a medical library available. Local bookstores may also have people on staff who can help you.

It's important to know that information is always changing and that new research results are reported every day. Be aware that if a book is written by only one person, you may only be getting that one person's view.

Questions to ask:

• Is the author an expert on this subject?

• Do you know anyone else who has read the book?

- Has the book been reviewed by other experts?
- Was it published in the past five years?
- Does the book offer different points of view, or does it seem to hold one opinion?
- Has the author researched the topic in full?
- Are the references listed in the back?

Magazine Articles

If you want to look for articles you can trust, ask your librarian to help you look for medical journals, books, and other research that has been done by experts.

Articles in popular magazines are usually not written by experts. Rather, the authors speak with experts, gather information, and then write the article. If claims about CAM are made in magazine articles, remember these points:

- The authors may not have expert knowledge in this area.
- They may not say where they found their information.
- The articles have not been reviewed by experts.
- The publisher may have ties to advertisers or other organizations. Therefore, the article may be one-sided.

When you read these articles, you can use the same process that the magazine writer uses:

- Speak with experts
- Ask lots of questions
- Then decide if the therapy is right for you

Resources

National Cancer Institute (NCI): Office of Cancer Complementary and Alternative Medicine (OCCAM), oversees NCI's projects in CAM, funds cancer CAM research, and provides information about CAM to health providers and the public:

- Visit: http://cancer.gov/cam

Cancer Information Service (CIS): Provides help finding NCI information on the internet, answers questions about cancer, provides printed materials from NCI, and gives referrals to clinical trials and other cancer-related services:

- Visit: http://cis.nci.nih.gov
- Chat online: http://www.cancer.gov (click on "Need Help?" then click on "LiveHelp")
- Toll-free: 800-4-CANCER (800-422-6237)
- TTY: 800-332-8615

PDQ®: Provides regularly updated information on most types of cancer and many related topics:

- Visit: http://www.cancer.gov/cancertopics/pdq

National Center for Complementary and Alternative Medicine (NCCAM): Funds CAM research and evaluates and provides information about CAM to health providers and the public:

- Visit: http://nccam.nih.gov
- Toll-free: 888-644-6226
- TTY: 866-464-3615

National Library of Medicine: The Directory of Information Resources Online (DIRLINE) contains locations of and information about a number of health organizations, including those that focus on CAM:

- Visit: http://dirline.nlm.nih.gov

Medline Plus: Provides access to reliable health information, including articles, organizations, directories, and answers to health questions:

- Visit: http://medlineplus.gov

PubMed: Has a free and easy-to-use search tool for finding scientific articles on CAM:

- Visit: http://www.ncbi.nlm.nih.gov/PubMed

Food and Drug Administration (FDA): Oversees safety of drugs and medical devices, provides information on many issues, including vitamins and pills, and informs people about how to look for health fraud:

- Visit: http://www.fda.gov
- Toll-free: 888-463-6332

Federal Trade Commission (FTC): Provides information about consumer protection laws and provides information about false advertising for foods and drugs:

- Visit: http://www.ftc.gov
- Toll-free: 877-FTC-HELP (877-382-4357)
- TTY: 866-653-4261

National Cancer Institute-Sponsored Cancer Centers: Many National Cancer Institute-sponsored cancer centers have CAM information available to you:

- Visit: http://www3.cancer.gov/cancercenters/centerslist.html
- Toll-free: 800-4-CANCER (800-422-6237). Ask for the cancer center list fact sheet.

Part Four

Special Concerns
Related to Recurrent or
Advanced Cancer

Chapter 85

If Cancer Returns

Adjusting to the News

Maybe in the back of your mind, you feared that your cancer might return. Now you might be thinking, "How can this be happening to me again? Haven't I been through enough?"

You may be feeling shocked, angry, sad, or scared. Many people have these feelings. But you have something now that you didn't have before—experience. You've lived through cancer once. You know a lot about what to expect and hope for.

Also remember that treatments may have improved since you had your first cancer. New drugs or methods may help with your treatment or in managing side effects. In fact, cancer is now often thought of as a chronic disease, one which people manage for many years.

Why and Where Cancer Returns

When cancer comes back, doctors call it a recurrence (or recurrent cancer). Some things you should know are:

- A recurrent cancer starts with cancer cells that the first treatment didn't fully remove or destroy. Some may have been too small to be seen in follow-up. This doesn't mean that the treatment you received was wrong. And it doesn't mean that you did anything

Excerpted from "When Cancer Returns," National Cancer Institute, August 23, 2005. The complete text of this document is available online at http://www .cancer.gov.

wrong, either. It just means that a small number of cancer cells survived the treatment. These cells grew over time into tumors or cancer that your doctor can now detect.

- When cancer comes back, it doesn't always show up in the same part of the body. For example, if you had colon cancer, it may come back in your liver. But the cancer is still called colon cancer. When the original cancer spreads to a new place, it is called a metastasis.

- It is possible to develop a completely new cancer that has nothing to do with your original cancer. But this doesn't happen very often. Recurrences are more common.

Where Cancer Can Return

Doctors define recurrent cancers by where they develop. The different types of recurrence are:

- **Local recurrence:** This means that the cancer is in the same place as the original cancer or is very close to it.

- **Regional recurrence:** This is when tumors grow in lymph nodes or tissues near the place of the original cancer.

- **Distant recurrence:** In these cases, the cancer has spread (metastasized) to organs or tissues far from the place of the original cancer.

Local cancer may be easier to treat than regional or distant cancer. But this can be different for each patient. Talk with your doctor about your options.

Taking Control: Your Care and Treatment

Cancer that returns can affect all parts of your life. You may feel weak and no longer in control. But you don't have to feel that way. You can take part in your care and in making decisions. You can also talk with your health care team and loved ones as you decide about your care. This may help you feel a sense of control and well-being.

Talking with Your Health Care Team

Many people have a treatment team of health providers who work together to help them. This team may include doctors, nurses, oncology social workers, dietitians, or other specialists. Some people don't like to ask about treatment choices or side effects. They think that doctors don't like being questioned. But this is not true. Most doctors want their patients to be involved in their own care. They want patients to discuss concerns with them.

Here are a few topics you may want to discuss with your health care team:

- **Pain or other symptoms:** Be honest and open about how you feel. Tell your doctors if you have pain and where. Tell them what you expect in the way of pain relief.

- **Communication:** Some people want to know details about their care. Others prefer to know as little as possible. Some people with cancer want their family members to make most of their decisions. What would you prefer? Decide what you want to know, how much you want to know, and when you've heard enough. Choose what is most comfortable for you. Then tell your doctor and family members. Ask that they follow through with your wishes.

- **Family wishes:** Some family members may have trouble dealing with cancer. They don't want to know how far the disease has advanced. Find out from your family members how much they want to know. And be sure to tell your doctors and nurses. Do this as soon as possible. It will help avoid conflicts or distress among your loved ones.

Other Tips for Talking with Your Health Care Team

- Speak openly about your needs, questions, and concerns. Don't be embarrassed to ask your doctor to repeat or explain something.

- Keep a file or notebook of all the papers and test results that your doctor has given you. Take this file to your visits. Also keep records or a diary of all your visits. List the drugs and tests you have taken. Then you can refer to your records when you need to. Many patients say this is helpful, especially when you meet with a new doctor for the first time.

- Write down your questions before you see your doctors so you will remember them.

- Ask a family member or friend to go to the doctor's office with you. They can help you ask questions to get a clear sense of what to expect. This can be an emotional time. You may have trouble focusing on what the doctor says. It may be easier for someone else to take notes. Then you can review them later.

- Ask your doctor if it's okay to tape-record your talks.

- Tell your doctor if you want to get dressed before talking about your results. Wearing a gown or robe is distracting for some patients. They find it harder to focus on what the doctor is saying.

Second Opinions

Some patients worry that doctors will be offended if they ask for a second opinion. Usually the opposite is true. Most doctors welcome a second opinion. And many health insurance companies will pay for them.

If you get a second opinion, the doctor may agree with your first doctor's treatment plan. Or the second doctor may suggest another approach. Either way, you have more information and perhaps a greater sense of control. You can feel more confident about the decisions you make, knowing that you've looked at your options.

Clinical Trials

Treatment clinical trials are research studies that try to find better ways to treat cancer. Every day, cancer researchers learn more about treatment options from clinical trials.

Each study has rules about who can take part. These rules include the person's age and type of cancer. They also cover earlier treatments and where the cancer has returned.

Clinical trials have both benefits and risks. Your doctor should tell you about them before you make any decisions about taking part.

There are different phases of clinical trials:

- Phase I trials test what dose of a treatment is safe and how it should be given.

- Phase II trials discover how cancer responds to a new drug or treatment.

- Phase III trials compare an accepted cancer treatment (standard treatment) with a new treatment that researchers hope is better.

Taking part in a clinical trial could help you and others who get cancer in the future. But insurance and managed care plans do not always cover the costs. What they cover varies by plan and by study. If you want to learn more about clinical trials, talk with your health care team.

Your Feelings

People feel so many emotions when they find out that their cancer has come back. Shock, fear, anger, and denial are just a few. The new diagnosis hits them as hard as it did the first time, or even harder.

Regardless of your first reaction, starting cancer treatment again can place even more demands on your mind and spirit. You'll have good days and bad days. So just remember that it's okay to feel a lot of different emotions.

Some of these emotions may be ones you have had at other times in your life. But you may be feeling them more intensely. If you have dealt with them in the past, you may be able to cope with them now, too. If some of the feelings are new, or are so strong that it is hard to get through everyday activities, you may want to ask for help.

There are many people who may be able to help you. These include health psychologists, oncology social workers, other mental health experts, and leaders in your faith or spiritual community. They know many ways to help you cope with your feelings.

Ways You Can Cope

Your feelings will come and go, just like they always have. If you have some strategies to deal with them, you have already taken a step in the right direction.

Know that many other people have been where you are. Some do better when they join a support group. It helps them to talk with others who are facing the same challenges. You may prefer to join an online support group. That way you can chat with people from home. Be sure to check the privacy issues before you join.

If support groups don't appeal to you, there are many experts who are trained to give cancer support. These include oncology social workers, psychologists or health psychologists, counselors, or members of your faith or spiritual community.

You may be able to continue many of your regular activities, even though some may be more difficult than before. Whatever you do, remember to conserve your strength for the things you really want to do. Don't plan too many things for one day. Also try to stagger them during the day.

Setting Goals

Cancer treatment can take up a lot of your time and energy. It helps to plan something that takes your mind off the disease each day. Aim for small goals each day. Here are some ideas:

• Exercising

- Completing tasks you've been wanting to do
- Making phone calls
- Having lunch with a friend
- Reading one chapter of a book or doing a puzzle
- Listening to music or a relaxation tape

Many people with cancer also set longer-term goals. They say that they do much better if they set goals or look forward to something special. It could be an anniversary, the birth of a child or grandchild, a wedding, a graduation, or a vacation. But if you set a long-term goal, make sure you are realistic about how you will achieve it.

Remember, too, that being flexible is important. You may have to change your plans if your energy level drops. You may have to adjust your goals if the cancer causes new challenges. Whatever your goals, try to spend your time in a way that you enjoy.

Family and Friends

Your loved ones may need time to adjust to the news that your cancer has returned. They need to come to terms with their own feelings. These may include confusion, shock, helplessness, anger, and other feelings. Let family members and friends know that they can offer comfort just by doing things like this:

- Being themselves
- Listening and not trying to solve problems
- Being at ease with you

Being able to comfort you can help them cope with their feelings.

Bear in mind that not everyone can handle the return of cancer. Sometimes a friend or family member can't face the idea that you might not get better. Some people may not know what to say or do for you. As a result, relationships may change, but not because of you. They may change because others can't cope with their own feelings and pain. If you can, remind your loved ones that you are still the same person you always were. Let them know if it's all right to ask questions or tell you how they feel. Sometimes just reminding them to be there for you is enough.

It's also okay if you don't feel comfortable talking about your cancer. Some topics are hard to talk about with people you are close to. In this case, you may want to talk with a member of your health care team or a trained counselor. You might want to attend a support group where people meet to share common concerns.

Family Meetings

Some families have trouble expressing their needs to each other. Other families simply do not get along. If you don't feel comfortable talking with family members, ask a member of your health care team to help. You could also ask a social worker or other professional to hold a family meeting. This may help family members feel that they can safely express their feelings. It can also be a time for you and your family to meet with your entire health care team to solve problems and set goals. Although it can be very hard to talk about these things, studies show that cancer care is a smoother process when everyone remains open and talks about the issues.

People Close to You

Often, talking with someone close to you is harder than talking with anyone else. Here's some advice on talking with loved ones during tough times.

Spouses and Partners

- Try as much as you can to keep your relationship as it was before you got sick.

- Talk things over. This may be hard for you or your spouse or partner. If so, ask a counselor or social worker to talk with both of you together.

- Be realistic about demands. Your spouse or partner may feel guilty about your illness. They may feel guilty about any time spent away from you. They also may be under stress due to changing family roles.

- Spend some time apart. Your spouse or partner needs time to address their own needs. If these needs are neglected, your loved one may have less energy and support to give. Remember, you didn't spend 24 hours a day together before you got sick.

- Body changes and emotional concerns may affect your sex life. Talking openly and honestly is key. But if you can't talk about these issues, you might want to talk with a professional. Don't be afraid to seek help or advice if you need it.

Children

Keeping your children's trust is very important at this time. Children can sense when things are wrong. So it's best to be as open as you can about your cancer. They may worry that they did something to cause the cancer. They may be afraid that no one will take care of them. They may also feel that you are not spending as much time with them as you used to. Although you can't protect them from what they might feel, you can prepare them for these feelings.

Some children become clingy. Others get into trouble at school or at home. It helps to keep the lines of communication open. Here are some tips to try:

- Be honest. Tell them you are sick and that the doctors are working to make you better.

- Let them know that nothing they did or said caused the cancer. And make sure that they know that they can't catch it from you.

- Reassure them that you love them.

- Encourage them to talk about their feelings.

- Tell them it's okay to be upset, angry, or scared.

- Be clear and simple when you talk, since children can focus only briefly. Use words they can understand.

- Let them know they will be taken care of and loved.

Let them know that it's okay to ask questions. Tell them that you will answer them as honestly as you can. In fact, children who aren't told the truth about an illness can become even more scared. They often depend on their imagination and fears to explain the changes around them.

Teenagers

Teenagers have some of the same needs as those of younger children. They need to hear the truth about an illness. This helps keep them from feeling needless guilt and stress. But be aware that they may try to avoid the subject. They may become angry, act out, or get into trouble as a way of coping. Others simply withdraw. Try these suggestions to help teens:

- Give them the space they need. This is especially important if you are relying on them more to help with family needs.

- Give them time to deal with their feelings, alone or with friends.

- Let them know that they should still go to school and take part in sports and other fun activities.

If you have trouble explaining your cancer, you might want to ask for help. A close friend, relative, healthcare worker, or trusted coach or teacher could help answer your teenager's questions. Your support group, social worker, or doctor can also help you find a counselor or psychologist.

Adult Children

Your relationship with your adult children may change now that you have cancer again. You may have to rely on them more. And it may be hard for you to ask for support. After all, you may be used to giving support rather than getting it.

Adult children have their concerns, too. They may start to think about their own mortality. They may feel guilt, because of the many demands on them as parents, children, and employees. Some may live far away or have other duties. They may feel bad that they can't spend as much time with you as they would like. These types of things often help:

- Share decision-making with your children.

- Involve them in issues that are important to you. These may include treatment choices, plans for the future, or activities that you want to continue.

- If they aren't able to be there with you, keep them updated on your progress.

- Make the most of the time you have. Share your feelings with them.

Try to reach out to your adult children. Openly sharing your feelings, goals, and wishes will help them adjust. It will also help prevent problems in the future. Remember, just as parents want the best for their children, children want the best for their parents. They want to see your needs met effectively and with compassion. Your children don't want to see you suffer.

Looking for Meaning

At different times in life, it's natural for people to look for meaning in their lives. And many people with recurrent cancer find this search for meaning important. They want to understand their purpose in life.

They often reflect on what they have gone through. Some look for a sense of peace or a bond with others. Some seek to forgive themselves or others for past actions. Some look for answers and strength through religion or spirituality.

Being spiritual means different things to different people. It's a very personal issue. Everyone has their own beliefs about the meaning of life. Some people find it through religion or faith. Some find it by teaching or through volunteer work. Others find it in other ways. Having cancer may cause you to think about what you believe—about God, an afterlife, or the connections between living things. This can bring a sense of peace, a lot of questions, or both.

You may have already given a lot of thought to these issues. Still, you might find comfort by exploring more deeply what is meaningful to you. You could do this with someone close to you, a member of your faith or spiritual community, a counselor, or a trusted friend. Or you may find that talking to others at gatherings and services at places of worship is helpful.

Or you may just want to take time for yourself. You may want to reflect on your experiences and relationships. Writing in a journal or reading also helps some people find comfort and meaning. Others find that prayer or meditation helps them.

Many people also find that cancer changes their values. The things you own and your daily duties may seem less important. You may decide to spend more time with loved ones or helping others. You may want to do more things outdoors or learn something new.

A Time to Reflect

This is a hard time in your life. Living with cancer is tough, especially when it has come back. You battled the disease once, and now you must face it again. But you're more experienced this time around.

Use this knowledge to your advantage. Try to remember what you did before to cope. Reflect on what you might have done differently. By looking back in this way, the hope is that you may find new strength. And that this strength can help carry you through each day, and through the coming weeks and months.

Chapter 86

Advanced Cancer

Chapter Contents

Section 86.1

Making Choices about Your Care when You Have Advanced Cancer

Excerpted from "Coping with Advanced Cancer,"
National Cancer Institute, September 20, 2005.

You've struggled with the diagnosis, treatment, and maybe the recurrence of cancer. Now doctors may have told you that you have advanced cancer. They may have said that your cancer is not responding to treatment and that long-term remission is no longer likely. Or they may have said they have run out of standard treatment options. However you learn the news, it can be devastating to you and your loved ones.

Try to remember that you are still in charge of your life. It may be hard to do this with all that you are going through. You may have trouble coping with your feelings from time to time. Or you may be grieving that your life has gone a different way than you had hoped. It's natural to feel negative at times. You'll have ups and downs. We hope this chapter will help you. Our goal is to help you stay in control as much as you can, and make the rest of your life fulfilling and satisfying. You can still have hope and joy in your life, even as you cope with what lies ahead.

Making Choices about Care

People have different goals for care when dealing with advanced cancer. And your goals for care may be changing. Perhaps you had been hoping for a remission. Yet now you need to think more about controlling the spread or growth of the cancer. Your decisions about treatment will be very personal. You will want to seek the help of your loved ones and health care providers. But only you can decide what to do. Your desire to avoid future regrets should be measured against the positives and negatives of treatment.

It is important to ask your health care team what to expect in the future. It's also important to be clear with them about how much information you want to receive from them.

Comfort Care

You have a right to comfort care both during and after treatment. This kind of care is often called palliative care. It includes treating or preventing cancer symptoms and the side effects caused by treatment. Comfort care can also mean getting help with emotional and spiritual problems during and after cancer treatment. Sometimes patients don't want to tell the doctor about their symptoms. They only want to focus on the cancer. Yet you can improve your quality of life with comfort care.

People once thought of palliative care as a way to comfort those dying of cancer. Doctors now offer this care to all cancer patients, beginning when the cancer is diagnosed. You should receive palliative care through treatment, survival, and advanced disease. Your oncologist may be able to help you. But a palliative care specialist may be the best person to treat some problems. Ask your doctor or nurse if there is a specialist you can go to.

Your Choices

You have a number of options for your care. These depend on the type of cancer you have and the goals you have for your care. Your health care team should tell you about any procedures and treatments available, as well as the benefits and risks of those treatments. Options include the following:

- Clinical trials
- Palliative radiation, chemotherapy, or surgery
- Hospice care
- Home care

Many patients choose more than one option. Ask all the questions you need to.

Try to base your decision on your own feelings about life and death, and the pros and cons of cancer treatment. If you choose not to receive any more active cancer treatment, it does not necessarily mean a quick decline and death. It also does not mean you will stop being given palliative care. Your health care team can offer information and advice on options. You also may want to talk about these options with family members and others who are close to you.

Clinical Trials

Treatment clinical trials are research studies that try to find better ways to treat cancer. Every day, cancer researchers learn more about treatment options from clinical trials. If you decide to try a clinical trial, the trial you choose will depend on the type of cancer you have. It will also depend on the treatments you have already received. Each study has rules about who can take part. These rules may include the patient's age, health, and type of cancer. Clinical trials have both benefits and risks. Your doctor and the study doctors should tell you about these before you make any decisions.

Taking part in a clinical trial could help you and help others who get cancer in the future. But insurance and managed care plans do not always cover costs. What they cover varies by plan and by study. Talk with your health care team to learn more about coverage for clinical trials for your type of cancer.

For more information about clinical trials talk to the NCI's Cancer Information Service at 800-422-6237 (800-4-CANCER).

Palliative Radiation, Chemotherapy, or Surgery

Some palliative chemotherapy and palliative radiation may help relieve pain and other symptoms. In this way, they may improve your quality of life even if they don't stop your cancer. These treatments may be given to remove or shrink a tumor. Or they may be given to slow down a tumor's spread. Palliative surgery is sometimes used to relieve pain or other problems.

Hospice

Hospice care is an option if you feel you are no longer benefiting from cancer treatments. Choosing hospice care doesn't mean that you've given up. It just means the treatment goals are different at this point. It does not mean giving up hope, but rather changing what you hope for. But be sure to check with the hospice you use to learn what treatments and services are covered. Check with your insurance company also.

The goal of hospice is to help patients live each day to the fullest by making them comfortable and lessen their symptoms. Hospice doctors, nurses, spiritual leaders, social workers, and volunteers are specially trained. They are dedicated to supporting their patients' and families' emotional, social, and spiritual needs as well as dealing with patients' medical symptoms.

People usually qualify for hospice services when their doctor signs a statement that says that patients with their type and stage of disease, on average, aren't likely to survive beyond six months. Many people don't realize that they can use hospice services for a number of months, not just a few weeks. In fact, many say they wish they had gotten hospice care much sooner than they did. They were surprised by the expert care and understanding that they got. Often, control of symptoms not only improves quality of life but also helps people live longer. You will be reviewed periodically to see if hospice care is still right for you. Services may include the following:

- Doctor services (You may still keep your own doctors, too.)

- Nursing care

- Medical supplies and equipment

- Drugs to manage cancer-related symptoms and pain

- Short-term in-patient care

- Homemaker and home health aide services

- Respite (relief) services for caregivers. This means someone else helps with care for awhile, so the caregiver can take a break.

- Counseling

- Social work services

- Spiritual care

- Bereavement (grief) counseling and support

- Volunteer services

You can get hospice services at home, in special facilities, in hospitals, and in nursing homes. They have specialists to help guide care. They also have nurses on call 24 hours a day in case you need advice. And they have many volunteers who help families care for their loved one. Some hospices will give palliative chemotherapy at home as well. Hospice care doesn't seek to treat cancer, but it does treat reversible problems with brief hospital stays if needed. An example might be pneumonia or a bladder infection. Medicare, Medicaid, and most private insurers cover hospice services. For those without coverage and in financial need, many hospices provide care for free. To learn more about hospice care, call the National Hospice and Palliative Care Organization at 800-658-8898. Or visit their website at http://www.nhpco.org. The website can also help you find a hospice in your community.

Hospice and home care professionals can help you and your family work through some tough emotional issues. A social worker can offer emotional support, help in planning hospice or home care, and ease the move between types of care. Many people prefer the comfort of their own home, familiar surroundings, and having friends and family members nearby. Getting health care at home gives family members, friends, and neighbors the chance to spend time with you and help with your care.

Home Care

Home care services are for people who are at home rather than in a hospital. Home care services may include the following:

- Monitoring care
- Managing symptoms
- Providing medical equipment
- Physical and other therapies

You may have to pay for home care services yourself. Check with your insurance company. Medicare, Medicaid, and private insurance will sometimes cover home care services when ordered by your doctor. But some rules apply. So talk to your social worker and other members of your health care team to find out more.

Talking with Your Health Care Team

As your disease advances, it's still important to give feedback to your doctor. That's the only way he or she can know what is working for you. Many people have a treatment team of health providers who work together to help them. This team may include doctors, nurses, oncology social workers, dietitians, and other specialists. They need to fully know your desires during treatment and at the end of your life. Let them know about any discomfort you have. You have a right to live your remaining days with dignity and peace of mind. So it's important to have a relationship and an understanding with those who will be caring for you.

Here are just a few topics you may want to discuss with your doctor or other members of your health care team:

- **Pain or other symptoms:** Be honest and open about how you feel. Tell your doctor if you have pain and where. Also tell him or her what you expect in the way of pain relief.

- **Communication:** Some people want to know details about their care. Others prefer to know as little as possible. Some patients want their family members to make most of their decisions. What would you prefer? Decide what you want to know, how much you want to know, and when you've heard enough. Choose what is most comfortable for you, then tell your doctor and family members. Ask that they follow through with your wishes.

- **Family wishes.** Some family members may have trouble dealing with cancer. They don't want to know how far the disease has advanced or how much time doctors think you have. Find out from your family members how much they want to know, and tell your health care team their wishes. Do this as soon as possible. It will help avoid conflicts or distress among your loved ones.

Remember that only you and those closest to you can answer many of these questions. Having answers to your questions can help you know what to expect now and in the future.

Tips for Meeting with Your Health Care Team

- Make a list of your questions before each appointment.

- Bring a family member or trusted friend with you to your medical visits. This person can help you remember what the doctor or nurse said, and talk with you about it after the visit.

- Ask all your questions. If you do not understand an answer, keep asking until you do. There is no such thing as a "stupid" question.

- Take notes. You can do this or you can ask a family member or friend to take them for you. Or you can ask if it's okay to use a tape recorder.

- Get a phone number of someone to call with follow-up questions.

- Keep a file or notebook of all the papers and test results that your doctor has given you. Take this with you to your visits. Also keep records or a diary of all your visits. List the drugs and tests you have taken.

- Keep a record of any upsetting symptoms or side effects you have. Note when and where they occur. Take this with you on your visits.

- Find out what to do in an emergency. This includes whom to call, how to reach them, and where to go.

No One Knows the Future

It's normal for people to want to know how long they will have to live. It's also natural to want to prepare for what lies ahead. You may want to prepare emotionally as well as to make certain arrangements and plans.

But predicting how long someone will live is not exact. Your doctor may be able to give you an estimate, but keep in mind that it's a guess. Every patient is different. Your doctor has to take into account your type of cancer, treatment, past illnesses, and other factors.

Some patients live long past the time the doctor first predicted. Others live a shorter time. Also, an infection or other complication could happen and change things. Your doctor may know your situation best, but even he or she cannot know the answer for sure. And doctors don't always feel comfortable trying to give you an answer.

In truth, none of us knows when we are going to die. Unexpected events happen every day. The best we can do is to try to live fully and for today.

Section 86.2

Managing the Symptoms of Advanced Cancer

Excerpted from "Coping with Advanced Cancer,"
National Cancer Institute, September 20, 2005.

Getting Help for Your Symptoms

Sometimes people assume their symptoms will get worse as their cancer progresses. But with good supports in place and good care, your symptoms should always be managed. So don't downplay your symptoms if you're having them. It's important to report how you are feeling. Tell your doctor, members of your health care team, and your loved ones. If you feel very sick or tired, your doctor may be able to adjust your treatment or give you other medicine.

Following are some of the symptoms you may have.

Pain

Having cancer doesn't always mean that you'll have pain. But if you do, you shouldn't accept pain as normal. Most types of pain can be treated. Your doctor can control pain with different medicines and treatments.

You may want to ask your doctor if you can talk to a pain specialist. Many hospitals have doctors on staff who are experts at treating pain. They may also have palliative medicine specialists.

Managing your pain helps you sleep and eat better. It makes it easier to enjoy your family and friends and focus on what gives you joy.

There are a few different ways to take pain medicine, including the following:

- By mouth
- Through the skin (like with a patch)
- By shots
- Through an I.V. (intravenous) or an S.C. (subcutaneous) pump

951

Your medicine, and how you take it, will depend on the type of pain and its cause. For example, for constant pain you may need a steady dose of medicine over a long period of time. You might use a patch placed on the skin or a slow-release pill.

You should have regular talks with your health care team about the type and extent of your pain. That's because pain can change throughout your illness. Let them know the kind of pain you have, how bad it is, and where it hurts.

You may want to keep a "pain diary." Include the time of day that the pain occurred and what you were doing. Rate the pain on a scale of 0 to 10. (Zero means no pain, and 10 is the worst pain you could have.) Use the diary when you talk to your doctor about your pain.

Unlike other medicines, there is no "right" dose for many pain medicines. Yours may be larger or smaller than someone else's. The right dose is the one that relieves your pain and makes you feel better.

Describing pain: When describing pain to your doctor, be as detailed as you can. Your doctor may ask:

- Where exactly is your pain? Does it move from one spot to another?
- How does the pain feel—dull, sharp, burning?
- How often does your pain occur?
- How long does it last?
- Does it start at a certain time—morning, afternoon, night?
- What makes the pain better? What makes it worse?

Pain medications: People with cancer often need strong medicine to help control their pain. Don't be afraid to ask for pain medicine or for larger doses if you need them. The drugs will help you stay as comfortable as you can be.

When treating pain in people with cancer, addiction is not an issue. Sadly, fears of addiction sometimes prevent people from taking medicine for pain. The same fears also prompt family members to encourage loved ones to "hold off" between doses. But people in pain get the most relief when they take their medicines and treatments on a regular schedule.

Other ways to treat pain: Cancer pain is usually treated with medicine and other therapies. But there are also some non-drug treatments. They are forms of complementary and alternative medicine

(CAM). Many people have found the methods listed below helpful. But talk with your health care team before trying any of them. Make sure they are safe and won't interfere with your cancer treatment.

- Acupuncture is a form of Chinese medicine that stimulates certain points on the body using small needles. It may help treat nausea and control pain. Before using acupuncture, ask your health care team if it is safe for your type of cancer.

- Imagery is imagining scenes, pictures, or experiences to feel calmer or perhaps to help the body heal.

- Relaxation techniques include deep breathing and exercises to relax your muscles.

- Hypnosis is a state of relaxed and focused attention. One focuses on a certain feeling, idea, or suggestion.

- Biofeedback is the use of a special machine to help the patient learn how to control certain body functions. These are things that we are normally not aware of (such as heart rate).

- Massage therapy brings relaxation and a sense of well-being by the gentle rubbing of different body parts or muscles. Before you try this, you need to check with your doctor. Massage is not recommended for some kinds of cancer.

These methods may also help manage stress. Again, talk to your health care team before using anything new, no matter how safe it may seem. Ask your health care team for more information about where to get these treatments.

Anxiety

Cancer takes a toll on both your body and your mind. You are coping with many different things now. You may feel overwhelmed. Pain and medicines for pain can also make you feel anxious or depressed. And you may be more likely to feel this way if you have had these feelings before.

Here are some signs of anxiety:

- Feeling very tense and nervous
- Racing heartbeat
- Sweating a lot
- Trouble breathing or catching your breath

- A lump in your throat or a knot in your stomach
- Sudden fear

Feeling anxious can be normal. But if it begins disrupting your daily life, ask for help from the members of your health care team. They can recommend someone for you to talk to. Counseling from a mental health professional has been shown to help many people cope with anxiety. Your doctor can also give you medicines that will help. Some of the complementary and alternative medicine choices for pain may work for your anxiety as well. Art therapy and music therapy have also helped people cope.

Fatigue

Fatigue is more than feeling tired. Fatigue is exhaustion—not being able to do even the small things you used to do. A number of things can cause fatigue. Besides cancer and its treatment, they include anxiety, stress, and changes in your diet or sleeping patterns. If you are having some of these problems, you might want to take some of these steps:

- Tell your health care team at your next visit. Some medicines can help with fatigue.
- Ask about your nutrition needs.
- Plan your daily activities. Do only what you really must do.
- Hand over tasks to others who are willing to help you.
- Include short periods of rest and relaxation every day.
- Take naps (no longer than 15–30 minutes).
- Ask others for help, especially when you are feeling fatigued.
- Do light exercises that are practical for you.

Nausea and Vomiting

Nausea and vomiting may be a problem for cancer patients. Both can make you feel very tired. They can also make it hard to get treatments or to care for yourself. If you feel sick to your stomach or are throwing up, there are many drugs to help you. Ask your health care team which medicines might work best for your nausea and vomiting.

Here are some tips you may want to try:

- Make small changes in your diet. Eat small amounts 5–6 times a day.

- Avoid foods that are sweet, fatty, salty, spicy, or have strong smells. These may make nausea and vomiting worse.

- Drink as much liquid as possible. You'll want to keep your body from getting dried out (dehydrated). Water, broth, juices, clear soft drinks, ice cream, and watermelon are good choices.

- Choose cool foods, which may help more than hot ones.

- Try acupuncture.

Constipation

Constipation is a problem in which stool becomes hard, dry, and difficult to pass, and bowel movements do not happen very often. Other symptoms may include painful bowel movements, and feeling bloated, uncomfortable, and sluggish. Chemotherapy, as well as other medicines (especially those used for pain), can cause constipation. It can also happen when people become less active and spend more time sitting or lying down.

Here are some ways to help manage constipation:

- Drink plenty of fluids each day. Many people find that drinking warm or hot fluids helps with bowel movements.

- Be active. You can be active by walking, doing water aerobics, or yoga. If you cannot walk, talk with your doctor or nurse about ways you can be active, such as doing exercises in bed or a chair.

- Ask your doctor, nurse, or dietitian if you should eat more fiber. He or she may suggest you eat bran, whole wheat bread and cereal, raw or cooked vegetables, fresh and dried fruit, nuts, and popcorn and other high-fiber foods.

- Let your doctor or nurse know if you are in pain or discomfort from not having a bowel movement. He or she may suggest you use an enema or take a laxative or stool softener. Check with your doctor or nurse before using any of these.

- Ask your doctor about giving you laxatives when you start to take pain medications. Taking a stool softener at the same time you start taking pain drugs may prevent the problem.

Loss of Appetite and Body Changes

Eating and appetite changes are common in the later stages of cancer. As your cancer progresses, your appetite may become poor.

On the other hand, you may be eating enough, but your body can't absorb the nutrients. This can cause you to lose weight, fat, and muscle.

Nutrition goals may become less important at this time. Even if your family members think you should have food, let your body be the judge. The goal should not be weight gain or improving your eating but rather comfort and symptom relief.

Your nurse, dietitian, and other members of your health care team can help. They can help you decide on changes to your diet that may be needed to keep you as healthy as possible. There are also new drugs to improve appetite and get rid of nausea. Ask your health care team about them.

Sleep Problems

Illness, pain, drugs, being in the hospital, and stress can cause sleep problems. Sleep problems may include having trouble falling asleep, sleeping only in short amounts of time, waking up in the middle of the night, or having trouble getting back to sleep. To help with your sleep problem, you may want to try some of these suggestions:

- Reduce noise, dim the lights, make the room warmer or cooler, and use pillows to support your body.

- Dress in soft, loose clothing.

- Go to the bathroom before bed.

- Eat a high-protein snack 2 hours before bedtime (such as peanut butter, cheese, nuts, or some sliced chicken or turkey).

- Avoid caffeine (coffee, teas, colas, hot cocoa).

- Keep regular sleep hours (avoid naps longer than 15–30 minutes).

- Talk with your health care team about drugs to help you sleep. These may give relief on a short-term basis.

Confusion

You may start noticing signs that you feel confused. This can occur in some people with advanced stage cancer. It can also be caused by some medicines. Confusion may begin suddenly or come and go during the day. Possible signs include the following:

- Sudden changes in feelings (such as feeling calm then suddenly becoming angry).

- Having trouble paying attention or concentrating (such as feeling easily distracted, having trouble answering questions, or finding it harder to do tasks that involve logic, such as math problems).

- Memory and awareness problems (such as forgetting where you are and what day it is or forgetting recent events).

If you notice these signs, talk to your health care team to try to find out the cause. Meanwhile, try one or more of the following to help relieve confusion:

- Go to a quiet, well-lit room with familiar objects.

- Reduce noise.

- Have family or loved ones nearby.

- Put a clock or calendar where it can be seen.

- Limit changes in caregivers.

- Ask your health care team about drugs that may help.

Section 86.3

Mental and Emotional Issues Related to Advanced Cancer

Excerpted from "Coping with Advanced Cancer,"
National Cancer Institute, September 20, 2005.

Coping with Your Feelings

You've probably felt a range of feelings during your cancer experience. You may have had these feelings at other times in your life, too, but they may be more intense now.

There is no right or wrong way to feel. And there is no right or wrong way to react to your feelings. Do what is most comfortable and useful for you.

You may relate to all of the feelings below or just a few. You may feel them at different times, with some days being better than others. It may help to know that others have felt the same way that you do.

Hope

You can feel a sense of hope, despite your cancer. But what you hope for changes with time. If you have been told that remission may not be possible, you can hope for other things. These may include comfort, peace, acceptance, even joy. Hoping may give you a sense of purpose. This, in itself, may help you feel better.

To build a sense of hope, set goals to look forward to each day. Plan something to get your mind off the cancer. Here are some tips from others with advanced stage cancer:

- Plan your days as you've always done.
- Don't stop doing the things you like to do just because you have cancer.
- Find small things in life to look forward to each day.

You can also set dates and events to look forward to. Don't limit yourself. Look for reasons to hope, while staying aware of what's at hand.

Inner Strength

People with cancer find strength they didn't know they had. You may have felt overwhelmed when you first learned that your doctors couldn't control your cancer. And now you aren't coping as well as you did in the past. But your feelings of helplessness may change. You may find physical and emotional reserves you didn't know you had. Calling on your inner strength can help revive your spirit.

Some people find it helpful to focus on the present instead of the past or future. They start a new daily routine. They accept that it may have to be different from the old routine. Others like to plan ahead and set goals. With places to go and things to do, life stretches out before them. Others focus on the relationships they have with people close to them. Inner strength is different for each person. So draw on the things in your life that are meaningful to you. Look at other sections in this chapter for ways to tap into your inner strength.

Sadness and Depression

It's normal to feel sad. You may have no energy or not want to eat. It's okay to cry or express your sadness in another way. You don't have to be upbeat all the time or pretend to be cheerful in front of others.

Pretending to feel okay when you don't doesn't help you feel better. And it may even create barriers between you and your loved ones. So don't hold it in. Do what feels natural to you.

Depression can happen if sadness or despair seems to take over your life. Some of the signs below are normal during a time like this. Talk to your doctor if they last for more than two weeks. Some symptoms could be due to physical problems. It's important to tell someone on your health care team about them. Here are some common signs of depression:

- Feeling helpless or hopeless, or that life has no meaning
- Having no interest in family, friends, hobbies, or things you used to enjoy
- Losing your appetite
- Feeling short-tempered and grouchy
- Not being able to get certain thoughts out of your mind
- Crying for long periods of time or many times each day
- Thinking about hurting or killing yourself
- Feeling "wired," having racing thoughts or panic attacks

959

- Having sleep problems, such as not being able to sleep, having nightmares, or sleeping too much

Your doctor can treat depression with medicine. He or she also may suggest that you talk about your feelings. You can do this with a psychologist or counselor. Or you may want to join a support group.

Grief

We all cope with loss or the threat of loss in different ways. You may feel sadness, loneliness, anger, fear, and guilt. Or you may find the way you think changes from time to time. For example, you may get easily confused or feel lost. Or your thoughts may repeat themselves over and over again. You may also find yourself low in energy. You may not want to do things or see people. These are all normal reactions to grief.

What you grieve for is as varied as how you think and feel. You may be grieving for the loss of your body as it used to be. You may grieve for the things you used to be able to do. You also may grieve losing what you have left: yourself, your family, your friends, your future.

It's okay to take time for yourself and look inward. It's also okay to surround yourself with people who are close to you. Let your loved ones know if you want to talk. Let them know if you just want to sit quietly with them. There is no right or wrong way to grieve.

Often people who go through major change and loss need extra help. You can talk with a member of your health care team, a member of your faith community, or a mental health professional. You don't have to go through this alone.

Denial

It's hard to accept the news that your cancer has spread or can no longer be controlled. And it's natural to need some time to adjust. But this can become a serious problem if it lasts longer than a few weeks. It can keep you from getting the care you need or talking about your treatment choices. As time passes, try to keep an open mind. Listen to what others around you suggest for your care.

Anger

The feeling of "No, not me!" often changes to "Why me?" or "What's next?" You have a lot to deal with right now. It's normal and healthy to feel angry. You don't have to pretend that everything is okay. You may be mad at your doctor, family members, neighbors, and even yourself. Some people get angry with God and question their faith.

At first, anger can help by moving you to take action. You may decide to learn more about different treatment options. Or you may become more involved in the care you are getting. But anger doesn't help if you hold it in too long or take it out on others. Often the people closest to us are the ones who have to deal with our anger, whether we want that or not.

It may help to figure out why you are angry. This isn't always easy. Sometimes anger comes from feelings that are hard to show, such as fear, panic, worry, or helplessness. But being open and dealing with your anger may help you let go of it. Anger is also a form of energy. It may help to express this energy through exercise or physical activity, art, or even just hitting the bed with a pillow.

Stress

Everyone has stress, but most likely you're having a lot more now. After all, you're dealing with many changes. Sometimes, you may not even notice that you're stressed. But your family and friends may see a change.

Anything that helps you feel calm or relaxed may help you. Try to think of things that you enjoy. Some people say it helps to do these things:

- Exercise or take a walk
- Write thoughts and feelings in a journal
- Meditate, pray, or do relaxation exercises
- Talk with someone about your stress
- Do yoga or gentle stretching
- Listen to soothing music
- Express yourself through art

Fear and Worry

Facing the unknown is very hard. At times, you may feel scared of losing control of your life. You may be afraid of becoming dependent on other people. You may be afraid of dying.

If you struggle with these fears, remember that many others have felt the same way. Some people worry about what will happen to their loved ones in the future. Others worry about money. Many people fear being in pain or feeling sick. All these fears are normal.

961

Sometimes patients or family members worry that talking about their fears will make the cancer worse. This is not true. Thinking about getting sicker or dying is not going to make your health worse. But it's good to be hopeful and positive. It's better for your health to express your feelings, rather than hold them in.

Some people say it helps if you:

- Know what to expect. Learn more about your illness and treatment options by asking questions of your healthcare team.

- Update your affairs. If you have not already done so, make sure your will and other legal paperwork are in order. Then you won't have to worry about it.

- Try to work through your feelings. If you can, talk with someone you trust.

If you feel overwhelmed by fear, remember that others have felt this way, too. It's okay to ask for help.

Guilt and Regret

It's normal for people with cancer to wonder if they did anything to add to their situation. They may blame themselves for lifestyle choices. They may feel guilty because treatment didn't work. They may regret ignoring a symptom and waiting too long to go to the doctor. Others worry that they didn't follow the doctor's orders in the right way.

It's important to remember that the treatment failed you. You didn't fail the treatment. We can't know why cancer happens to some people and not others. In any case, feeling guilty won't help; it can even stop you from taking action and getting the treatment you need. So, it's important for you to:

- Try to let go of any mistakes you think you may have made;

- Focus on things worthy of your time and energy;

- Forgive yourself.

You may want to share these feelings with your loved ones. Some people blame themselves for upsetting the people they love. Others worry that they'll be a burden on their families. If you feel this way too, take comfort in this: many family members have said it is an honor and a privilege to care for their loved one. Many consider it a time when they can share experiences and become closer to one another. Others say that caring for someone else makes them take life more seriously and causes them to rethink their priorities.

Maybe you feel that you can't talk openly about these things with your loved ones. If so, counseling or a support group may be an option for you. Let your health care team know if you would like to talk with someone.

Loneliness

You may feel alone, even if you have lots of people around you who care. You may feel that no one really understands what you're going through. And as the cancer progresses, you may see family, friends, or coworkers less often. You may find yourself alone more than you would like. Some people may even distance themselves from you because they have a hard time coping with your cancer. This can make you feel really alone.

Although some days may be harder than others, remember that you aren't alone. Keep doing the things you've always done the best you can. If you want to, tell people that you don't want to be alone. Let them know that you welcome their visits.

More than likely, your loved ones are feeling many of the same things you are. They, too, may feel cut off from you if they can't talk with you. You may also want to try joining a support group. There you can talk with others who share your feelings.

Finding Humor

Laughter can help you relax. Even a smile can fight off stressful thoughts. Of course, you may not always feel like laughing, but other people have found these ideas can help:

- Enjoy funny things children and pets do.

- Watch funny movies or TV shows.

- Read a joke book or look at jokes on the internet. If you don't own a computer, use one at your local library. Or ask a friend to print some for you.

- Listen to comedy tapes.

- Read the comics in the newspaper or the cartoons and quotes in magazines.

- Look in the humor section in the library or book store.

Getting Support

Your feelings will come and go, just as they always have in your life. It helps to have some strategies to deal with them.

First, know that you aren't alone. Many people have been in your situation. Some choose to confide in friends and family members. Others do better when they join a support group. It helps them to talk with others who are facing the same challenges. You may prefer to join an online support group, so you can chat with people from your home.

If support groups don't appeal to you, there are many experts who are trained to work in cancer care. These include oncology social workers, health psychologists, or counselors.

Many people also find faith as their source of support. They may seek comfort from the different members of their faith community. Or they may find that talking to a leader in their religious or spiritual community can be helpful. If you need help finding faith-based support, many hospitals have a staff chaplain who can give support to people of all faiths and religions. Your health care team may also be able to tell you about faith-based organizations in the area.

Ways You Can Cope

You may be able to keep doing many of your regular activities, even though some may be harder to do. Just remember to save your strength for the things you really want to do. Don't plan too many events for one day. Also, try to stagger things throughout the day.

Section 86.4

Directing Your Personal Affairs: Information for Patients with Advanced Cancer

Excerpted from "Coping with Advanced Cancer,"
National Cancer Institute, September 30, 2005.

Advance Planning

This section outlines some things you can do to ensure your wishes are understood. This can help relieve the burden on your loved ones later.

Advance Directives

It's important to start talking about your wishes with the people who matter most to you. There may come a time when you can't tell your health care team what you need. Some people prefer to let their doctor or their family members make decisions for them. But often people with cancer feel better once they have made their desires known.

Advance directives are legal papers that tell your loved ones and doctors what to do if you can't tell them yourself. The papers let you decide ahead of time how you want to be treated. They may include a living will and a durable power of attorney for health care. Think about giving someone you trust the right to make medical decisions for you. This is one of the most important things you can do.

A living will lets people know what kind of medical care you want if you are terminally ill (dying). It states in writing your wishes about being kept alive by artificial means or extreme measures (such as a breathing machine or feeding tube). Some states allow you to give other instructions as well.

A durable power of attorney for health care names a person to make medical decisions for you when you can't make them yourself. (In some places, you can appoint this person to make decisions when you no longer want to.) This person is called a health care proxy.

965

Choose a person you can trust to carry out your decisions and follow your preferences. Be sure to discuss this in-depth with the person you choose. They need to know they could be called upon. They should understand your wishes and any religious concerns you have.

Setting up an advance directive is not the same as giving up. Making decisions now keeps you in control. You are making your wishes known for all to follow. This can help you worry less about the future and live each day to the fullest.

It's hard to talk about these issues. But it often comforts family members to know what you want. And it saves them having to bring up the subject themselves. You may also gain peace of mind. You are making hard choices for yourself instead of leaving them to your loved ones.

Make copies of your advance directives. Give them to your family members, your health care team, and your hospital medical records department. This will ensure that everyone knows your decisions.

Other Legal Papers

Here are some other legal papers that are not part of the advance directives:

- A will divides your property among your heirs.

- A trust is when a person you appoint oversees, invests, or pays out money to those named in the trust.

- Legal power of attorney—you appoint a person to make financial decisions for you when you can't make them yourself.

Following State Laws

You do not always need a lawyer present to fill out these documents. But you may need a notary public. Each state has its own laws concerning living wills and durable powers of attorney. These laws can vary in important details. In some states, a living will or durable power of attorney signed in another state isn't legal. Talk with your lawyer or social worker to get more details. Or look at your state's government website.

Planning for Your Family

Careful planning reduces the financial, legal, and emotional burden your family and friends will face after you're gone. For many people, it's hard bringing up these subjects. But talking about them now can avoid problems later.

Maybe you don't feel comfortable bringing up the subject with loved ones. Or maybe your family simply doesn't talk about these things. In either case, seek help from a member of your health care team. They may be able to help your family understand.

- **Clearing up insurance issues:** Contact your health insurance company if you decide to try a new treatment or go into hospice. Most insurance plans cover hospice. They also cover brief home visits from a nurse or a home health aide several times a week. But it's wise to ask in advance. This may prevent payment problems later.

- **Putting your affairs in order:** You can help your family by organizing records, insurance policies, documents, and instructions. You may want to call your bank to make sure you have taken all the right steps in doing these things.

- **Making funeral arrangements:** You may want to help your family plan a funeral or memorial service that has your personal touch. Some people plan services that are celebrations. Talk with your family about how you want others to remember you.

A Checklist for Organizing Your Affairs

- If you can't physically gather important papers, make a list of where your family can find them.

- Keep your papers in a fireproof box or with your lawyer.

- If you keep your important papers in a safety deposit box, make sure that a family member or friend has access to the box.

- Although original documents are needed for legal purposes, give family members photocopies.

Personal Affairs Checklist

You can help family members deal with your personal affairs after you're gone by reviewing this checklist with them. You may wish to write it down. This will help them cope with your death and find comfort in knowing your needs and wishes were met. Try to keep it updated and in a safe place. Make sure that only those you trust have access to it.

Include a list of contact information and what needs to be done for each of the following:

- Banks, savings and loans
- Life insurance company
- Health insurance company
- Disability insurance company
- Homeowners' or renters' insurance company
- Burial insurance company
- Unions and fraternal organizations
- Attorney
- Accountant
- Executor of the estate
- Internal Revenue Service
- Social Security office
- Pension or retirement plans
- Department of Veterans Affairs
- Investment companies
- Mortgage companies
- Credit card companies
- All other lenders
- Employer
- Faith or spiritual leader/organization
- Safety deposit box keys and box location
- Safe, lock combinations
- Location of other important items (such as jewelry)

Talking with Special People

Your loved ones may need time to adjust to the new stage of your illness. They need to come to terms with their own feelings. These may include confusion, shock, helplessness, or anger. Let them know that they can offer comfort just by being themselves and by being at ease with you. Ask them to listen when you need it, rather than try to solve every problem.

Knowing that people cope with bad news in their own way will help you and your loved ones deal with their emotions. Many people are reassured and comforted by sharing feelings and taking the time to say what they need to.

Bear in mind that not everyone can handle the thought that they might lose you. Or some people may not know what to say or do for you. As a result, relationships may change. This isn't because of you, but because others have trouble coping with their own painful feelings.

If you can, remind them that you are still the same person you always were. Let them know if it's all right to ask questions or tell you how they feel. Sometimes just reminding them to be there for you is enough. But it's also okay if you don't feel comfortable talking about it either. Sometimes certain topics are hard to talk about with others. If this is the case, you may want to talk by yourself with a member of your medical team or a trained counselor. You also may want to attend a support group where people meet to share common concerns.

Some families have trouble expressing their needs to each other. Other families simply do not get along with each other. If you don't feel comfortable talking with family members, ask a member of your health care team to help. You could also ask a social worker or other professional to hold a family meeting. This may help family members feel safer to express their feelings openly. It can also be a time for you and your family to meet with your team to problem-solve and set goals.

It can be very hard to talk about these things. But studies show that cancer care goes more smoothly when everyone stays open and talks about the issues.

Often, talking with the people closest to you is harder than talking with anyone else. Here's some advice on talking with loved ones during tough times.

Spouses and Partners

Some relationships grow stronger during cancer treatment, but others are weakened. It's very common for patients and their partners to feel more stress than usual as a couple. There is often stress about these types of issues:

- Knowing how to give and get support
- Coping with new feelings that have come up
- Figuring out how to communicate

- Having money problems
- Making decisions
- Changing roles
- Having changes in social life
- Coping with changes in daily routines

Some people feel more comfortable talking about serious issues than others. Only you and your loved one know how you communicate. Here are some things to think about:

- **Talk things over:** This may be hard for you or your partner. If so, ask a counselor or social worker to talk to both of you together.

- **Be realistic about demands:** Your spouse or partner may feel guilty about your illness. They may feel guilty about any time spent away from you. They also may be under stress due to changing family roles.

- **Spend some time apart:** Your partner needs time to address his or her own needs. If these needs are neglected, your loved one may have less energy and support to give. Remember, you didn't spend 24 hours a day together before you got sick.

- **Know that it's normal for body changes and emotional concerns to affect your sex life:** Talking openly and honestly is key. But if you can't talk about these issues, you might want to talk with a professional. Don't be afraid to seek help or advice if you need it.

Small Children

Keeping your children's and grandchildren's trust is still very important at this time. Children can sense when things are wrong. It's best to be as open as you can about your cancer. They may worry that they did something to cause the cancer. They may be afraid that no one will take care of them. They may also feel that you are not spending as much time with them as you used to. Although you can't protect them from what they may feel, you can prepare them.

Some children become very clingy. Others get into trouble in school or at home. Let the teacher or guidance counselor know what is going on. And with your kids, it helps to keep the lines of communication open. Try to follow these suggestions:

- Be honest. Tell them you are sick and that the doctors are working to help you feel comfortable.

- Let them know that nothing they did or said caused the cancer. And make sure they know that they can't catch it from others.

- Tell them you love them.

- Tell them it's okay to be upset, angry, or scared. Encourage them to talk.

- Be clear and simple, since children do not have the focus of adults. Use words they can understand.

- Let them know that they will be taken care of and loved.

- Let them know that it's okay to ask questions. Tell them you will answer them as honestly as you can. In fact, children who aren't told the truth about an illness can become even more scared. They often use their imagination and fears to explain the changes around them.

Teenagers

Many of the things listed above also apply to teenagers. They need to hear the truth about an illness. This helps keep them from feeling guilt and stress. But be aware that they may try to avoid the subject. They may become angry, act out, or get into trouble as a way of coping. Others simply withdraw. Try to:

- Give teenagers the space they need. This is especially important if you rely on them more than before to help with family needs.

- Give them time to deal with their feelings, alone or with friends.

- Let your teenager know that they should still go to school and take part in sports and other fun activities.

If you have trouble explaining your illness, you might want to ask for help. Try asking a close friend, relative, or health care provider for advice. You could also go to a trusted coach, teacher, or youth minister. Your social worker or doctor can help you find a good counselor.

Adult Children

Your relationship with your adult children may change now that you have advanced cancer. You may have to rely on them more for different needs. It may be hard for you to ask for support. After all, you may be used to giving support rather than getting it. Or it may be hard for other reasons; perhaps your relationship with them has been distant.

Adult children have their concerns, too. They may become fearful of their own mortality. They may feel guilty because they feel that they can't meet the many demands on their lives as parents, children, and employees.

As your illness progresses, it helps to:

- Share decision-making with your children.

- Involve them in issues that are important to you. These may include treatment choices, plans for the future, or types of activities you want to continue.

- Reaching out to your children and openly sharing your feelings, goals, and wishes may help them cope with your disease. It may also help lessen fears and conflict between siblings when other important decisions need to be made.

Looking for Meaning

Many people who have advanced cancer look more deeply for meaning in their lives. They want to understand their purpose and their legacy. They want to examine the things they have gone through in life. Some look for a sense of peace or a bond with others. Some seek to forgive themselves or others for past actions. Some look for answers and strength through religion or spirituality.

Being spiritual can mean different things to different people. It can be a very personal issue. Everyone has their own beliefs about the meaning of life. Some people find it through religion or faith. Some people find it by teaching, or through volunteer work. Others find it in different ways. Having cancer may cause you to think about what you believe. You may think about God, an afterlife, about the connections made between living things. This can bring a sense of peace, a lot of questions, or both.

Like some people, you may also find that cancer changes your values. Having the disease may help you learn what is most important to you. The things you own and your daily duties may seem less important. You may decide to spend more time with loved ones or helping others. You may want to do more things in the outdoors, or learn something new.

You may have already given a lot of thought to these issues. Still, you might find comfort by exploring more deeply what is meaningful to you. You could do this with someone close to you, a member of your faith community, or a mental health professional.

Or you may just want to take time for yourself. You may want to reflect on your experiences and relationships. Writing in a journal or reading also helps some people find comfort and meaning. Many people find that prayer, meditation, or talking with others has helped them cope and explore their lives.

Celebrating Your Life

Having advanced cancer often gives people a chance to look back on life and all they have done. They like to look at the different roles they have played throughout life. They think about what something meant at the time, and what it means now. Some gather things that have meaning to them to give to their loved ones. Others share memories or projects with loved ones.

Doing these things is often called "making a legacy" for yourself. It can be whatever you want. Don't limit yourself! And you can do these things alone or with others close to you. Here are some examples of ways people have celebrated their lives:

- Making a video of special memories
- Reviewing or arranging family photo albums
- Charting or writing down your family's history or family tree
- Keeping a daily journal of your feelings and experiences
- Making a scrapbook
- Writing notes or letters to loved ones and children
- Reading or writing poetry
- Creating artwork, knitting, or making jewelry
- Giving meaningful objects or mementos to loved ones
- Writing down or recording funny or meaningful stories from your past
- Planting a garden
- Making a tape or CD of favorite songs
- Gathering favorite recipes into a cookbook

You can do whatever you want that brings joy and meaning to you. Some people with cancer also make what is called an "ethical will." It's not a legal paper. It's something you write yourself to share with your loved ones. Many ethical wills contain the person's thoughts on his or her values, memories, and hopes. They may also talk about the lessons learned in life or other things that are meaningful. It can say anything you want, in any way you want.

Closing Thoughts

Living with advanced stage cancer may bring many challenges and hardships. But it can also be a time of fulfillment and joy.

As you think about the issues raised in this chapter, keep in mind that survival statistics are just numbers. The numbers that really mean the most for any of us are quite different. They measure the good days, the comfortable nights, and the hours of happiness and joy. Keep living your life the best that you can and in the fullest way possible.

Chapter 87

When Someone You Love Has Advanced Cancer

Terms Used: This chapter uses the terms "loved one" and "patient" throughout to describe the person you are caring for. In addition, for ease of reading, we alternate using the pronouns "he" and "she" when referring to the person with cancer.

Getting Support

You may be faced with new challenges and concerns now that your loved one has advanced cancer. If the illness has been going on for a long time, these challenges may wear you down even more. Many caregivers say that, looking back, they took on too much themselves. Or they wish they had asked for help sooner in sharing tasks or seeking support. Take an honest look at what you can and can't do. What things are you good at or need to do yourself? What tasks can you give to or share with others? Be willing to let go of things that others can do.

Many people probably want to help but don't know what you need or whether you want help. And as the cancer progresses, you may see changes in the support you get from others:

- People who have helped before may not help now.

- Others who have helped before may want to help in new ways now.

Excerpted from "When Someone You Love Has Advanced Cancer: Support for Caregivers," National Cancer Institute, 2005.

- People who haven't helped before may start helping now.
- Agencies that couldn't help before may offer services now.

Why Getting Help Is Important

Many people don't want support when they need it most. You may pull back from your regular social life and people in general. You may feel that it's just too much work to ask for help. Some caregivers have said that more people helped them in the beginning. But as time went on, they felt abandoned.

Accepting help from other people isn't always easy. When tough things happen, some people tend to pull away. They think, "We can handle this on our own." But things can get harder as your loved one continues to go through treatment. You may need to change your schedule and take on new tasks. Many caregivers have said, "There's just too much on my plate." They feel stretched to the point that they can't do it anymore. As simple as it sounds, it's good to remind others that you still need help.

Remember that getting help for yourself can also help your loved one, as well as other friends and family.

- You may stay healthier.
- Your loved one may feel less guilty about all the things that you're doing.
- Some of your helpers may offer time and skills that you don't have.
- Having a support system is a way of taking care of your family. The idea is to remove some tasks so that you can focus on those that you can do.

Talk with someone you trust, such as a friend, member of your faith community, or counselor. Other people may be able to help you sort out your thoughts and feelings. They may also be able to help you find other ways to get support.

How Others Can Help You

Many people want to help, but they don't know what you need or how to offer help. It's okay for you to take the first step. Ask for what you need and for those things that would help you most. For instance, you may want someone to help you in these areas:

- Help with household chores, including cooking, cleaning, shopping, yard work, and childcare or eldercare
- Talk and share your feelings
- Drive your loved one to appointments
- Pick up a child from school or activities
- Pick up a prescription
- Look up information you need
- Be the contact person and help keep others updated on your loved one

Be Prepared for Some People to Say "No"

Some people may choose not to help. This may hurt your feelings or make you angry. It's especially hard coming from those you expected to help you. You might wonder why someone wouldn't help you. There are a lot of reasons. Here are some common ones:

- Some may be coping with their own problems. Or they may not have enough time.
- Some people are afraid of cancer or may have already had a bad experience with cancer. They don't want to get involved and feel that pain again.
- Some believe it's best to keep a distance when people are struggling.
- Some people may not realize how hard things are for you. Or they may not understand that you need help unless you ask for it directly.
- Some people feel awkward because they don't know how to show they care.

If people choose not to help, you may want to explain your needs to them and be direct about what you are asking. Or you can just let it go. But if the relationship is important, you may want to tell the person how you feel. This can help prevent resentment or stress from building up. These feelings could hurt your relationship in the long run.

Long-Distance Caregiving

It can be really tough to be away from your loved one with cancer. You may feel like you're always a step behind in knowing what's happening with care. Yet even if you live far away, it's possible for you to give support and be a care coordinator.

Caregivers who live more than an hour away often rely on the telephone or e-mail as their link. Try to create a support network of people who live nearby. These should be people who you could call day or night and count on in times of crisis. You may also want them to check in with your loved one from time to time. Ask a local family member or friend to update you daily by e-mail. Or, consider creating a website to share news about your loved one's condition and needs.

Life Planning

It's common to feel sad, angry, or worried about lifestyle changes that happen because of your loved one's cancer. You may also be making major decisions that will affect your job or your finances. Finding ways to cope with these issues can bring some peace of mind.

Handling Money Worries

The financial challenges that people with cancer and their families face are very real. During an illness, you may find it hard to find the time or energy to review your options. Yet it's important to keep your family financially healthy.

For hospital bills, you or your loved one may want to talk with a hospital financial counselor. You may be able to work out a monthly payment plan or even get a reduced rate. You may also want to stay in touch with the insurance company to make sure certain treatment costs are covered.

For information about resources that are available you may want to order the National Cancer Institute (NCI) fact sheet, "Financial Assistance for Cancer Care," at www.cancer.gov (search for the terms "financial assistance"), or call toll-free 800-4-CANCER (800-422-6237) to ask for a free copy.

Coping with Work Issues

One of the greatest sources of strain is trying to balance work demands with providing care and support. The stress of caregiving can affect your work life in many ways, including challenges such as these:

- Having mood swings that leave coworkers confused or reluctant to work with you

- Being distracted or less productive

- Being late or calling in sick because of stress

- Feeling pressure from being the sole provider for your family if your spouse or partner is unable to work

- Feeling pressure to keep working, even though retirement may have been approaching

It's a good idea to check into your company's rules and policies related to a loved one's illness. See if there are any support programs for employees. Many companies have employee assistance programs with work-life counselors for you to talk with. Some companies have eldercare policies or other employee benefit programs that can help support you. Your employer may let you use your paid sick leave or leave without pay.

If your employer doesn't have any policies in place, you could try to arrange something informally. Examples include flex-time, switching shifts with coworkers, adjusting your schedule, or telecommuting as needed.

The Family and Medical Leave Act may apply to your situation. Covered employers must give eligible employees up to 12 work weeks of unpaid leave during a 12-month period to care for an immediate family member with a serious health condition. Visit www.dol.gov/esa/whd/fmla/ for more information.

Talking with Family and Friends

Talking about serious issues is never easy. It's hard to face an uncertain future and the potential death of your loved one. Often people are uncomfortable talking about it, or just don't know what to say. But you will need to talk to your loved one or others about a number of issues. These might include the seriousness of the cancer, preparing for the future, fears of death, or wishes at the end of life.

Some families talk openly about things. Others don't. There is no right or wrong way to communicate. But studies show that families who talk things out feel better about the care they get and the decisions they make.

Talking with Your Loved One Who Has Advanced Cancer

It's likely that you and your loved one are both having the same thoughts and fears about the end of life. It's natural to want to protect each other. But talking about death does not cause someone to die. And keeping things to yourself doesn't make them live longer.

You and your loved one can still have hope for longer life or an unexpected recovery. But it's also a good idea to talk about what's happening and the fact that the future is uncertain. And keeping the truth from each other is not healthy. Avoiding important issues only makes them harder to deal with later. You may find that you both are thinking the same things. Or you may find you're thinking very different things. This makes it all the more important to get them out in the open. Talking over your concerns can be very healing for all involved.

Sometimes the best way to communicate with someone is to just listen. This is one of the main ways of showing that you are there for them. It may be one of the most valuable things you can do. And it's important to be supportive of whatever your loved one wants to say. It's his life and his cancer. He needs to process his thoughts and fears in his own time and his own way. You can always ask whether he is willing to think about the issue and talk another time. He may even prefer to talk to someone else about the topic.

Bringing Up Hard Topics

Bringing up difficult subjects is draining. You may think, for example, that your loved one needs to try a different treatment or see a different doctor. Or she may be worrying about losing independence, being seen as weak, or being a burden to you.

What is important to remember is that your loved one has the right to choose how to live the rest of her life. Although you may have strong opinions about what she should do, the decision is hers to make. Here are some tips on how to bring up hard topics:

- Practice what you'll say in advance.
- Find a quiet time. Ask if it's an okay time to talk.
- Be clear on what your aims are. What do you want as the result?
- Speak from your heart.
- Allow time for your loved one to talk. Listen and try not to interrupt.
- Don't feel the need to settle things after one talk.
- You don't always have to say, "It'll be okay."

Some people won't start a conversation themselves, but may respond if you start first. Also, you can ask other caregivers how they have handled hard topics.

If you continue to have trouble talking about painful issues, ask for help from a mental health professional. One may be able to explore issues that you didn't feel you could yourself. But if your loved one doesn't want to go, you can always make an appointment to go by yourself. You may pick up some ideas for how to bring up these topics. You can also talk about other concerns and feelings that you are dealing with right now.

Talking with Children and Teens

Children as young as 18 months begin to think about and understand the world around them. And if someone close to them has advanced cancer, their world may be changing monthly, weekly, or daily.

Table 87.1: Words to Try

When You Think You Want to Say:	Try This Instead:
Dad, you are going to be just fine.	Dad, are there some things that worry you?
Don't talk like that! You can beat this!	It must be hard to come to terms with all this.
I can't see how anyone can help.	We will be there for you always.
I just can't talk about this.	I am feeling a little overwhelmed right now. Can we take this up later tonight?
What do the doctors know? You might live forever.	Do you think the doctors are right? How does it seem to you?
Please don't give up. I need you here.	I need you here. I will miss you terribly. But we will get through somehow.
There has to be something more to do.	Let's be sure to get the best of medical treatments, but let's be together when we have done all we can.
Don't be glum. You'll get well.	It must be hard. Can I just sit with you for a while?

Source: Reprinted from Joanne Lynn, MD and Joan Harrold, MD, *Handbook for Mortals: Guidance for People Facing Serious Illness*, 1999, by permission of Oxford University Press, Inc.

That's why it's important to be honest with them and prepare them each step of the way. Children need to be reassured that they will be taken care of no matter what happens.

Your own daily stresses and fears can affect how you act with your kids. You may be torn between wanting to give time to your kids, and knowing your loved one with cancer also needs your time. That's why it's good to let children know how you are feeling, as well as to find out how they are feeling. And never assume you know what your children are thinking. You don't know how they will react to information, either. Experts say that telling children the truth about the cancer is better than letting them imagine the worst.

Although it's a very hard chapter in a family's life, children can continue to grow and learn during this time. Dealing with cancer honestly and openly can teach them how to handle uncertainty for the rest of their lives. Making the most of the present is an important lesson to learn for everyone.

Understand your children's actions and feelings. Children react to their loved one's cancer in many different ways. They may:

- Be confused, scared, angry, lonely, or overwhelmed;
- Be scared or unsure how to act when they see the treatment's effects on the patient;
- Act clingy or miss all the attention they used to get;
- Feel responsible or guilty;
- Get angry if they're asked to do more chores around the house;
- Get into trouble at school and neglect their homework;
- Have trouble eating, sleeping, keeping up with schoolwork, or relating to friends;
- Be angry that someone else is taking care of them now.

No matter how your children are reacting, it's usually easier to deal with their feelings before other problems appear. If you notice changes, you may want to ask for help from your pediatrician who knows your family already. You could also seek advice from a school counselor or social worker. Or, your child may prefer to talk to someone outside the family, such as a trusted teacher or coach. A pediatrician or social worker may also be able to suggest a mental health professional for your children to talk to.

It is very normal for some children to show signs of regression. They may begin acting younger than their years, resuming behaviors that they had stopped. Or they may lose skills they had mastered recently. This is usually a sign of stress. It's telling you that your children need more attention. It's a way for them to express their feelings and, in their own way, ask for support. Recognize that they are needier right now. Be patient as you work with them to get them back to their normal behavior. But don't hesitate to seek help from a social worker or other professional if you feel you need more advice.

Ask open-ended questions: For some families, talking about serious issues is very hard. As hard as it may be, not talking about it can be worse. Try to ask open-ended questions, instead of "yes" or "no" questions. Here are some things you might want to say. They are fine for children of any age.

- "No matter what happens, you will always be taken care of."

- "Nothing you did caused the cancer. And there is nothing you can do to take it away either."

- "People may act differently around you because they're worried about you or worried about all of us."

- "You can ask me anything anytime."

- "Are you okay talking with me about this? Or would you rather talk to Mrs. Jones at school?"

- "It is okay to be upset, angry, scared, or sad about all this. You may feel lots of feelings throughout this time. You'll probably feel happy sometimes, too. It's okay to feel all those things."

Encourage children to share their feelings and questions: Let children know that they're not alone, and it's normal to have mixed emotions. Help them find ways to talk about their feelings. Young children may be able to show you how they're feeling by playing with dolls or drawing pictures. Other forms of art can help older children express themselves. Keep encouraging them to ask questions throughout caregiving. Keep in mind that young children may ask the same question over and over. This is normal, and you should calmly answer the question each time.

Find bits of time to connect: Come up with new ways to connect. Make a point of tucking them in at bedtime, eating together, talking on the phone or by e-mail. Talk to them while you fold clothes or do the dishes. Have a set time when your children do homework while you do something else in the same room. Or take a walk together. Going to the grocery store can even be "together time." Just five minutes alone with each child without interruptions can make a world of difference.

Talking with teens: Teens may ask very tough questions, or questions for which you don't have answers. They may ask the "what if" questions and what cancer means for the future. As always, keep being honest with them. Even more important, listen to what they have to say. As with adults, sometimes it's the listening that counts, not the words you speak to them.

Older children, especially teenagers, may feel uncomfortable sharing their feelings with you. They may try to ignore or avoid topics. Encourage them to talk with others. Also let them know that it's okay if they don't know what they're feeling right now. Many older children also find comfort in just spending time together, without talking about the situation. Hugs and letting your children know that you understand can help. With teenagers, problems may be less obvious or more complicated than with younger children.

Preparing children for visits: If your children don't live with the person who has cancer, it's helpful to prepare them before they visit. The decision of whether or not to let them visit is up to you, your loved one, and perhaps other family members. However, children should have the choice about whether or not they want to go see the patient. If she is in a hospital or other facility, explain what the area and the room looks like. Tell them who might be there and what they might see. Also explain gently if her physical condition or personality has changed.

For a younger child, you might say something like this:

- "Grandma is very sick. When you see her, she will be in bed. She is a little bit smaller, but all of her is still there. She also doesn't have any hair on her head—kind of like Daddy."

- "Mom may be sleeping while you're there. Or she may be awake but won't talk because she's resting. But she'll know and be happy that you're there. She loves you!"

- "Don't worry if you are visiting Uncle Bill and he says things that don't make sense. Sometimes the medicine he takes makes him do that. If it happens, we can tell his doctor about it to make sure he's okay."

Sometimes children don't want to visit, or can't for other reasons. In that case, there are other ways of showing they care. They can write a letter or do artwork. They can call the patient up or leave messages or songs on an answering machine. Encourage them to show love and support in any way they want.

Talking to children about death: Children deserve to be told the truth about a poor prognosis. Hiding the truth from them only prolongs the grief they will feel. And if you don't talk about it or don't tell the truth about it, you risk your children having difficulty trusting others when they grow up. Also, if you don't talk about it, you can't help your children prepare, nor can you help them cope with what is happening. They will need the time to accept the eventual loss of their loved one.

Children of all ages may wonder about dying, life after death, and what happens to the body. It's important to answer all their questions. If not, they may imagine the worst. Let them know that everything is being done to keep their loved one comfortable. Tell them that you will keep them updated. And let them say goodbye.

Counselors and oncology social workers can suggest ways of handling these questions, too. They may know of programs offered for children. Or they may suggest books, videos, and websites that explore these topics.

Communicating with Your Partner with Cancer

Some couples feel more comfortable talking about serious issues than others. Only you and your partner know how you feel about it.

Some things that cause stress for you and your partner can't be solved right now. Sometimes talking about these things can be helpful. You may want to say up front, "I know we can't solve this today. But I'd like to just talk some about how it's going and how we're feeling."

Topics to explore may include how each person:

- Copes with change and the unknown;
- Feels about being a caregiver or being cared for;
- Handles changing roles in the relationship or home;
- Would like to be connected to one another;

- Sees what issues may be straining the relationship;
- Feels, or would like to feel, cared for and appreciated;
- Feels thankful for the other person.

As your loved one becomes sicker, you may also want to share more practical issues. These may include which decisions you should share together, and which you should make alone. Along with this, you may want to talk about the different tasks you can each handle right now.

Find ways to say thanks: Maybe your partner used to do a lot to keep your family going. And now you're trying to get used to less help. It also may be hard to notice the small things your partner is doing to get through this hard time. There's just too much going on. But when you can, try to look for these things and thank your partner for doing them.

Often it doesn't take much to put a bright spot in someone's day. Bringing your partner a cool drink, giving him a card, or calling to check in can show him that you care. Showing a little gratitude can make both of you feel better.

Find ways to be intimate: You may find that your sex life with your partner is different than it used to be. Many things could be affecting it. However, you can still have an intimate relationship in spite of these issues. Intimacy isn't just physical. It also involves feelings. Here are some ways to keep your intimate relationship:

- Talk about it. Focus on how you can renew your connection.

- Try not to judge. If your partner isn't performing, try not to read meaning into it. Let your partner tell you what he or she needs.

- Protect your time together to reconnect. Plan an hour or so to be together without trying to have sex. For example, you may want to play special music or take a walk. Take it slow.

- Try new touch. Cancer treatment or surgery can change your partner's body. Areas where touch used to feel good may now be numb or painful. For now, you can figure out together what kind of touch feels good, such as holding, hugging, and cuddling.

Communicating with Other Family Members and Friends

Any problems your family may have had before the cancer diagnosis are likely to be more intense now. This is true whether you are caring for a young child, an adult child, a parent, or a spouse. Your caregiver role can often trigger feelings and role changes that affect your family in ways you never expected. And relatives you don't know very well or who live far away may be present more often, which may complicate things.

It's very common for families to argue over a number of things at this time. While everyone may be trying to do what's best for your loved one, some family members may disagree as to what this means. Everyone brings their own set of beliefs and values to the table, which makes these decisions hard. It is often during these times that families ask their health care team to hold a family meeting. Meetings can be used to:

- Have the health care team explain the overall goals for care;
- Let the family state their wishes for care;
- Give everyone an open forum in which to express their feelings;
- Clarify caregiving tasks.

How to Communicate when Support Is Not Helpful

Sometimes, people may be eager to help you because they want to feel useful. At times, this assistance is not helpful. You may not need it yet, or you may simply want to spend time alone with your sick loved one. Other people may offer unwanted advice on parenting, medical care, or any number of other things.

If people offer help that you don't need or want, thank them for their concern. Let them know you'll contact them if you need anything. You can tell them that it always helps to send cards and letters. Or they can pray or send good thoughts.

Caring for Yourself

You may find yourself so busy and concerned about your loved one that you don't pay attention to your own health. But it's very important that you take care of yourself. Taking care of yourself will give you strength to help others. Even though you are putting your loved one's needs first, it's important to:

- Keep up with your own checkups, screenings, and other medical needs.
- Try to remember to take your medicines as prescribed. Ask your doctor to give you extra refills to save trips. Find out if your grocery store or pharmacy delivers.

- Try to eat healthy meals. Eating well will help you keep up your strength. If your loved one is in the hospital or has long doctor's appointments, bring easy-to-prepare food from home.

- Get enough rest. Listening to soft music or doing breathing exercises may help you fall asleep. Short naps can energize you if you aren't getting enough sleep. But talk with your doctor if lack of sleep becomes an ongoing problem.

- Exercise. Walking, swimming, running, or bike riding are only a few ways to get your body moving. Any kind of exercise (including working in the garden, cleaning, mowing, or going up stairs) can help you keep your body healthy. Finding at least 15–30 minutes a day to exercise may make you feel better and help manage your stress.

- Take time to recharge your own body, mind, and spirit. Caring for your own needs, hopes, and desires is important to give you the strength to carry on. Giving yourself an outlet to cope with your thoughts and feelings is important, too. And if you are sick or injured yourself, it's even more important that you take care of yourself. Try to think about what would help give you a lift.

Caring for Your Mind and Spirit

Find comfort: Your mind needs a break from the demands of caregiving. Think about what gives you comfort or helps you relax. Caregivers say that even a few minutes a day without interruptions helps them to cope and focus.

Take 15–30 minutes each day to do something for yourself, no matter how small it is. For example, caregivers often find that they feel less tired and stressed after light exercise. Try to make time for taking a walk, going for a run, riding a bike, or doing gentle stretches.

You may find that it's hard to relax even when you have time for it. Some caregivers find it helpful to do exercises designed to help you relax, such as stretching or yoga. Other relaxing activities include taking deep breaths or just sitting still.

Look for positives: It can be hard finding positive moments when you're busy caregiving. Caregivers say that looking for the good things in life helps them feel better. Each day, try to think about something that you find rewarding about caregiving. You also might take a moment to feel good about anything else from the day that is positive—a nice sunset, a hug, or something funny that you heard or read.

Find acceptance: You're on your own path toward accepting the fact that your loved one may die. Although it may take time, acceptance can bring feelings of peace. You may find that cancer helps you value life more. You may feel that you live each day more fully, even though the future is unknown.

Feel thankful: You may feel thankful that you can be there for your loved one. You may be glad for a chance to do something positive and give to another person in a way you never knew you could. Some caregivers feel that they've been given the chance to build or strengthen a relationship. This doesn't mean that caregiving is easy or stress-free. But finding meaning in caregiving can make it easier to manage.

Connect with other people: Studies show that connecting with people is very important for most caregivers. It's especially helpful when you feel overwhelmed. Sometimes you want to say things that you just can't say to your loved one.

Try to find someone you can really open up to about your feelings or fears. You may find it helpful to talk with someone outside the situation. Some caregivers have an informal network of people to contact. If you're concerned about a caregiving issue, you may want to talk with your loved one's health care team. Knowledge often helps reduce fears.

Let yourself laugh: It's okay to laugh, even if your loved one has advanced cancer. In fact, it's healthy. Laughter releases tension and makes you feel better. You can read funny columns and comics, watch comedy shows, or talk with upbeat friends. Or remember funny things that have happened to you in the past. Keeping your sense of humor is a good coping skill.

Write in a journal: It can be a tricky balance between thinking too much about the cancer and not thinking enough about it. Research shows that writing in a journal can relieve negative thoughts and feelings. It can also help improve your health. You can write about any topic. You might write about your most stressful experiences. Or you may want to express your deepest thoughts and feelings. You can also write about things that make you feel good.

Confront your anger or frustration: You may find that you are getting more and more angry and frustrated as the person you are caring for gets sicker. It may help to try to diffuse these feelings as they happen, rather than hold them in. Ask yourself what's really causing the anger. Are you tired? Frustrated with medical care? Does your loved one seem demanding? If you can, try to let some time pass before bringing up your feelings. It may also help you to express your anger through exercise, art, or even hitting the bed with a pillow.

Let go of your guilt: If you are feeling guilty, here are some things you can do:

- **Let go of mistakes.** You can't be perfect. No one is. The best we can do is learn from our mistakes and move on. Continue to do the best you can. And try not to expect too much from yourself.

- **Put your energy into the things that matter to you.** Focus on the things you feel are worth your time and energy. Let the other things go for now. For example, don't fold the clothes when you're tired. Go ahead and rest instead.

- **Forgive yourself and others.** Chances are good that people are doing what they can. That includes you. Each new moment and new day gives you a chance to try again.

Join a support group: Support groups can meet in person, by phone, or over the internet. They may help you gain new insight into what's happening, give you ideas about how to cope, and help you know that you're not alone.

In a support group, people may talk about their feelings and what they have gone through. They may trade advice with each other and help others who are dealing with the same kinds of issues. Some people like to go and just listen. And others prefer not to join support groups at all. Some people aren't comfortable with this kind of sharing.

If you feel like you would benefit from outside support such as this, but can't get to a group in your area, try a support group on the internet. Some caregivers say websites with support groups have helped them a lot.

Use respite help: Many caregivers say that they wish they had gotten respite help sooner. Some say that they waited out of pride or guilt. Others just didn't think of it earlier.

Respite providers spend time with the patient so you can rest, see friends, run errands, or do whatever you'd like to do. Respite services can also help with the physical demands of caregiving, like lifting your loved one into bed or a chair. If this service sounds useful, you may want to:

- Talk with your loved one about having someone come into your home to help out from time to time. If she seems to resist this request, you may want to ask a friend or family member to help explain why this could help both of you.

- Get referrals from friends or health care professionals. Your local agency on aging should also have suggestions.

- Ask the respite helpers what types of tasks they do.

- You can get respite help from family, friends, neighbors, coworkers, members of your faith community, government agencies, or nonprofit groups. Whatever you do, remember that you haven't failed as a caregiver if you need help and relief.

Finding Meaning

Many caregivers find that the cancer experience causes them to look for meaning in their lives. Taking time to think about your life and your relationship with your loved one may help you feel a sense of closure, accomplishment, and meaning. You may want to share your thoughts with your loved one or others, or you may just want to write them down or tape-record them for yourself.

Here are some questions to ask yourself or your loved one:

- What are the happiest and saddest times we have shared together?

- What are the defining or most important moments of our life together?

- What have we taught each other?

- How has being a caregiver affected my life?

Once you get over the shock and fear, you may want to step back and take a further look at life together. When someone you love has cancer, you may begin to rethink the things that are important to you. Some caregivers and their loved ones may do things together that they had always planned to do. Others may not make a lot of changes. Instead, they enjoy the life they have together much more. Life can become more about the person, not the disease.

Faith and spirituality: For some, meaning can be found in religion. Others look to another kind of higher power. Some caregivers wonder why they have to go through this experience. Others feel that they've been blessed by it. Some caregivers feel both these things.

Being spiritual is very personal and means something different for everyone. As you look at life in new ways, you may find a spiritual path helpful.

Chapter 88

Cardiopulmonary Syndromes in Advanced Cancer

Cardiopulmonary syndromes are heart and lung symptoms, such as dyspnea (shortness of breath), cough, chest pain, irregular heartbeats, and excess fluid around the lungs (pleural effusion) or heart (pericardial effusion). These may be caused by cancer or by other conditions.

Dyspnea and Coughing during Advanced Cancer

Dyspnea is difficult, painful breathing or shortness of breath. Patients may use different words to describe the feeling of breathlessness; terms such as "tightness in the chest" and "suffocating" are sometimes used. The distress caused by dyspnea is different for each patient, from mild discomfort in one patient to severe discomfort in another. Dyspnea is common in patients with advanced cancer, lung cancer, and in the last six weeks of life.

Causes of Dyspnea and Coughing

Many conditions may cause dyspnea and coughing. In cancer patients, causes may include the following:

- A tumor that spreads to the chest cavity, lung, airway, or vein that carries blood through the chest to the heart

Excerpted from PDQ® Cancer Information Summary. National Cancer Institute; Bethesda, MD. Cardiopulmonary Syndromes (PDQ®): Supportive Care - Patient. Updated 11/2005. Available at: http://cancer.gov. Accessed April 30, 2006.

- Blood clots or tumor cells that break loose and block a blood vessel in the lungs

- Pneumonia, an infection of the lung. Anticancer therapy increases a patient's risk of developing infections

- Scarring of the lung by radiation therapy or chemotherapy

- Weakening of the heart by chemotherapy

- Other conditions the patient may have, such as chronic obstructive airway disease, congestive heart failure, other lung or heart diseases, weakened breathing muscles, or malnutrition

- A history of smoking

Diagnosis of Dyspnea and Coughing

A diagnosis of the cause of the patient's dyspnea and coughing is helpful in planning treatment. In addition to a physical exam and history and chest x-ray, diagnostic tests and procedures may include the following:

CT (computed tomography) scan: A procedure that makes a series of detailed pictures of areas inside the body, taken from different angles. The pictures are made by a computer linked to an x-ray machine. A dye may be injected into a vein or swallowed to help the organs or tissues show up more clearly.

Complete blood count: A procedure in which a sample of blood is drawn and checked for the following:

- The number of red blood cells, white blood cells, and platelets

- The amount of hemoglobin (the protein that carries oxygen) in the red blood cells

- The portion of the blood sample made of red blood cells

Oxygen saturation test: A procedure to determine the amount of oxygen being carried by the red blood cells. A lower than normal amount of oxygen may be a sign of lung disease or other medical conditions. One method uses a device clipped to the finger. The device senses the amount of oxygen in the blood flowing through the finger. Another method uses a sample of blood drawn from an artery, usually in the wrist, and tested for the amount of oxygen.

Maximum inspiratory pressure (MIP) test: The MIP is the highest pressure that can be generated while breathing in. The MIP test measures this pressure and the strength of the muscles used to breathe. The patient breathes through a device called a manometer, which measures the pressure and sends the information to a computer.

Managing Dyspnea and Coughing

It may be possible to identify and treat the causes of dyspnea. Treatment may include the following:

- Treatment to shrink or destroy the tumor with radiation therapy, hormone therapy, or chemotherapy. Laser therapy or cauterization may be used to treat tumors inside large airways. Laser therapy uses a narrow beam of intense light as a knife to remove the tumor. Cauterization uses a hot instrument, electric current, or caustic substance to destroy the tumor.

- Stent placement: If a large airway is blocked by a tumor that is pressing on it from the outside, surgery may be done to place a stent (a thin tube) within the airway to keep it open.

- Medications may include: steroid drugs (to reduce the inflammation and swelling of lymph vessels in the lungs); bronchodilators (medicines that open up small airways in the lungs); diuretics and other drugs for heart failure; antibiotics for chest infections (these may be combined with chest physical therapy).

- Procedures to remove fluid that has built up around the lungs or in the abdominal cavity.

- Blood transfusions for anemia

Management of the symptoms of dyspnea may include the following:

Oxygen therapy: Patients who cannot breathe enough oxygen from the air may be given supplemental oxygen to inhale from tanks or cylinders. Devices that concentrate oxygen already in the air may also be prescribed.

Medicines: Pain medicines may reduce physical and mental distress and exhaustion, and improve the patient's quality of life. Other drugs may be used to treat dyspnea that is related to panic disorder or severe anxiety.

Support and counseling: Supportive measures may be effective for some patients. These measures include new breathing techniques, cold air directed across the cheek, meditation, relaxation training, biofeedback, and psychotherapy.

In some patients, chronic (long-term) coughing causes pain, interferes with sleep, and worsens dyspnea and fatigue. Treatments include the following:

• Cough-suppressing medicine

• Medicines that break down mucus

• An inhaled drug for chronic coughing related to lung cancer

Malignant Pleural Effusions

The pleural cavity is the space surrounding each lung in the chest. The pleura is the thin layer of tissue that covers the outer surface of each lung and lines the interior wall of the chest cavity, creating a sac that encloses the pleural cavity. Pleural tissue normally produces a small amount of fluid that helps the lungs move smoothly in the chest while a person is breathing. A pleural effusion is an increased amount of fluid in the pleural cavity, which then presses on the lungs and makes breathing difficult.

Causes of Malignant Pleural Effusions

Pleural effusions may be malignant (caused by cancer) or nonmalignant (caused by a condition that is not cancer). Malignant effusions are a common complication of cancer. Lung cancer, breast cancer, lymphoma, and leukemia cause most malignant effusions. Effusions caused by cancer treatment, such as radiation therapy or chemotherapy, are called paramalignant effusions.

Not all pleural effusions found in cancer patients are malignant. Cancer patients often develop conditions such as congestive heart failure, pneumonia, pulmonary embolism, and malnutrition, and these conditions may cause pleural effusions to occur.

The following symptoms may be caused by malignant pleural effusion: dyspnea, cough, and chest pain.

The management of a malignant pleural effusion is different from the management of a nonmalignant effusion, so an accurate diagnosis is important. In addition to chest x-rays or CT scans, diagnostic tests may include the following:

- **Thoracentesis:** The removal of fluid from the pleural cavity using a needle inserted between the ribs. This procedure may be used to reduce pressure on the lungs and/or to check the fluid under a microscope to see if cancer cells are present.

- **Biopsy:** The removal of cells or tissues so they can be viewed under a microscope to check for signs of cancer. If thoracentesis is not possible, a biopsy may be done during a thoracoscopy, a surgical procedure to look at the organs inside the chest to check for abnormal areas. An incision (cut) is made between two ribs and a thoracoscope (a thin, lighted tube) is inserted into the chest. Samples are then taken for biopsy.

Managing Malignant Pleural Effusions

Malignant pleural effusions often occur in advanced or unresectable cancer or in the last few weeks of life. The goal of treatment is usually palliative, to relieve the symptoms and improve the quality of life. The goals of therapy will depend on a number of factors, including the following:

- The prognosis (chance of recovery)

- The patient's preferences in regard to the risks and benefits of treatment

- The patient's ability to perform activities of daily living

- The type of primary cancer

- The number and type of previous treatments. For example, patients whose cancer has not responded to chemotherapy are unlikely to obtain symptom relief with additional chemotherapy.

Treatment of the symptoms of malignant pleural effusion may include the following:

Thoracentesis: Removal of fluid from the pleural cavity using a needle may help to alleviate severe symptoms in the short-term. A few days after thoracentesis, the effusion will begin to reform. Repeated thoracentesis has risks, however, including bleeding, infection, collapsed lung, fluid in the lungs, and low blood pressure.

Pleurodesis: This is a procedure to close the pleural sac so that fluid cannot collect there. Fluid is first removed by thoracentesis. A drug or chemical that causes the sac to close is then inserted into the space through a chest tube. Chemical agents such as bleomycin or talc may be used.

Surgery: Surgery may be done to implant a shunt (tube) to transfer the fluid from the pleural cavity to the peritoneal (abdominal) cavity, where the fluid can be more easily removed. Another option is pleurectomy, removal of the part of the pleura that lines the chest.

Malignant Pericardial Effusions

Pericardial effusion is an increased amount of fluid inside the pericardium, the thin layer of tissue that forms a sac surrounding the heart. The excess fluid causes pressure on the heart, which prevents it from pumping blood normally. Lymph vessels may also be blocked, and bacterial or viral infections often develop. If fluid builds up very quickly, a condition called cardiac tamponade may occur, in which the pressure on the heart becomes life-threatening and must be treated promptly.

Causes of Malignant Pericardial Effusions

Pericardial effusions may be malignant or nonmalignant. Malignant pericardial effusions are caused by cancer that begins in the pericardium or the heart muscle, or by cancer that has spread there from the lung, esophagus, thymus, or lymph system. Malignant pericardial effusions are commonly caused by lung cancer in males and breast cancer in females. Nonmalignant causes include infection of the pericardium, heart attack, underactive thyroid gland, lupus, injury, surgery, and AIDS. Infection of the pericardium is a possible side effect of radiation therapy or chemotherapy.

Diagnosis of Malignant Pericardial Effusion

The following symptoms may be caused by malignant pericardial effusions:

- Dyspnea
- Cough
- Chest pain
- Difficulty breathing while lying flat
- Swelling in the upper abdomen

- Hiccups
- Extreme tiredness and weakness

Because pericardial effusions usually occur in advanced cancer or in the last few weeks of life, extensive diagnostic testing may be less important than relief of symptoms. In addition to chest x-rays, the following tests and procedure may be used to diagnose pericardial effusion:

- **Echocardiography:** A procedure in which high-energy sound waves (ultrasound) are bounced off internal tissues or organs of the chest. The echoes form a picture of the heart's position, motion of the walls, and internal parts such as the valves.

- **Electrocardiogram (EKG or ECG):** A recording of the heart's electrical activity to evaluate its rate and rhythm. A number of small pads (electrodes) are placed on the patient's chest, arms, and legs, and are connected by wires to the electrocardiograph machine. Heart activity is then recorded as a line graph on paper. Electrical activity that is faster or slower than normal may be a sign of heart disease or damage.

- **Pericardiocentesis:** The removal of fluid from the pericardium using a needle inserted through the chest wall. The physician may use an echocardiogram to view the movement of the needle inside the chest. This procedure can be used to drain fluid from an effusion and reduce pressure on the heart. To diagnose malignant pericardial effusion, the fluid is examined under a microscope to check for cancer cells. The fluid may also be checked for signs of infection.

Managing Malignant Pericardial Effusions

Large malignant pericardial effusions are managed by draining the fluid, unless the goals of therapy are to use a less invasive approach that may improve quality of life but not help the patient live longer. The goals of therapy depend on a number of factors, including the patient's prognosis; the cost, risks, and invasiveness of treatment; whether treatment will relieve symptoms and improve the patient's quality of life; and whether treatment will shorten the patient's hospital stay. Treatment options include the following:

Pericardiocentesis: In some patients, fluid may again collect in the pericardium after pericardiocentesis. A catheter may be inserted and left in place to allow continued drainage. This procedure may be used for patients with advanced cancer instead of more invasive surgery.

Pericardial sclerosis: A procedure to close the pericardium so fluid cannot collect in the cavity. Fluid is first removed by pericardiocentesis. A drug or chemical that causes the pericardium to close is then injected through a catheter into the pericardial space. Three or more treatments may be needed to completely close the pericardium.

Pericardotomy: A surgical incision is made in the chest and then in the pericardium to insert a drainage tube. This increases the quantity of fluid that can be drained from the pericardium.

Pericardiectomy: Surgery to remove part of the pericardium. This may be done when there are chronic infections of the pericardium or to drain fluid quickly when cardiac tamponade occurs. This surgery is also called pericardial window.

Balloon pericardiostomy: A catheter with a balloon tip is inserted through the chest and into the pericardium. The balloon is then inflated to enlarge the pericardial opening and allow fluid to drain into the pleural cavity. This may be used when an effusion has recurred (come back) after pericardiocentesis or as an alternative to more invasive surgery.

Superior Vena Cava Syndrome

Superior vena cava syndrome (SVCS) is a group of symptoms that occur when the superior vena cava becomes partially blocked.

The right atrium (chamber) of the heart receives blood from two major veins: the superior (upper) vena cava and the inferior (lower) vena cava. The superior vena cava returns blood from the upper body to the heart. The inferior vena cava returns the blood from the lower body to the heart.

The superior vena cava is thin-walled, and the blood is under low pressure. If a tumor forms in the chest or nearby lymph nodes become swollen (as from lymphoma), the superior vena cava can be squeezed. Blood flow slows. Complete blockage of the vein can occur. Sometimes, the other veins can become larger and take over for the superior vena cava if it is blocked, but this takes time. Superior vena cava syndrome (SVCS) is the group of symptoms that occur when this vein is partially blocked.

The location of the blocked area and how fast the blockage occurs affect the symptoms. The symptoms will be more severe if the vein becomes blocked quickly. This is because the other veins do not have time to widen and take over the increased blood flow from the superior vena cava.

The location of the blocked area also affects how severe the symptoms will be:

- If the blockage is above where the superior and inferior vena cava veins join, other veins can become larger over time and take over the increased blood flow. The symptoms may be milder.

- If the blockage occurs below where the superior vena cava and inferior vena cava meet, the blood must be returned to the heart by the veins in the upper abdomen and the inferior vena cava, which require higher pressure. Symptoms may be more severe.

The most common symptoms are problems breathing, coughing, and swollen face, neck, upper body, and arms. Less common symptoms include hoarse voice, chest pain, problems swallowing and/or talking, coughing up blood, swollen veins in the chest or neck, bluish color to the skin, and drooping eyelid.

Diagnosis of Superior Vena Cava Syndrome

Chest x-rays, CT scans, and the following tests may be done to diagnose SVCS and find the location of the blockage:

- **Venography:** A procedure to x-ray veins. A contrast dye is injected into the veins to outline them on the x-rays.

- **MRI (magnetic resonance imaging):** A procedure that uses a magnet, radio waves, and a computer to make a series of detailed pictures of areas inside the body. This procedure is also called nuclear magnetic resonance imaging (NMRI).

- **Ultrasound:** A procedure in which high-energy sound waves (ultrasound) are bounced off internal tissues or organs and make echoes. The echoes form a picture of body tissues called a sonogram.

The type of cancer can affect the type of treatment needed; for this reason, a diagnosis of suspected cancer should be made before treatment of SVCS is begun. Unless the airway is blocked or the brain is swelling, waiting to start treatment while a diagnosis is made usually presents no problem in adults. If lung cancer is suspected, a sputum sample and a biopsy may be taken.

Managing Superior Vena Cava Syndrome

Treatment of SVCS may include the following:

Watchful waiting: Watchful waiting is closely monitoring a patient's condition without giving any treatment unless symptoms appear or change. A patient who has good blood flow through other veins and mild symptoms may not need treatment.

The following may be used to relieve symptoms and keep the patient comfortable:

- Keeping the upper body raised higher than the lower body
- Corticosteroids (drugs that reduce swelling)
- Diuretics (drugs that make excess fluid pass from the body in urine). Patients taking diuretics are closely monitored because these drugs can cause dehydration (loss of too much fluid from the body).

Radiation therapy: If the blockage of the superior vena cava is caused by a tumor that is not sensitive to chemotherapy, radiation therapy may be given. Radiation therapy uses high-energy x-rays or other types of radiation to kill cancer cells. There are two types of radiation therapy. External radiation therapy uses a machine outside the body to send radiation toward the cancer. Internal radiation therapy uses a radioactive substance sealed in needles, seeds, wires, or catheters that are placed directly into or near the cancer.

Chemotherapy: Chemotherapy is the usual treatment for tumors that respond to anticancer drugs, including small cell lung cancer and lymphoma. This treatment would not be changed for patients who have SVCS. Chemotherapy uses drugs to stop the growth of cancer cells, either by killing the cells or by stopping the cells from dividing. When chemotherapy is taken by mouth or injected into a vein or muscle, the drugs enter the bloodstream and can reach cancer cells throughout the body (systemic chemotherapy). When chemotherapy is placed directly into the spinal column, an organ, or a body cavity such as the abdomen, the drugs mainly affect cancer cells in those areas (regional chemotherapy).

Thrombolysis: SVCS may occur when a thrombus (blood clot) forms in a partially blocked vein. Thrombolysis is a method used to break up and remove blood clots. This may done using a drug put directly into the clot, through a catheter, or by a thrombectomy (the use of a device inserted into the vein).

Stent placement: A stent may be used to open up the blocked vein. A stent is a tube-like device that is inserted into the blocked area of a vein to allow blood to pass through. This helps most patients. Patients may also receive an anticoagulant to keep more blood clots from forming.

Surgery: Surgery to bypass (go around) the blocked part of the vein is sometimes used for cancer patients, but is used more often for patients without cancer.

Social Considerations of Superior Vena Cava Syndrome

Superior vena cava syndrome is serious and the symptoms can be upsetting to the patient and family. It is important that patients and family members receive information about the causes of superior vena cava syndrome and how to treat it. This can help relieve anxiety over symptoms such as swelling, trouble swallowing, coughing, and hoarseness.

When a patient has chosen not to receive aggressive treatment because of terminal cancer, palliative treatment can help keep the patient comfortable by relieving symptoms. Patients and family members can be taught how to provide palliative care to relieve symptoms and improve quality of life.

Chapter 89

End-of-Life Care: Questions and Answers

When a patient's health care team determines that the cancer can no longer be controlled, medical testing and cancer treatment often stop. But the patient's care continues. The care focuses on making the patient comfortable. The patient receives medications and treatments to control pain and other symptoms, such as constipation, nausea, and shortness of breath. Some patients remain at home during this time, while others enter a hospital or other facility. Either way, services are available to help patients and their families with the medical, psychological, and spiritual issues surrounding dying. A hospice often provides such services.

The time at the end of life is different for each person. Each individual has unique needs for information and support. The patient's and family's questions and concerns about the end of life should be discussed with the health care team as they arise.

The following information can help answer some of the questions that many patients, their family members, and caregivers have about the end of life.

How long is the patient expected to live?

Patients and their family members often want to know how long a person is expected to live. This is a hard question to answer. Factors such as where the cancer is located and whether the patient has other

"End of Life Care: Questions and Answers," National Cancer Institute, October 30, 2002.

illnesses can affect what will happen. Although doctors may be able to make an estimate based on what they know about the patient, they might be hesitant to do so. Doctors may be concerned about over or under-estimating the patient's life span. They also might be fearful of instilling false hope or destroying a person's hope.

When caring for the patient at home, when should the caregiver call for professional help?

When caring for a patient at home, there may be times when the caregiver needs assistance from the patient's health care team. A caregiver can contact the patient's doctor or nurse for help in any of the following situations:

- The patient is in pain that is not relieved by the prescribed dose of pain medication
- The patient shows discomfort, such as grimacing or moaning
- The patient is having trouble breathing and seems upset
- The patient is unable to urinate or empty the bowels
- The patient has fallen
- The patient is very depressed or talking about committing suicide
- The caregiver has difficulty giving medication to the patient
- The caregiver is overwhelmed by caring for the patient, or is too grieved or afraid to be with the patient
- At any time the caregiver does not know how to handle a situation

What are some ways that caregivers can provide emotional comfort to the patient?

Everyone has different needs, but some emotions are common to most dying patients. These include fear of abandonment and fear of being a burden. They also have concerns about loss of dignity and loss of control. Some ways caregivers can provide comfort are as follows:

- Keep the person company—talk, watch movies, read, or just be with the person.
- Allow the person to express fears and concerns about dying, such as leaving family and friends behind. Be prepared to listen.

- Be willing to reminisce about the person's life.

- Avoid withholding difficult information. Most patients prefer to be included in discussions about issues that concern them.

- Reassure the patient that you will honor advance directives, such as living wills.

- Ask if there is anything you can do.

- Respect the person's need for privacy.

What are the signs that death is approaching? What can the caregiver do to make the patient comfortable?

Certain signs and symptoms can help a caregiver anticipate when death is near. They are described below, along with suggestions for managing them. It is important to remember that not every patient experiences each of the signs and symptoms. In addition, the presence of one or more of these symptoms does not necessarily indicate that the patient is close to death. A member of the patient's health care team can give family members and caregivers more information about what to expect.

Drowsiness, increased sleep, and/or unresponsiveness (caused by changes in the patient's metabolism): The caregiver and family members can plan visits and activities for times when the patient is alert. It is important to speak directly to the patient and talk as if the person can hear, even if there is no response. Most patients are still able to hear after they are no longer able to speak. Patients should not be shaken if they do not respond.

Confusion about time, place, and/or identity of loved ones; restlessness; visions of people and places that are not present; pulling at bed linens or clothing (caused in part by changes in the patient's metabolism). Gently remind the patient of the time, date, and people who are with them. If the patient is agitated, do not attempt to restrain the patient. Be calm and reassuring. Speaking calmly may help to re-orient the patient.

Decreased socialization and withdrawal: This is caused by decreased oxygen to the brain, decreased blood flow, and mental preparation for dying. Speak to the patient directly. Let the patient know you are there for them. The patient may be aware and able to hear, but unable to respond. Professionals advise that giving the patient permission to "let go" can be helpful.

Decreased need for food and fluids, and loss of appetite (caused by the body's need to conserve energy and its decreasing ability to use food and fluids properly): Allow the patient to choose if and when to eat or drink. Ice chips, water, or juice may be refreshing if the patient can swallow. Keep the patient's mouth and lips moist with products such as glycerin swabs and lip balm.

Loss of bladder or bowel control (caused by the relaxing of muscles in the pelvic area): Keep the patient as clean, dry, and comfortable as possible. Place disposable pads on the bed beneath the patient and remove them when they become soiled.

Darkened urine or decreased amount of urine (caused by slowing of kidney function and/or decreased fluid intake): Caregivers can consult a member of the patient's health care team about the need to insert a catheter to avoid blockage. A member of the health care team can teach the caregiver how to take care of the catheter if one is needed.

Skin becomes cool to the touch, particularly the hands and feet; skin may become bluish in color, especially on the underside of the body (caused by decreased circulation to the extremities): Blankets can be used to warm the patient. Although the skin may be cool, patients are usually not aware of feeling cold. Caregivers should avoid warming the patient with electric blankets or heating pads, which can cause burns.

Rattling or gurgling sounds while breathing, which may be loud; breathing that is irregular and shallow; decreased number of breaths per minute; breathing that alternates between rapid and slow (caused by congestion from decreased fluid consumption, a buildup of waste products in the body, and/or a decrease in circulation to the organs): Breathing may be easier if the patient's body is turned to the side and pillows are placed beneath the head and behind the back. Although labored breathing can sound very distressing to the caregiver, gurgling and rattling sounds do not cause discomfort to the patient. An external source of oxygen may benefit some patients. If the patient is able to swallow, ice chips also may help. In addition, a cool mist humidifier may help make the patient's breathing more comfortable.

Turning the head toward a light source (caused by decreasing vision): Leave soft, indirect lights on in the room.

Increased difficulty controlling pain (caused by progression of the disease): It is important to provide pain medications as the patient's doctor has prescribed. The caregiver should contact the doctor if the prescribed dose does not seem adequate. With the help of the health care team, caregivers can also explore methods such as massage and relaxation techniques to help with pain.

Involuntary movements (called myoclonus), changes in heart rate, and loss of reflexes in the legs and arms are additional signs that the end of life is near.

What are the signs that the patient has died?

- There is no breathing or pulse.

- The eyes do not move or blink, and the pupils are dilated (enlarged). The eyelids may be slightly open.

- The jaw is relaxed and the mouth is slightly open.

- The body releases the bowel and bladder contents.

- The patient does not respond to being touched or spoken to.

What needs to be done after the patient has died?

After the patient has passed away, there is no need to hurry with arrangements. Family members and caregivers may wish to sit with the patient, talk, or pray. When the family is ready, the following steps can be taken.

- Place the body on its back with one pillow under the head. If necessary, caregivers or family members may wish to put the patient's dentures or other artificial parts in place.

- If the patient is in a hospice program, follow the guidelines provided by the program. A caregiver or family member can request a hospice nurse to verify the patient's death.

- Contact the appropriate authorities in accordance with local regulations. If the patient has requested not to be resuscitated through a do-not-resuscitate (DNR) order or other mechanism, do not call 911.

- Contact the patient's doctor and funeral home.

- When the patient's family is ready, call other family members, friends, and clergy.

- Provide or obtain emotional support for family members and friends to cope with their loss.

Part Five

Additional Help and Information

Chapter 90

Dictionary of Cancer Terms

acute: Symptoms or signs that begin and worsen quickly; not chronic.

acute leukemia: A rapidly progressing cancer that starts in blood-forming tissue such as the bone marrow, and causes large numbers of white blood cells to be produced and enter the blood stream.

acute lymphocytic leukemia (ALL): A fast-growing type of leukemia (blood cancer) in which too many lymphoblasts (immature white blood cells) are found in the blood and bone marrow. It is also called acute lymphoblastic leukemia.

adenoid cystic cancer: A rare type of cancer that usually begins in the salivary glands.

adenoma: A noncancerous tumor.

adenopathy: Large or swollen lymph glands.

adrenocortical cancer: A rare cancer that forms in the outer layer of tissue of the adrenal gland (a small organ on top of each kidney that makes steroid hormones, adrenaline, and noradrenaline to control heart rate, blood pressure, and other body functions). It is also called adrenocortical carcinoma and cancer of the adrenal cortex.

adult T-cell leukemia/lymphoma (ATLL): An aggressive (fast-growing) type of T-cell non-Hodgkin lymphoma caused by the human

---

Excerpted from "Dictionary of Cancer Terms," National Cancer Institute (www.cancer.gov/dictionary), 2006.

T-cell leukemia virus type 1 (HTLV-1). It is marked by bone and skin lesions, high calcium levels, and enlarged lymph nodes, spleen, and liver.

allogeneic bone marrow transplantation: A procedure in which a person receives stem cells (cells from which all blood cells develop) from a genetically similar, but not identical, donor.

allogeneic stem cell transplantation: A procedure in which a person receives blood-forming stem cells (cells from which all blood cells develop) from a genetically similar, but not identical, donor. This is often a sister or brother, but could be an unrelated donor.

amelanotic melanoma: A type of skin cancer in which the cells do not make melanin. Skin lesions are often irregular and may be pink, red, or have light brown, tan, or gray at the edges.

anal cancer: Cancer that forms in tissues of the anus. The anus is the opening of the rectum (last part of the large intestine) to the outside of the body.

anaplastic thyroid cancer: A rare, aggressive type of thyroid cancer in which the malignant (cancer) cells look very different from normal thyroid cells.

androblastoma: A rare type of ovarian tumor in which the tumor cells secrete a male sex hormone. This may cause virilization (the appearance of male physical characteristics in females). It is also called arrhenoblastoma and Sertoli-Leydig cell tumor of the ovary.

anemia: A condition in which the number of red blood cells is below normal.

anesthetic: A substance that causes loss of feeling or awareness. Local anesthetics cause loss of feeling in a part of the body. General anesthetics put the person to sleep.

angioimmunoblastic T-cell lymphoma: An aggressive (fast-growing) type of T-cell non-Hodgkin lymphoma marked by enlarged lymph nodes and hypergammaglobulinemia (increased antibodies in the blood). Other symptoms may include a skin rash, fever, weight loss, or night sweats.

antioxidant: A substance that protects cells from the damage caused by free radicals (unstable molecules made by the process of oxidation during normal metabolism). Free radicals may play a part in cancer, heart disease, stroke, and other diseases of aging. Antioxidants include beta-carotene, lycopene, vitamins A, C, and E, and other natural and manufactured substances.

aspiration: Removal of fluid or tissue through a needle. Also, the accidental breathing in of food or fluid into the lungs.

astrocytoma: A tumor that begins in the brain or spinal cord in small, star-shaped cells called astrocytes.

B cell: A white blood cell that comes from bone marrow. As part of the immune system, B cells make antibodies and help fight infections. It is also called B lymphocyte.

B lymphocyte: A white blood cell that comes from bone marrow. As part of the immune system, B lymphocytes make antibodies and help fight infections. It is also called B cell.

barium swallow: A series of x-rays of the esophagus. The x-ray pictures are taken after the person drinks a solution that contains barium. The barium coats and outlines the esophagus on the x-ray. It is also called an esophagram and upper GI series.

basal cell carcinoma: A type of skin cancer that arises from the basal cells, small round cells found in the lower part (or base) of the epidermis, the outer layer of the skin.

basal cell nevus syndrome: A genetic condition that causes unusual facial features and disorders of the skin, bones, nervous system, eyes, and endocrine glands. People with this syndrome have a higher risk of basal cell carcinoma. It is also called Gorlin syndrome and nevoid basal cell carcinoma syndrome.

benign: Not cancerous. Benign tumors may grow larger but do not spread to other parts of the body.

bilateral: Affecting both the right and left sides of the body.

biofeedback: A method of learning to voluntarily control certain body functions such as heartbeat, blood pressure, and muscle tension with the help of a special machine. This method can help control pain.

biomedicine: A system in which medical doctors and other health-care professionals (such as nurses, pharmacists, and therapists) treat symptoms and diseases using drugs, radiation, or surgery. It is also called conventional medicine, Western medicine, mainstream medicine, orthodox medicine, and allopathic medicine.

biopsy: The removal of cells or tissues for examination by a pathologist. The pathologist may study the tissue under a microscope or perform other tests on the cells or tissue. When only a sample of tissue is removed, the procedure is called an incisional biopsy. When an entire lump or suspicious area is removed, the procedure is called an excisional biopsy. When a sample of tissue or fluid is removed with a needle, the procedure is called a needle biopsy, core biopsy, or fine-needle aspiration.

bladder cancer: Cancer that forms in tissues of the bladder (the organ that stores urine). Most bladder cancers are transitional cell carcinomas (cancer that forms in cells in the innermost tissue layer of the bladder). Other types include squamous cell carcinoma (cancer that begins in flat cells lining the inside of the bladder) and adenocarcinoma (cancer that begins in cells that make and release mucus and other fluids).

body mass index (BMI): A measure that relates body weight to height. BMI is sometimes used to measure total body fat and whether a person is a healthy weight. Excess body fat is linked to an increased risk of some diseases including heart disease and some cancers.

bone cancer: Primary bone cancer is cancer that forms in cells of the bone. Some types of primary bone cancer are osteosarcoma, Ewing sarcoma, malignant fibrous histiocytoma, and chondrosarcoma. Secondary bone cancer is cancer that spreads to the bone from another part of the body (such as the prostate, breast, or lung).

bone marrow: The soft, sponge-like tissue in the center of most bones. It produces white blood cells, red blood cells, and platelets.

brain tumor: The growth of abnormal cells in the tissues of the brain. Brain tumors can be benign (non-cancerous) or malignant (cancerous).

breast cancer: Cancer that forms in tissues of the breast, usually the ducts (tubes that carry milk to the nipple) and lobules (glands that make milk). It occurs in both men and women, although male breast cancer is rare.

bronchoscope: A thin, tube-like instrument used to examine the inside of the trachea, bronchi (air passages that lead to the lungs), and lungs. A bronchoscope has a light and a lens for viewing, and may have a tool to remove tissue.

Burkitt lymphoma: An aggressive (fast-growing) type of B-cell non-Hodgkin lymphoma that occurs most often in children and young adults. The disease may affect the jaw, central nervous system, bowel, kidneys, ovaries, or other organs. There are three main types of Burkitt lymphoma (sporadic, endemic, and immunodeficiency related). Sporadic Burkitt lymphoma occurs throughout the world, and endemic Burkitt lymphoma occurs in Africa. Immunodeficiency-related Burkitt lymphoma is most often seen in AIDS patients.

C cell: A type of cell in the thyroid. C cells make calcitonin, a hormone that helps control the calcium level in the blood.

cancer of unknown primary origin: A case in which cancer cells are found in the body, but the place where the cells first started growing (the origin or primary site) cannot be determined.

carcinoma: Cancer that begins in the skin or in tissues that line or cover internal organs.

carcinoma in situ: Cancer that involves only cells in the tissue in which it began and that has not spread to nearby tissues.

carcinomatosis: A condition in which cancer is spread widely throughout the body, or, in some cases, to a relatively large region of the body. It is also called carcinosis.

carcinostatic: Pertaining to slowing or stopping the growth of cancer.

central nervous system tumor (CNS tumor): A tumor of the central nervous system (CNS), including brain stem glioma, craniopharyngioma, medulloblastoma, and meningioma.

cervical cancer: Cancer that forms in tissues of the cervix (organ connecting the uterus and vagina). It is usually a slow-growing cancer that may not have symptoms, but can be found with regular Pap smears.

Chamberlain procedure: A procedure in which a tube is inserted into the chest to view the tissues and organs in the area between the lungs and between the breastbone and heart. The tube is inserted through an incision next to the breastbone. This procedure is usually used to get a tissue sample from the lymph nodes on the left side of the chest. It is also called anterior mediastinotomy.

chemoembolization: A procedure in which the blood supply to the tumor is blocked surgically or mechanically and anticancer drugs are administered directly into the tumor. This permits a higher concentration of drug to be in contact with the tumor for a longer period of time.

chemotherapy: Treatment with drugs that kill cancer cells.

chronic: A disease or condition that persists or progresses over a long period of time.

chronic leukemia: A slowly progressing cancer that starts in blood-forming tissues such as the bone marrow, and causes large numbers of white blood cells to be produced and enter the blood stream.

chronic pain: Pain that can range from mild to severe, and persists or progresses over a long period of time.

cleaved: Having to do with the appearance of cells when viewed under a microscope. The nucleus of cleaved cells appears divided or segmented.

clinical trial: A type of research study that tests how well new medical approaches work in people. These studies test new methods of screening, prevention, diagnosis, or treatment of a disease. It is also called a clinical study.

computerized axial tomography scan (CT scan or CAT scan): A series of detailed pictures of areas inside the body, taken from different angles; the pictures are created by a computer linked to an x-ray machine. It is also called computed tomography (CT scan) or computerized tomography.

cytotoxic T cell: A type of white blood cell that can directly destroy specific cells. T cells can be separated from other blood cells, grown in the laboratory, and then given to a patient to destroy tumor cells. Certain cytokines can also be given to a patient to help form cytotoxic T cells in the patient's body.

dose-dense chemotherapy: A chemotherapy treatment plan in which drugs are given with less time between treatments than in a standard chemotherapy treatment plan.

dysplastic nevus: An atypical mole; a mole whose appearance is different from that of a common mole. A dysplastic nevus is generally larger than an ordinary mole and has irregular and indistinct borders. Its color frequently is not uniform and ranges from pink to dark brown; it is usually flat, but parts may be raised above the skin surface.

early-stage breast cancer: Breast cancer that has not spread beyond the breast or the axillary lymph nodes. This includes ductal carcinoma in situ and stage I, stage IIA, stage IIB, and stage IIIA breast cancers.

endocrine cancer: Cancer that occurs in endocrine tissue, the tissue in the body that secretes hormones.

endometrial cancer: Cancer that forms in the tissue lining the uterus. Most endometrial cancers are adenocarcinomas (cancers that begin in cells that make and release mucus and other fluids).

endoscopy: A procedure that uses an endoscope to examine the inside of the body. An endoscope is a thin, tube-like instrument with a light and a lens for viewing. It may also have a tool to remove tissue to be checked under a microscope for signs of disease.

epithelial carcinoma: Cancer that begins in the cells that line an organ.

esophageal cancer: Cancer that forms in tissues lining the esophagus (the muscular tube through which food passes from the throat to the stomach). Two types of esophageal cancer are squamous cell carcinoma (cancer that begins in flat cells lining the esophagus) and adenocarcinoma (cancer that begins in cells that make and release mucus and other fluids).

Ewing sarcoma: A type of bone cancer that usually forms in the middle (shaft) of large bones. It is also called Ewing sarcoma/primitive neuroectodermal tumor (PNET).

external radiation: Radiation therapy that uses a machine to aim high-energy rays at the cancer. It is also called external-beam radiation.

eye cancer: Cancer that forms in tissues of and around the eye. Some of the cancers that may affect the eye include melanoma (a rare cancer that begins in cells that make the pigment melanin in the eye), carcinoma (cancer that begins in tissues that cover structures in the eye), lymphoma (cancer that begins in immune system cells), and retinoblastoma (cancer that begins in the retina and usually occurs in children younger than 5 years).

familial cancer: Cancer that occurs in families more often than would be expected by chance. These cancers often occur at an early age, and may indicate the presence of a gene mutation that increases the risk of cancer. They may also be a sign of shared environmental or lifestyle factors.

gallbladder cancer: Cancer that forms in tissues of the gallbladder. The gallbladder is a pear-shaped organ below the liver that collects and stores bile (a fluid made by the liver to digest fat). Gallbladder cancer begins in the innermost layer of tissue and spreads through the outer layers as it grows.

gamma scanning: A procedure to find areas in the body where cells, such as tumor cells, are dividing rapidly. A small amount of radioactive material is injected into a vein or swallowed, and travels through the bloodstream. A machine called a scanner measures the radioactivity and produces pictures (scans) of internal parts of the body. The pictures can show abnormal changes in the area of the body containing the radioactive material. Examples of gamma scans include PET scans, gallium scans, and bone scans. It is also called radionuclide scanning.

graft: Healthy skin, bone, or other tissue taken from one part of the body and used to replace diseased or injured tissue removed from another part of the body.

gynecologic cancer: Cancer of the female reproductive tract, including the cervix, endometrium, fallopian tubes, ovaries, uterus, and vagina.

hairy cell leukemia: A rare type of leukemia in which abnormal B-lymphocytes (a type of white blood cell) are present in the bone marrow, spleen, and peripheral blood. When viewed under a microscope, these cells appear to be covered with tiny hair-like projections.

head and neck cancer: Cancer that arises in the head or neck region (in the nasal cavity, sinuses, lip, mouth, salivary glands, throat, or larynx).

heart cancer: A rare cancer that develops in tissues of the heart. It is also called cardiac sarcoma.

hematologic malignancy: A cancer of the blood or bone marrow, such as leukemia or lymphoma. It is also called hematologic cancer.

high-risk cancer: Cancer that is likely to recur (come back), or spread.

Hodgkin disease: A cancer of the immune system that is marked by the presence of a type of cell called the Reed Sternberg cell. Symptoms include the painless enlarged lymph nodes, spleen, or other immune tissue. Other symptoms include fever, weight loss, fatigue, or night sweats. It is also called Hodgkin lymphoma.

hysterectomy: Surgery to remove the uterus and, sometimes, the cervix. When the uterus and part, or all, of the cervix are removed, it is called a total hysterectomy. When only the uterus is removed, it is called a partial hysterectomy.

immunity: The condition of being protected against an infectious disease. Immunity can be caused by a vaccine, previous infection with the same agent, or by transfer of immune substances from another person or animal.

in situ cancer: Early cancer that has not spread to neighboring tissue.

in vitro: In the laboratory (outside the body). The opposite of in vivo (in the body).

in vivo: In the body. The opposite of in vitro (outside the body or in the laboratory).

indolent lymphoma: A type of lymphoma that tends to grow and spread slowly, and has few symptoms. It is also called low-grade lymphoma.

infertility: The inability to produce children.

infiltrating ductal carcinoma: The most common type of invasive breast cancer. It starts in the cells that line the milk ducts in the breast, grows outside the ducts, and often spreads to the lymph nodes.

intraocular melanoma: A rare cancer of melanocytes (cells that produce the pigment melanin) found in the eye. It is also called ocular melanoma.

invasive cancer: Cancer that has spread beyond the layer of tissue in which it developed and is growing into surrounding, healthy tissues. It is also called infiltrating cancer.

invasive hydatidiform mole: A type of cancer that grows into the muscular wall of the uterus. It is formed after conception (fertilization of an egg by a sperm). It may spread to other parts of the body, such as the vagina, vulva, and lung. It is also called chorioadenoma destruens.

invasive procedure: A medical procedure that invades (enters) the body, usually by cutting or puncturing the skin or by inserting instruments into the body.

inverted papilloma: A type of tumor in which surface epithelial cells grow downward into the underlying supportive tissue. It may occur in the nose or sinuses or in the urinary tract (bladder, renal pelvis, ureter, urethra). When it occurs in the nose or sinuses, it may cause symptoms similar to those caused by sinusitis, such as nasal congestion. When it occurs in the urinary tract, it may cause blood in the urine.

jaundice: A condition in which the skin and the whites of the eyes become yellow, urine darkens, and the color of stool becomes lighter than normal. Jaundice occurs when the liver is not working properly or when a bile duct is blocked.

Kaposi sarcoma-associated herpesvirus: A type of herpesvirus that may cause Kaposi sarcoma (a rare cancer that can cause skin lesions) and a type of lymphoma (cancer that begins in the lymph system), especially in patients who have a weak immune system. It is also called human herpesvirus 8 (HHV8).

keratoacanthoma: A benign (noncancerous), rapidly growing skin tumor that usually occurs on sun-exposed areas of the skin and that can go away without treatment.

kidney cancer: Cancer that forms in tissues of the kidneys. Kidney cancer includes renal cell carcinoma (cancer that forms in the lining of very small tubes in the kidney that filter the blood and remove waste products) and renal pelvis carcinoma (cancer that forms in the center of the kidney where urine collects). It also includes Wilms tumor, which is a type of kidney cancer that usually develops in children under the age of five.

laryngeal cancer: Cancer that forms in tissues of the larynx (area of the throat that contains the vocal cords and is used for breathing, swallowing, and talking). Most laryngeal cancers are squamous cell carcinomas (cancer that begins in flat cells lining the larynx).

larynx: The area of the throat containing the vocal cords and used for breathing, swallowing, and talking. It is also called the voice box.

laser therapy: The use of an intensely powerful beam of light to kill cancer cells.

leukemia: Cancer that starts in blood-forming tissue such as the bone marrow, and causes large numbers of blood cells to be produced and enter the bloodstream.

leukoplakia: An abnormal patch of white tissue that forms on mucous membranes in the mouth and other areas of the body. It may become cancerous. Tobacco (smoking and chewing) and alcohol may increase the risk of leukoplakia in the mouth.

liver cancer: A disease in which malignant (cancer) cells are found in the tissues of the liver.

local cancer: An invasive malignant cancer confined entirely to the organ where the cancer began.

localized malignant mesothelioma: Cancer is found in the lining of the chest wall and may also be found in the lining of the lung, the lining of the diaphragm (the thin muscle below the lungs and heart that separates the chest from the abdomen), or the lining of the sac that covers the heart on the same side of the chest. It is also called stage I malignant mesothelioma.

locally advanced cancer: Cancer that has spread only to nearby tissues or lymph nodes.

low grade: When referring to cancerous and precancerous growths, a term used to describe cells that look nearly normal under a microscope. These cells are less likely to grow and spread quickly than cells in high-grade cancerous or precancerous growths.

lung cancer: Cancer that forms in tissues of the lung, usually in the cells lining air passages. The two main types are small cell lung cancer and non-small cell lung cancer. These types are diagnosed based on how the cells look under a microscope.

lymphatic system: The tissues and organs that produce, store, and carry white blood cells that fight infections and other diseases. This system includes the bone marrow, spleen, thymus, lymph nodes, and lymphatic vessels (a network of thin tubes that carry lymph and white blood cells). Lymphatic vessels branch, like blood vessels, into all the tissues of the body.

lymphocytic leukemia: A type of cancer in which the bone marrow makes too many lymphocytes (white blood cells).

lymphoma: Cancer that begins in cells of the immune system. There are two basic categories of lymphomas. One kind is Hodgkin lymphoma, which is marked by the presence of a type of cell called the Reed-Sternberg cell. The other category is non-Hodgkin lymphomas, which includes a large, diverse group of cancers of immune system cells. Non-Hodgkin lymphomas can be further divided into cancers that have an indolent (slow-growing) course and those that have an aggressive (fast-growing) course. These subtypes behave and respond to treatment differently. Both Hodgkin and non-Hodgkin lymphomas can occur in children and adults, and prognosis and treatment depend on the stage and the type of cancer.

magnetic resonance imaging (MRI): A procedure in which radio waves and a powerful magnet linked to a computer are used to create detailed pictures of areas inside the body. These pictures can show the difference between normal and diseased tissue. MRI makes better images of organs and soft tissue than other scanning techniques, such as CT or x-ray. MRI is especially useful for imaging the brain, spine, the soft tissue of joints, and the inside of bones. It is also called nuclear magnetic resonance imaging.

malignant: Cancerous. Malignant tumors can invade and destroy nearby tissue and spread to other parts of the body.

medullary breast carcinoma: A rare type of breast cancer that often can be treated successfully. It is marked by lymphocytes (a type of white blood cell) in and around the tumor that can be seen when viewed under a microscope.

medullary thyroid cancer: Cancer that develops in C cells of the thyroid. The C cells make a hormone (calcitonin) that helps maintain a healthy level of calcium in the blood.

menopause: The time of life when a woman's menstrual periods stop. A woman is in menopause when she hasn't had a period for 12 months in a row. It is also called "change of life."

mesonephroma: A rare type of tumor, usually of the female genital tract, in which the inside of the cells looks clear when viewed under a microscope. It is also called clear cell carcinoma and clear cell adenocarcinoma.

metastatic cancer: Cancer that has spread from the place in which it started to other parts of the body.

mutation: Any change in the DNA of a cell. Mutations may be caused by mistakes during cell division, or they may be caused by exposure to DNA-damaging agents in the environment. Mutations can be harmful, beneficial, or have no effect. If they occur in cells that make eggs or sperm, they can be inherited; if mutations occur in other types of cells, they are not inherited. Certain mutations may lead to cancer or other diseases.

nasopharyngeal cancer: Cancer that forms in tissues of the nasopharynx (upper part of the throat behind the nose). Most nasopharyngeal cancers are squamous cell carcinomas (cancer that begins in flat cells lining the nasopharynx).

non-Hodgkin lymphoma (NHL): Any of a large group of cancers of the immune system. NHLs can occur at any age, and are often marked by enlarged lymph nodes, fever, and weight loss. There are many different types of NHL, and they can be divided into aggressive (fast-growing) and indolent (slow-growing) types, and are classified as either B-cell or T-cell NHL. B-cell NHLs include Burkitt lymphoma, diffuse large B-cell lymphoma, follicular lymphoma, immunoblastic large cell lymphoma, precursor B-lymphoblastic lymphoma, and mantle cell lymphoma. T-cell NHLs include mycosis fungoides, anaplastic large cell lymphoma, and precursor T-lymphoblastic lymphoma. Lymphomas related to lymphoproliferative disorders following bone marrow or stem cell transplantation are usually B-cell NHLs. Prognosis and treatment depend on the stage and type of disease.

nuclear magnetic resonance imaging (NMRI): A procedure in which radio waves and a powerful magnet linked to a computer are used to create detailed pictures of areas inside the body. These pictures can show the difference between normal and diseased tissue. NMRI makes better images of organs and soft tissue than other scanning techniques, such as CT or x-ray. NMRI is especially useful for imaging the brain, spine, the soft tissue of joints, and the inside of bones. It is also called magnetic resonance imaging (MRI).

oat cell cancer: An aggressive (fast-growing) cancer that usually forms in tissues of the lung and spreads to other parts of the body. The cancer cells look small and oval-shaped when looked at under a microscope. It is also called small cell lung cancer.

occult primary tumor: Cancer in which the site of the primary (original) tumor cannot be found. Most metastases from occult primary tumors are found in the head and neck.

occult stage non-small cell lung cancer: Cancer cells are found in sputum (mucus coughed up from the lungs), but no tumor can be found in the lung by imaging or bronchoscopy, or the primary tumor is too small to be assessed.

oral cancer: Cancer that forms in tissues of the lip or mouth. This includes the front two thirds of the tongue, the upper and lower gums, the lining inside the cheeks and lips, the bottom of the mouth under the tongue, the bony top of the mouth, and the small area behind the wisdom teeth.

orchiectomy: Surgery to remove one or both testicles. It is also called orchidectomy.

oropharyngeal cancer: Cancer that forms in tissues of the oropharynx (the part of the throat at the back of the mouth, including the soft palate, the base of the tongue, and the tonsils). Most oropharyngeal cancers are squamous cell carcinomas (cancer that begins in flat cells lining the oropharynx).

osteosarcoma: A cancer of the bone that usually affects the large bones of the arm or leg. It occurs most commonly in young people and affects more males than females. It is also called osteogenic sarcoma.

ostomy: An operation to create an opening (a stoma) from an area inside the body to the outside. Colostomy and urostomy are types of ostomies.

ovarian cancer: Cancer that forms in tissues of the ovary. Most ovarian cancers are either ovarian epithelial carcinomas (cancer that begins in the cells on the surface of the ovary) or malignant germ cell tumors (cancer that begins in egg cells).

pancreatic cancer: A disease in which malignant (cancer) cells are found in the tissues of the pancreas. It is also called exocrine cancer.

papillary serous carcinoma: An aggressive cancer that usually affects the uterus/endometrium, peritoneum, or ovary.

papillary thyroid cancer: Cancer that forms in cells in the thyroid and grows in small finger-like shapes. It grows slowly, is more common in women than in men, and often occurs before age 40. It is the most common type of thyroid cancer.

penile cancer: A rare cancer that forms in the penis (the external male reproductive organ). Most penile cancers are squamous cell carcinomas (cancer that begins in flat cells lining the penis).

positron emission tomography scan (PET scan): A procedure in which a small amount of radioactive glucose (sugar) is injected into a vein, and a scanner is used to make detailed, computerized pictures of areas inside the body where the glucose is used. Because cancer cells often use more glucose than normal cells, the pictures can be used to find cancer cells in the body.

pulmonary sulcus tumor: A type of lung cancer that begins in the upper part of a lung and spreads to nearby tissues such as the ribs and vertebrae. Most pulmonary sulcus tumors are non-small cell cancers. It is also called Pancoast tumor.

radiation therapy: The use of high-energy radiation from x-rays, gamma rays, neutrons, and other sources to kill cancer cells and shrink tumors. Radiation may come from a machine outside the body (external-beam radiation therapy), or it may come from radioactive material placed in the body near cancer cells (internal radiation therapy, implant radiation, or brachytherapy). Systemic radiation therapy uses a radioactive substance, such as a radiolabeled monoclonal antibody, that circulates throughout the body. It is also called radiotherapy.

recurrent cancer: Cancer that has returned after a period of time during which the cancer could not be detected. The cancer may come back to the same place as the original (primary) tumor or to another place in the body. It is also called recurrence.

salivary gland cancer: A rare cancer that forms in tissues of a salivary gland (gland in the mouth that makes saliva). Most salivary gland cancers occur in older people.

sarcoma: A cancer of the bone, cartilage, fat, muscle, blood vessels, or other connective or supportive tissue.

skin cancer: Cancer that forms in tissues of the skin. When cancer forms in cells that make pigment, it is called melanoma. When cancer forms in cells that do not make pigment it may begin in basal cells (small, round cells in the base of the outer layer of skin) or squamous cells (flat cells that form the surface of the skin). Both types of skin cancer usually occur in skin that has been exposed to sunlight, such as the skin on the face, neck, hands, and arms.

small intestine cancer: A rare cancer that forms in tissues of the small intestine (the part of the digestive tract between the stomach and the large intestine). The most common type is adenocarcinoma (cancer that begins in cells that make and release mucus and other fluids). Other types of small intestine cancer include sarcoma (cancer that begins in connective or supportive tissue), carcinoid tumor (a slow-growing type of cancer), gastrointestinal stromal tumor (a type of soft tissue sarcoma), and lymphoma (cancer that begins in immune system cells).

squamous cell: Flat cell that looks like a fish scale under a microscope. These cells cover inside and outside surfaces of the body. They are found in the tissues that form the surface of the skin, the lining of the hollow organs of the body (such as the bladder, kidney, and uterus), and the passages of the respiratory and digestive tracts.

stem cell transplantation: A method of replacing immature blood-forming cells that were destroyed by cancer treatment. The stem cells are given to the person after treatment to help the bone marrow recover and continue producing healthy blood cells.

testicular cancer: Cancer that forms in tissues of the testis (one of two egg-shaped glands inside the scrotum that make sperm and male hormones). Testicular cancer usually occurs in young or middle aged men. Two main types of testicular cancer are seminomas (cancers that grow slowly and are sensitive to radiation therapy), and nonseminomas (different cell types that grow more quickly than seminomas).

thyroid cancer: Cancer that forms in the thyroid gland (an organ at the base of the throat that makes hormones that help control heart rate, blood pressure, body temperature, and weight). Four main types of thyroid cancer are papillary, follicular, medullary, and anaplastic thyroid cancer. The four types are based on how the cancer cells look under a microscope.

urethral cancer: A rare cancer that forms in tissues of the urethra (the tube through which urine empties the bladder and leaves the body). Types of urethral cancer include transitional cell carcinoma (cancer that begins in cells that can change shape and stretch without breaking apart), squamous cell carcinoma (cancer that begins in flat cells lining the urethra), and adenocarcinoma (cancer that begins in cells that make and release mucus and other fluids).

uterine cancer: Cancer that forms in tissues of the uterus (small, hollow, pear-shaped organ in a woman's pelvis in which a baby grows). Two types of uterine cancer are endometrial cancer (cancer that begins in cells lining the uterus), and uterine sarcoma (a rare cancer that begins in muscle or other tissues in the uterus).

white blood cell (WBC): Refers to a blood cell that does not contain hemoglobin. White blood cells include lymphocytes, neutrophils, eosinophils, macrophages, and mast cells. These cells are made by bone marrow and help the body fight infection and other diseases.

Chapter 91

Resources for Information about Cancer

General Cancer Information

**American Academy of
Family Physicians**
11400 Tomahawk Creek Parkway
Leawood, KS 66211-2672
Toll-Free: 800-274-2237
Phone: 913-906-6000
Website: http://www.aafp.org
E-mail: fp@aafp.org

American Cancer Society
1599 Clifton Road, NE
Atlanta, GA 30329-4251
Phone: 404-320-3333
Toll-Free: 800-227-2345
Website: http://www.cancer.org

**American College of
Physicians**
190 N Independence Mall West
Philadelphia, PA 19106-1572
Toll-Free: 800-523-1546
Phone: 215-351-2600
Website: http://
www.acponline.org

**American Institute for
Cancer Research**
1759 R Street, NW
Washington, DC 20009
Toll-Free: 800-843-8114
Phone: 202-328-7744
Website: http://www.aicr.org
E-mail: aicrweb@aicr.org

Information in this chapter was compiled from many sources deemed reliable. Inclusion does not constitute endorsement and omission does not imply disapproval. All contact information was updated and verified in October 2006.

Canadian Cancer Society
565 W. 10th Ave.
Vancouver, BC V5Z 4J4
Tel: 604-872-4400
Website: www.bc.cancer.ca
E-mail: inquiries@bc.cancer.ca

Cancer Project
5100 Wisconsin Avenue
Suite 400
Washington, DC 20016
Phone: 202-244-5038
Website: http://
www.CancerProject.org
E-mail: info@CancerProject.org

Cancer Research and Prevention Foundation
1600 Duke Street
Suite 500
Alexandria, VA 22314
Phone: 703-836-4412
Toll-Free: 800-227-2732
Website: http://
www.preventcancer.org
E-mail: info@preventcancer.org

CancerBACUP
3 Bath Place
Rivington Street
London EC2A 3JR
United Kingdom
Phone: 011-44-20-7-696-9003
Fax: 011-44-20-7-696-9002
Website: http://
www.cancerbacup.org.uk

CancerEducation.com
Website: http://
www.cancereducation.com

Cancervive
11636 Chayote Street
Los Angeles, CA 90049
Toll-Free: 800-4-TO-CURE
(486-2873)
Phone: 310-203-9232
Fax: 310-471-4618
Website: www.cancervive.org
E-mail: cancervivr@aol.com

CancerWise
Website: http://
www.cancerwise.org

Cleveland Clinic
9500 Euclid Avenue NA31
Cleveland, OH 44195
Toll-Free: 800-223-2273
Phone: 216-444-2200
TTY: 216-444-0261
Website: http://
www.clevelandclinic.org
E-mail: healthl@ccf.org

Facing Our Risk of Cancer Empowered (FORCE)
16057 Tampa Palms Blvd. W,
PMB #373
Tampa, FL 33647
Toll-Free: 866-824-RISK or
866-824-7475
Phone: 954-255-8732
Website: www.facingourrisk.org
E-mail: info@facingourrisk.org

Intercultural Cancer Council
1720 Dryden, PMB 25
Houston, TX 77030
Phone: 713-798-4617
Website: http://iccnetwork.org
E-mail: info@iccnetwork.org

International Union Against Cancer
62 Route de Frontenex
1205 Geneva
Switzerland
Phone: + 41 22 809 18 11
Website: http://www.uicc.org

Johns Hopkins Cancer Information Center
Website: http://
www.hopkinscancercenter.org

Mayo Foundation for Medical Education and Research
200 First Street SW
Rochester, MN 55905
Website: http://
www.mayoclinic.com
E-mail:
comments@mayoclinic.com

Memorial Sloan-Kettering Cancer Center
1275 York Avenue
New York, NY 10021
Toll-free: 800-525-2225
Phone: 212-639-2000
Website: www.mskcc.org

National Association for Proton Therapy
1301 Highland Drive
Silver Spring, MD 20910
Phone: 301-587-6100
Website: http://
www.proton-therapy.org

National Cancer Institute (NCI)
Public Inquiries Office
Suite 3036A
6116 Executive Boulevard,
MSC8322
Bethesda, MD 20892-8322
Toll-Free: 800-4-CANCER
(800-422-6237)
TTY: 800-332-8615
Website: http://www.cancer.gov

National Women's Health Information Center
8270 Willow Oaks Corporate Dr.
Fairfax, VA 22031
Toll-Free: 800-994-WOMAN
(994-9662)
TTY: 888-220-5446
Website: http://www.4woman.gov

Novartis Oncology
Novartis Pharmaceuticals
Corporation
One Health Plaza
East Hanover, NJ 07936-1080
Toll-Free: 888-669-6682
Website: http://
www.us.novartisoncology.com

OncoLink
Abramson Cancer Center of the
University of Pennsylvania
3400 Spruce Street, 2 Donner
Philadelphia, PA 19104-4283
Fax: 215-349-5445
Website: http://
www.oncolink.com

Oncologychannel.com
Healthcommunities, Inc.
Website: http://
www.oncologychannel.com

University of Texas
M.D. Anderson Cancer Center
1515 Holcombe Blvd.
Houston, TX 77030
Toll-Free: 800-392-1611
Phone: 713-792-6161
Website: http://
www.mdanderson.org

Information about Specific Cancers

To make it easier to find information about cancer in specific sites, the organizations listed in this section are alphabetized by key word.

Bladder Cancer Advocacy
Network
Website: http://www.bcan.org

National **Bladder** Foundation
Website: http://www.bladder.org

Orthopedic Oncology [**Bone
Cancer**]
Website: http://
www.bonecancer.org

American Association of Neurological Surgeons [**Brain Tumor**]
Website: http://
www.neurosurgerytoday.org

American **Brain Tumor**
Association
2720 River Road
Des Plaines, IL 60018
Toll-Free: 800-886-2282
Phone: 847-827-9910
Website: http://www.abta.org
E-mail: info@abta.org

Brain Tumor Society
124 Watertown Street, Suite 3-H
Watertown, MA 02472
Phone: 617-924-9997
Toll-Free: 800-770-8287
Website: http://www.tbts.org
E-mail: info@tbts.org

Children's **Brain Tumor**
Foundation
274 Madison Avenue, Suite 1004
New York, NY 10016
Toll-Free: 866-228-4673
Phone: 212-448-9494
Website: http://www.cbtf.org
E-mail: info@cbtf.org

National **Brain Tumor**
Foundation
22 Battery Street, Suite 612
San Francisco, CA 94111-5520
Phone: 415-834-9970
Toll-Free: 800-934-2873
Website: http://
www.braintumor.org
E-mail: nbtf@braintumor.org

American **Breast Cancer**
Foundation
1220 B East Joppa Road
Suite 332
Baltimore, MD 21286
Toll-Free: 877-539-2543
Phone: 410-825-9388
Fax: 410-825-4395
Website: www.abcf.org
E-mail: contact@abcf.org

BreastCancer.org
Website: www.breastcancer.org

Breast Cancer Action
55 New Montgomery, Suite 323
San Francisco, CA 94105
Toll-Free: 877-278-6722
Phone: 415-243-9301
Fax: 415-243-3996
Website: http://www.bcaction.org
E-mail: info@bcaction.org

Imaginis [**Breast Cancer**]
Website: www.imaginis.com
E-mail: learnmore@imaginis.com

Susan G. Komen **Breast
Cancer** Foundation
5005 LBJ Freeway, Suite 250
Dallas, TX 75244
Phone: 972-855-1600
Toll-Free: 800-462-9273
E-mail: helpline@komen.org
Website: http://
www.breastcancerinfo.com

Rose Kushner **Breast Cancer**
Advisory Center
P.O. Box 757
Malaga, CA 90274
Website: www.rkbcac.org

National **Breast Cancer**
Coalition
1101 17th Street, NW
Suite 1300
Washington, DC 20036
Toll-Free: 800-622-2838
Phone: 202-296-7477
Website: http://
www.stopbreastcancer.org
E-mail:
info@stopbreastcancer.org

Women's Information Network
against **Breast Cancer**
536 S Second Ave., Suite K
Covina, CA 91723-3043
Fax: 626-332-2585
Website: http://
www.healthywomen.org
E-mail: mail@winabc.org

Y-ME National **Breast Cancer**
Organization, Inc.
212 West Van Buren Street,
Suite 1000
Chicago, IL 60607
Phone: 312-986-8338
Toll-Free (English):
800-221-2141
Toll-Free (Spanish):
800-986-9505
E-mail (English):
askyme@y-me.org
E-mail (Spanish)
latino@y-me.org
Website: http://www.y-me.org

Carcinoid Cancer Foundation
333 Mamaroneck Avenue # 492
White Plains, NY 10605
Phone: 888-722-3132
Website: http://www.carcinoid.org

Caring for **Carcinoid** Foundation
One Kendall Square, MPB 180
Cambridge, Ma 02139
Phone: 857-222-5492
Website: http://
www.caringforcarcinoid.org

Net Tumor Advisor [**Carcinoid Tumors**]
Website: http://
www.netumoradvisor.org

Alliance for **Cervical Cancer** Prevention
Website: http://
www.alliance-cxca.org
E-mail: accp@path.org

National **Cervical Cancer** Coalition
7247 Hayvenhurst Avenue, Suite A-7
Van Nuys, CA 91406
Toll-Free: 800-685-5531
Phone: 818-909-3849
Fax: 818-780-8199
Website: http://
www.nccc-online.org
E-mail: info@nccc-online.org

National HPV and **Cervical Cancer** Prevention Resource Center
P.O. Box 13827
Research Triangle Park, NC 27713
Website: http://www.ashastd.org/hpvccrc

Colon Cancer Alliance
1440 Coral Ridge Drive
Suite 386
Coral Springs, FL 33071
Toll-Free: 877-422-2030
Phone: 212-627-7451
Website: http://
www.ccalliance.org
E-mail: info@ccalliance.org

American Gastroenterological Association [**Colorectal Cancer**]
4930 Del Ray Avenue
Bethesda, MD 20814
Phone: 301-654-2055
Fax: 301-654-5920
Website: http://www.gastro.org
E-mail: member@gstro.org

C3: **Colorectal Cancer** Coalition
4301 Connecticut Avenue NW, Suite 404
Washington DC 20008
Phone: 202-244-2906
Website: http://www.c-three.org
E-mail: info@c-three.org

Colorectal Cancer Network
P.O. Box 182
Kensington, MD 20895-0182
Phone: 301-879-1500
Website: http://
www.colorectal-cancer.net
E-mail: ccnetwork @colorectal-cancer.net

Bascom Palmer **Eye** Institute
University of Miami School of
Medicine
900 Northwest 17th Street
Miami, FL 33136
Toll-Free: 800-329-7000
Phone: 305-326-6000
Fax: 305-326-6417
Website: http://
www.eyecancermd.org

Eye Cancer Network
115 East 61st street
New York City, NY 10021
Phone: 212-832-8170
Website: http://
www.eyecancer.com

Gynecologic Cancer Founda-
tion/Women's Cancer Network
230 W. Monroe, Suite 2528
Chicago, IL 60606
Phone: 312-578-1439
Website: http://www.wcn.org
E-mail: info@thegcf.org

International **Gynecologic
Cancer** Society
P.O. Box 6387
Louisville, KY 40206
Phone: 502-891-4460
Fax: 502-891-4461
Website: http://www.igcs.org
E-mail: adminoffice@igcs.org

American Academy of Otolaryn-
gology-**Head and Neck** Surgery
One Prince Street
Alexandria, VA 22314-3357
Phone: 703-836-4444
Website: www.entnet.org
E-mail: webmaster@entnet.org

National Institute of Dental and
Craniofacial Research [**Head
and Neck Cancer**]
One NOHIC Way
Bethesda, MD 20892-3500
Telephone: 301-402-7364
E-mail: nidcrinfo@mail.nih.gov
Website: http://
www.nidcr.nih.gov

American Association of **Kidney**
Patients
3505 E. Frontage Rd., Suite 315
Tampa, FL 33607
Phone: 800-749-2257
Fax: 813-636-8122
Website: http://www.aakp.org
E-mail: info@aakp.org

Kidney Cancer Association
1234 Sherman Avenue
Suite 203
Evanston, IL 60202-1375
Phone: 847-332-1051
Toll-Free: 800-850-9132
Website: http://
www.curekidneycancer.org
E-mail:
office@curekidneycancer.org

National Institute of Diabetes
and Digestive and **Kidney**
Diseases
National Institutes of Health
Building 31, Room 9A06
31 Center Drive, MSC 2560
Bethesda, MD 20892-2560
NIDDK Information Clearing-
house Toll-Free: 800-891-5390
Website: http://www.niddk.nih.gov
E-mail: dkwebmaster@extra
.niddk.nih.gov

National **Kidney** Foundation
30 East 33rd Street
New York, NY 10016
Phone: 212-889-2210
Toll Free: 800-622-9010
Website: http://www.kidney.org

Leukemia and **Lymphoma**
Society
1311 Mamaroneck Avenue
White Plains, NY 10605-5221
Phone: 914-949-5213
Toll-Free: 800-955-4572
Website: http://www.leukemia-lymphoma.org
E-mail: infocenter@leukemia-lymphoma.org

American **Liver** Foundation
75 Maiden Lane, Suite 603
New York, NY 10038
Toll-Free: 800-GO-Liver
(465-4837)
Phone: 212-668-1000
Fax: 212-483-8179
Website: http://www.liverfoundation.org

LiverTumor.org
Website: http://www.livertumor.org

American **Lung** Association
61 Broadway, 6th Floor
New York, NY 10006
Toll-Free: 800-LUNGUSA
(586-4872)
Phone: 213-315-8700
Website: http://www.lungusa.org

Lung Cancer Alliance
888 16th Street, NW, Suite 800
Washington, DC 20006
Phone: 202-463-2080
Toll-Free: 800-298-2436
Website: http://www.lungcanceralliance.org
E-mail: info@lungcanceralliance.org

Lung Cancer Online Foundation
P.O. Box 762
East Setauket, NY 11733
Phone: 631-689-2754
Website: http://www.lungcanceronline.org
E-mail: kparles@lungcanceronline.org

LungCancer.org
Website: http://www.lungcancer.org

Lymphoma Foundation of
America
1100 North Main Street
Ann Arbor, MI 48104
Phone: 734-222-1133
Toll-Free: 800-385-1060
E-mail: LFA@lymphomahelp.org
Website: http://www.lymphomahelp.org

Lymphoma Research
Foundation
8800 Venice Boulevard
Suite 207
Los Angeles, CA 90034
Toll-Free: 800-500-9976
Phone: 310-204-7040
Website: http://
www.lymphoma.org
E-mail for general information:
LRF@lymphoma.org
E-mail for patient services:
helpline@lymphoma.org

American **Melanoma** Foundation
2160 Fletcher Parkway, Suite O
El Cajon, CA 92020
Phone: 619-448-0991
Fax: 619-448-2902
Website: http://
www.melanomafoundation.org
E-mail: sunsmartz@
melanomafoundation.org

Melanoma Education
Foundation
P.O. Box 2023
Peabody, MA 01960
Phone: 978-535-3080
Fax: 978-535-5602
Website: http://
www.skincheck.org
E-mail: mef@skincheck.org

Asbestos Disease Awareness
Organization [**Mesothelioma**]
Website: http://www
.asbestosdiseaseawareness.org

Mesothelioma Applied
Research Foundation
Website: http://www.marf.org

Mesothelioma Information and
Resource Group
Coady Law Firm
205 Portland Street
Boston, MA 02114
Website: http://www.mirg.org

Multiple Myeloma Research
Foundation
383 Main Ave, 5th floor
Norwalk, CT 06851
Phone: 203-972-1250
Website: http://
www.multiplemyeloma.org
E-mail: info@themmrf.org

International **Myeloma**
Foundation (IMF)
12650 Riverside Drive
Suite 206
North Hollywood, CA 91607-3421
Phone: 818-487-7455
Toll-Free: 800-452-2873
E-mail: TheIMF@myeloma.org
Website: http://
www.myeloma.org

Oral Cancer Foundation
3419 Via Lido, Number 205
Newport Beach, CA 92663
Phone: 949-646-8000
Website: http://
www.oralcancerfoundation.org
E-mail:
info@oralcancerfoundation.org

Osteosarcoma Online
Website: http://
iucc.iu.edu/osteosarcoma

National **Ovarian Cancer**
Association
101-145 Front Street East
Toronto, Ontario M5A 1E3
Canada
Toll-Free: 877-413-7970
Phone: 416-962-2700
Fax: 416-962-2701
Website: http://
www.ovariancanada.org
E-mail: noca@ovariancanada.org

National **Ovarian Cancer**
Coalition
500 Northeast Spanish River
Boulevard, Suite 8
Boca Raton, FL 33431
Toll-Free: 888-682-7426
Phone: 561-393-0005
Website: http://www.ovarian.org
E-mail: NOCC@ovarian.org

Ovarian Cancer National
Alliance
910 17th Street, NW, Suite 1190
Washington, DC 20006
Phone: 202-331-1332
Website: http://
www.ovariancancer.org
E-mail: ocna@ovariancancer.org

Ovarian Cancer Research
Fund, Inc.
14 Pennsylvania Plaza
Suite 1400
New York, NY 10122
Toll-Free: 800-873-9569
Phone: 212-268-1002
Fax: 212-947-5652
Website: http://www.ocrf.org
E-mail: info@ocrf.org

Hirshberg Foundation for
Pancreatic Cancer Research
375 Homewood Road
Los Angeles, CA 90049
Phone: 310-472-6310
Fax: 310-471-1020
Website: http://
www.pancreatic.org

Lustgarten Foundation for
Pancreatic Cancer Research
1111 Stewart Avenue
Bethpage, NY 11714
Phone: 516-803-2304
Toll-Free: 866-789-1000
Website: http://
www.lustgartenfoundation.org

Pancreatic Cancer Action
Network (PanCAN)
241 Rosecrans Avenue
Suite 7000
El Segundo, CA 90245
Toll-Free: 877-272-6226
Phone: 310-725-0025
Website: http://www.pancan.org
E-mail: information@pancan.org

Hormone Foundation
[Pituitary Tumor]
8401 Connecticut Avenue
Suit 900
Chevy Chase, MD 20815-5817
Phone: 1-800-Hormone
Website: http://www.hormone.org
E-mail: hormone
@endo-society.org

Pituitary Network Association
Website: http://
www.pituitary.com

American **Prostate** Society
P.O. Box 870
Hanover, MD 21076
Toll-Free: 800-308-1106
Fax: 410-850-0818
Website: http://
www.ameripros.org

Canadian **Prostate Cancer**
Network
P.O. Box 1253
Lakefield, ON K0L 2H0
Canada
Toll-Free: 866-810-2726
Francais: 800-363-0063
TTY: 705-652-9200
Website: http://www.cpcn.org

National **Prostate Cancer**
Coalition
1154 Fifteenth Street, NW
Washington, DC 20005
Toll-Free: 888-245-9455
Phone: 202-463-9455
Fax: 202-463-9456
Website: http://
www.pcacoalition.org
E-mail:
info@fightprotatecancer.org

Prostate Cancer Foundation
1250 Fourth Street
Santa Monica, CA 90401
Phone: 310-570-4700
Toll-Free: 800-757-2873
Website: http://www
.prostatecancerfoundation.org
E-mail: info
@prostatecancerfoundation.org

Prostate Cancer Foundation of
Australia
P.O. Box 1332
Lane Cove, NSW 1595
Australia
Phone: 011 61 2 9418 7942
Fax: 011 61 2 9420 3635
Website: http://
www.prostate.org.au
E-mail:
enquiries@prostate.org.au

Prostate Cancer Research
Institute
5777 W. Century Blvd.
Suite 800
Los Angeles, CA 90045
Toll-Free Helpline: 800-641-PCRI
Phone: 310-743-2116
Fax: 310-743-2113
Website: http://www.prostate-
cancer.org
E-mail: info@pcri.org

American Academy of
Dermatology [**Skin Cancer**]
P.O. Box 4014
Schaumburg, IL 60173
Toll-Free: 888-462- 3376
Phone: 847-330-0230
Fax: 847-330-0050
Website: http://www.aad.org

National Institute of Arthritis
and Musculoskeletal and **Skin**
Diseases
1 AMS Circle
Bethesda, MD 20892-3675
Toll-Free: 877-226-4267
Phone: 301-495-4484
TTY: 301-565-2966
Fax: 301-718-6366
Website: http://
www.niams.nih.gov
E-mail: niamsinfo@mail.nih.gov

New Zealand Dermatological
Society, Inc. [**Skin Cancer**]
Website: http://dermnetnz.org

Skin Cancer Foundation
149 Madison, Suite 901
New York, NY 10016
Phone: 212-725-5176
Toll-Free: 800-754-6490
E-mail: info@skincancer.org
Website: http://
www.skincancer.org

Testicular Cancer Resource
Center
Website: http://tcrc.acor.org

American **Thyroid** Association
6066 Leesburg Pike, Suite 550
Falls Church, VA 22041
Phone: 703-998-8890
Fax: 703-998-8893
E-mail: admin@thyroid.org
Website: http://www.thyroid.org

Thyroid Cancer Survivors'
Association, Inc.
P.O. Box 1545
New York, NY 10159-1545
Toll-Free: 877-588-7904
Website: http://www.thyca.org
E-mail: thyca@thyca.org

Thyroid Foundation of
America, Inc.
One Longfellow Place
Suite 1518
Boston, MA 02114
Toll-Free: 800-832-8321
Fax: 617-534-1515
Website: http://www.tsh.org
E-mail: info@allthyroid.org

American **Urological** Associa-
tion Foundation
1000 Corporate Boulevard
Suite 410
Linthicum, MD 21090
Toll-Free: 800-828-7866
Phone: 410-689-3990
Website: http://www.afud.org

International **Waldenström's
Macroglobulinemia** Founda-
tion
3932 D Swift Road
Sarasota, FL 34231
Phone: 941-927-4963
Website: http://www.iwmf.com
E-mail: info@iwmf.com

Chapter 92

Cancer Information Available in Spanish

Recursos Informativos del Instituto Nacional del Cáncer

Tal vez desee más información para usted, para su familia y su médico. Los siguientes servicios del Instituto Nacional del Cáncer (NCI) están a su disposición para ayudarle.

Información por Teléfono

Servicio de Información sobre el Cáncer (CIS): El Servicio de Información sobre el Cáncer del NCI ofrece servicio telefónico en español. En Estados Unidos y sus territorios, llame al 800-4-CANCER (800-422-6237), de lunes a viernes, de las nueve de la mañana a las cuatro treinta de la tarde hora local. Las personas sordas o con problemas de audición que cuentan con equipo TTY pueden llamar al 800-332-8615.

No podemos responder a preguntas específicas de medicina, ni dar referencias o consultas. El médico familiarizado con el estado del paciente es el más indicado para responder a preguntas específicas de medicina.

Internet

Estos sitios de la web pueden ser útiles: http://www.cancer.gov. El sitio de la web del Instituto Nacional del Cáncer Cancer.gov™ proporciona

Information in this chapter is excerpted from "Documentos sobre en cáncer: información en Español" and "Hoja informativa: En Español," National Cancer Institute (http://www.cancer.gov); accessed May 12, 2006.

información de numerosas fuentes del NCI, incluyendo PDQ®, el banco de datos de información del NCI sobre el cáncer. PDQ contiene información actual sobre la prevención, los exámenes selectivos de detección, diagnóstico, tratamiento, genética, cuidados médicos de apoyo y estudios clínicos en curso. Se puede tener acceso a Cancer.gov en http://www.cancer.gov.

Folletos del Instituto Nacional del Cáncer

Las publicaciones del Instituto Nacional del Cáncer (NCI) se pueden pedir escribiendo a la dirección de abajo, y algunas se pueden ver y descargar del sitio https://cissecure.nci.nih.gov/ncipubs.

Publications Ordering Service
National Cancer Institute
Suite 3036A
6116 Executive Boulevard, MSC 8322
Bethesda, MD 20892-8322

Además, si usted está en Estados Unidos o en uno de sus territorios, usted puede pedir estos folletos del NCI y otras publicaciones si llama al Servicio de Información sobre el Cáncer (CIS) al 800-4-CANCER. Es posible también pedir publicaciones en línea en https://cissecure .nci.nih.gov/ncipubs.

Hojas Informativas del NCI

Las hojas informativas del NCI, constituyen una colección de documentos que tratan sobre diversos tópicos relacionados con el cáncer y son elaboradas por el Servicio de Información sobre el Cáncer (CIS) del NCI. Estas hojas informativas se revisan y actualizan con frecuencia de acuerdo a las últimas investigaciones sobre el cáncer. Se puede tener acceso a las hojas informativas en http://www.cancer .gov/espanol/hojasinformativas.

Hoja Informativa

Atención en el hogar para pacientes con cáncer (Revisión: 02/15/2005): Hoja informativa acerca de los diversos servicios que proporcionan las agencias de atención en el hogar y la ayuda económica disponible por parte de agencias públicas, privadas y del gobierno (hoja informativa 8.5s).

Ayuda económica para gastos relacionados con el cáncer (Revisión: 09/08/2004): Hoja informativa que contiene la lista de organizaciones que pueden ayudar a los pacientes y a sus familias con ayuda económica durante el tratamiento (hoja informativa 8.3s).

Cáncer metastático: preguntas y respuestas (Revisión: 01/03/2005): Hoja informativa acerca del diagnóstico y tratamiento del cáncer que se ha diseminado (hoja informativa 6.20s).

Cáncer ovárico: preguntas y respuestas (Actualización: 07/05/2002, Revisión: 02/29/2000): Hoja informativa acerca de los factores de riesgo, síntomas, diagnóstico y tratamiento del cáncer de ovario (hoja informativa 6.33s).

Cáncer temprano de próstata: preguntas y respuestas (Revisión: 01/03/2005): Hoja informativa que describe los factores de riesgo para cáncer de próstata y los síntomas y las opciones de tratamiento para la enfermedad localizada. Discute los exámenes selectivos de detección a disposición (hoja informativa 5.23s).

Cómo encontrar a un doctor o un establecimiento de tratamiento si usted tiene cáncer (Revisión: 12/16/2004): Esta hoja informativa ofrece sugerencias para escoger a un médico y un establecimiento para el tratamiento de cáncer (hoja informativa 6.47s).

Cómo encontrar recursos en su comunidad si usted tiene cáncer (Revisión: 12/08/1999): Hoja informativa que discute los tipos de ayuda que están disponibles para gente con cáncer y en dónde encontrar estos servicios (hoja informativa 8.9s).

Cambios en el seno y el riesgo de desarrollar cáncer (Publicación: 09/22/2000): Hoja informativa que explica los varios tipos de cambios en los senos que experimentan las mujeres, y da un resumen de los métodos usados para distinguir entre cambios benignos y cambios que pueden ser cancerosos (hoja informativa 3.69s).

Cuidados paliativos (Revisión: 10/17/2002): Hoja informativa acerca de las organizaciones que proporcionan cuidados paliativos; también discute la cobertura del seguro médico (hoja informativa 8.6s).

El análisis del antígeno prostático específico (PSA): preguntas y respuestas (Revisión: 12/30/2004): Hoja informativa que define el antígeno prostático específico (PSA) y los exámenes selectivos de detección para cáncer de próstata, y describe los beneficios y las limitaciones de la prueba (hoja informativa 5.29s).

El cáncer de hígado: preguntas y respuestas (Revisión: 10/23/2001): Hoja informativa acerca de los factores de riesgo, síntomas, diagnóstico y tratamiento del cáncer que se desarrolla en el hígado (hoja informativa 6.28s).

El cáncer de hueso: preguntas y respuestas (Revisión: 04/24/2002): Hoja informativa acerca del diagnóstico y tratamiento de los cánceres que se presentan en los huesos (hoja informativa 6.26s).

El cáncer de pulmón (Revisión: 10/23/2002): Esta hoja informativa sobre el cáncer de pulmón (en español) habla de los síntomas, diagnóstico, tratamiento, asuntos emocionales y preguntas para hacer al doctor. Incluye una lista de otros recursos (hoja informativa 6.41s).

El cáncer de testículo: preguntas y respuestas (Revisión: 03/01/2006): Hoja informativa acerca del cáncer de testículo, los factores de riesgo, síntomas, diagnóstico, tratamiento y cuidados de seguimiento (hoja informativa 6.34s).

El cáncer: preguntas y respuestas (Revisión: 09/23/2005): Hoja informativa acerca de la prevención, síntomas, diagnóstico y tratamiento del cáncer (hoja informativa 6.7s).

El cuidado para niños y adolescentes con cáncer: preguntas y respuestas (Revisión: 06/28/2005): Hoja informativa acerca de los centros oncológicos para niños, y sobre enfoques de cuidados médicos, incluyendo estudios clínicos para niños con cáncer (hoja informativa 1.21s).

El equipo de atención médica: el médico es sólo el principio (Publicación: 08/15/2000): Hoja informativa que describe a los especialistas incluidos en el tratamiento y atención; pone el énfasis en que el paciente es el miembro más importante del equipo de cuidados médicos (hoja informativa 8.1s).

El Estudio del Tamoxifeno y del Raloxifeno (STAR): preguntas y respuestas (Revisión: 08/16/2004): Hoja informativa acerca de un estudio clínico que compara la efectividad y seguridad de dos fármacos, tamoxifeno y raloxifeno, para la prevención del cáncer de seno (hoja informativa 4.19s).

El Instituto Nacional del Cáncer de Estados Unidos (Revisión: 03/26/2003): Hoja informativa acerca del Instituto Nacional del Cáncer, un componente de los Institutos Nacionales de la Salud (hoja informativa 1.23s).

El Servicio de Información sobre el Cáncer del Instituto Nacional del Cáncer: preguntas y respuestas (Revisión: 04/12/2005): Hoja informativa acerca del Servicio de Información sobre el Cáncer del NCI, un recurso que proporciona la información más actual y precisa del cáncer a los pacientes y sus familias, al público y a los profesionales de la salud (hoja informativa 2.5s).

El trasplante de médula ósea y el trasplante de células madre de sangre periférica: preguntas y respuestas (Revisión: 05/25/2005): Hoja informativa que explica paso a paso los procedimientos de dos tipos de trasplantes que se usan con quimioterapia de dosis elevadas e incluye sus riesgos y beneficios (hoja informativa 7.41s).

Estudio del Selenio y la Vitamina E para Prevenir el Cáncer (SELECT): preguntas y respuestas (Revisión: 06/28/2005): Esta es la versión en español de una hoja informativa que responde preguntas acerca de un estudio clínico para ver si el selenio o la vitamina previenen el cáncer de próstata (hoja informativa 4.20s).

Estudios clínicos de cáncer en el Centro Clínico de los Institutos Nacionales de la Salud: preguntas y respuestas (Revisión: 12/12/2005): Hoja informativa acerca de los estudios clínicos que se llevan a cabo en el Centro Clínico de los NIH en Bethesda, Maryland (hoja informativa 1.22s).

Estudios clínicos: preguntas y respuestas (Revisión: 08/26/2005): Esta es la versión en español de una hoja informativa del Instituto Nacional del Cáncer que responde preguntas acerca del estudios clínicos (hoja informativa 2.11s).

Etapa del cáncer: preguntas y respuestas (Revisión: 08/30/2004): Esta es la versión en español de una hoja informativa del Instituto Nacional del Cáncer que explica el proceso de agrupar los casos de cáncer en categorías (etapas) en base al tamaño del tumor y la extensión del tumor en el cuerpo (hoja informativa 5.32s).

Exámenes selectivos de detección de cáncer colorrectal: preguntas y respuestas (Revisión: 09/08/2004): Esta hoja informativa habla de las ventajas y desventajas de varios exámenes selectivos de detección de cáncer colorrectal (hoja informativa 5.31s).

Fumar cigarrillos y el cáncer: preguntas y respuestas (Revisión: 03/05/2004): Hoja informativa que trata de los riesgos para la salud causados por fumar cigarrillos; incluye el hecho que el fumar cigarrillos es responsable directamente de al menos una tercera parte de las muertes por cáncer en los Estados Unidos (hoja informativa 10.14s).

Grado de un tumor: preguntas y respuestas (Revisión: 09/02/2004): Hoja informativa que define los tumores de alto y bajo grado y su papel en el pronóstico. Explica algunos conceptos como la biología normal de las células y la diferenciación celular (hoja informativa 5.9s).

La interpretación de los pronósticos y las estadísticas del cáncer (Revisión: 01/28/2005): Hoja informativa que describe la importancia de la predicción del resultado y recuperación de una enferemedad y cómo la estadística ayuda a los médicos a calcular un pronóstico (hoja informativa 8.2s).

La medicina complementaria y alternativa en el tratamiento del cáncer: preguntas y respuestas (Revisión: 10/07/2003): Hoja informativa que describe métodos complementarios y alternativos del tratamiento de cáncer (hoja informativa 7.50s).

La prueba de Papanicolaou: preguntas y respuestas (Revisión: 01/04/2005): Hoja informativa que describe el procedimiento de la prueba de Papanicolaou, los resultados posibles y la conexión entre el papilomavirus humano (PVH) y el cáncer de cérvix (hoja informativa 5.16s).

Las píldoras anticonceptivas y el riesgo de cáncer (Revisión: 01/30/2004): Hoja informativa acerca de la investigación sobre el riesgo de desarrollar cáncer de seno, cérvix, hígado y de ovario por el uso de anticonceptivos orales (hoja informativa 3.13s).

Los virus del papiloma humano y el cáncer: preguntas y respuestas (Revisión: 08/09/2004): Hoja informativa acerca de la conexión entre la infección de papilomavirus humano (PVH) y el cáncer (hoja informativa 3.20s).

Mamografías selectivas de detección: preguntas y respuestas (Revisión: 06/06/2002): Hoja informativa que define las mamografías selectivas de detección y sus ventajas y límites. Contiene una lista de las tasas de incidencia y factores de riesgo para cáncer de seno (hoja informativa 5.28s).

Marcadores tumorales (Revisión: 08/20/1999): Hoja informativa que contiene una lista de ejemplos de marcadores tumorales en la sangre y describe cómo pueden ser utilizados para ayudar en el diagnóstico y tratamiento (hoja informativa 5.18s).

Obesidad y cáncer: preguntas y respuestas (Revisión: 11/22/2004): Hoja informativa que resume la investigación sobre la posible conexión entre la obesidad y el riesgo de cáncer (hoja informativa 3.70s).

Organizaciones nacionales que brindan servicios a las personas con cáncer y a sus familias (Revisión: 02/07/2006): Hoja informativa que contiene una lista de organizaciones que proporcionan apoyo financiero y emocional, defensa e información a pacientes con cáncer y a sus familias (hoja informativa 8.1s).

PDQ®: preguntas y respuestas (Revisión: 07/07/2005): Hoja informativa acerca del banco de datos PDQ del Instituto Nacional del Cáncer (hoja informativa 2.2s.

Preguntas y respuestas sobre dejar de fumar (Publicación: 12/27/2000): Hoja informativa que contiene una lista de los métodos para dejar de fumar, los beneficios a corto y a largo plazo de dejar de fumar y las organizaciones que pueden ayudar (hoja informativa 10.19s).

Programa de Centros Oncológicos del Instituto Nacional del Cáncer (Revisión: 04/24/2006): Hoja informativa acerca de los centros oncológicos subvencionados por el Instituto Nacional del Cáncer (hoja informativa 1.2s).

Tamoxifeno: preguntas y respuestas (Revisión: 05/17/2002): Hoja informativa que describe la acción, los riesgos, beneficios y efectos secundarios del tamoxifeno, un fármaco que interrumpe la conexión de la hormona estrógeno al cáncer de seno (hoja informativa 7.16s).

Terapia adyuvante para el cáncer de seno: preguntas y respuestas (Revisión: 05/17/2002): Hoja informativa que explica los tipos de terapias adyuvantes (tratamiento que se administra además de la terapia primaria). Discute los efectos secundarios, los riesgos y beneficios de la terapia adyuvante (hoja informativa 7.20s).

Terapias biológicas del cáncer: preguntas y respuestas (Revisión: 02/22/2005): Una hoja informativa que proporciona una vista general de cómo funciona el sistema inmune y describe las terapias biológicas disponibles (hoja informativa 7.2s).

Sumarios de Información sobre el Cáncer (PDQ®)

Están escritos con claridad y contienen la información más reciente sobre el cáncer, la cual es revisada y actualizada mensualmente por los expertos. Desde enero de 2005, el NCI ha añadido ilustraciones a varios de los sumarios.

- Tratamiento del cáncer en adultos (http://www.cancer.gov/espanol/pdq/tratamientoadultos): Opciones de tratamiento para cánceres en adultos.

- Tratamiento del cáncer pediátrico (http://www.cancer.gov/espanol/pdq/tratamientopediátrico): Opciones de tratamiento para cánceres pediátricos.

- Cuidados médicos de apoyo (cómo superar los efectos del cáncer) (http://www.cancer.gov/espanol/pdq/cuidadosdeapoyo): Efectos secundarios del tratamiento del cáncer, manejo de sus complicaciones y preocupaciones de tipo psicosocial.

- La medicina complementaria y alternativa en el tratamiento del cáncer (PDQ®) (http://www.cancer.gov/espanol/pdq/mca/mca-cancer-tratamiento): Resumen de información revisada por expertos acerca del uso de la medicina complementaria y alternativa como tratamiento del cáncer.

Estudios Clínicos

Existen aproximadamente 2,000 estudios abiertos o activos y unos 14,000 cerrados relacionados con el tratamiento, exámenes de detección, prevención, genética y cuidados médicos de apoyo.

- Búsqueda de estudios clínicos (http://www.cancer.gov/clinicaltrials): Acceso directo a la base de datos del PDQ con estudios clínicos. Esta información sólo está disponible en inglés.

Chapter 93

Resources for End-of-Life Issues

Administration on Aging
Washington, DC 20201
Phone: 202-619-0724
Fax: 202-357-3556
Website: http://www.aoa.gov
E-mail: aoainfo@aoa.gov

American Academy of Hospice and Palliative Medicine
4700 W. Lake Ave.
Glenview IL 60025
Phone: 847-375-4712
Fax: 877-734-8671
Website: http://www.aahpm.org
E-mail: info@aahpm.org

American Chronic Pain Association
P.O. Box 850
Rocklin, CA 95677
Toll-Free: 800-533-3231
Fax: 916-632-3208
Website: http://www.theacpa.org

American Hospice Foundation
2120 L Street, NW
Suite 200
Washington, DC 20037
Phone: 202-223-0204
Fax: 202-223-0208
Website: http://www.americanhospice.org
E-mail: ahf@americanhospice.org

Information in this chapter was compiled from many sources deemed reliable. Inclusion does not constitute endorsement and omission does not imply disapproval. All contact information was updated and verified in October 2006.

American Pain Foundation
201 N. Charles St.
Suite 710
Baltimore, MD 21201-4111
Toll-Free: 888-615-7246 (message line)
Website: http://
www.painfoundation.org
E-mail: info@painfoundation.org

American Pain Society
4700 W. Lake Ave.
Glenview IL 60025
Phone: 847-375-4715
Website: http://
www.ampainsoc.org
E-mail: info@ampainsoc.org

Americans for Better Care of the Dying
1700 Diagonal Rd.
Suite 625
Alexandria, VA 22314
Phone: 703-647-8505
Fax: 703-837-1233
Website: http://
www.abcd-caring.org
E-mail: info@abcd-caring.org

Children's Hospice International
1101 King Street
Suite 360
Alexandria, VA 22314
Toll-Free: 800-242-4453
Phone: 703-684-0330
Website: http://
www.chionline.org
E-mail: info@chionline.org

Compassion and Choices
P.O. Box 101810
Denver, CO 80250-1810
Toll-Free: 800-247-7421
Fax: 303-639-1224
Website: http://
www.compassionandchoices.org

Death with Dignity
520 SW 6th Avenue, Suite 1030
Portland, OR 97204
Phone: 503-228-4415
Fax: 503-228-7454
Website: http://
www.deathwithdignity.org

Family Caregiver Alliance
180 Montgomery St., Suite 1100
San Francisco, CA 94104
Toll-Free: 800-445-8106
Phone: 415-434-3388
Website: http://caregiver.org
E-mail: info@caregiver.org

Hospice Association of America
228 Seventh Street, SE
Washington, DC 20003
Phone: 202-546-4759
Fax: 202-547-3540
Fax-On-Demand: 202-547-6638
Website: http://www.nahc.org

Hospice Education Institute
Three Unity Square
P.O. Box 98
Machiasport, ME 04655-0098
Phone: 207-255-8800
Toll-Free: 800-331-1620
Website: http://
www.hospiceworld.org
E-mail: info@hospiceworld.org

Hospice Foundation of America
1621 Connecticut Ave., NW, Suite 300
Washington, DC 20009
Toll-Free: 800-854-3402
Fax: 202-638-5312
Website: http://www.hospicefoundation.org
E-mail: info@hospicefoundation.org

Hospice Net
401 Bowling Avenue, Suite 51
Nashville, TN 37205-5124
Website: http://www.hospicenet.org
E-mail: info@hospicenet.org

Hospice Patients Alliance
Website: http://www.hospicepatients.org

National Association for Home Care
228 Seventh Street, SE
Washington, DC 20003
Phone: 202-547-7424
Website: http://www.nahc.org

National Family Caregivers
10400 Connecticut Ave., Suite 500
Kensington, MD 20895-3944
Toll-Free: 800-896-3650
Phone: 301-942-6430
Fax: 301-942-2302
Website: http://www.thefamilycaregiver.org
E-mail: info@thefamilycaregiver.org

National Hospice and Palliative Care Organization
1700 Diagonal Road
Suite 625
Alexandria, VA 22314
Toll-Free: 800-658-8898 (helpline)
Phone: 703-837-1500
Website: http://www.nhpco.org
E-mail: info@nhpco.org

National Institute on Aging (NIA)
Bldg. 31, Room 5C27
31 Center Dr., MSC 2292
Bethesda, MD 20892
Toll-Free: 800-222-2225
Fax: 301-495-3334
Toll-Free TTY: 800-222-4225
Website: http://www.nia.nih.gov

Visiting Nurse Associations of America
99 Summer St.
Suite 1700
Boston, MA 02110
Phone: 617-737-3200
Fax: 617-737-1144
Website: http://www.vnaa.org.
E-mail: vnaa@vnaa.org

Index

Index

Page numbers followed by 'n' indicate a footnote. Page numbers in *italics* indicate a table or illustration.

American Urological Association
Foundation, contact information
1040
amino acids
asparagine 76
tyrosine 101
aminoglutethimide 582
amitriptyline *392*
AML *see* acute myelogenous leukemia
amosite 167
amphiboles, described 167
amputation
sarcomas 773, 775–76
soft tissue sarcomas 789–90
anal cancer
defined 1014
human papillomavirus 162
overview 465–72
statistics 189–90
anaplastic astrocytomas
described 298
grade *286*
anaplastic ependymoma, grade *286*
anaplastic gangliogliomas, described
282
anaplastic large cell lymphoma,
described 1025
anaplastic oligodendroglioma, grade
286
anaplastic thyroid cancer
defined 1014
described 716–18
Anaprox *392*
anastomosis
gastrointestinal carcinoid
tumors 404
small intestine cancer 432
M.D. Anderson Cancer Center,
publications
non-rhabdomyosarcoma soft
tissue sarcoma 795n
pediatric germ cell tumors 555n
androblastoma, defined 1014
anemia
chemotherapy 835–36
colon cancer 438
defined 1014
leukemia 586
anesthetic, defined 1014

anger, coping strategies 960–61
angiograms, gastrointestinal
carcinoid tumors 402
angioimmunoblastic T-cell
lymphoma, defined 1014
angiosarcomas
liver 787
overview 798–800
animal studies
artificial sweeteners 78
colorectal cancer 441
fluoridated water 81
formaldehyde exposure 180
magnetic field exposure 136
phthalates 83
red wine 89
anoscopy, anal cancer 467
Ansaid *392*
anterior exenteration, urethral
cancer 503
anterior mediastinotomy, defined
1017
anthophyllite 167
anticancer medication *see*
chemotherapy
antidiuretic hormone (ADH),
described 682–83
antigens, described 898
antioxidants
colorectal cancer 444
defined 1014–15
red wine 88
anus, described 465
anxiety, coping strategies 953–54
APC *see* adenomatous polyposis coli
apheresis, described 883
Aplastic Anemia and MDS
International Foundation, contact
information 614
apoptosis-inducing medications 911
appendectomy, gastrointestinal
carcinoid tumors 404
appendix, described 399
appetite loss, coping strategies
955–56
arrhenoblastoma, defined 1014
arsenic, lung cancer 314
Arthrotec *392*
artificial sweeteners, cancer risk 77–80

glioblastomas, described 298
gliomas
  astrocytomas 297–99
  RF energy 141–42
glomus jugulare tumors, described 282
glottis
  depicted *251*
  described 249
glucagonoma, described 396
Gorlin syndrome, defined 1015
goserelin 582
grafts, defined 1020
graft *versus* host disease (GVHD)
  leukemia 880
  stem cell transplantation 17, 881,
    884–85
grief, coping strategies 960
growth factors
  cancer formation 910
  colorectal cancer 437, 449
  male breast cancer 535
  multiple myeloma 619
growth hormone (GH), described 682
guaiac stool test, described 24
guilt, coping strategies 962–63
gum disease, smokeless tobacco 51
GVHD *see* graft *versus* host disease
Gynecologic Cancer Foundation,
  reproductive organ cancers
  publication 541n
Gynecologic Cancer Foundation/
  Women's Cancer Network,
  contact information 1035
gynecologic cancers
  defined 1020
  overview 541–48
  see also cervical cancer; ovarian
    cancer; uterine cancer; vaginal
    cancer; vulva cancer

H

HAART *see* highly-active
  antiretroviral therapy
Hafez, Bahaa E. 296
hair loss
  chemotherapy 15, 834–35
  radiation therapy 867–68

hairy cell leukemia
  defined 1020
  overview 602–4
hard palate, described 215
HBV *see* hepatitis B virus
HCA *see* heterocyclic amines
HCV *see* hepatitis C virus
head and neck cancer, defined 1020
heart, localized malignant
  mesothelioma 1023
heart cancer
  defined 1020
  statistics 210–11
heart disease
  advanced cancer 993–1003
  environmental tobacco smoke 54
  tobacco use 314
heating, ventilation, and air
  conditioning (HVAC),
  environmental tobacco smoke 55
helical low-dose CT scan, lung
  cancer 316
Helicobacter pylori
  cancer risk factor 6
  non-Hodgkin lymphoma 650
  stomach cancer 354–55
helper T cells, described 898
hemangioblastomas, described 285
hemangiomas, described 265
hematologic malignancy, defined 1020
hematopoietic stem cells, described
  879
hemihypertrophy, Wilms tumor 482
hemilaryngectomy, laryngeal
  cancer 255
hepatectomy
  liver cancer 414
  pediatric liver cancer 425
hepatic artery embolization, gastrointestinal carcinoid tumors 404
hepatic artery ligation, gastrointestinal carcinoid tumors 404
hepatic bile ducts, described 371
hepatic resection, gastrointestinal
  carcinoid tumors 404
hepatitis B virus (HBV)
  cancer risk factor 5, 29
  hepatocellular carcinoma 420
  liver cancer 409

Health Reference Series
COMPLETE CATALOG
List price $87 per volume. **School and library price $78 per volume.**

Adolescent Health Sourcebook, 2nd Edition

Basic Consumer Health Information about the Physical, Mental, and Emotional Growth and Development of Adolescents, Including Medical Care, Nutritional and Physical Activity Requirements, Puberty, Sexual Activity, Acne, Tanning, Body Piercing, Common Physical Illnesses and Disorders, Eating Disorders, Attention Deficit Hyperactivity Disorder, Depression, Bullying, Hazing, and Adolescent Injuries Related to Sports, Driving, and Work

Along with Substance Abuse Information about Nicotine, Alcohol, and Drug Use, a Glossary, and Directory of Additional Resources

Edited by Joyce Brennfleck Shannon. 683 pages. 2006. 978-0-7808-0943-7.

"It is written in clear, nontechnical language aimed at general readers. . . . Recommended for public libraries, community colleges, and other agencies serving health care consumers."
— *American Reference Books Annual, 2003*

"Recommended for school and public libraries. Parents and professionals dealing with teens will appreciate the easy-to-follow format and the clearly written text. This could become a 'must have' for every high school teacher." — *E-Streams, Jan '03*

"A good starting point for information related to common medical, mental, and emotional concerns of adolescents." — *School Library Journal, Nov '02*

"This book provides accurate information in an easy to access format. It addresses topics that parents and caregivers might not be aware of and provides practical, useable information."
— *Doody's Health Sciences Book Review Journal, Sep-Oct '02*

"Recommended reference source."
— *Booklist, American Library Association, Sep '02*

AIDS Sourcebook, 3rd Edition

Basic Consumer Health Information about Acquired Immune Deficiency Syndrome (AIDS) and Human Immunodeficiency Virus (HIV) Infection, Including Facts about Transmission, Prevention, Diagnosis, Treatment, Opportunistic Infections, and Other Complications, with a Section for Women and Children, Including Details about Associated Gynecological Concerns, Pregnancy, and Pediatric Care

Along with Updated Statistical Information, Reports on Current Research Initiatives, a Glossary, and Directories of Internet, Hotline, and Other Resources

Edited by Dawn D. Matthews. 664 pages. 2003. 978-0-7808-0631-3.

"The 3rd edition of the *AIDS Sourcebook*, part of Omnigraphics' *Health Reference Series*, is a welcome update. . . . This resource is highly recommended for academic and public libraries."
— *American Reference Books Annual, 2004*

"Excellent sourcebook. This continues to be a highly recommended book. There is no other book that provides as much information as this book provides."
— *AIDS Book Review Journal, Dec-Jan '00*

"Recommended reference source."
— *Booklist, American Library Association, Dec '99*

Alcoholism Sourcebook, 2nd Edition

Basic Consumer Health Information about Alcohol Use, Abuse, and Dependence, Featuring Facts about the Physical, Mental, and Social Health Effects of Alcohol Addiction, Including Alcoholic Liver Disease, Pancreatic Disease, Cardiovascular Disease, Neurological Disorders, and the Effects of Drinking during Pregnancy

Along with Information about Alcohol Treatment, Medications, and Recovery Programs, in Addition to Tips for Reducing the Prevalence of Underage Drinking, Statistics about Alcohol Use, a Glossary of Related Terms, and Directories of Resources for More Help and Information

Edited by Amy L. Sutton. 653 pages. 2006. 978-0-7808-0942-0.

"This title is one of the few reference works on alcoholism for general readers. For some readers this will be a welcome complement to the many self-help books on the market. Recommended for collections serving general readers and consumer health collections."
— *E-Streams, Mar '01*

"This book is an excellent choice for public and academic libraries."
— *American Reference Books Annual, 2001*

"Recommended reference source."
— *Booklist, American Library Association, Dec '00*

"Presents a wealth of information on alcohol use and abuse and its effects on the body and mind, treatment, and prevention." — *SciTech Book News, Dec '00*

"Important new health guide which packs in the latest consumer information about the problems of alcoholism." — *Reviewer's Bookwatch, Nov '00*

SEE ALSO *Drug Abuse Sourcebook*

Allergies Sourcebook, 2nd Edition

Basic Consumer Health Information about Allergic Disorders, Triggers, Reactions, and Related Symptoms, Including Anaphylaxis, Rhinitis, Sinusitis, Asthma, Dermatitis, Conjunctivitis, and Multiple Chemical Sensitivity

Along with Tips on Diagnosis, Prevention, and Treatment, Statistical Data, a Glossary, and a Directory of Sources for Further Help and Information

Edited by Annemarie S. Muth. 598 pages. 2002. 978-0-7808-0376-3.

"This book brings a great deal of useful material together. . . . This is an excellent addition to public and consumer health library collections."
— *American Reference Books Annual, 2003*

"This second edition would be useful to laypersons with little or advanced knowledge of the subject matter. This book would also serve as a resource for nursing and other health care professions students. It would be useful in public, academic, and hospital libraries with consumer health collections." — *E-Streams, Jul '02*

Alternative Medicine Sourcebook

SEE *Complementary & Alternative Medicine Sourcebook*

Alzheimer's Disease Sourcebook, 3rd Edition

Basic Consumer Health Information about Alzheimer's Disease, Other Dementias, and Related Disorders, Including Multi-Infarct Dementia, AIDS Dementia Complex, Dementia with Lewy Bodies, Huntington's Disease, Wernicke-Korsakoff Syndrome (Alcohol-Related Dementia), Delirium, and Confusional States

Along with Information for People Newly Diagnosed with Alzheimer's Disease and Caregivers, Reports Detailing Current Research Efforts in Prevention, Diagnosis, and Treatment, Facts about Long-Term Care Issues, and Listings of Sources for Additional Information

Edited by Karen Bellenir. 645 pages. 2003. 978-0-7808-0666-5.

"This very informative and valuable tool will be a great addition to any library serving consumers, students and health care workers."
— *American Reference Books Annual, 2004*

"This is a valuable resource for people affected by dementias such as Alzheimer's. It is easy to navigate and includes important information and resources."
— *Doody's Review Service, Feb '04*

"Recommended reference source."
— *Booklist, American Library Association, Oct '99*

SEE ALSO *Brain Disorders Sourcebook*

Arthritis Sourcebook, 2nd Edition

Basic Consumer Health Information about Osteoarthritis, Rheumatoid Arthritis, Other Rheumatic Disorders, Infectious Forms of Arthritis, and Diseases with Symptoms Linked to Arthritis, Featuring Facts about Diagnosis, Pain Management, and Surgical Therapies

Along with Coping Strategies, Research Updates, a Glossary, and Resources for Additional Help and Information

Edited by Amy L. Sutton. 593 pages. 2004. 978-0-7808-0667-2.

"This easy-to-read volume is recommended for consumer health collections within public or academic libraries." — *E-Streams, May '05*

"As expected, this updated edition continues the excellent reputation of this series in providing sound, usable health information. . . . Highly recommended."
— *American Reference Books Annual, 2005*

"Excellent reference." — *The Bookwatch, Jan '05*

Asthma Sourcebook, 2nd Edition

Basic Consumer Health Information about the Causes, Symptoms, Diagnosis, and Treatment of Asthma in Infants, Children, Teenagers, and Adults, Including Facts about Different Types of Asthma, Common Co-Occurring Conditions, Asthma Management Plans, Triggers, Medications, and Medication Delivery Devices

Along with Asthma Statistics, Research Updates, a Glossary, a Directory of Asthma-Related Resources, and More

Edited by Karen Bellenir. 609 pages. 2006. 978-0-7808-0866-9.

"A worthwhile reference acquisition for public libraries and academic medical libraries whose readers desire a quick introduction to the wide range of asthma information." — *Choice, Association of College & Research Libraries, Jun '01*

"Recommended reference source."
— *Booklist, American Library Association, Feb '01*

"Highly recommended." — *The Bookwatch, Jan '01*

"There is much good information for patients and their families who deal with asthma daily."
— *American Medical Writers Association Journal, Winter '01*

"This informative text is recommended for consumer health collections in public, secondary school, and community college libraries and the libraries of universities with a large undergraduate population."
— *American Reference Books Annual, 2001*

Attention Deficit Disorder Sourcebook

Basic Consumer Health Information about Attention Deficit/Hyperactivity Disorder in Children and Adults,

Including Facts about Causes, Symptoms, Diagnostic Criteria, and Treatment Options Such as Medications, Behavior Therapy, Coaching, and Homeopathy

Along with Reports on Current Research Initiatives, Legal Issues, and Government Regulations, and Featuring a Glossary of Related Terms, Internet Resources, and a List of Additional Reading Material

Edited by Dawn D. Matthews. 470 pages. 2002. 978-0-7808-0624-5.

"Recommended reference source."
— Booklist, American Library Association, Jan '03

"This book is recommended for all school libraries and the reference or consumer health sections of public libraries." — American Reference Books Annual, 2003

Back & Neck Sourcebook, 2nd Edition

Basic Consumer Health Information about Spinal Pain, Spinal Cord Injuries, and Related Disorders, Such as Degenerative Disk Disease, Osteoarthritis, Scoliosis, Sciatica, Spina Bifida, and Spinal Stenosis, and Featuring Facts about Maintaining Spinal Health, Self-Care, Pain Management, Rehabilitative Care, Chiropractic Care, Spinal Surgeries, and Complementary Therapies

Along with Suggestions for Preventing Back and Neck Pain, a Glossary of Related Terms, and a Directory of Resources

Edited by Amy L. Sutton. 633 pages. 2004. 978-0-7808-0738-9.

"Recommended . . . an easy to use, comprehensive medical reference book." — E-Streams, Sep '05

"The strength of this work is its basic, easy-to-read format. Recommended." — Reference and User Services Quarterly, American Library Association, Winter '97

Blood & Circulatory Disorders Sourcebook, 2nd Edition

Basic Consumer Health Information about the Blood and Circulatory System and Related Disorders, Such as Anemia and Other Hemoglobin Diseases, Cancer of the Blood and Associated Bone Marrow Disorders, Clotting and Bleeding Problems, and Conditions That Affect the Veins, Blood Vessels, and Arteries, Including Facts about the Donation and Transplantation of Bone Marrow, Stem Cells, and Blood and Tips for Keeping the Blood and Circulatory System Healthy

Along with a Glossary of Related Terms and Resources for Additional Help and Information

Edited by Amy L. Sutton. 659 pages. 2005. 978-0-7808-0746-4.

"Highly recommended pick for basic consumer health reference holdings at all levels."
— The Bookwatch, Aug '05

"Recommended reference source."
— Booklist, American Library Association, Feb '99

"An important reference sourcebook written in simple language for everyday, non-technical users. "
— Reviewer's Bookwatch, Jan '99

Brain Disorders Sourcebook, 2nd Edition

Basic Consumer Health Information about Acquired and Traumatic Brain Injuries, Infections of the Brain, Epilepsy and Seizure Disorders, Cerebral Palsy, and Degenerative Neurological Disorders, Including Amyotrophic Lateral Sclerosis (ALS), Dementias, Multiple Sclerosis, and More

Along with Information on the Brain's Structure and Function, Treatment and Rehabilitation Options, Reports on Current Research Initiatives, a Glossary of Terms Related to Brain Disorders and Injuries, and a Directory of Sources for Further Help and Information

Edited by Sandra J. Judd. 625 pages. 2005. 978-0-7808-0744-0.

"Highly recommended pick for basic consumer health reference holdings at all levels."
— The Bookwatch, Aug '05

"Belongs on the shelves of any library with a consumer health collection." — E-Streams, Mar '00

"Recommended reference source."
— Booklist, American Library Association, Oct '99

SEE ALSO Alzheimer's Disease Sourcebook

Breast Cancer Sourcebook, 2nd Edition

Basic Consumer Health Information about Breast Cancer, Including Facts about Risk Factors, Prevention, Screening and Diagnostic Methods, Treatment Options, Complementary and Alternative Therapies, Post-Treatment Concerns, Clinical Trials, Special Risk Populations, and New Developments in Breast Cancer Research

Along with Breast Cancer Statistics, a Glossary of Related Terms, and a Directory of Resources for Additional Help and Information

Edited by Sandra J. Judd. 595 pages. 2004. 978-0-7808-0668-9.

"This book will be an excellent addition to public, community college, medical, and academic libraries."
— American Reference Books Annual, 2006

"It would be a useful reference book in a library or on loan to women in a support group."
— Cancer Forum, Mar '03

"Recommended reference source."
— Booklist, American Library Association, Jan '02

"This reference source is highly recommended. It is quite informative, comprehensive and detailed in nature, and yet it offers practical advice in easy-to-read language. It could be thought of as the 'bible' of breast cancer for the consumer." — *E-Streams, Jan '02*

"From the pros and cons of different screening methods and results to treatment options, *Breast Cancer Sourcebook* provides the latest information on the subject."
— *Library Bookwatch, Dec '01*

"This thoroughgoing, very readable reference covers all aspects of breast health and cancer.... Readers will find much to consider here. Recommended for all public and patient health collections."
— *Library Journal, Sep '01*

SEE ALSO Cancer Sourcebook for Women, Women's Health Concerns Sourcebook

■

Breastfeeding Sourcebook

Basic Consumer Health Information about the Benefits of Breastmilk, Preparing to Breastfeed, Breastfeeding as a Baby Grows, Nutrition, and More, Including Information on Special Situations and Concerns Such as Mastitis, Illness, Medications, Allergies, Multiple Births, Prematurity, Special Needs, and Adoption

Along with a Glossary and Resources for Additional Help and Information

Edited by Jenni Lynn Colson. 388 pages. 2002. 978-0-7808-0332-9.

"Particularly useful is the information about professional lactation services and chapters on breastfeeding when returning to work.... *Breastfeeding Sourcebook* will be useful for public libraries, consumer health libraries, and technical schools offering nurse assistant training, especially in areas where Internet access is problematic."
— *American Reference Books Annual, 2003*

SEE ALSO Pregnancy & Birth Sourcebook

■

Burns Sourcebook

Basic Consumer Health Information about Various Types of Burns and Scalds, Including Flame, Heat, Cold, Electrical, Chemical, and Sun Burns

Along with Information on Short-Term and Long-Term Treatments, Tissue Reconstruction, Plastic Surgery, Prevention Suggestions, and First Aid

Edited by Allan R. Cook. 604 pages. 1999. 978-0-7808-0204-9.

"This is an exceptional addition to the series and is highly recommended for all consumer health collections, hospital libraries, and academic medical centers."
— *E-Streams, Mar '00*

"This key reference guide is an invaluable addition to all health care and public libraries in confronting this ongoing health issue."
— *American Reference Books Annual, 2000*

"Recommended reference source."
— *Booklist, American Library Association, Dec '99*

SEE ALSO Dermatological Disorders Sourcebook

Cancer Sourcebook, 5th Edition

Basic Consumer Health Information about Major Forms and Stages of Cancer, Featuring Facts about Head and Neck Cancers, Lung Cancers, Gastrointestinal Cancers, Genitourinary Cancers, Lymphomas, Blood Cell Cancers, Endocrine Cancers, Skin Cancers, Bone Cancers, Metastatic Cancers, and More

Along with Facts about Cancer Treatments, Cancer Risks and Prevention, a Glossary of Related Terms, Statistical Data, and a Directory of Resources for Additional Information

Edited by Karen Bellenir. 1,133 pages. 2007. 978-0-7808-0947-5.

"With cancer being the second leading cause of death for Americans, a prodigious work such as this one, which locates centrally so much cancer-related information, is clearly an asset to this nation's citizens and others."
— *Journal of the National Medical Association, 2004*

"This title is recommended for health sciences and public libraries with consumer health collections."
— *E-Streams, Feb '01*

"... can be effectively used by cancer patients and their families who are looking for answers in a language they can understand. Public and hospital libraries should have it on their shelves."
— *American Reference Books Annual, 2001*

"Recommended reference source."
— *Booklist, American Library Association, Dec '00*

SEE ALSO Breast Cancer Sourcebook, Cancer Sourcebook for Women, Pediatric Cancer Sourcebook, Prostate Cancer Sourcebook

■

Cancer Sourcebook for Women, 3rd Edition

Basic Consumer Health Information about Leading Causes of Cancer in Women, Featuring Facts about Gynecologic Cancers and Related Concerns, Such as Breast Cancer, Cervical Cancer, Endometrial Cancer, Uterine Sarcoma, Vaginal Cancer, Vulvar Cancer, and Common Non-Cancerous Gynecologic Conditions, in Addition to Facts about Lung Cancer, Colorectal Cancer, and Thyroid Cancer in Women

Along with Information about Cancer Risk Factors, Screening and Prevention, Treatment Options, and Tips on Coping with Life after Cancer Treatment, a Glossary of Cancer Terms, and a Directory of Resources for Additional Help and Information

Edited by Amy L. Sutton. 715 pages. 2006. 978-0-7808-0867-6.

"An excellent addition to collections in public, consumer health, and women's health libraries."
— *American Reference Books Annual, 2003*

"Overall, the information is excellent, and complex topics are clearly explained. As a reference book for the consumer it is a valuable resource to assist them to make informed decisions about cancer and its treatments."
— *Cancer Forum, Nov '02*

SEE ALSO Breast Cancer Sourcebook, Women's Health Concerns Sourcebook

Cancer Survivorship Sourcebook

Basic Consumer Health Information about the Physical, Educational, Emotional, Social, and Financial Needs of Cancer Patients from Diagnosis, through Cancer Treatment, and Beyond, Including Facts about Researching Specific Types of Cancer and Learning about Clinical Trials and Treatment Options, and Featuring Tips for Coping with the Side Effects of Cancer Treatments and Adjusting to Life after Cancer Treatment Concludes

Along with Suggestions for Caregivers, Friends, and Family Members of Cancer Patients, a Glossary of Cancer Care Terms, and Directories of Related Resources

Edited by Karen Bellenir. 650 pages. 2007. 978-0-7808-0985-7.

Cardiovascular Diseases & Disorders Sourcebook, 3rd Edition

Basic Consumer Health Information about Heart and Vascular Diseases and Disorders, Such as Angina, Heart Attacks, Arrhythmias, Cardiomyopathy, Valve Disease, Atherosclerosis, and Aneurysms, with Information about Managing Cardiovascular Risk Factors and Maintaining Heart Health, Medications and Procedures Used to Treat Cardiovascular Disorders, and Concerns of Special Significance to Women

Along with Reports on Current Research Initiatives, a Glossary of Related Medical Terms, and a Directory of Sources for Further Help and Information

Edited by Sandra J. Judd. 713 pages. 2005. 978-0-7808-0739-6.

Caregiving Sourcebook

Basic Consumer Health Information for Caregivers, Including a Profile of Caregivers, Caregiving Responsibilities and Concerns, Tips for Specific Conditions, Care Environments, and the Effects of Caregiving

Along with Facts about Legal Issues, Financial Information, and Future Planning, a Glossary, and a Listing of Additional Resources

Edited by Joyce Brennfleck Shannon. 600 pages. 2001. 978-0-7808-0331-2.

Child Abuse Sourcebook

Basic Consumer Health Information about the Physical, Sexual, and Emotional Abuse of Children, with Additional Facts about Neglect, Munchausen Syndrome by Proxy (MSBP), Shaken Baby Syndrome, and Controversial Issues Related to Child Abuse, Such as Withholding Medical Care, Corporal Punishment, and Child Maltreatment in Youth Sports, and Featuring Facts about Child Protective Services, Foster Care, Adoption, Parenting Challenges, and Other Abuse Prevention Efforts

Along with a Glossary of Related Terms and Resources for Additional Help and Information

Edited by Dawn D. Matthews. 620 pages. 2004. 978-0-7808-0705-1.

SEE ALSO: Domestic Violence Sourcebook

Childhood Diseases & Disorders Sourcebook

Basic Consumer Health Information about Medical Problems Often Encountered in Pre-Adolescent Children, Including Respiratory Tract Ailments, Ear Infections, Sore Throats, Disorders of the Skin and Scalp, Digestive and Genitourinary Diseases, Infectious Diseases, Inflammatory Disorders, Chronic Physical and Developmental Disorders, Allergies, and More

Along with Information about Diagnostic Tests, Common Childhood Surgeries, and Frequently Used Medications, with a Glossary of Important Terms and Resource Directory

Edited by Chad T. Kimball. 662 pages. 2003. 978-0-7808-0458-6.

"This is an excellent book for new parents and should be included in all health care and public libraries."
—*American Reference Books Annual, 2004*

SEE ALSO: Healthy Children Sourcebook

■

Colds, Flu & Other Common Ailments Sourcebook

Basic Consumer Health Information about Common Ailments and Injuries, Including Colds, Coughs, the Flu, Sinus Problems, Headaches, Fever, Nausea and Vomiting, Menstrual Cramps, Diarrhea, Constipation, Hemorrhoids, Back Pain, Dandruff, Dry and Itchy Skin, Cuts, Scrapes, Sprains, Bruises, and More

Along with Information about Prevention, Self-Care, Choosing a Doctor, Over-the-Counter Medications, Folk Remedies, and Alternative Therapies, and Including a Glossary of Important Terms and a Directory of Resources for Further Help and Information

Edited by Chad T. Kimball. 638 pages. 2001. 978-0-7808-0435-7.

"A good starting point for research on common illnesses. It will be a useful addition to public and consumer health library collections."
—*American Reference Books Annual, 2002*

"Will prove valuable to any library seeking to maintain a current, comprehensive reference collection of health resources. . . . Excellent reference."
—*The Bookwatch, Aug '01*

"Recommended reference source."
—*Booklist, American Library Association, Jul '01*

■

Communication Disorders Sourcebook

Basic Information about Deafness and Hearing Loss, Speech and Language Disorders, Voice Disorders, Balance and Vestibular Disorders, and Disorders of Smell, Taste, and Touch

Edited by Linda M. Ross. 533 pages. 1996. 978-0-7808-0077-9.

"This is skillfully edited and is a welcome resource for the layperson. It should be found in every public and medical library." —*Booklist Health Sciences Supplement, American Library Association, Oct '97*

■

Complementary & Alternative Medicine Sourcebook, 3rd Edition

Basic Consumer Health Information about Complementary and Alternative Medical Therapies, Including Acupuncture, Ayurveda, Traditional Chinese Medicine, Herbal Medicine, Homeopathy, Naturopathy, Biofeedback, Hypnotherapy, Yoga, Art Therapy, Aromatherapy, Clinical Nutrition, Vitamin and Mineral Supplements, Chiropractic, Massage, Reflexology, Crystal Therapy, Therapeutic Touch, and More

Along with Facts about Alternative and Complementary Treatments for Specific Conditions Such as Cancer, Diabetes, Osteoarthritis, Chronic Pain, Menopause, Gastrointestinal Disorders, Headaches, and Mental Illness, a Glossary, and a Resource List for Additional Help and Information

Edited by Sandra J. Judd. 657 pages. 2006. 978-0-7808-0864-5.

"Recommended for public, high school, and academic libraries that have consumer health collections. Hospital libraries that also serve the public will find this to be a useful resource." —*E-Streams, Feb '03*

"Recommended reference source."
—*Booklist, American Library Association, Jan '03*

"An important alternate health reference."
—*MBR Bookwatch, Oct '02*

"A great addition to the reference collection of every type of library." —*American Reference Books Annual, 2000*

■

Congenital Disorders Sourcebook, 2nd Edition

Basic Consumer Health Information about Nonhereditary Birth Defects and Disorders Related to Prematurity, Gestational Injuries, Congenital Infections, and Birth Complications, Including Heart Defects, Hydrocephalus, Spina Bifida, Cleft Lip and Palate, Cerebral Palsy, and More

Along with Facts about the Prevention of Birth Defects, Fetal Surgery and Other Treatment Options, Research Initiatives, a Glossary of Related Terms, and Resources for Additional Information and Support

Edited by Sandra J. Judd. 647 pages. 2006. 978-0-7808-0945-1.

"Recommended reference source."
—*Booklist, American Library Association, Oct '97*

SEE ALSO Pregnancy & Birth Sourcebook

■

Contagious Diseases Sourcebook

Basic Consumer Health Information about Infectious Diseases Spread by Person-to-Person Contact through

Direct Touch, Airborne Transmission, Sexual Contact, or Contact with Blood or Other Body Fluids, Including Hepatitis, Herpes, Influenza, Lice, Measles, Mumps, Pinworm, Ringworm, Severe Acute Respiratory Syndrome (SARS), Streptococcal Infections, Tuberculosis, and Others

Along with Facts about Disease Transmission, Antimicrobial Resistance, and Vaccines, with a Glossary and Directories of Resources for More Information

Edited by Karen Bellenir. 643 pages. 2004. 978-0-7808-0736-5.

"This easy-to-read volume is recommended for consumer health collections within public or academic libraries." — *E-Streams, May '05*

"This informative book is highly recommended for public libraries, consumer health collections, and secondary schools and undergraduate libraries." — *American Reference Books Annual, 2005*

"Excellent reference." — *The Bookwatch, Jan '05*

Death & Dying Sourcebook, 2nd Edition

Basic Consumer Health Information about End-of-Life Care and Related Perspectives and Ethical Issues, Including End-of-Life Symptoms and Treatments, Pain Management, Quality-of-Life Concerns, the Use of Life Support, Patients' Rights and Privacy Issues, Advance Directives, Physician-Assisted Suicide, Caregiving, Organ and Tissue Donation, Autopsies, Funeral Arrangements, and Grief

Along with Statistical Data, Information about the Leading Causes of Death, a Glossary, and Directories of Support Groups and Other Resources

Edited by Joyce Brennfleck Shannon. 653 pages. 2006. 978-0-7808-0871-3.

"Public libraries, medical libraries, and academic libraries will all find this sourcebook a useful addition to their collections." — *American Reference Books Annual, 2001*

"An extremely useful resource for those concerned with death and dying in the United States." — *Respiratory Care, Nov '00*

"Recommended reference source." — *Booklist, American Library Association, Aug '00*

"This book is a definite must for all those involved in end-of-life care." — *Doody's Review Service, 2000*

Dental Care & Oral Health Sourcebook, 2nd Edition

Basic Consumer Health Information about Dental Care, Including Oral Hygiene, Dental Visits, Pain Management, Cavities, Crowns, Bridges, Dental Implants, and Fillings, and Other Oral Health Concerns, Such as Gum Disease, Bad Breath, Dry Mouth, Genetic and Developmental Abnormalities, Oral Cancers, Orthodontics, and Temporomandibular Disorders

Along with Updates on Current Research in Oral Health, a Glossary, a Directory of Dental and Oral Health Organizations, and Resources for People with Dental and Oral Health Disorders

Edited by Amy L. Sutton. 609 pages. 2003. 978-0-7808-0634-4.

"This book could serve as a turning point in the battle to educate consumers in issues concerning oral health." — *American Reference Books Annual, 2004*

"Unique source which will fill a gap in dental sources for patients and the lay public. A valuable reference tool even in a library with thousands of books on dentistry. Comprehensive, clear, inexpensive, and easy to read and use. It fills an enormous gap in the health care literature." — *Reference & User Services Quarterly, American Library Association, Summer '98*

"Recommended reference source." — *Booklist, American Library Association, Dec '97*

Depression Sourcebook

Basic Consumer Health Information about Unipolar Depression, Bipolar Disorder, Postpartum Depression, Seasonal Affective Disorder, and Other Types of Depression in Children, Adolescents, Women, Men, the Elderly, and Other Selected Populations

Along with Facts about Causes, Risk Factors, Diagnostic Criteria, Treatment Options, Coping Strategies, Suicide Prevention, a Glossary, and a Directory of Sources for Additional Help and Information

Edited by Karen Bellenir. 602 pages. 2002. 978-0-7808-0611-5.

"*Depression Sourcebook* is of a very high standard. Its purpose, which is to serve as a reference source to the lay reader, is very well served." — *Journal of the National Medical Association, 2004*

"Invaluable reference for public and school library collections alike." — *Library Bookwatch, Apr '03*

"Recommended for purchase." — *American Reference Books Annual, 2003*

Dermatological Disorders Sourcebook, 2nd Edition

Basic Consumer Health Information about Conditions and Disorders Affecting the Skin, Hair, and Nails, Such as Acne, Rosacea, Rashes, Dermatitis, Pigmentation Disorders, Birthmarks, Skin Cancer, Skin Injuries, Psoriasis, Scleroderma, and Hair Loss, Including Facts about Medications and Treatments for Dermatological Disorders and Tips for Maintaining Healthy Skin, Hair, and Nails

Along with Information about How Aging Affects the Skin, a Glossary of Related Terms, and a Directory of Resources for Additional Help and Information

Edited by Amy L. Sutton. 645 pages. 2005. 978-0-7808-0795-2.

1113

∎

Diabetes Sourcebook, 3rd Edition

Basic Consumer Health Information about Type 1 Diabetes (Insulin-Dependent or Juvenile-Onset Diabetes), Type 2 Diabetes (Noninsulin-Dependent or Adult-Onset Diabetes), Gestational Diabetes, Impaired Glucose Tolerance (IGT), and Related Complications, Such as Amputation, Eye Disease, Gum Disease, Nerve Damage, and End-Stage Renal Disease, Including Facts about Insulin, Oral Diabetes Medications, Blood Sugar Testing, and the Role of Exercise and Nutrition in the Control of Diabetes

Along with a Glossary and Resources for Further Help and Information

Edited by Dawn D. Matthews. 622 pages. 2003. 978-0-7808-0629-0.

"This edition is even more helpful than earlier versions. . . . It is a truly valuable tool for anyone seeking readable and authoritative information on diabetes."
— *American Reference Books Annual, 2004*

"An invaluable reference." — *Library Journal, May '00*

Selected as one of the 250 "Best Health Sciences Books of 1999." — *Doody's Rating Service, Mar-Apr '00*

"Provides useful information for the general public."
— *Healthlines, University of Michigan Health Management Research Center, Sep/Oct '99*

". . . provides reliable mainstream medical information . . . belongs on the shelves of any library with a consumer health collection." — *E-Streams, Sep '99*

"Recommended reference source."
— *Booklist, American Library Association, Feb '99*

∎

Diet & Nutrition Sourcebook, 3rd Edition

Basic Consumer Health Information about Dietary Guidelines and the Food Guidance System, Recommended Daily Nutrient Intakes, Serving Proportions, Weight Control, Vitamins and Supplements, Nutrition Issues for Different Life Stages and Lifestyles, and the Needs of People with Specific Medical Concerns, Including Cancer, Celiac Disease, Diabetes, Eating Disorders, Food Allergies, and Cardiovascular Disease

Along with Facts about Federal Nutrition Support Programs, a Glossary of Nutrition and Dietary Terms, and Directories of Additional Resources for More Information about Nutrition

Edited by Joyce Brennfleck Shannon. 633 pages. 2006. 978-0-7808-0800-3.

"This book is an excellent source of basic diet and nutrition information." — *Booklist Health Sciences Supplement, American Library Association, Dec '00*

"This reference document should be in any public library, but it would be a very good guide for beginning students in the health sciences. If the other books in this publisher's series are as good as this, they should all be in the health sciences collections."
— *American Reference Books Annual, 2000*

"This book is an excellent general nutrition reference for consumers who desire to take an active role in their health care for prevention. Consumers of all ages who select this book can feel confident they are receiving current and accurate information." — *Journal of Nutrition for the Elderly, Vol. 19, No. 4, 2000*

SEE ALSO Digestive Diseases & Disorders Sourcebook, Eating Disorders Sourcebook, Gastrointestinal Diseases & Disorders Sourcebook, Vegetarian Sourcebook

∎

Digestive Diseases & Disorders Sourcebook

Basic Consumer Health Information about Diseases and Disorders that Impact the Upper and Lower Digestive System, Including Celiac Disease, Constipation, Crohn's Disease, Cyclic Vomiting Syndrome, Diarrhea, Diverticulosis and Diverticulitis, Gallstones, Heartburn, Hemorrhoids, Hernias, Indigestion (Dyspepsia), Irritable Bowel Syndrome, Lactose Intolerance, Ulcers, and More

Along with Information about Medications and Other Treatments, Tips for Maintaining a Healthy Digestive Tract, a Glossary, and Directory of Digestive Diseases Organizations

Edited by Karen Bellenir. 335 pages. 2000. 978-0-7808-0327-5.

"This title would be an excellent addition to all public or patient-research libraries."
— *American Reference Books Annual, 2001*

"This title is recommended for public, hospital, and health sciences libraries with consumer health collections." — *E-Streams, Jul-Aug '00*

"Recommended reference source."
— *Booklist, American Library Association, May '00*

SEE ALSO Eating Disorders Sourcebook, Gastrointestinal Diseases & Disorders Sourcebook

∎

Disabilities Sourcebook

Basic Consumer Health Information about Physical and Psychiatric Disabilities, Including Descriptions of Major Causes of Disability, Assistive and Adaptive Aids, Workplace Issues, and Accessibility Concerns

Along with Information about the Americans with Disabilities Act, a Glossary, and Resources for Additional Help and Information

Edited by Dawn D. Matthews. 616 pages. 2000. 978-0-7808-0389-3.

"It is a must for libraries with a consumer health section." — *American Reference Books Annual, 2002*

"A much needed addition to the Omnigraphics *Health Reference Series*. A current reference work to provide people with disabilities, their families, caregivers or those who work with them, a broad range of information in one volume, has not been available until now. . . . It is recommended for all public and academic library reference collections." — *E-Streams, May '01*

"An excellent source book in easy-to-read format covering many current topics; highly recommended for all libraries." — *Choice, Association of College & Research Libraries, Jan '01*

"Recommended reference source." — *Booklist, American Library Association, Jul '00*

■

Domestic Violence Sourcebook, 2nd Edition

Basic Consumer Health Information about the Causes and Consequences of Abusive Relationships, Including Physical Violence, Sexual Assault, Battery, Stalking, and Emotional Abuse, and Facts about the Effects of Violence on Women, Men, Young Adults, and the Elderly, with Reports about Domestic Violence in Selected Populations, and Featuring Facts about Medical Care, Victim Assistance and Protection, Prevention Strategies, Mental Health Services, and Legal Issues

Along with a Glossary of Related Terms and Resources for Additional Help and Information

Edited by Dawn D. Matthews. 628 pages. 2004. 978-0-7808-0669-6.

"Educators, clergy, medical professionals, police, and victims and their families will benefit from this realistic and easy-to-understand resource." — *American Reference Books Annual, 2005*

"Recommended for all collections supporting consumer health information. It should also be considered for any collection needing general, readable information on domestic violence." — *E-Streams, Jan '05*

"This sourcebook complements other books in its field, providing a one-stop resource . . . Recommended." — *Choice, Association of College & Research Libraries, Jan '05*

"Interested lay persons should find the book extremely beneficial. . . . A copy of *Domestic Violence and Child Abuse Sourcebook* should be in every public library in the United States." — *Social Science & Medicine, No. 56, 2003*

"This is important information. The Web has many resources but this sourcebook fills an important societal need. I am not aware of any other resources of this type." — *Doody's Review Service, Sep '01*

"Recommended reference source." — *Booklist, American Library Association, Apr '01*

"Important pick for college-level health reference libraries." — *The Bookwatch, Mar '01*

"Because this problem is so widespread and because this book includes a lot of issues within one volume, this work is recommended for all public libraries." — *American Reference Books Annual, 2001*

SEE ALSO *Child Abuse Sourcebook*

■

Drug Abuse Sourcebook, 2nd Edition

Basic Consumer Health Information about Illicit Substances of Abuse and the Misuse of Prescription and Over-the-Counter Medications, Including Depressants, Hallucinogens, Inhalants, Marijuana, Stimulants, and Anabolic Steroids

Along with Facts about Related Health Risks, Treatment Programs, Prevention Programs, a Glossary of Abuse and Addiction Terms, a Glossary of Drug-Related Street Terms, and a Directory of Resources for More Information

Edited by Catherine Ginther. 607 pages. 2004. 978-0-7808-0740-2.

"Commendable for organizing useful, normally scattered government and association-produced data into a logical sequence." — *American Reference Books Annual, 2006*

"This easy-to-read volume is recommended for consumer health collections within public or academic libraries." — *E-Streams, Sep '05*

"An excellent library reference." — *The Bookwatch, May '05*

"Containing a wealth of information, this book will be useful to the college student just beginning to explore the topic of substance abuse. This resource belongs in libraries that serve a lower-division undergraduate or community college clientele as well as the general public." — *Choice, Association of College & Research Libraries, Jun '01*

"Recommended reference source." — *Booklist, American Library Association, Feb '01*

SEE ALSO *Alcoholism Sourcebook*

■

Ear, Nose & Throat Disorders Sourcebook, 2nd Edition

Basic Consumer Health Information about Disorders of the Ears, Hearing Loss, Vestibular Disorders, Nasal and Sinus Problems, Throat and Vocal Cord Disorders, and Otolaryngologic Cancers, Including Facts about Ear Infections and Injuries, Genetic and Congenital Deafness, Sensorineural Hearing Disorders, Tinnitus, Vertigo, Ménière Disease, Rhinitis, Sinusitis, Snoring, Sore Throats, Hoarseness, and More

Along with Reports on Current Research Initiatives, a Glossary of Related Medical Terms, and a Directory of Sources for Further Help and Information

Edited by Sandra J. Judd. 659 pages. 2006. 978-0-7808-0872-0.

"Overall, this sourcebook is helpful for the consumer seeking information on ENT issues. It is recommended for public libraries."
— *American Reference Books Annual, 1999*

"Recommended reference source."
— *Booklist, American Library Association, Dec '98*

Eating Disorders Sourcebook, 2nd Edition

Basic Consumer Health Information about Anorexia Nervosa, Bulimia Nervosa, Binge Eating, Compulsive Exercise, Female Athlete Triad, and Other Eating Disorders, Including Facts about Body Image and Other Cultural and Age-Related Risk Factors, Prevention Efforts, Adverse Health Effects, Treatment Options, and the Recovery Process

Along with Guidelines for Healthy Weight Control, a Glossary, and Directories of Additional Resources

Edited by Joyce Brennfleck Shannon. 585 pages. 2007. 978-0-7808-0948-2.

"Recommended for health science libraries that are open to the public, as well as hospital libraries. This book is a good resource for the consumer who is concerned about eating disorders." — *E-Streams, Mar '02*

"This volume is another convenient collection of excerpted articles. Recommended for school and public library patrons; lower-division undergraduates; and two-year technical program students."
— *Choice, Association of College & Research Libraries, Jan '02*

"Recommended reference source."
— *Booklist, American Library Association, Oct '01*

SEE ALSO *Diet & Nutrition Sourcebook, Digestive Diseases & Disorders Sourcebook, Gastrointestinal Diseases & Disorders Sourcebook*

Emergency Medical Services Sourcebook

Basic Consumer Health Information about Preventing, Preparing for, and Managing Emergency Situations, When and Who to Call for Help, What to Expect in the Emergency Room, the Emergency Medical Team, Patient Issues, and Current Topics in Emergency Medicine

Along with Statistical Data, a Glossary, and Sources of Additional Help and Information

Edited by Jenni Lynn Colson. 494 pages. 2002. 978-0-7808-0420-3.

"Handy and convenient for home, public, school, and college libraries. Recommended."
— *Choice, Association of College & Research Libraries, Apr '03*

"This reference can provide the consumer with answers to most questions about emergency care in the United States, or it will direct them to a resource where the answer can be found."
— *American Reference Books Annual, 2003*

"Recommended reference source."
— *Booklist, American Library Association, Feb '03*

Endocrine & Metabolic Disorders Sourcebook

Basic Information for the Layperson about Pancreatic and Insulin-Related Disorders Such as Pancreatitis, Diabetes, and Hypoglycemia; Adrenal Gland Disorders Such as Cushing's Syndrome, Addison's Disease, and Congenital Adrenal Hyperplasia; Pituitary Gland Disorders Such as Growth Hormone Deficiency, Acromegaly, and Pituitary Tumors; Thyroid Disorders Such as Hypothyroidism, Graves' Disease, Hashimoto's Disease, and Goiter; Hyperparathyroidism; and Other Diseases and Syndromes of Hormone Imbalance or Metabolic Dysfunction

Along with Reports on Current Research Initiatives

Edited by Linda M. Shin. 574 pages. 1998. 978-0-7808-0207-0.

"Omnigraphics has produced another needed resource for health information consumers."
— *American Reference Books Annual, 2000*

"Recommended reference source."
— *Booklist, American Library Association, Dec '98*

Environmental Health Sourcebook, 2nd Edition

Basic Consumer Health Information about the Environment and Its Effect on Human Health, Including the Effects of Air Pollution, Water Pollution, Hazardous Chemicals, Food Hazards, Radiation Hazards, Biological Agents, Household Hazards, Such as Radon, Asbestos, Carbon Monoxide, and Mold, and Information about Associated Diseases and Disorders, Including Cancer, Allergies, Respiratory Problems, and Skin Disorders

Along with Information about Environmental Concerns for Specific Populations, a Glossary of Related Terms, and Resources for Further Help and Information

Edited by Dawn D. Matthews. 673 pages. 2003. 978-0-7808-0632-0.

"This recently updated edition continues the level of quality and the reputation of the numerous other volumes in Omnigraphics' *Health Reference Series*."
— *American Reference Books Annual, 2004*

"An excellent updated edition."
— *The Bookwatch, Oct '03*

"Recommended reference source."
— *Booklist, American Library Association, Sep '98*

"This book will be a useful addition to anyone's library." — *Choice Health Sciences Supplement, Association of College & Research Libraries, May '98*

". . . a good survey of numerous environmentally induced physical disorders . . . a useful addition to anyone's library."
— *Doody's Health Sciences Book Reviews, Jan '98*

Ethnic Diseases Sourcebook

Basic Consumer Health Information for Ethnic and Racial Minority Groups in the United States, Including General Health Indicators and Behaviors, Ethnic Diseases, Genetic Testing, the Impact of Chronic Diseases, Women's Health, Mental Health Issues, and Preventive Health Care Services

Along with a Glossary and a Listing of Additional Resources

Edited by Joyce Brennfleck Shannon. 664 pages. 2001. 978-0-7808-0336-7.

"Recommended for health sciences libraries where public health programs are a priority."
— *E-Streams, Jan '02*

"Not many books have been written on this topic to date, and the *Ethnic Diseases Sourcebook* is a strong addition to the list. It will be an important introductory resource for health consumers, students, health care personnel, and social scientists. It is recommended for public, academic, and large hospital libraries."
— *American Reference Books Annual, 2002*

"Recommended reference source."
— *Booklist, American Library Association, Oct '01*

"Will prove valuable to any library seeking to maintain a current, comprehensive reference collection of health resources. . . . An excellent source of health information about genetic disorders which affect particular ethnic and racial minorities in the U.S."
— *The Bookwatch, Aug '01*

Eye Care Sourcebook, 2nd Edition

Basic Consumer Health Information about Eye Care and Eye Disorders, Including Facts about the Diagnosis, Prevention, and Treatment of Common Refractive Problems Such as Myopia, Hyperopia, Astigmatism, and Presbyopia, and Eye Diseases, Including Glaucoma, Cataract, Age-Related Macular Degeneration, and Diabetic Retinopathy

Along with a Section on Vision Correction and Refractive Surgeries, Including LASIK and LASEK, a Glossary, and Directories of Resources for Additional Help and Information

Edited by Amy L. Sutton. 543 pages. 2003. 978-0-7808-0635-1.

". . . a solid reference tool for eye care and a valuable addition to a collection."
— *American Reference Books Annual, 2004*

Family Planning Sourcebook

Basic Consumer Health Information about Planning for Pregnancy and Contraception, Including Traditional Methods, Barrier Methods, Hormonal Methods, Permanent Methods, Future Methods, Emergency Contraception, and Birth Control Choices for Women at Each Stage of Life

Along with Statistics, a Glossary, and Sources of Additional Information

Edited by Amy Marcaccio Keyzer. 520 pages. 2001. 978-0-7808-0379-4.

"Recommended for public, health, and undergraduate libraries as part of the circulating collection."
— *E-Streams, Mar '02*

"Information is presented in an unbiased, readable manner, and the sourcebook will certainly be a necessary addition to those public and high school libraries where Internet access is restricted or otherwise problematic." — *American Reference Books Annual, 2002*

"Recommended reference source."
— *Booklist, American Library Association, Oct '01*

"Will prove valuable to any library seeking to maintain a current, comprehensive reference collection of health resources. . . . Excellent reference."
— *The Bookwatch, Aug '01*

SEE ALSO Pregnancy & Birth Sourcebook

Fitness & Exercise Sourcebook, 3rd Edition

Basic Consumer Health Information about the Physical and Mental Benefits of Fitness, Including Cardiorespiratory Endurance, Muscular Strength, Muscular Endurance, and Flexibility, with Facts about Sports Nutrition and Exercise-Related Injuries and Tips about Physical Activity and Exercises for People of All Ages and for People with Health Concerns

Along with Advice on Selecting and Using Exercise Equipment, Maintaining Exercise Motivation, a Glossary of Related Terms, and a Directory of Resources for More Help and Information

Edited by Amy L. Sutton. 663 pages. 2007. 978-0-7808-0946-8.

"This work is recommended for all general reference collections."
— *American Reference Books Annual, 2002*

"Highly recommended for public, consumer, and school grades fourth through college." — *E-Streams, Nov '01*

"Recommended reference source."
— *Booklist, American Library Association, Oct '01*

"The information appears quite comprehensive and is considered reliable. . . . This second edition is a welcomed addition to the series."
— *Doody's Review Service, Sep '01*

Food Safety Sourcebook

Basic Consumer Health Information about the Safe Handling of Meat, Poultry, Seafood, Eggs, Fruit Juices, and Other Food Items, and Facts about Pesticides, Drinking Water, Food Safety Overseas, and the Onset, Duration, and Symptoms of Foodborne Illnesses, Including Types of Pathogenic Bacteria, Parasitic Protozoa, Worms, Viruses, and Natural Toxins

Along with the Role of the Consumer, the Food Hand-ler, and the Government in Food Safety; a Glossary, and Resources for Additional Help and Information

Edited by Dawn D. Matthews. 339 pages. 1999. 978-0-7808-0326-8.

"This book is recommended for public libraries and universities with home economic and food science pro-grams." — E-Streams, Nov '00

"Recommended reference source."
— Booklist, American Library Association, May '00

"This book takes the complex issues of food safety and foodborne pathogens and presents them in an easily understood manner. [It does] an excellent job of cover-ing a large and often confusing topic."
— American Reference Books Annual, 2000

■

Forensic Medicine Sourcebook

Basic Consumer Information for the Layperson about Forensic Medicine, Including Crime Scene Investiga-tion, Evidence Collection and Analysis, Expert Testi-mony, Computer-Aided Criminal Identification, Digi-tal Imaging in the Courtroom, DNA Profiling, Acci-dent Reconstruction, Autopsies, Ballistics, Drugs and Explosives Detection, Latent Fingerprints, Product Tampering, and Questioned Document Examination

Along with Statistical Data, a Glossary of Forensics Terminology, and Listings of Sources for Further Help and Information

Edited by Annemarie S. Muth. 574 pages. 1999. 978-0-7808-0232-2.

"Given the expected widespread interest in its content and its easy to read style, this book is recommended for most public and all college and university libraries."
— E-Streams, Feb '01

"Recommended for public libraries."
— Reference & User Services Quarterly, American Library Association, Spring 2000

"Recommended reference source."
— Booklist, American Library Association, Feb '00

"A wealth of information, useful statistics, references are up-to-date and extremely complete. This wonderful collection of data will help students who are interested in a career in any type of forensic field. It is a great resource for attorneys who need information about types of expert witnesses needed in a particular case. It also offers useful information for fiction and nonfiction writers whose work involves a crime. A fascinating compilation. All levels."
— Choice, Association of College & Research Libraries, Jan '00

"There are several items that make this book attractive to consumers who are seeking certain forensic data. . . . This is a useful current source for those seeking gener-al forensic medical answers."
— American Reference Books Annual, 2000

Gastrointestinal Diseases & Disorders Sourcebook, 2nd Edition

Basic Consumer Health Information about the Upper and Lower Gastrointestinal (GI) Tract, Including the Esophagus, Stomach, Intestines, Rectum, Liver, and Pancreas, with Facts about Gastroesophageal Reflux Disease, Gastritis, Hernias, Ulcers, Celiac Disease, Diverticulitis, Irritable Bowel Syndrome, Hemorrhoids, Gastrointestinal Cancers, and Other Diseases and Dis-orders Related to the Digestive Process

Along with Information about Commonly Used Diagnostic and Surgical Procedures, Statistics, Reports on Current Research Initiatives and Clinical Trials, a Glossary, and Resources for Additional Help and Information

Edited by Sandra J. Judd. 681 pages. 2006. 978-0-7808-0798-3.

". . . very readable form. The successful editorial work that brought this material together into a useful and understandable reference makes accessible to all readers information that can help them more effectively under-stand and obtain help for digestive tract problems."
— Choice, Association of College & Research Libraries, Feb '97

SEE ALSO Diet & Nutrition Sourcebook, Digestive Diseases & Disorders Sourcebook, Eating Disorders Sourcebook

■

Genetic Disorders Sourcebook, 3rd Edition

Basic Consumer Health Information about Hereditary Diseases and Disorders, Including Facts about the Hu-man Genome, Genetic Inheritance Patterns, Disorders Associated with Specific Genes, Such as Sickle Cell Disease, Hemophilia, and Cystic Fibrosis, Chromo-some Disorders, Such as Down Syndrome, Fragile X Syndrome, and Turner Syndrome, and Complex Dis-eases and Disorders Resulting from the Interaction of Environmental and Genetic Factors, Such as Allergies, Cancer, and Obesity

Along with Facts about Genetic Testing, Suggestions for Parents of Children with Special Needs, Reports on Current Research Initiatives, a Glossary of Genetic Terminology, and Resources for Additional Help and Information

Edited by Karen Bellenir. 777 pages. 2004. 978-0-7808-0742-6.

"This text is recommended for any library with an interest in providing consumer health resources."
— E-Streams, Aug '05

"This is a valuable resource for anyone wishing to have an understandable description of any of the topics or disorders included. The editor succeeds in making com-plex genetic issues understandable."
— Doody's Book Review Service, May '05

"A good acquisition for public libraries."
— American Reference Books Annual, 2005

━

Head Trauma Sourcebook

Basic Information for the Layperson about Open-Head and Closed-Head Injuries, Treatment Advances, Recovery, and Rehabilitation

Along with Reports on Current Research Initiatives

Edited by Karen Bellenir. 414 pages. 1997. 978-0-7808-0208-7.

Headache Sourcebook

Basic Consumer Health Information about Migraine, Tension, Cluster, Rebound and Other Types of Headaches, with Facts about the Cause and Prevention of Headaches, the Effects of Stress and the Environment, Headaches during Pregnancy and Menopause, and Childhood Headaches

Along with a Glossary and Other Resources for Additional Help and Information

Edited by Dawn D. Matthews. 362 pages. 2002. 978-0-7808-0337-4.

━

Healthy Aging Sourcebook

Basic Consumer Health Information about Maintaining Health through the Aging Process, Including Advice on Nutrition, Exercise, and Sleep, Help in Making Decisions about Midlife Issues and Retirement, and Guidance Concerning Practical and Informed Choices in Health Consumerism

Along with Data Concerning the Theories of Aging, Different Experiences in Aging by Minority Groups, and Facts about Aging Now and Aging in the Future; and Featuring a Glossary, a Guide to Consumer Help, Additional Suggested Reading, and Practical Resource Directory

Edited by Jenifer Swanson. 536 pages. 1999. 978-0-7808-0390-9.

SEE ALSO *Physical & Mental Issues in Aging Sourcebook*

━

Healthy Children Sourcebook

Basic Consumer Health Information about the Physical and Mental Development of Children between the Ages of 3 and 12, Including Routine Health Care, Preventative Health Services, Safety and First Aid,

Healthy Sleep, Dental Care, Nutrition, and Fitness, and Featuring Parenting Tips on Such Topics as Bedwetting, Choosing Day Care, Monitoring TV and Other Media, and Establishing a Foundation for Substance Abuse Prevention

Along with a Glossary of Commonly Used Pediatric Terms and Resources for Additional Help and Information

Edited by Chad T. Kimball. 647 pages. 2003. 978-0-7808-0247-6.

SEE ALSO *Childhood Diseases & Disorders Sourcebook*

━

Healthy Heart Sourcebook for Women

Basic Consumer Health Information about Cardiac Issues Specific to Women, Including Facts about Major Risk Factors and Prevention, Treatment and Control Strategies, and Important Dietary Issues

Along with a Special Section Regarding the Pros and Cons of Hormone Replacement Therapy and Its Impact on Heart Health, and Additional Help, Including Recipes, a Glossary, and a Directory of Resources

Edited by Dawn D. Matthews. 336 pages. 2000. 978-0-7808-0329-9.

SEE ALSO *Cardiovascular Diseases & Disorders Sourcebook, Women's Health Concerns Sourcebook*

━

Hepatitis Sourcebook

Basic Consumer Health Information about Hepatitis A, Hepatitis B, Hepatitis C, and Other Forms of Hepatitis, Including Autoimmune Hepatitis, Alcoholic Hepatitis, Nonalcoholic Steatohepatitis, and Toxic Hepatitis, with

Facts about Risk Factors, Screening Methods, Diagnostic Tests, and Treatment Options

Along with Information on Liver Health, Tips for People Living with Chronic Hepatitis, Reports on Current Research Initiatives, a Glossary of Terms Related to Hepatitis, and a Directory of Sources for Further Help and Information

Edited by Sandra J. Judd. 597 pages. 2005. 978-0-7808-0749-5.

"Highly recommended."
— American Reference Books Annual, 2006

◼

Household Safety Sourcebook

Basic Consumer Health Information about Household Safety, Including Information about Poisons, Chemicals, Fire, and Water Hazards in the Home

Along with Advice about the Safe Use of Home Maintenance Equipment, Choosing Toys and Nursery Furniture, Holiday and Recreation Safety, a Glossary, and Resources for Further Help and Information

Edited by Dawn D. Matthews. 606 pages. 2002. 978-0-7808-0338-1.

"This work will be useful in public libraries with large consumer health and wellness departments."
— American Reference Books Annual, 2003

"As a sourcebook on household safety this book meets its mark. It is encyclopedic in scope and covers a wide range of safety issues that are commonly seen in the home."
— E-Streams, Jul '02

◼

Hypertension Sourcebook

Basic Consumer Health Information about the Causes, Diagnosis, and Treatment of High Blood Pressure, with Facts about Consequences, Complications, and Co-Occurring Disorders, Such as Coronary Heart Disease, Diabetes, Stroke, Kidney Disease, and Hypertensive Retinopathy, and Issues in Blood Pressure Control, Including Dietary Choices, Stress Management, and Medications

Along with Reports on Current Research Initiatives and Clinical Trials, a Glossary, and Resources for Additional Help and Information

Edited by Dawn D. Matthews and Karen Bellenir. 613 pages. 2004. 978-0-7808-0674-0.

"Academic, public, and medical libraries will want to add the Hypertension Sourcebook to their collections."
— E-Streams, Aug '05

"The strength of this source is the wide range of information given about hypertension."
— American Reference Books Annual, 2005

◼

Immune System Disorders Sourcebook, 2nd Edition

Basic Consumer Health Information about Disorders of the Immune System, Including Immune System Function and Response, Diagnosis of Immune Disorders, Information about Inherited Immune Disease, Acquired Immune Disease, and Autoimmune Diseases, Including Primary Immune Deficiency, Acquired Immunodeficiency Syndrome (AIDS), Lupus, Multiple Sclerosis, Type 1 Diabetes, Rheumatoid Arthritis, and Graves' Disease

Along with Treatments, Tips for Coping with Immune Disorders, a Glossary, and a Directory of Additional Resources.

Edited by Joyce Brennfleck Shannon. 671 pages. 2005. 978-0-7808-0748-8.

"Highly recommended for academic and public libraries." — American Reference Books Annual, 2006

"The updated second edition is a 'must' for any consumer health library seeking a solid resource covering the treatments, symptoms, and options for immune disorder sufferers. . . . An excellent guide."
— MBR Bookwatch, Jan '06

◼

Infant & Toddler Health Sourcebook

Basic Consumer Health Information about the Physical and Mental Development of Newborns, Infants, and Toddlers, Including Neonatal Concerns, Nutrition Recommendations, Immunization Schedules, Common Pediatric Disorders, Assessments and Milestones, Safety Tips, and Advice for Parents and Other Caregivers

Along with a Glossary of Terms and Resource Listings for Additional Help

Edited by Jenifer Swanson. 585 pages. 2000. 978-0-7808-0246-9.

"As a reference for the general public, this would be useful in any library." — E-Streams, May '01

"Recommended reference source."
— Booklist, American Library Association, Feb '01

"This is a good source for general use."
— American Reference Books Annual, 2001

◼

Infectious Diseases Sourcebook

Basic Consumer Health Information about Non-Contagious Bacterial, Viral, Prion, Fungal, and Parasitic Diseases Spread by Food and Water, Insects and Animals, or Environmental Contact, Including Botulism, E. Coli, Encephalitis, Legionnaires' Disease, Lyme Disease, Malaria, Plague, Rabies, Salmonella, Tetanus, and Others, and Facts about Newly Emerging Diseases, Such as Hantavirus, Mad Cow Disease, Monkeypox, and West Nile Virus

Along with Information about Preventing Disease Transmission, the Threat of Bioterrorism, and Current Research Initiatives, with a Glossary and Directory of Resources for More Information

Edited by Karen Bellenir. 634 pages. 2004. 978-0-7808-0675-7.

■

Injury & Trauma Sourcebook

Basic Consumer Health Information about the Impact of Injury, the Diagnosis and Treatment of Common and Traumatic Injuries, Emergency Care, and Specific Injuries Related to Home, Community, Workplace, Transportation, and Recreation

Along with Guidelines for Injury Prevention, a Glossary, and a Directory of Additional Resources

Edited by Joyce Brennfleck Shannon. 696 pages. 2002. 978-0-7808-0421-0.

■

Kidney & Urinary Tract Diseases & Disorders Sourcebook

SEE Urinary Tract & Kidney Diseases & Disorders Sourcebook

■

Learning Disabilities Sourcebook, 2nd Edition

Basic Consumer Health Information about Learning Disabilities, Including Dyslexia, Developmental Speech and Language Disabilities, Non-Verbal Learning Disorders, Developmental Arithmetic Disorder, Developmental Writing Disorder, and Other Conditions That Impede Learning Such as Attention Deficit/Hyperactivity Disorder, Brain Injury, Hearing Impairment, Klinefelter Syndrome, Dyspraxia, and Tourette's Syndrome

Along with Facts about Educational Issues and Assistive Technology, Coping Strategies, a Glossary of Related Terms, and Resources for Further Help and Information

Edited by Dawn D. Matthews. 621 pages. 2003. 978-0-7808-0626-9.

■

Leukemia Sourcebook

Basic Consumer Health Information about Adult and Childhood Leukemias, Including Acute Lymphocytic Leukemia (ALL), Chronic Lymphocytic Leukemia (CLL), Acute Myelogenous Leukemia (AML), Chronic Myelogenous Leukemia (CML), and Hairy Cell Leukemia, and Treatments Such as Chemotherapy, Radiation Therapy, Peripheral Blood Stem Cell and Marrow Transplantation, and Immunotherapy

Along with Tips for Life During and After Treatment, a Glossary, and Directories of Additional Resources

Edited by Joyce Brennfleck Shannon. 587 pages. 2003. 978-0-7808-0627-6.

Liver Disorders Sourcebook

Basic Consumer Health Information about the Liver and How It Works; Liver Diseases, Including Cancer, Cirrhosis, Hepatitis, and Toxic and Drug Related Diseases; Tips for Maintaining a Healthy Liver; Laboratory Tests, Radiology Tests, and Facts about Liver Transplantation

Along with a Section on Support Groups, a Glossary, and Resource Listings

Edited by Joyce Brennfleck Shannon. 591 pages. 2000. 978-0-7808-0383-1.

"A valuable resource."
— *American Reference Books Annual, 2001*

"This title is recommended for health sciences and public libraries with consumer health collections."
— *E-Streams, Oct '00*

"Recommended reference source."
— *Booklist, American Library Association, Jun '00*

■

Lung Disorders Sourcebook

Basic Consumer Health Information about Emphysema, Pneumonia, Tuberculosis, Asthma, Cystic Fibrosis, and Other Lung Disorders, Including Facts about Diagnostic Procedures, Treatment Strategies, Disease Prevention Efforts, and Such Risk Factors as Smoking, Air Pollution, and Exposure to Asbestos, Radon, and Other Agents

Along with a Glossary and Resources for Additional Help and Information

Edited by Dawn D. Matthews. 678 pages. 2002. 978-0-7808-0339-8.

"This title is a great addition for public and school libraries because it provides concise health information on the lungs."
— *American Reference Books Annual, 2003*

"Highly recommended for academic and medical reference collections." — *Library Bookwatch, Sep '02*

SEE ALSO *Respiratory Diseases & Disorders Sourcebook*

■

Medical Tests Sourcebook, 2nd Edition

Basic Consumer Health Information about Medical Tests, Including Age-Specific Health Tests, Important Health Screenings and Exams, Home-Use Tests, Blood and Specimen Tests, Electrical Tests, Scope Tests, Genetic Testing, and Imaging Tests, Such as X-Rays, Ultrasound, Computed Tomography, Magnetic Resonance Imaging, Angiography, and Nuclear Medicine

Along with a Glossary and Directory of Additional Resources

Edited by Joyce Brennfleck Shannon. 654 pages. 2004. 978-0-7808-0670-2.

"Recommended for hospital and health sciences

libraries with consumer health collections."
— *E-Streams, Mar '00*

"This is an overall excellent reference with a wealth of general knowledge that may aid those who are reluctant to get vital tests performed."
— *Today's Librarian, Jan '00*

"A valuable reference guide."
— *American Reference Books Annual, 2000*

■

Men's Health Concerns Sourcebook, 2nd Edition

Basic Consumer Health Information about the Medical and Mental Concerns of Men, Including Theories about the Shorter Male Lifespan, the Leading Causes of Death and Disability, Physical Concerns of Special Significance to Men, Reproductive and Sexual Concerns, Sexually Transmitted Diseases, Men's Mental and Emotional Health, and Lifestyle Choices That Affect Wellness, Such as Nutrition, Fitness, and Substance Use

Along with a Glossary of Related Terms and a Directory of Organizational Resources in Men's Health

Edited by Robert Aquinas McNally. 644 pages. 2004. 978-0-7808-0671-9.

"A very accessible reference for non-specialist general readers and consumers." — *The Bookwatch, Jun '04*

"This comprehensive resource and the series are highly recommended."
— *American Reference Books Annual, 2000*

"Recommended reference source."
— *Booklist, American Library Association, Dec '98*

■

Mental Health Disorders Sourcebook, 3rd Edition

Basic Consumer Health Information about Mental and Emotional Health and Mental Illness, Including Facts about Depression, Bipolar Disorder, and Other Mood Disorders, Phobias, Post-Traumatic Stress Disorder (PTSD), Obsessive-Compulsive Disorder, and Other Anxiety Disorders, Impulse Control Disorders, Eating Disorders, Personality Disorders, and Psychotic Disorders, Including Schizophrenia and Dissociative Disorders

Along with Statistical Information, a Special Section Concerning Mental Health Issues in Children and Adolescents, a Glossary, and Directories of Resources for Additional Help and Information

Edited by Karen Bellenir. 661 pages. 2005. 978-0-7808-0747-1.

"Recommended for public libraries and academic libraries with an undergraduate program in psychology."
— *American Reference Books Annual, 2006*

"Recommended reference source."
— *Booklist, American Library Association, Jun '00*

Mental Retardation Sourcebook

Basic Consumer Health Information about Mental Retardation and Its Causes, Including Down Syndrome, Fetal Alcohol Syndrome, Fragile X Syndrome, Genetic Conditions, Injury, and Environmental Sources

Along with Preventive Strategies, Parenting Issues, Educational Implications, Health Care Needs, Employment and Economic Matters, Legal Issues, a Glossary, and a Resource Listing for Additional Help and Information

Edited by Joyce Brennfleck Shannon. 642 pages. 2000. 978-0-7808-0377-0.

"Public libraries will find the book useful for reference and as a beginning research point for students, parents, and caregivers."
— *American Reference Books Annual, 2001*

"The strength of this work is that it compiles many basic fact sheets and addresses for further information in one volume. It is intended and suitable for the general public. This sourcebook is relevant to any collection providing health information to the general public."
— *E-Streams, Nov '00*

"From preventing retardation to parenting and family challenges, this covers health, social and legal issues and will prove an invaluable overview."
— *Reviewer's Bookwatch, Jul '00*

■

Movement Disorders Sourcebook

Basic Consumer Health Information about Neurological Movement Disorders, Including Essential Tremor, Parkinson's Disease, Dystonia, Cerebral Palsy, Huntington's Disease, Myasthenia Gravis, Multiple Sclerosis, and Other Early-Onset and Adult-Onset Movement Disorders, Their Symptoms and Causes, Diagnostic Tests, and Treatments

Along with Mobility and Assistive Technology Information, a Glossary, and a Directory of Additional Resources

Edited by Joyce Brennfleck Shannon. 655 pages. 2003. 978-0-7808-0628-3.

". . . a good resource for consumers and recommended for public, community college and undergraduate libraries." — *American Reference Books Annual, 2004*

■

Muscular Dystrophy Sourcebook

Basic Consumer Health Information about Congenital, Childhood-Onset, and Adult-Onset Forms of Muscular Dystrophy, Such as Duchenne, Becker, Emery-Dreifuss, Distal, Limb-Girdle, Facioscapulohumeral (FSHD), Myotonic, and Ophthalmoplegic Muscular Dystrophies, Including Facts about Diagnostic Tests, Medical and Physical Therapies, Management of Co-Occurring Conditions, and Parenting Guidelines

Along with Practical Tips for Home Care, a Glossary, and Directories of Additional Resources

Edited by Joyce Brennfleck Shannon. 577 pages. 2004. 978-0-7808-0676-4.

"This book is highly recommended for public and academic libraries as well as health care offices that support the information needs of patients and their families."
— *E-Streams, Apr '05*

"Excellent reference." — *The Bookwatch, Jan '05*

■

Obesity Sourcebook

Basic Consumer Health Information about Diseases and Other Problems Associated with Obesity, and Including Facts about Risk Factors, Prevention Issues, and Management Approaches

Along with Statistical and Demographic Data, Information about Special Populations, Research Updates, a Glossary, and Source Listings for Further Help and Information

Edited by Wilma Caldwell and Chad T. Kimball. 376 pages. 2001. 978-0-7808-0333-6.

"The book synthesizes the reliable medical literature on obesity into one easy-to-read and useful resource for the general public."
— *American Reference Books Annual, 2002*

"This is a very useful resource book for the lay public."
— *Doody's Review Service, Nov '01*

"Well suited for the health reference collection of a public library or an academic health science library that serves the general population." — *E-Streams, Sep '01*

"Recommended reference source."
— *Booklist, American Library Association, Apr '01*

"Recommended pick both for specialty health library collections and any general consumer health reference collection." — *The Bookwatch, Apr '01*

■

Oral Health Sourcebook

SEE Dental Care & Oral Health Sourcebook

■

Osteoporosis Sourcebook

Basic Consumer Health Information about Primary and Secondary Osteoporosis and Juvenile Osteoporosis and Related Conditions, Including Fibrous Dysplasia, Gaucher Disease, Hyperthyroidism, Hypophosphatasia, Myeloma, Osteopetrosis, Osteogenesis Imperfecta, and Paget's Disease

Along with Information about Risk Factors, Treatments, Traditional and Non-Traditional Pain Management, a Glossary of Related Terms, and a Directory of Resources

Edited by Allan R. Cook. 584 pages. 2001. 978-0-7808-0239-1.

"This would be a book to be kept in a staff or patient library. The targeted audience is the layperson, but the therapist who needs a quick bit of information on a particular topic will also find the book useful."
— *Physical Therapy, Jan '02*

"This resource is recommended as a great reference source for public, health, and academic libraries, and is another triumph for the editors of Omnigraphics."
— *American Reference Books Annual, 2002*

"Recommended for all public libraries and general health collections, especially those supporting patient education or consumer health programs."
— *E-Streams, Nov '01*

"Will prove valuable to any library seeking to maintain a current, comprehensive reference collection of health resources. . . . From prevention to treatment and associated conditions, this provides an excellent survey."
— *The Bookwatch, Aug '01*

"Recommended reference source."
— *Booklist, American Library Association, Jul '01*

SEE ALSO *Healthy Aging Sourcebook, Physical & Mental Issues in Aging Sourcebook, Women's Health Concerns Sourcebook*

■

Pain Sourcebook, 2nd Edition

Basic Consumer Health Information about Specific Forms of Acute and Chronic Pain, Including Muscle and Skeletal Pain, Nerve Pain, Cancer Pain, and Disorders Characterized by Pain, Such as Fibromyalgia, Shingles, Angina, Arthritis, and Headaches

Along with Information about Pain Medications and Management Techniques, Complementary and Alternative Pain Relief Options, Tips for People Living with Chronic Pain, a Glossary, and a Directory of Sources for Further Information

Edited by Karen Bellenir. 670 pages. 2002. 978-0-7808-0612-2.

"A source of valuable information. . . . This book offers help to nonmedical people who need information about pain and pain management. It is also an excellent reference for those who participate in patient education."
— *Doody's Review Service, Sep '02*

"Highly recommended for academic and medical reference collections." — *Library Bookwatch, Sep '02*

"The text is readable, easily understood, and well indexed. This excellent volume belongs in all patient education libraries, consumer health sections of public libraries, and many personal collections."
— *American Reference Books Annual, 1999*

"The information is basic in terms of scholarship and is appropriate for general readers. Written in journalistic style . . . intended for non-professionals. Quite thorough in its coverage of different pain conditions and summarizes the latest clinical information regarding pain treatment." — *Choice, Association of College and Research Libraries, Jun '98*

"Recommended reference source."
— *Booklist, American Library Association, Mar '98*

■

Pediatric Cancer Sourcebook

Basic Consumer Health Information about Leukemias, Brain Tumors, Sarcomas, Lymphomas, and Other Cancers in Infants, Children, and Adolescents, Including Descriptions of Cancers, Treatments, and Coping Strategies

Along with Suggestions for Parents, Caregivers, and Concerned Relatives, a Glossary of Cancer Terms, and Resource Listings

Edited by Edward J. Prucha. 587 pages. 1999. 978-0-7808-0245-2.

"An excellent source of information. Recommended for public, hospital, and health science libraries with consumer health collections." — *E-Streams, Jun '00*

"Recommended reference source."
— *Booklist, American Library Association, Feb '00*

"A valuable addition to all libraries specializing in health services and many public libraries."
— *American Reference Books Annual, 2000*

SEE ALSO *Childhood Diseases & Disorders Sourcebook, Healthy Children Sourcebook*

■

Physical & Mental Issues in Aging Sourcebook

Basic Consumer Health Information on Physical and Mental Disorders Associated with the Aging Process, Including Concerns about Cardiovascular Disease, Pulmonary Disease, Oral Health, Digestive Disorders, Musculoskeletal and Skin Disorders, Metabolic Changes, Sexual and Reproductive Issues, and Changes in Vision, Hearing, and Other Senses

Along with Data about Longevity and Causes of Death, Information on Acute and Chronic Pain, Descriptions of Mental Concerns, a Glossary of Terms, and Resource Listings for Additional Help

Edited by Jenifer Swanson. 660 pages. 1999. 978-0-7808-0233-9.

"This is a treasure of health information for the layperson." — *Choice Health Sciences Supplement, Association of College & Research Libraries, May '00*

"Recommended for public libraries."
— *American Reference Books Annual, 2000*

"Recommended reference source."
— *Booklist, American Library Association, Oct '99*

SEE ALSO *Healthy Aging Sourcebook*

■

Podiatry Sourcebook, 2nd Edition

Basic Consumer Health Information about Disorders, Diseases, Deformities, and Injuries that Affect the Foot and Ankle, Including Sprains, Corns, Calluses, Bunions, Plantar Warts, Plantar Fasciitis, Neuromas, Clubfoot, Flat Feet, Achilles Tendonitis, and Much More

Along with Information about Selecting a Foot Care Specialist, Foot Fitness, Shoes and Socks, Diagnostic Tests and Corrective Procedures, Financial Assistance for Corrective Devices, a Glossary of Related Terms, and a Directory of Resources for Additional Help and Information

Edited by Ivy L. Alexander. 543 pages. 2007. 978-0-7808-0944-4.

"Recommended reference source."
— *Booklist, American Library Association, Feb '02*

"There is a lot of information presented here on a topic that is usually only covered sparingly in most larger comprehensive medical encyclopedias."
— *American Reference Books Annual, 2002*

Pregnancy & Birth Sourcebook, 2nd Edition

Basic Consumer Health Information about Conception and Pregnancy, Including Facts about Fertility, Infertility, Pregnancy Symptoms and Complications, Fetal Growth and Development, Labor, Delivery, and the Postpartum Period, as Well as Information about Maintaining Health and Wellness during Pregnancy and Caring for a Newborn

Along with Information about Public Health Assistance for Low-Income Pregnant Women, a Glossary, and Directories of Agencies and Organizations Providing Help and Support

Edited by Amy L. Sutton. 626 pages. 2004. 978-0-7808-0672-6.

"Will appeal to public and school reference collections strong in medicine and women's health. . . . Deserves a spot on any medical reference shelf."
— *The Bookwatch, Jul '04*

"A well-organized handbook. Recommended."
— *Choice, Association of College & Research Libraries, Apr '98*

"Recommended reference source."
— *Booklist, American Library Association, Mar '98*

"Recommended for public libraries."
— *American Reference Books Annual, 1998*

SEE ALSO *Breastfeeding Sourcebook, Congenital Disorders Sourcebook, Family Planning Sourcebook*

Prostate & Urological Disorders Sourcebook

Basic Consumer Health Information about Urogenital and Sexual Disorders in Men, Including Prostate and Other Andrological Cancers, Prostatitis, Benign Prostatic Hyperplasia, Testicular and Penile Trauma, Cryptorchidism, Peyronie Disease, Erectile Dysfunction, and Male Factor Infertility, and Facts about Commonly Used Tests and Procedures, Such as Prostatectomy, Vasectomy, Vasectomy Reversal, Penile Implants, and Semen Analysis

Along with a Glossary of Andrological Terms and a Directory of Resources for Additional Information

Edited by Karen Bellenir. 631 pages. 2005. 978-0-7808-0797-6.

Prostate Cancer Sourcebook

Basic Consumer Health Information about Prostate Cancer, Including Information about the Associated Risk Factors, Detection, Diagnosis, and Treatment of Prostate Cancer

Along with Information on Non-Malignant Prostate Conditions, and Featuring a Section Listing Support and Treatment Centers and a Glossary of Related Terms

Edited by Dawn D. Matthews. 358 pages. 2001. 978-0-7808-0324-4.

"Recommended reference source."
— *Booklist, American Library Association, Jan '02*

"A valuable resource for health care consumers seeking information on the subject. . . . All text is written in a clear, easy-to-understand language that avoids technical jargon. Any library that collects consumer health resources would strengthen their collection with the addition of the *Prostate Cancer Sourcebook*."
— *American Reference Books Annual, 2002*

SEE ALSO *Men's Health Concerns Sourcebook*

Reconstructive & Cosmetic Surgery Sourcebook

Basic Consumer Health Information on Cosmetic and Reconstructive Plastic Surgery, Including Statistical Information about Different Surgical Procedures, Things to Consider Prior to Surgery, Plastic Surgery Techniques and Tools, Emotional and Psychological Considerations, and Procedure-Specific Information

Along with a Glossary of Terms and a Listing of Resources for Additional Help and Information

Edited by M. Lisa Weatherford. 374 pages. 2001. 978-0-7808-0214-8.

"An excellent reference that addresses cosmetic and medically necessary reconstructive surgeries. . . . The style of the prose is calm and reassuring, discussing the many positive outcomes now available due to advances in surgical techniques."
— *American Reference Books Annual, 2002*

"Recommended for health science libraries that are open to the public, as well as hospital libraries that are open to the patients. This book is a good resource for the consumer interested in plastic surgery."
— *E-Streams, Dec '01*

"Recommended reference source."
— *Booklist, American Library Association, Jul '01*

Rehabilitation Sourcebook

Basic Consumer Health Information about Rehabilitation for People Recovering from Heart Surgery, Spinal Cord Injury, Stroke, Orthopedic Impairments, Amputation, Pulmonary Impairments, Traumatic Injury, and More, Including Physical Therapy, Occupational Therapy, Speech/Language Therapy, Massage Therapy, Dance Therapy, Art Therapy, and Recreational Therapy

Along with Information on Assistive and Adaptive Devices, a Glossary, and Resources for Additional Help and Information

Edited by Dawn D. Matthews. 531 pages. 1999. 978-0-7808-0236-0.

"This is an excellent resource for public library reference and health collections."
— American Reference Books Annual, 2001

"Recommended reference source."
— Booklist, American Library Association, May '00

■

Respiratory Diseases & Disorders Sourcebook

Basic Information about Respiratory Diseases and Disorders, Including Asthma, Cystic Fibrosis, Pneumonia, the Common Cold, Influenza, and Others, Featuring Facts about the Respiratory System, Statistical and Demographic Data, Treatments, Self-Help Management Suggestions, and Current Research Initiatives

Edited by Allan R. Cook and Peter D. Dresser. 771 pages. 1995. 978-0-7808-0037-3.

"Designed for the layperson and for patients and their families coping with respiratory illness. . . . an extensive array of information on diagnosis, treatment, management, and prevention of respiratory illnesses for the general reader." — Choice, Association of College & Research Libraries, Jun '96

"A highly recommended text for all collections. It is a comforting reminder of the power of knowledge that good books carry between their covers."
— Academic Library Book Review, Spring '96

"A comprehensive collection of authoritative information presented in a nontechnical, humanitarian style for patients, families, and caregivers."
— Association of Operating Room Nurses, Sep/Oct '95

SEE ALSO Lung Disorders Sourcebook

■

Sexually Transmitted Diseases Sourcebook, 3rd Edition

Basic Consumer Health Information about Chlamydial Infections, Gonorrhea, Hepatitis, Herpes, HIV/AIDS, Human Papillomavirus, Pubic Lice, Scabies, Syphilis, Trichomoniasis, Vaginal Infections, and Other Sexually Transmitted Diseases, Including Facts about Risk Factors, Symptoms, Diagnosis, Treatment, and the Prevention of Sexually Transmitted Infections

Along with Updates on Current Research Initiatives, a Glossary of Related Terms, and Resources for Additional Help and Information

Edited by Amy L. Sutton. 629 pages. 2006. 978-0-7808-0824-9.

"Recommended for consumer health collections in public libraries, and secondary school and community college libraries."
— American Reference Books Annual, 2002

"Every school and public library should have a copy of this comprehensive and user-friendly reference book."
— Choice, Association of College & Research Libraries, Sep '01

"This is a highly recommended book. This is an especially important book for all school and public libraries."
— AIDS Book Review Journal, Jul-Aug '01

"Recommended reference source."
— Booklist, American Library Association, Apr '01

■

Sleep Disorders Sourcebook, 2nd Edition

Basic Consumer Health Information about Sleep and Sleep Disorders, Including Insomnia, Sleep Apnea, Restless Legs Syndrome, Narcolepsy, Parasomnias, and Other Health Problems That Affect Sleep, Plus Facts about Diagnostic Procedures, Treatment Strategies, Sleep Medications, and Tips for Improving Sleep Quality

Along with a Glossary of Related Terms and Resources for Additional Help and Information

Edited by Amy L. Sutton. 567 pages. 2005. 978-0-7808-0743-3.

"This book will be useful for just about everybody, especially the 40 million Americans with sleep disorders."
— American Reference Books Annual, 2006

"Recommended for public libraries and libraries supporting health care professionals." — E-Streams, Sep '05

". . . key medical library acquisition."
— The Bookwatch, Jun '05

■

Smoking Concerns Sourcebook

Basic Consumer Health Information about Nicotine Addiction and Smoking Cessation, Featuring Facts about the Health Effects of Tobacco Use, Including Lung and Other Cancers, Heart Disease, Stroke, and Respiratory Disorders, Such as Emphysema and Chronic Bronchitis

Along with Information about Smoking Prevention Programs, Suggestions for Achieving and Maintaining a Smoke-Free Lifestyle, Statistics about Tobacco Use, Reports on Current Research Initiatives, a Glossary of Related Terms, and Directories of Resources for Additional Help and Information

Edited by Karen Bellenir. 621 pages. 2004. 978-0-7808-0323-7.

"Provides everything needed for the student or general reader seeking practical details on the effects of tobacco use." — The Bookwatch, Mar '05

"Public libraries and consumer health care libraries will find this work useful."
— American Reference Books Annual, 2005

Sports Injuries Sourcebook, 2nd Edition

Basic Consumer Health Information about the Diagnosis, Treatment, and Rehabilitation of Common Sports-Related Injuries in Children and Adults

Along with Suggestions for Conditioning and Training, Information and Prevention Tips for Injuries Frequently Associated with Specific Sports and Special Populations, a Glossary, and a Directory of Additional Resources

Edited by Joyce Brennfleck Shannon. 614 pages. 2002. 978-0-7808-0604-7.

"This is an excellent reference for consumers and it is recommended for public, community college, and undergraduate libraries."
— American Reference Books Annual, 2003

"Recommended reference source."
— Booklist, American Library Association, Feb '03

■

Stress-Related Disorders Sourcebook

Basic Consumer Health Information about Stress and Stress-Related Disorders, Including Stress Origins and Signals, Environmental Stress at Work and Home, Mental and Emotional Stress Associated with Depression, Post-Traumatic Stress Disorder, Panic Disorder, Suicide, and the Physical Effects of Stress on the Cardiovascular, Immune, and Nervous Systems

Along with Stress Management Techniques, a Glossary, and a Listing of Additional Resources

Edited by Joyce Brennfleck Shannon. 610 pages. 2002. 978-0-7808-0560-6.

"Well written for a general readership, the *Stress-Related Disorders Sourcebook* is a useful addition to the health reference literature."
— American Reference Books Annual, 2003

"I am impressed by the amount of information. It offers a thorough overview of the causes and consequences of stress for the layperson. . . . A well-done and thorough reference guide for professionals and nonprofessionals alike."
— Doody's Review Service, Dec '02

■

Stroke Sourcebook

Basic Consumer Health Information about Stroke, Including Ischemic, Hemorrhagic, Transient Ischemic Attack (TIA), and Pediatric Stroke, Stroke Triggers and Risks, Diagnostic Tests, Treatments, and Rehabilitation Information

Along with Stroke Prevention Guidelines, Legal and Financial Information, a Glossary, and a Directory of Additional Resources

Edited by Joyce Brennfleck Shannon. 606 pages. 2003. 978-0-7808-0630-6.

"This volume is highly recommended and should be in every medical, hospital, and public library."
— American Reference Books Annual, 2004

"Highly recommended for the amount and variety of topics and information covered." — Choice, Nov '03

Surgery Sourcebook

Basic Consumer Health Information about Inpatient and Outpatient Surgeries, Including Cardiac, Vascular, Orthopedic, Ocular, Reconstructive, Cosmetic, Gynecologic, and Ear, Nose, and Throat Procedures and More

Along with Information about Operating Room Policies and Instruments, Laser Surgery Techniques, Hospital Errors, Statistical Data, a Glossary, and Listings of Sources for Further Help and Information

Edited by Annemarie S. Muth and Karen Bellenir. 596 pages. 2002. 978-0-7808-0380-0.

"Large public libraries and medical libraries would benefit from this material in their reference collections."
— American Reference Books Annual, 2004

"Invaluable reference for public and school library collections alike." — Library Bookwatch, Apr '03

■

Thyroid Disorders Sourcebook

Basic Consumer Health Information about Disorders of the Thyroid and Parathyroid Glands, Including Hypothyroidism, Hyperthyroidism, Graves Disease, Hashimoto Thyroiditis, Thyroid Cancer, and Parathyroid Disorders, Featuring Facts about Symptoms, Risk Factors, Tests, and Treatments

Along with Information about the Effects of Thyroid Imbalance on Other Body Systems, Environmental Factors That Affect the Thyroid Gland, a Glossary, and a Directory of Additional Resources

Edited by Joyce Brennfleck Shannon. 599 pages. 2005. 978-0-7808-0745-7.

"Recommended for consumer health collections."
— American Reference Books Annual, 2006

"Highly recommended pick for basic consumer health reference holdings at all levels."
— The Bookwatch, Aug '05

■

Transplantation Sourcebook

Basic Consumer Health Information about Organ and Tissue Transplantation, Including Physical and Financial Preparations, Procedures and Issues Relating to Specific Solid Organ and Tissue Transplants, Rehabilitation, Pediatric Transplant Information, the Future of Transplantation, and Organ and Tissue Donation

Along with a Glossary and Listings of Additional Resources

Edited by Joyce Brennfleck Shannon. 628 pages. 2002. 978-0-7808-0322-0.

"Along with these advances [in transplantation technology] have come a number of daunting questions for potential transplant patients, their families, and their health care providers. This reference text is the best single tool to address many of these questions. . . . It will be a much-needed addition to the reference collections in health care, academic, and large public libraries."
— American Reference Books Annual, 2003

Traveler's Health Sourcebook

Basic Consumer Health Information for Travelers, Including Physical and Medical Preparations, Transportation Health and Safety, Essential Information about Food and Water, Sun Exposure, Insect and Snake Bites, Camping and Wilderness Medicine, and Travel with Physical or Medical Disabilities

Along with International Travel Tips, Vaccination Recommendations, Geographical Health Issues, Disease Risks, a Glossary, and a Listing of Additional Resources

Edited by Joyce Brennfleck Shannon. 613 pages. 2000. 978-0-7808-0384-8.

SEE ALSO Worldwide Health Sourcebook

Urinary Tract & Kidney Diseases & Disorders Sourcebook, 2nd Edition

Basic Consumer Health Information about the Urinary System, Including the Bladder, Urethra, Ureters, and Kidneys, with Facts about Urinary Tract Infections, Incontinence, Congenital Disorders, Kidney Stones, Cancers of the Urinary Tract and Kidneys, Kidney Failure, Dialysis, and Kidney Transplantation

Along with Statistical and Demographic Information, Reports on Current Research in Kidney and Urologic Health, a Summary of Commonly Used Diagnostic Tests, a Glossary of Related Terms, and a Directory of Resources for Additional Help and Information

Edited by Ivy L. Alexander. 649 pages. 2005. 978-0-7808-0750-1.

Vegetarian Sourcebook

Basic Consumer Health Information about Vegetarian Diets, Lifestyle, and Philosophy, Including Definitions of Vegetarianism and Veganism, Tips about Adopting Vegetarianism, Creating a Vegetarian Pantry, and Meeting Nutritional Needs of Vegetarians, with Facts Regarding Vegetarianism's Effect on Pregnant and Lactating Women, Children, Athletes, and Senior Citizens

Along with a Glossary of Commonly Used Vegetarian Terms and Resources for Additional Help and Information

Edited by Chad T. Kimball. 360 pages. 2002. 978-0-7808-0439-5.

SEE ALSO Diet & Nutrition Sourcebook

Women's Health Concerns Sourcebook, 2nd Edition

Basic Consumer Health Information about the Medical and Mental Concerns of Women, Including Maintaining Health and Wellness, Gynecological Concerns, Breast Health, Sexuality and Reproductive Issues, Menopause, Cancer in Women, Leading Causes of Death and Disability among Women, Physical Concerns of Special Significance to Women, and Women's Mental and Emotional Health

Along with a Glossary of Related Terms and Directories of Resources for Additional Help and Information

Edited by Amy L. Sutton. 746 pages. 2004. 978-0-7808-0673-3.

SEE ALSO Breast Cancer Sourcebook, Cancer Sourcebook for Women, Healthy Heart Sourcebook for Women, Osteoporosis Sourcebook

Workplace Health & Safety Sourcebook

Basic Consumer Health Information about Workplace Health and Safety, Including the Effect of Workplace Hazards on the Lungs, Skin, Heart, Ears, Eyes, Brain,

Reproductive Organs, Musculoskeletal System, and Other Organs and Body Parts

Along with Information about Occupational Cancer, Personal Protective Equipment, Toxic and Hazardous Chemicals, Child Labor, Stress, and Workplace Violence

Edited by Chad T. Kimball. 626 pages. 2000. 978-0-7808-0231-5.

"As a reference for the general public, this would be useful in any library."   *— E-Streams, Jun '01*

"Provides helpful information for primary care physicians and other caregivers interested in occupational medicine. . . . General readers; professionals."
— Choice, Association of College & Research Libraries, May '01

"Recommended reference source."
— Booklist, American Library Association, Feb '01

"Highly recommended."   *— The Bookwatch, Jan '01*

■

Worldwide Health Sourcebook

Basic Information about Global Health Issues, Including Malnutrition, Reproductive Health, Disease Dispersion and Prevention, Emerging Diseases, Risky Health Behaviors, and the Leading Causes of Death

Along with Global Health Concerns for Children, Women, and the Elderly, Mental Health Issues, Research and Technology Advancements, and Economic, Environmental, and Political Health Implications, a Glossary, and a Resource Listing for Additional Help and Information

Edited by Joyce Brennfleck Shannon. 614 pages. 2001. 978-0-7808-0330-5.

"Named an Outstanding Academic Title."
— Choice, Association of College & Research Libraries, Jan '02

"Yet another handy but also unique compilation in the extensive *Health Reference Series*, this is a useful work because many of the international publications reprinted or excerpted are not readily available. Highly recommended."   *— Choice, Association of College & Research Libraries, Nov '01*

"Recommended reference source."
— Booklist, American Library Association, Oct '01

SEE ALSO Traveler's Health Sourcebook

Teen Health Series
Helping Young Adults Understand, Manage, and Avoid Serious Illness

List price $65 per volume. **School and library price $58 per volume.**

Alcohol Information for Teens
Health Tips about Alcohol and Alcoholism

Including Facts about Underage Drinking, Preventing Teen Alcohol Use, Alcohol's Effects on the Brain and the Body, Alcohol Abuse Treatment, Help for Children of Alcoholics, and More

Edited by Joyce Brennfleck Shannon. 370 pages. 2005. 978-0-7808-0741-9.

"Boxed facts and tips add visual interest to the well-researched and clearly written text."
— *Curriculum Connection, Apr '06*

Allergy Information for Teens
Health Tips about Allergic Reactions Such as Anaphylaxis, Respiratory Problems, and Rashes

Including Facts about Identifying and Managing Allergies to Food, Pollen, Mold, Animals, Chemicals, Drugs, and Other Substances

Edited by Karen Bellenir. 410 pages. 2006. 978-0-7808-0799-0.

Asthma Information for Teens
Health Tips about Managing Asthma and Related Concerns

Including Facts about Asthma Causes, Triggers, Symptoms, Diagnosis, and Treatment

Edited by Karen Bellenir. 386 pages. 2005. 978-0-7808-0770-9.

"Highly recommended for medical libraries, public school libraries, and public libraries."
— *American Reference Books Annual, 2006*

"It is so clearly written and well organized that even hesitant readers will be able to find the facts they need, whether for reports or personal information. . . . A succinct but complete resource."
— *School Library Journal, Sep '05*

Body Information for Teens
Health Tips about Maintaining Well-Being for a Lifetime

Including Facts about the Development and Functioning of the Body's Systems, Organs, and Structures and the Health Impact of Lifestyle Choices

Edited by Sandra Augustyn Lawton. 458 pages. 2007. 978-0-7808-0443-2.

Cancer Information for Teens
Health Tips about Cancer Awareness, Prevention, Diagnosis, and Treatment

Including Facts about Frequently Occurring Cancers, Cancer Risk Factors, and Coping Strategies for Teens Fighting Cancer or Dealing with Cancer in Friends or Family Members

Edited by Wilma R. Caldwell. 428 pages. 2004. 978-0-7808-0678-8.

"Recommended for school libraries, or consumer libraries that see a lot of use by teens."
— *E-Streams, May '05*

"A valuable educational tool."
— *American Reference Books Annual, 2005*

"Young adults and their parents alike will find this new addition to the *Teen Health Series* an important reference to cancer in teens."
— *Children's Bookwatch, Feb '05*

Complementary and Alternative Medicine Information for Teens
Health Tips about Non-Traditional and Non-Western Medical Practices

Including Information about Acupuncture, Chiropractic Medicine, Dietary and Herbal Supplements, Hypnosis, Massage Therapy, Prayer and Spirituality, Reflexology, Yoga, and More

Edited by Sandra Augustyn Lawton. 405 pages. 2006. 978-0-7808-0966-6.

Diabetes Information for Teens
Health Tips about Managing Diabetes and Preventing Related Complications

Including Information about Insulin, Glucose Control, Healthy Eating, Physical Activity, and Learning to Live with Diabetes

Edited by Sandra Augustyn Lawton. 410 pages. 2006. 978-0-7808-0811-9.

Diet Information for Teens, 2nd Edition

Health Tips about Diet and Nutrition

Including Facts about Dietary Guidelines, Food Groups, Nutrients, Healthy Meals, Snacks, Weight Control, Medical Concerns Related to Diet, and More

Edited by Karen Bellenir. 432 pages. 2006. 978-0-7808-0820-1.

"Full of helpful insights and facts throughout the book. . . . An excellent resource to be placed in public libraries or even in personal collections."
— *American Reference Books Annual, 2002*

"Recommended for middle and high school libraries and media centers as well as academic libraries that educate future teachers of teenagers. It is also a suitable addition to health science libraries that serve patrons who are interested in teen health promotion and education."
— *E-Streams, Oct '01*

"This comprehensive book would be beneficial to collections that need information about nutrition, dietary guidelines, meal planning, and weight control. . . . This reference is so easy to use that its purchase is recommended."
— *The Book Report, Sep-Oct '01*

"This book is written in an easy to understand format describing issues that many teens face every day, and then provides thoughtful explanations so that teens can make informed decisions. This is an interesting book that provides important facts and information for today's teens."
— *Doody's Health Sciences Book Review Journal, Jul-Aug '01*

"A comprehensive compendium of diet and nutrition. The information is presented in a straightforward, plain-spoken manner. This title will be useful to those working on reports on a variety of topics, as well as to general readers concerned about their dietary health."
— *School Library Journal, Jun '01*

Drug Information for Teens, 2nd Edition

Health Tips about the Physical and Mental Effects of Substance Abuse

Including Information about Marijuana, Inhalants, Club Drugs, Stimulants, Hallucinogens, Opiates, Prescription and Over-the-Counter Drugs, Herbal Products, Tobacco, Alcohol, and More

Edited by Sandra Augustyn Lawton. 468 pages. 2006. 978-0-7808-0862-1.

"A clearly written resource for general readers and researchers alike."
— *School Library Journal*

"This book is well-balanced. . . . a must for public and school libraries."
— *VOYA: Voice of Youth Advocates, Dec '03*

"The chapters are quick to make a connection to their teenage reading audience. The prose is straightforward and the book lends itself to spot reading. It should be useful both for practical information and for research, and it is suitable for public and school libraries."
— *American Reference Books Annual, 2003*

"Recommended reference source."
— *Booklist, American Library Association, Feb '03*

"This is an excellent resource for teens and their parents. Education about drugs and substances is key to discouraging teen drug abuse and this book provides this much needed information in a way that is interesting and factual."
— *Doody's Review Service, Dec '02*

Eating Disorders Information for Teens

Health Tips about Anorexia, Bulimia, Binge Eating, and Other Eating Disorders

Including Information on the Causes, Prevention, and Treatment of Eating Disorders, and Such Other Issues as Maintaining Healthy Eating and Exercise Habits

Edited by Sandra Augustyn Lawton. 337 pages. 2005. 978-0-7808-0783-9.

"An excellent resource for teens and those who work with them."
— *VOYA: Voice of Youth Advocates, Apr '06*

"A welcome addition to high school and undergraduate libraries." — *American Reference Books Annual, 2006*

"This book covers the topic in a lucid manner but delves deeper into every aspect of an eating disorder. A solid addition for any nonfiction or reference collection."
— *School Library Journal, Dec '05*

Fitness Information for Teens

Health Tips about Exercise, Physical Well-Being, and Health Maintenance

Including Facts about Aerobic and Anaerobic Conditioning, Stretching, Body Shape and Body Image, Sports Training, Nutrition, and Activities for Non-Athletes

Edited by Karen Bellenir. 425 pages. 2004. 978-0-7808-0679-5.

"Another excellent offering from Omnigraphics in their *Teen Health Series*. . . . This book will be a great addition to any public, junior high, senior high, or secondary school library."
— *American Reference Books Annual, 2005*

Learning Disabilities Information for Teens

Health Tips about Academic Skills Disorders and Other Disabilities That Affect Learning

Including Information about Common Signs of Learning Disabilities, School Issues, Learning to Live with a Learning Disability, and Other Related Issues

Edited by Sandra Augustyn Lawton. 337 pages. 2005. 978-0-7808-0796-9.

"This book provides a wealth of information for any reader interested in the signs, causes, and consequences

of learning disabilities, as well as related legal rights and educational interventions. . . . Public and academic libraries should want this title for both students and general readers."
— *American Reference Books Annual, 2006*

■

Mental Health Information for Teens, 2nd Edition
Health Tips about Mental Wellness and Mental Illness

Including Facts about Mental and Emotional Health, Depression and Other Mood Disorders, Anxiety Disorders, Behavior Disorders, Self-Injury, Psychosis, Schizophrenia, and More

Edited by Karen Bellenir. 400 pages. 2006. 978-0-7808-0863-8.

"In both language and approach, this user-friendly entry in the *Teen Health Series* is on target for teens needing information on mental health concerns."
— *Booklist, American Library Association, Jan '02*

"Readers will find the material accessible and informative, with the shaded notes, facts, and embedded glossary insets adding appropriately to the already interesting and succinct presentation."
— *School Library Journal, Jan '02*

"This title is highly recommended for any library that serves adolescents and parents/caregivers of adolescents."
— *E-Streams, Jan '02*

"Recommended for high school libraries and young adult collections in public libraries. Both health professionals and teenagers will find this book useful."
— *American Reference Books Annual, 2002*

"This is a nice book written to enlighten the society, primarily teenagers, about common teen mental health issues. It is highly recommended to teachers and parents as well as adolescents."
— *Doody's Review Service, Dec '01*

■

Sexual Health Information for Teens
Health Tips about Sexual Development, Human Reproduction, and Sexually Transmitted Diseases

Including Facts about Puberty, Reproductive Health, Chlamydia, Human Papillomavirus, Pelvic Inflammatory Disease, Herpes, AIDS, Contraception, Pregnancy, and More

Edited by Deborah A. Stanley. 391 pages. 2003. 978-0-7808-0445-6.

"This work should be included in all high school libraries and many larger public libraries. . . . highly recommended."
— *American Reference Books Annual, 2004*

"*Sexual Health* approaches its subject with appropriate seriousness and offers easily accessible advice and information."
— *School Library Journal, Feb '04*

Skin Health Information for Teens
Health Tips about Dermatological Concerns and Skin Cancer Risks

Including Facts about Acne, Warts, Hives, and Other Conditions and Lifestyle Choices, Such as Tanning, Tattooing, and Piercing, That Affect the Skin, Nails, Scalp, and Hair

Edited by Robert Aquinas McNally. 429 pages. 2003. 978-0-7808-0446-3.

"This volume, as with others in the series, will be a useful addition to school and public library collections."
— *American Reference Books Annual, 2004*

"There is no doubt that this reference tool is valuable."
— *VOYA: Voice of Youth Advocates, Feb '04*

"This volume serves as a one-stop source and should be a necessity for any health collection."
— *Library Media Connection*

■

Sports Injuries Information for Teens
Health Tips about Sports Injuries and Injury Protection

Including Facts about Specific Injuries, Emergency Treatment, Rehabilitation, Sports Safety, Competition Stress, Fitness, Sports Nutrition, Steroid Risks, and More

Edited by Joyce Brennfleck Shannon. 405 pages. 2003. 978-0-7808-0447-0.

"This work will be useful in the young adult collections of public libraries as well as high school libraries."
— *American Reference Books Annual, 2004*

■

Suicide Information for Teens
Health Tips about Suicide Causes and Prevention

Including Facts about Depression, Risk Factors, Getting Help, Survivor Support, and More

Edited by Joyce Brennfleck Shannon. 368 pages. 2005. 978-0-7808-0737-2.

■

Tobacco Information for Teens
Health Tips about the Hazards of Using Cigarettes, Smokeless Tobacco, and Other Nicotine Products

Including Facts about Nicotine Addiction, Immediate and Long-Term Health Effects of Tobacco Use, Related Cancers, Smoking Cessation, Tobacco Use Prevention, and Tobacco Use Statistics

Edited by Karen Bellenir. 440 pages. 2007. 978-0-7808-0976-5.

Health Reference Series